FEVERS, FEUDS, AND DIAMONDS

FEVERS, FEUDS, AND DIAMONDS

EBOLA AND THE RAVAGES OF HISTORY

Paul Farmer

FARRAR, STRAUS AND GIROUX | NEW YORK

Farrar, Straus and Giroux
120 Broadway, New York 10271

Owing to limitations of space, all acknowledgments for permission to reprint
previously published material can be found on page 655.

Maps and tree illustration by Katy Farmer.

Library of Congress Cataloging-in-Publication Data
Names: Farmer, Paul, 1959– author.
Title: Fevers, feuds, and diamonds : Ebola and the ravages of history / Paul Farmer.
Description: First edition. | New York : Farrar, Straus and Giroux, 2020. | Includes
    bibliographical references and index.
Identifiers: LCCN 2020027255 | ISBN 9780374234324 (hardcover)
Subjects: LCSH: Ebola virus disease—History. | Epidemics.
Classification: LCC RC140.5 .F37 2020 | DDC 614.5/7—dc23
LC record available at https://lccn.loc.gov/2020027255

Designed by Richard Oriolo

Our books may be purchased in bulk for promotional, educational, or business
use. Please contact your local bookseller or the Macmillan Corporate and
Premium Sales Department at 1-800-221-7945, extension 5442, or by e-mail at
MacmillanSpecialMarkets@macmillan.com.

www.fsgbooks.com
www.twitter.com/fsgbooks • www.facebook.com/fsgbooks

10 9 8 7 6 5 4 3 2 1

To Humarr and Martin, who didn't make it;

to Ibrahim and Yabom, who did;

to all the caregivers;

and to Ronda and Bill, who helped us join them

There's a thread you follow. It goes among

things that change. But it doesn't change.

People wonder about what you are pursuing.

You have to explain about the thread.

But it is hard for others to see.

While you hold it you can't get lost.

Tragedies happen; people get hurt

or die; and you suffer and get old.

Nothing you do can stop time's unfolding.

You don't ever let go of the thread.

—William Stafford, "The Way It Is," 1993

CONTENTS

PREFACE: THE CAREGIVERS' DISEASE xi

Part I: Ebola Hits Home

1. The Twenty-Fifth Epidemic? 3
2. Tough Calls 46
3. Ibrahim's Second Chance 96
4. The Two Ordeals of Yabom 144

Interlude I: Down the Rabbit Hole 177

Part II: Fevers, Feuds, and Diamonds

5. The Upper Guinea Coast and the World the Slaves Made 191
6. The Great Scramble and the Rise of the Pasteurians 237
7. A World at War: The Making of a Clinical Desert 280
8. Things Fall Apart: Civil War and Its Aftermath 355

Interlude II: The Crisis Caravan 419

Part III: Death and Life After Ebola

9. How Ebola Kills: An Exercise in Social Medicine 435
10. The Silly Things and the Fever Next Time 492

Epilogue: The Color of COVID 515

NOTES 527
ACKNOWLEDGMENTS 621
INDEX 627

Preface:
The Caregivers' Disease

IN OCTOBER 2014, HAVING SIGNED UP TO HELP RESPOND TO AN EXPLOSIVE Ebola epidemic, I traveled to West Africa in the company of colleagues. The disease had spread from the eaves of a shrinking forest, where the eastern reaches of Sierra Leone, Liberia, and Guinea meet in a narrow firth of land. By the time we arrived, all three countries faced an increasingly urban epidemic with no end in sight. There are no hard borders, and for months the afflicted had crossed watery ones, or traversed frontiers along hidden paths, in search of care. It hadn't taken long for Ebola, hidden in human hosts, to reach capital cities on the Atlantic—about as far west as the virus could go without boarding a boat or a plane.

Across the region, many medical facilities had been shuttered by October. That's because Ebola spreads easily in hospitals, clinics, and other places where the sick seek care; indeed, a significant fraction of the stricken had been health professionals, already in short supply when the virus struck. Its westward surge had just taken out the health-care systems of Liberia and Sierra Leone. Since then, those suffering from injuries or illnesses unrelated to Ebola were denied even the most basic medical services. This was a replay of the mortal drama of the previous decade, when civil war shut down or destroyed what clinics and hospitals there were in these countries. The forested region of Guinea, as it's termed, was spared some of this violence, but had received hundreds of thousands of war refugees from its neighbors.

We knew little of this when we touched down in Monrovia, Liberia's capital, in mid-October. A few days earlier, in Sierra Leone, we'd been assigned to reopen several idle clinics and hospitals and were awaiting a similar assignment in Liberia. But we had yet to lay eyes on the interior of a functioning Ebola treatment unit—an ETU—much less provide medical care for a single victim of the disease. We couldn't have known what we were in for. Though many had been assigned to *contain* the outbreak, fewer had signed up for the messy and dangerous work of *caring for*, rather than quarantining or isolating, the already afflicted. In order to learn more about how to provide care without becoming casualties ourselves, three friends and I were invited to spend an afternoon in an ETU in Monrovia, just then overrun by Ebola.

The facility had been erected on the campus of a mission hospital, which earlier that summer had prepared for the viral assault on the city by converting its chapel into an Ebola ward. In short order, several working there—including a couple of missionaries—had themselves fallen ill. Much of the campus had since been overhauled by the world's largest, and most Ebola-savvy, medical humanitarian organization. The ETU was by the time of our visit an impressive operation, with new open-air wards laid out under canvas awnings. These design features could not reduce the baking heat, which verged on intolerable for staff obliged to wear biohazard suits. I kept thinking, "How on earth is it possible to last more than fifteen minutes here in protective gear?"

Hazmat suits were only the most visible reminders of the ETU's sharp focus on infection control. The facility was divided into two zones, separated by flimsy waist-high orange mesh barriers: a red zone for patients confirmed to have Ebola and a green zone for patients deemed Ebola-free. Visitors were steered away from the barriers and instructed not to touch any surfaces, even on the "safe" side of the mesh.[1] Having known a couple of the nurses and doctors who'd fallen ill in previous weeks, the four of us welcomed the general climate of caution that prevailed within the unit. It wasn't long, however, before its basic premise—that the primary purpose of the ETU was isolation, rather than treatment—began to make the two of us who were clinicians feel uncomfortable. There was too little T in the ETU.

Our delegation broke into smaller groups shortly after the tour began. My doctor friend (an Italian infectious-disease specialist) and I stuck tight to our guide (also a compassionate and knowledgeable Italian physician). Both of us hoped our host might answer the questions we had about how best to care for the sickest subset of the Ebola-afflicted. Most of them were termed "wet" patients, because their gastrointestinal symptoms usually included vomiting and diarrhea. (Contrary to received wisdom, Ebola's clinical course is highly variable, with patients regularly reclassified as wet or dry during their illness.) These contaminated body fluids posed a great risk to those who had to clean up after the sick, but their loss posed an immediate threat to the afflicted: both fluids and electrolytes need to be replaced in order for patients to survive. Such replacement therapy, which is prescribed for pathologies ranging from gastroenteritis to gunshot wounds, has likely saved more lives than any other.

Replacement therapy requires estimating the volume of what comes out as liquid stool, vomit, urine, blood, and even sweat. In the United States, health professionals refer to what's replaced and lost as "ins" and "outs"—I's and O's, for short. Nurses and nursing aides are usually the ones measuring losses in order to replace them, but doctors all learn the basics. There are several ways to replace fluids and electrolytes, including their infusion into the abdomen or even through the marrow of the body's bigger bones. For almost a century, however, the most important methods of replacing the O's have been by mouth and by vein. The oral approach is preferred for all patients old enough and awake enough to drink what's called ORS, short for "oral rehydration salts." You probably call it Pedialyte.

As any mother knows, even thirsty, dehydrated children don't—or can't—always take ORS as instructed. It's not only small kids who have that problem: my friend and our host knew several professional caregivers stricken by Ebola who'd been unable to keep down ORS. I had two of them on my mind that day, both of them doctors who had become wet patients. The first was a Sierra Leonean physician, a much-lauded researcher and colleague whom I admired greatly. He'd died on July 29 in an ETU that had been set up and run by the same group now hosting us in Monrovia. No one in that unit had charted the precise volume of his losses to diarrhea, vomiting, and fever, but I'd heard they'd been substantial.

The second person on my mind that day was an American doctor who'd fallen ill after he had taken over for my deceased friend. We knew a lot more about the American's clinical course, as he'd been airlifted to Atlanta and was still a patient there on the day we inspected the Monrovia unit. He had been about as sick as you can get, losing up to ten liters of fluid per day, but a colleague caring for him at Emory University Hospital had just let me know they thought he'd make it. If he did, it would be in part because the team in Atlanta was carefully replacing the fluids and electrolytes he lost during the wet phase of the disease, which in some cases was accompanied by kidney failure. The doctor-patient had required renal dialysis, which permitted even more carefully calibrated replacement of his losses. He'd also required a breathing machine. In essence, these basic interventions allowed him to live long enough for his immune system to launch a counterassault on this virus.

Two other Americans—a missionary doctor and one of his assistants—had also survived Ebola after being airlifted to Atlanta from the same campus we were visiting that day. A handful of Europeans who'd fallen ill elsewhere in West Africa had been medevacked and survived. This was good news, not only for their friends and family but for clinicians hesitating to step up to the plate because they'd been informed by public-health experts that Ebola was untreatable. But good news from the United States and Europe seemed to make little difference to patients in West African ETUs, who were being provided with the bare minimum—right then and there, only cups of ORS, which many were unable to keep down. Most were dying.

Admittedly, it wasn't crystal-clear why. My Italian colleague and I had stored up several clinical questions that we hoped to discuss with our guide as we made our way through the green zone. Before either of us could pose our questions, we encountered two brothers who were leaving the triage area, just a few yards from where we stood.

Tall and thin, the brothers were inside the red zone but not yet patients: they still had to reach their beds, but could barely walk and looked disoriented. The older one, retching uncontrollably as watery stool ran down his legs, was the first Ebola patient my friend and I had seen shrivel up before us. His sunken eyes and withered skin made him look elderly, but I guessed him to be in his early thirties, maybe younger. We saw him sink into a squat while his brother struggled to hoist him back to his feet. The younger man, who couldn't have been much more than twenty, was covered with vomit, which I'd assumed was his brother's. But then he, too, began to gag and heave, even as he tried to steady his trembling, stumbling sibling. As we watched, paralyzed, the sicker man collapsed on a chlorine-scorched patch of grass and gravel outside one of the tents. His brother squatted beside him, weeping loudly but tearlessly—probably because he was too dehydrated to make tears.

Our guide called loudly for assistance from within the red zone, exchanging a few words with someone on the other side of the barrier. A few minutes later (it seemed like forever) the prostrate man was clumsily hoisted up by three staff in protective gear and hauled over to a "bed"—a flat slab without a pillow positioned under the white canvas and dark green mesh covering the confirmed-cases ward. The younger brother followed, swaying unsteadily as a fourth similarly outfitted person walked over with a cup of ORS. I thought this was a nurse's aide or a nurse but couldn't be sure. The space-suited Samaritans were Liberian, we surmised, but we couldn't make out what they were saying. The brothers, for their part, didn't say a thing; the one on the slab probably couldn't. He lifted his head while the presumed nurse tried to get him to drink some ORS. He gagged and sprayed it on them and on himself, moaning loudly enough that we could hear him.

I turned from this spectacle to look for my friends in the other group. With equal horror, they were watching a girl of about six years being hauled kicking and screaming into the confirmed ward by two women in protective garb. But the man we'd just seen collapse had no fight left in him. Without replacement of lost fluids and electrolytes, he would likely die of hypovolemic shock; his brother might be right behind him if he kept vomiting. The whole scene was excruciating for us and our guide to watch, because we knew that the treatment for the brothers' immediate emergency—the loss of fluids and electrolytes—had been worked out during the world war that had started exactly a century previously. We looked on, fearing that yet another early twenty-first-century family was being undone by a failure to deliver early twentieth-century therapies.

At first, I said nothing; my coworker was also uncharacteristically silent. What could we add? Surely this failure to deliver would be regarded as such by all involved, including our guide? Watching the young Liberians collapse while standing at his side challenged our camaraderie. It seemed somehow indelicate to ask questions about the spectacle. But hadn't that been the point of matching us with a fellow clinician for an informational tour?

Both of us turned away from the drama in the tent and toward the Virgil leading us through this inferno, a doctor whose life's work we knew well. All three of us had long been engaged in treating AIDS and drug-resistant tuberculosis in southern Africa and other places where treatment of these afflictions had once been declared impossible, impracticable, unsustainable, and (in the jargon of the day) not cost-effective. Those pilot projects, as they were termed, had brought our organizations closer together. We'd jointly published papers in medical journals and were then poised to launch a major new effort to provide novel antituberculous drugs—the first developed in over forty years—to thousands of patients sick from highly drug-resistant strains of the disease. With so much connecting us, we felt we knew each other well. In fact, we'd just met in person that day.

I knew that I had to say something about the dying man in front of us, and struggled to find just the right tone. "How long has he been sick like that?" I asked, pointing to the inert man. "He looks like a patient with really bad cholera." All three of us had extensive experience treating that disease.

"Three days," our Italian guide replied, "according to the intake team."

I braced myself to launch a couple of rhetorical questions. "Surely he's headed toward hypovolemic shock? If he's been doing that for three days, he's lost half his bodily fluids, right?"

Although shock isn't the only way to die of Ebola, it's one of them. The desperately ill man might have already lost more than twenty liters of electrolyte-rich effluent—not only from vomiting and diarrhea but also from what are termed "insensate losses" due to sweating and fever. These had been hastened and heightened by Monrovia's torrid heat.

All three of us knew that the sicker of the two brothers might not live long unless he received rapid fluid resuscitation. Usually provided through intravenous lines, fluid resuscitation is typically thought of as basic supportive care. During the West African Ebola epidemic, however, putting in an intravenous line had become controversial, primarily because any therapies involving needles or sustained contact with the afflicted increased the risks of accidental transmission to nurses and other caregivers. It was a tough situation, because Ebola was by then already the number one killer of health professionals in this part of West Africa. But regardless of who was afflicted, a smallish number of questions would matter. Chief among them: How will I, or my loved ones, fare?

This was surely the primary question running through the minds of the stricken brothers, but it couldn't be answered without laboratory data. Just a bit of routine information could steer anxious and imperiled clinicians to the sickest patients—and the right balance of fluid and electrolytes. As my colleague strained to watch the hazmat-suited workers continue to press one brother to drink, and to get the other onto his cot, I pulled closer to our guide: "Do we have any labs on the critically ill patients? What about electrolytes? Liver or renal function?" He stiffly replied that the headquarters of his organization had announced there would be no blood draws and no laboratory tests except for one: a polymerase chain reaction, or "PCR," test for the Zaire species of Ebola. (That was the species on the loose in West Africa and long alleged to be the most lethal.) "But if you're going to draw blood for one test," I protested mildly, "why not use part of the sample for basic labs—electrolytes, say, or lactic acid, to give you a sense of who needs more supportive care?"

He hesitated, then replied, "It's not in the protocol."

Our guide offered this in a tone that suggested the protocol was wrong, an order issued by generals too far from the front lines. The doctor then fell silent, looking at me with what I judged to be pain tinged by shame.

That look alone suggested that there was, already, a deep internal rift within his organization, one of a few that had committed to helping victims of the West African outbreak and with experience doing so elsewhere on the continent. Our host had sacrificed his vacation time to take up a dangerous post, but the organization he worked for had felt so overwhelmed and iso- lated that it had decided against trying to rehydrate patients with intravenous fluids and electrolytes. Since our guide was a superb and principled doctor, I didn't want to make him uncomfortable. Besides, we had similar feelings of pain and shame: by the second week of October, our team had yet to treat anyone with Ebola, even though we should have been at it for weeks.

My own Italian colleague and friend was uncharacteristically silent as the three of us turned away from the mortal dramas unfolding in the red zone and rejoined the others. I stopped asking questions about clinical manage- ment and returned to infection control, the safe topic of the day. We watched the complex decontamination proceedings and marveled at how many people it took to run the unit—our hosts reckoned they'd soon have seven hundred employees, mostly Liberians—and how smoothly much of it worked. We beamed at one sturdy young man who was clearly going to recover. He lifted his hands up in a hearty if mistaken tribute to us visitors, rather than to the valiant staff who'd seen him through his illness. He looked as healthy as any of the young employees. We felt like cheering, and probably did.

The three of us rejoined our colleagues, and the tour continued for a couple more hours. The sun began to set, and the oppressive heat abated. A welcome breeze hit our sweaty backs, wafting the smell of shit and vomit away from us, along with the sting of chlorine. As the light dwindled, the medical campus briefly seemed an orderly haven, though the crematorium's stench lingered. I tried to keep my mind on all we were learning and to express my appreciation for our guide and for the woman who'd organized the visit, a friend who'd also worked for years in southern Africa. We'd taken up their time with questions they'd surely heard a hundred times before. We left the ETU grateful for the hospitality shown us, and for the courage of our hosts.

That night, however, I couldn't get the young brothers out of my head. I kept seeing images of the sicker one, a man whose life might have been saved with a few liters of the right intravenous solution.

I wrote this book before the coronavirus pandemic of 2020. A novel pathogen's rapid diffusion has suddenly made many of the dilemmas discussed in these pages familiar around the world; in a brief epilogue, I consider the implications of West Africa's Ebola crisis for today, as we confront another disease that disproportionately afflicts caregivers. For although there are many differences between this strictly regional epidemic and a truly global pandemic—for starters, one pathogen is spread through direct contact while the other is a respiratory virus—there are many lessons to be learned from Ebola, and obvious implications for our response to COVID-19.

The Ebola epidemic that this book examines—the longest and largest in recorded history—began in southeastern Guinea in 2013. The book is part memoir, since I was often in this part of West Africa during the epidemic and thereafter, and wrote most of it in Sierra Leone. It's part biography, with a couple of long chapters about the lives of two former patients now counted as friends. There are also shorter inserted narratives about a handful of professional caregivers from Sierra Leone who didn't survive Ebola, and some who did. All told, close to a thousand professional health-care workers from Liberia, Sierra Leone, and Guinea fell ill with Ebola. More than half of them died.

Whether health professionals or not, tens of thousands contracted Ebola in the course of caring for the sick or carrying out caregiving's final act, preparing the dead for burial. They did so without the safeguards and assistance—pragmatic measures that can stop the spread of Ebola once the virus has been introduced into the human family—that most of us take for granted. But as the epidemic erupted into global consciousness, often in the form of breathless journalistic accounts, few in the public conversation mentioned the link between the epidemic and the dearth of trained and equipped medical professionals in the affected regions. Nor was there much mention of the absence of undertakers, morticians, or others to whom the last act of caregiving is outsourced by those affluent enough to pay for their services.

As with COVID-19, the disease caused by a novel coronavirus, a lot of published or broadcast Ebola commentary did, however, discuss where the epidemic had originated and hypothesized about how it had spread. The latter was never a mystery: for centuries, footpaths and river crossings, along with shared languages and cultures and family ties, have bound the eastern reaches of Sierra Leone, Liberia, and Guinea into a single ecological and social zone sometimes termed "Upper West Africa." The epidemic was fueled and sustained within this three-country region by everyday acts of caregiving, the mundane yet sacred obligations people felt to nurse the sick and bury the dead—without the PPE, or personal protective equipment, that such duties often require. But many commentators couldn't resist titillating diverse audiences with exotic explanations, alleging that Ebola's spread was hastened by bizarre healing and sexual practices, arcane funerary rituals, "secret societies" practicing scarification and all sorts of weird juju, and—especially—the consumption of "bushmeat." You call it game.

Like COVID-19, Ebola is a zoonosis, meaning it's caused by a pathogen that jumps from animals to humans. This is termed, in the jargon of epidemiology, a "spillover event." The natural hosts of both viruses are believed to be bats, but even that's uncertain. Humans living in or near what remains of equatorial Africa's once-great forests are bound to bump into, and sometimes eat, animals that are the hosts of Ebola and related pathogens. But that doesn't mean that human–animal contact defines epidemics, which occur among and between people.[2]

You wouldn't know it from much of what I heard on both sides of the Atlantic, where the animal part of the connection enthralled. One anthropologist summed up views commonly held in the United States in the latter half of 2014, as Ebola's toll mounted on the far side of the Atlantic:

> The formula had become predictable by August: Ebola is contained in exotic animals + West Africans eat these animals = a pandemic that kills its victims by causing their internal organs to liquefy. The oft-cited clichés of people bleeding from every orifice, a 90% mortality rate, and reality TV-style examples of "they eat *that*?!" gave the story the added sensational punch.[3]

Perhaps the most outrageous claims staked in those early months of the epidemic were that the afflicted and their caregivers obstinately refused to follow sound advice or accept modern medical care. People who should have known better—public-health authorities, humanitarians, and journalists—kept making variants of this claim. But few received sound advice, and almost nobody was offered modern care.

This book is thus also a reflection on how erroneous and misleading claims about Ebola echo across an increasingly fragmented media ecosystem—among alt-right Internet trolls and purveyors of fake news, as you might expect, but also among urban elites, politicians, and public authorities from all three nations, and many others. These entitled speakers, purporting to explain Ebola's sudden West African debut, invoked a host of exotic practices and beliefs held to be common in this part of the world. But variations of these practices (eating game, having babies, nursing the sick, respecting and transmitting traditions about last rites and burial) are encountered across the world, and Ebola's putative natural host or hosts also have a wide distribution zone. As a result, explanations that underline the deficiencies of the victims' culture didn't throw much light on the particulars of the disease's catastrophic spread across Upper West Africa. Too rarely was it noted that similar outbreaks elsewhere in Africa have typically occurred near shrinking forests and in the aftermath of armed conflict—problems of our own making that more closely approach the nature of an explanation.

The claim that Ebola's spread was hastened by "traditional" burial practices did have some merit. But it's absurd to characterize those practices—family members washing the bodies of their loved ones, laying them out for burial, and interring them with religious rites—as exotic. Until very recently, these practices were almost universal in human society, and they're still practiced in much of the world. In her caustic 1963 book, *The American Way of Death*, Jessica Mitford reminds us that this was long the way of it in the United States: "Simplicity to the point of starkness, the plain pine box, the laying out of the dead by friends and family who also bore the coffin to the grave—these were the hallmarks of the traditional funeral until the end of the nineteenth century."[4]

What happened in previous centuries is not irrelevant to the study of today's epidemics and social responses to them. Discussions of epidemic disease in Africa make frequent use of the colonial era's exoticizing language: game becomes "bushmeat," burials become "funerary rituals," and the terms "traditional" and "native" appear regularly, in proximity to each other, as code for "primitive." Many of these myths and mystifications, much of the vocabulary, and a good deal of armed conflict were brought to West Africa by colonial rule; so were martial disease-control efforts. What European colonialism didn't bring to the region was health care.

The game-eating, caregiving natives of this part of West Africa might not be acquainted with modern medical care, but they are quite familiar with colonialism's primary purpose: to rip riches from the earth and export them for profit. That's because West Africans have endured the extractive trades, and the many myths that obscured them, for so long. For centuries, a stream of commerce has moved commodities—initially, slaves and gold, and then rubber, iron ore, oil, bauxite, hardwoods, diamonds, and more—from West Africa to the Americas and Europe. It doesn't take much digging to learn that the natives, especially in the three most Ebola-affected countries, are still caught up in the aftermath of extractive colonialism.

Not that much effort is invested in hiding the ongoing project of extraction. A single visit to the eastern Sierra Leonean town of Koidu, a place discussed often in this book, suffices to remind even the casual observer that artisanal mining of alluvial diamonds turns once verdant rice paddies into a landscape pockmarked by pools of standing orange water—inhospitable to fish or plant life, but luxury resorts for mosquitoes and other vectors of disease. And that's before visitors note numerous giant slag heaps bordering the war-torn town or the vast funnels of the industrial diamond pits a few miles away.

The precipitate extraction of wealth from earth and forest profoundly disrupted the region's ecology, and in ways that have contributed acutely to the Ebola crisis. Whether by panning or river dredging or excavations that rival the visuals of Mordor, mining spells ecological ruin. It has sparked the rapid, hazardous development of cities and towns where once tiny villages and small farms stood. But mining, urbanization, and deforestation occur across Africa, and indeed the world. So why was this particular Ebola epidemic so much larger than any other yet described? How and why did it spread to cities? And why should such a readily transmitted and lethal pathogen have confined its toll almost exclusively to three countries among more than a dozen in close proximity?

The legacy of violence offers at least a part of the answer. When readily portable diamonds were the object of panning and dredging and digging, mining fueled armed conflict before and long after the end of colonial rule. Only a few years before Ebola erupted from the forest districts of eastern Guinea, civil war in Liberia and Sierra Leone pushed millions of refugees into camps, most of them in eastern Guinea or in crowded slums of the three capitals. As the fires of war depleted the hamlets and gardens that once fed these nations, flight and hunger created fertile terrain for explosive epidemics, of which Ebola is only the latest. Accordingly, this study of Ebola can't be only about recent events; West Africa has long been ground zero for stripping, feuds, and fevers.[5] Nor can this book sidestep a more remote history of armed conflict; at least a third of it seeks to record some of the spectacular mayhem that invariably followed in the wake of pillage: centuries of conflict and epidemics on both sides of the Atlantic.

I wasn't around for any of these events, or for the recent civil strife that rolled out the red carpet for Ebola's rapid spread from the forest villages of Upper West Africa to its coastal cities. During the region's recent spate of wars—or the long continuous war, depending on your views—I was splitting my time between Haiti, Peru, and Harvard Medical School. I knew next to nothing about the cultures and everyday lives of those inhabiting the areas where Ebola took its toll, although by the time it erupted I'd spent much of the previous decade in Rwanda. Once we began working to reopen West African clinics and hospitals, and to care for Ebola patients, I didn't learn any of the two dozen or so local languages spoken in the region. Nor did I have the time or inclination to conduct ethnographic research in the midst of a medical emergency. To learn more about the social complexity of this region, I relied on the published work of others—anthropologists and historians who came by this sort of deep knowledge the hard way.

Formal training in infectious disease and anthropology did, however, help me write this book. By directly providing clinical care and other pragmatic assistance to victims of the Ebola epidemic, and by engaging on other fronts in the fight against a host of other pathogens and pathogenic forces, I got to know many Ebola survivors—and what was left of their families—well enough to write about them. Partners In Health, a nongovernmental organization founded more than thirty years ago in order to directly address the needs of the destitute sick, afforded me this type of engagement. Anthropology, for its part, taught me to distrust confident claims about local culture as *the* chief determinant of recurrent suffering and early death, even as it taught me that culture and context are always and everywhere important in facing unequally distributed misfortune; whatever the fates deal out, culture invariably shapes social responses to it.

Writing this book also required an understanding of how this virus and other microbes kill some while sparing others. The relative explanatory importance of varied factors—from biological susceptibility to newly introduced pathogens to the impact of conquest, extractive colonialism, and the inequalities and conflicts that ensued—has for centuries triggered debates about health disparities, many of them registered between the descendants of the conquerors and conquered. Understanding such disparities, along with holistic and historical understanding of human affliction and responses to it, is the goal of social medicine, a regrettably obscure branch of the profession. It's in this tradition that I offer this account.

Much of this book is, in other words, a synthesis of other people's knowledge and an account of other people's suffering. But it's a synthesis informed by direct service to the afflicted. This account is also informed by years of friendship with several people who have survived Ebola.

Previous books about the disease written for the general reader have made it sound as if there would be few survivors left to befriend. Richard Preston's *The Hot Zone*, the best-known and bestselling such book, set the tone—and widespread expectations—over the past couple of decades:

> As Ebola sweeps through you, your immune system fails, and
> you seem to lose your ability to respond to viral attack. Your
> body becomes a city under siege, with its gates thrown open and
> hostile armies pouring in, making camp in the public squares
> and setting everything on fire; and from the moment Ebola enters
> your bloodstream, the war is already lost; you are almost certainly
> doomed.[6]

I'm pleased to report that this is hyperbole. (Preston, I have no doubt, is pleased, too.) In the past few years, many thousands have survived infection with the species of Ebola that he names the deadliest. As regards those who did not survive, two related questions must be raised. How many of these deaths were caused more by the virulence of social conditions than by the virulence of the pathogen? If it came down solely to the virulence of a particular strain or species, as is still commonly alleged, then why have mortality rates varied so widely among people infected with the same variants of Ebola? With the exception of one Liberian-born U.S. citizen, every American who fell ill from the strains circulating in West Africa survived. So did most Europeans.[7]

That's because they were medevacked out of the clinical desert, fell ill shortly after returning from it, or were among the handful of professional caregivers infected beyond its borders.

Meanwhile, back in Upper West Africa, mortality rates at the close of the epidemic—when we should have had on hand more of the staff, stuff, and space needed to improve the quality of care—were unchanged from its early months. (The staff in question would include nurses, doctors, and other clinicians unambivalent about caregiving; the stuff includes everything from gowns and gloves to IV fluids; the space includes ETUs.) This high mortality rate was widely alleged to result from the population's deep distrust of authoritarian disease-control efforts and of authority in general. But it's also because what became the world's largest public-health endeavor always remained a clinically paltry one.

Overweening disease-control efforts that are clinically paltry are nothing new since the late nineteenth-century rise of germ theory and its application in an increasingly unequal world. But this rise and its colonial rollout happened simultaneously, and with peculiar force, in West Africa. I didn't know any of the details when I first traveled to Sierra Leone in June 2014. The historical chapters that constitute the middle of this book are also its heart, and they're meant to distill an unfolding astonishment I hope to share with the reader. There are several reasons for this foray into history, and into material that is unlikely to figure prominently in other first-person accounts of the Ebola epidemic.

First, West African epidemics and social responses to them can't be fully comprehended without knowledge of the region's long entanglement with Europe and the Americas. This is the story of how our world—the Atlantic world that's long been the nucleus of the global economy—came to be as it is. It's the story of the all-too-little-recognized precursors to Ebola: slavery and the extractive trades, the feuds they engendered or worsened in West Africa, and their links to diverse epidemics affecting this long-disrupted region.

Second, much of this story—the transatlantic slave trade, the late nineteenth-century European partition of Africa, the harsh colonial rule that endured until the early years of the Cold War, the diamond-fueled hot wars that ended in this century, the epidemics that erupted throughout—is simply startling. Again and again, as I learned more of the details, my reaction was, *How could I not have known this?* These epiphanies were humbling, in that I've long worked in and written about Haiti, peopled almost exclusively by descendants of those who passed through the Door of No Return on or near what was once called the Upper Guinea Coast.

A third reason is restorative. Down the oubliette had gone rich if confused colonial-era accounts of febrile disease, the famed fevers of the "fever coast," as it was termed before being redubbed the "White Man's Grave." These accounts represent a rich trove of victim-blaming and self-exculpation, shot through with self-serving sensationalism and old-school racism, a brand of history writing and storytelling that in many ways has defined what we tell ourselves about much of the formerly colonial world and its troubles today. They also presage a more material legacy. This includes, as noted, entrenched health disparities, explosive pandemics, weak health systems, and widespread lack of confidence in them. These, more than any specific disease, are the ranking public health problems of our times. Their roots, too, are to be found in the colonial era.

Also standard, at least in West Africa under European rule, were the punitive practices of public-health authorities. Once termed sanitarians or (as an homage to the French father of microbiology) Pasteurians, they were often the architects and implementers of the control-over-care paradigm. Their twentieth-century endeavors—sometimes based on harebrained notions of epidemiology or microbiology, often racist, and rarely effective—met with resistance, often vigorous, from the populations they targeted. What motivated much resistance wasn't ignorance but the knowledge that disease-control efforts led by physicians in the colonial medical services were rarely linked to medical care: French and British Pasteurians pasteurized caregiving right out of their practice.

Many colonial health authorities surely had the best of intentions, but this is not a study of Pasteurian motivations; it's a study of their actions and inaction. It's absurd to assume that those who endured authoritarian public-health endeavors for over a century would have forgotten them—even though so many of Europe's African subjects were themselves forgotten by professional caregivers. Despite colonial boasts of a civilizing mission, and despite the presence of the sanitarians, care of the critically ill and injured in rural areas, like assistance during childbirth, remained the lonely and often terrifying responsibility of family members and of a diverse group of practitioners and diviners called "traditional healers." It was the same in Liberia, the only part of West Africa not subjected to European (meaning white) rule, and remained the case after civil war finished off its health system, and Sierra Leone's, while crippling Guinea's. Armed conflict left this part of West Africa both a public-health desert, which is why Ebola spread, and a clinical desert, which is why Ebola killed.

I'm not arguing that providing effective care for those sick with Ebola requires familiarity with the long and sorry history of the extractive trades and of armed conflict in West Africa. In preference to historical consciousness, that neglected task requires staff, stuff, space, and attention to infection control. But historical understanding can help us in many ways. It can help us decipher unfamiliar and often hostile responses to disease-control efforts. It can help us call out outlandish claims from experts and novices alike. Historical understanding can even help us show respect for people native to West Africa. And if history can enlighten us in these ways, we might do better the next time around. As regards the Ebola epidemic, there was never any doubt that there would be one. What recently unfolded in the eastern Congo—another conflict-ridden and parched patch of the postcolonial desert—is proof of that. But there will be, on our ecologically deranged planet, many other reminders of the need to look back on previous epidemics and social responses to them.

One of these reminders is the COVID-19 crisis that is currently roiling the world. This global pandemic now afflicts those living far from the medical desert, which will no doubt give rise to new cultural complexities and new challenges. Most of them, however, will be the same ones described in these pages.

PART I

EBOLA HITS HOME

Everybody knows that pestilences have a way of recurring in the world; yet somehow we find it hard to believe in ones that crash down on our heads from a blue sky. There have been as many plagues as wars in history; yet always plagues and wars take people equally by surprise.

—Albert Camus, *The Plague*, 1947

Outbreaks are inevitable. Pandemics are optional.

—Dr. Larry Brilliant on Ebola, 2014

1.

The Twenty-Fifth Epidemic?

This is the first time the disease has been detected in West Africa, and the outbreak has now spread to the American and European continents.
—World Health Organization, October 24, 2014

Serologic results provide evidence that ebolaviruses are circulating and infecting humans in West Africa. This extends the ebolavirus geographic region to Sierra Leone and the surrounding region.
—Dr. Humarr Khan and colleagues, in reference to blood samples collected in eastern Sierra Leone over the decade prior to 2014

THE REGIONS USUALLY AFFECTED BY THE EBOLA VIRUS—IN OR NEAR THE receding forests of central and eastern Africa—have long been the theater of explosive if uncharted epidemics. When these plagues kill, as they're apt to do in a medical desert, surviving family don't receive any official report of cause of death. No labs or health systems have tracked the disease while treating it; nobody can say for sure what the culprit pathogens are. To echo Albert Camus, nobody knows what's come crashing down on them. Survivors and their families come up with their own explanations. So do epidemiologists, medical journalists, and public-health authorities of every stripe.

West Africa's Ebola outbreak, the largest in recorded history, is widely held by expert opinion to have its origins in the eastern reaches of Guinea, Liberia, and Sierra Leone, which converge in a bit of turf known as the Kissi Triangle. For centuries this "trizone" region—in which the virus, we're assured repeatedly, was unknown until 2013—was largely covered by a mosaic of forest and savannah, tended by a large and mobile population of farmers, traders, and hunters of diverse origins. (Guineans often call them *forestiers*.) In recent decades, commercial logging, small-scale charcoal production, mining, and war have greatly reduced the forest and its wildlife. From this disrupted real estate, Ebola snaked its tendrils into several other nations. But it was in Guinea, Liberia, and Sierra Leone, and really only there, that the epidemic blanketed the land.

Why? All documented Ebola outbreaks—the World Health Organization (WHO) pronounced this one the world's twenty-fifth—have been registered in settings of profound poverty. By most criteria, that's an apt description of what one finds in Guinea, Liberia, and Sierra Leone. But in terms of gross domestic product per capita, these three countries were growing faster than the United States or Europe throughout the decade prior to the outbreak. Measured only by this tired calculus, Sierra Leone boasted the world's highest rate of economic growth in 2013.[1]

The engines of this specious boom remain the extractive industries—logging, along with the quest for oil, minerals, precious metals, diamonds, and rubber latex. But profits from these industries rarely remained in the vicinity, and they were almost never invested in public goods, such as robust health systems able to contain epidemics—or to flatten their curves and surges—while caring for the afflicted. Maybe in Norway, but not in West Africa: For all their natural wealth, Guinea, Liberia, and Sierra Leone rank among the most medically impoverished nations on the face of the earth; for all their rainfall, their citizens are stranded in the medical desert. In this desert, a diagnosis—and answers to the who-when-why-how questions—is more likely to come from a diviner or other traditional healer than from a laboratory, or is produced by authorities well after the fact and on a basis other than firsthand observations. This raises a corollary question. When an epidemic occurs in a public-health desert, who decides when and where it begins or ends?

To understand the how and the why of the West African Ebola epidemic, you have to turn first to the specifics of who, when, and where. Since Ebola is a zoonosis, a disease caused by a pathogen able to leap from its natural hosts to humans, the people posing these questions tend to search for an outbreak's first human victims. Epidemiologists, health authorities, and journalists look for "Patient Zero" and seek to trace subsequent paths of spread. But Ebola origin stories can rarely be confirmed, since most stricken by Ebola in the clinical desert die. Blood samples aren't often collected prior to death, nor are postmortem studies performed.

Here, with ready acknowledgment of uncertainty, is the dominant origin story of the Ebola epidemic believed to have begun at the close of 2013 in southeastern Guinea.

In early December, or maybe a couple of weeks later, a toddler named Émile fell ill in the tiny upland village of Meliandou.[2] He's said to be one year old in some accounts, in others two, and usually somewhere in between. Émile's mother, then heavily pregnant, noted the boy was running a fever and had diarrhea. (In some versions of the story, this was black or bloody stool.) Although such signs and symptoms aren't rare occurrences in Meliandou, she was worried enough to move back to her own mother's house in the same village.

Recollections and reports are discrepant regarding not only Émile's age and symptoms but also what care he received, and from whom. One takedown of Meliandou origin stories insists that he was diagnosed with malaria by a "doctor" in the village's "community health clinic," but Guinean villages with a few hundred residents don't boast any of these, not in the sense implied by the terms.[3] The family's interventions, whatever they may have been, were in vain. When Émile died—on December 6 in early versions of the story and on December 28 in later ones—no red flags were raised beyond the village or beyond its families, which counted many scattered in towns and cities across the region. It's doubtful that health authorities in nearby Guéckédou, the district capital, were alerted. A toddler's death, exceedingly rare in the wealthier parts of the world, occurs all too often in rural Guinea, where malaria is the most common culprit. Nor was any official fuss made when Émile's four-year-old sister—sometimes said to be three, which would imply unusual fecundity if the boy was two and their mother eight months pregnant—perished eight days after he did.

Their mother was the next to mount a fever. In her case, it was accompanied by signs of early labor, including passage of blood clots. (Other iterations assert she'd received an injection for hip pain, which triggered hemorrhage from the injection site.) In the course of a stillbirth, the young woman began bleeding out. Her husband desperately sought help from a "village midwife," who wasn't formally trained as a midwife and certainly not supplied with the tools of the trade—gloves, aprons, sutures, pads and dressings, sterile razors, clamps, and blood for such emergencies. She and another birth attendant, who were related to Émile by marriage or blood, did their best. But Émile's mother died that night in her mother's home, or, according to some accounts, her own.

As if these losses weren't enough to make any family feel cursed, Émile's maternal grandmother was soon sick with fever, nausea, and abdominal pain. According to a report bearing the imprimatur of the World Health Organization, she hedged any bets on curses and other supernatural etiologies by seeking care in Guéckédou, where she knew a nurse at its public hospital. Guéckédou, too, is all over the map in these origin stories: sometimes it's a forest village, sometimes a town, sometimes a city. It's in fact a small city and the capital of the district of the same name, and its ragged edges extend to a few miles away from an unpaved track leading to Meliandou. The village can be reached, as is clear from photographs illustrating scores of articles and reports about Patient Zero, by jeeps and the like.

Even critically ill or injured villagers didn't have ready access to such transport. When they made it to hospitals, it was on foot, by motorcycle taxi, or on handcrafted stretchers carried by kin. Émile's grandmother took a moto taxi to Guéckédou's district hospital, which, according to a hand-lettered billboard at the facility, had benefited from a "health-systems strengthening program" funded by a large international aid agency. But said health system hadn't been strengthened nearly enough: After a harried and rapid exchange, which didn't include more than a cursory examination, the forty-six-year-old grandmother was judged to have malaria or some other infection common on the outskirts of the forest. She went home and died there in mid-January 2014. Other kin were sickened at about the same time, and several perished.

The decimation of this extended family and several others was attributed to Ebola by a retrospective study of transmission chains leading from subsequent patients back to Meliandou, and back to Émile. But since Ebola is a zoonosis, another species must be implicated in the fevered quest for Patient Zero. Bats are likely culprits, and there were plenty of those flitting about Meliandou. The ones alleged (by some experts) to be Ebola's natural hosts have lovely names: Franquet's epauletted fruit bat, the hammer-headed fruit bat, the little-collared fruit bat, the little free-tailed bat. Generous helpings of speculation prop up the assertion that Émile had fallen ill a few days after eating a bat-gnawed mango, or maybe a plum, or the fruit of a palm tree well liked by bats.

Some experts reported that Meliandou's toddlers were pleased to snack on bats as well as fruit. The journalist Laurie Garrett offered up the following scenario (starring yet another bat species with different dietary habits) in the now-dominant origin story. It draws on scientific authority of the German variety:

> At the edge of a great rainforest where Guinea, Liberia, and Sierra Leone meet, a two-year-old boy named Émile crawled about a water-soaked tree stump with other toddlers and discovered a bunch of little, furry winged creatures. Grabbing at them and poking them with a stick, Émile reportedly played with the nest of *lolibelo*—the name locals use to describe musk-smelling, dark gray bats with bodies about the size of a child's open hand. Many months later, a team of German anthropologists and biologists would visit the Guinean village of Meliandou and determine that Émile's *lolibelo*

were Angolan free-tailed bats or perhaps members of a similar species of mammal found across most of sub-Saharan Africa. Surviving children in the village told visiting scientists and reporters that youngsters had smoked *lolibelo* out of the tree, filled up sacks with the flying mammals, and eaten them.[4]

One problem with this sort of scientific authority is that the Germans' eight days in Meliandou didn't turn up much in the way of evidence to support such an origin story: None of the sacks of bats they sampled—including eighty-eight captured in the village—had evidence of Ebola infection.[5]

More classically defined monkey business also shows up in many Ebola origin stories. Nonhuman primates are sickened or killed by the viral strains that sicken humans and thus unlikely to be natural hosts, but they reliably play at least a part in these tales. As regards the spillover event in Guinea, the German team and local ones were unable to document a recent die-off of nonhuman primates or other fauna, as had been described during prior Ebola outbreaks in the Congo. None of this tempered the need for an authoritative origin story—and a Patient Zero—in the absence of solid evidence. That's why some of these stories allege that villagers in Meliandou kept monkeys as pets or, in another trending version, that Émile's family was among those whose diets included monkey: even if the toddler was too young to chew on monkey meat, he might have been splashed by blood-spatter as it was being butchered or prepared for dinner.

More free-range speculation in the race to identify Patient Zero posited that Émile had received an injection with an unsterilized syringe. This marked an unconventional twist in an Ebola origin story, since he would no longer be a contender for the title unless he shared needles with another species. As babies are unlikely to hunt, gather, dress, smoke out, or poke at animals, or to eat them uncooked, Émile makes a less compelling Patient Zero than might older kids in Meliandou. His grieving father—likely weary of interrogation, impoverished by funeral expenses, and having concluded his family was cursed by more than German scientists and journalists—later said as much: "It wasn't Émile that started it. Émile was too young to eat bats, and he was too small to be playing in the bush all on his own. He was always with his mother."[6]

A boy dies of an unknown fever, followed by his mother and other close kin: this is among the oldest, saddest, and most common stories of the fever coast and what remains of its brooding inland forest. In the year or so that followed, close to a third of Meliandou's inhabitants died, were sickened, or fled. But the tragedies in Meliandou, though investigated by local authorities

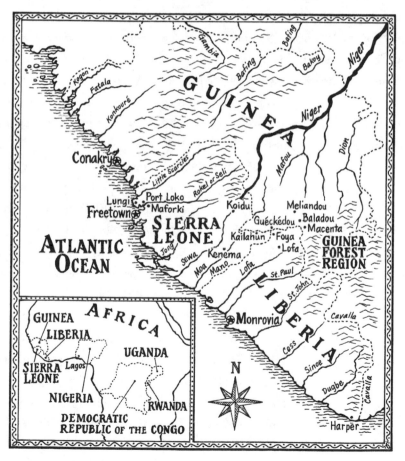

Upper West Africa

and reported to national ones, did not announce the Ebola nightmare. That happened after the region's professional caregivers began to sicken and die.

Although Émile's immediate family was decimated within a month or two of his demise, the events in Meliandou might have gone unnoticed beyond Guinea's forest districts, or forgotten as quickly as his grandmother's miserable visit to a miserable outpatient clinic in a miserably staffed and stocked hospital. No international alarms were sounded when other kin and neighbors—those who'd cared for or cleaned up after the sick, or buried them—were felled in the first weeks of the new year. Casualties included the birth attendants who'd assisted Émile's mother the night she died, as well as another of their peers. By then, however, Guinea's local health authorities had taken note.

Shortly after Émile's grandmother perished, a doctor in a town not far away saw three patients die in the span of two days, laid low by diarrhea, vomiting, and severe dehydration. He suspected cholera. When the physician realized all three were from Meliandou, which counted fewer than forty households, he reported these deaths to his superiors in Guéckédou. They in turn reported them to provincial authorities in N'Zérékoré, another city in the Kissi Triangle. Along with Macenta, these cities and their surrounding districts had received the great majority of war refugees during the early years of the civil wars that wracked Liberia and Sierra Leone; not long before the Ebola outbreak, there were more Liberian refugees than native *forestiers* living in Guinea's patch of the triangle. Health authorities in the Kissi Triangle were, in other words, accustomed to responding to transnational epidemics in the region.

When Guéckédou's health authorities kicked the report up to Conakry, the capital of Guinea, they also dispatched a small team to investigate the rash of unexplained febrile deaths in Meliandou and among folks from or visiting it. Members of this team knew there were clinical reasons to doubt the diagnosis of cholera: most deaths had followed high fevers, which would be an atypical presentation of the disease. But as cholera outbreaks weren't rare in the region, the team from Guéckédou settled on it as the likely culprit. At least its members allowed they were far from sure—a rare modesty in the crafting of outbreak narratives.

Medical modesty is warranted in considering outbreaks of Ebola, since the disease is spread by acts of caregiving: it's when a patient or health professional is confirmed to have been stricken with Ebola *within* a health facility that the international containment whistle usually blows. That's what came to pass in Guinea. The alarm was sounded not long after the sudden death of a nurse within another forest-district hospital was revealed as a link in the chain leading to Meliandou.

This was the same nurse, a young man, who saw Émile's grandmother in Guéckédou's hospital. In early February 2014, he fell ill with fever, muscle aches, and profound weakness. When diarrhea and nausea kicked in, he sought care from a doctor friend living in the neighboring district of Macenta. By the time he reached its capital, the city of Macenta, the nurse was critically ill. The doctor urged him to report at once to the district hospital for laboratory tests. But as it was late and the lab was closed, he opened up his home to the stricken man, who shared a room with the doctor's son. It must have been a sleepless night: the nurse retched uncontrollably, and his diarrhea did not let up. The next day—February 10 in most reports—he died in the waiting room of the hospital's laboratory.

Shaken, and at a loss to identify the cause of his friend's demise, the physician from Macenta reported the death to regional authorities in the city of N'Zérékoré. A week or two later, he fell ill with a similar constellation of signs and symptoms and set off for Conakry, on the other side of the country, in search of more advanced care and a diagnosis. He received neither, dying on the road on March 7. In the Kissi Triangle, women and girls do most of the caregiving, nursing the sick and cleaning up after them, but men usually prepare men for last rites and interment. In the case of the fallen physician, his brothers prepared his body for burial in his hometown, the trizone city of Kissidougou. At least two of them then fell ill with similar symptoms. Both died in March, and so did the doctor's son and a lab worker from Macenta's hospital.

Within a couple months of Émile's death, Ebola had spread in a widening circle on at least two sides of the Kissi Triangle, from Meliandou to towns and cities across the forest districts. Widening circles are by definition not linear, which is why it was unsurprising to later learn that several of the

Ebola-afflicted, in their quest for care or to give it, trod the soil of all three countries before dying or recovering. People in the Kissi Triangle, as elsewhere in this part of West Africa, move freely across frontiers, which often are marked only by rivers, or blazes on a footpath. These frontiers are so porous that hundreds of thousands of war refugees moved across them in recent decades.[7] Needless to say, the virus did the same.

By mid-February, Ebola had spread east through the forest to the town of Baladou, near the Liberian border. It had also spread west across four hundred miles of difficult terrain to Guinea's capital, a ramshackle coastal city of close to two million. Subsequent investigations of the Meliandou transmission chains suggested that a nephew of Émile's grandmother, moving back and forth between city and village to attend funerals, died in Conakry on February 5. Even before that, these links led to Sierra Leone, where at least two women in these chains perished toward the close of January. None of these connections were made at the time, at least not by health authorities.

Who's to know who died, and how, in those first months of the epidemic? Even if intrepid contact tracers, journalists, and researchers had been able to identify all close contacts of the alleged Patient Zero and his caregivers, and to determine their whereabouts, on this earth or under it, it would be difficult to trace with certainty the fates of all those afflicted. The dimensions of the epidemic eventually prompted several high-profile assessments of what went wrong with an array of "outbreak warning systems" designed to contain lethal epidemics. But local warnings clearly did spread: that's why so many Meliandou residents cleared out. It was the *global* alarm that didn't sound early in the game.

Not that much would probably have changed if it had. When international alarms are sounded, it's rarely as a summons to international caregivers to rush in with medical supplies and relief. It's more like the grim peal of the leper's bell. Clinicians and other hospital staff fear these alarms, and not only because they themselves stand in harm's way: since person-to-person spread within clinics and hospitals is almost always implicated in Ebola outbreaks, such events trigger calls to shut down hospitals and clinics. No one wants to be blamed for "nosocomial spread"—transmission of disease within a health facility. In previous outbreaks of Ebola and of the closely related and similarly spread Marburg virus—the first identified member of the filovirus family—bad report cards regarding infection control had been issued but had little positive effect.

Bad marks didn't prompt more than cursory training of staff, when and if staff were even on hand to train; they often stigmatized health facilities, towns, and sometimes entire countries. What they didn't do was elicit sustained remedial efforts to improve supply chains and install and equip better labs. And when it came to ongoing protection for African caregivers, a failing grade didn't prompt much beyond exhortations to avoid contact with the sick—an impractical and unethical aspiration for health professionals in the absence of meaningful alternatives, and a socially untenable one for family caregivers. After previous outbreaks, a clean bill of health was issued only after an outbreak had, in the crass lingo of epidemiology, "burned itself out." What often didn't flame out quickly after documented outbreaks of Ebola and Marburg was the blame heaped on African caregivers and on the afflicted themselves.

Villagers in Meliandou had their own complex calculus of responsibility, which initially (it would seem) had little to do with doctors or health authorities, invoking instead curses, unpropitiated ancestors, vengeful neighbors, malign spirits, and (of course) microbes. As the outbreaks spread, the various parties concerning themselves with control of communicable disease tended to blame either refractory patients or one another. This, not surprisingly, fanned mistrust among the locals, which in turn led them to hide sick family members and to resist contact tracing, voluntary isolation, travel restrictions, and funeral bans. Uncontested, these measures might have made the epidemic easier to control. But they were vigorously contested, further compounding misguided attempts to blame patients and their caregivers— many of whom soon became patients themselves—for their affliction.

Other experts and pundits blamed the failure of early attempts to contain Ebola on its tardy identification. A stack of lessons-learned reports later bemoaned the fact that three months into the epidemic, no one suspected Ebola as the culprit. But health authorities based in Conakry knew by early March that something terrible was afoot in the forest districts and suspected that the events in Guéckédou and Macenta were part of a single outbreak. They just didn't know what might be causing it. Malaria, a parasitic affliction often causing similar symptoms, was omnipresent. The bacterial diseases cholera and typhoid were often invoked, since gastrointestinal symptoms were present, but the signs and symptoms seen in these outbreaks could have been provoked by a large number of viruses, bacteria, and parasites. Without the right lab facilities, it was impossible to say.

Since many infectious pathogens could trigger the nonspecific signs and symptoms registered in the first months of 2014, reasoned Guéckédou's health authorities, perhaps the pattern of spread might help identify the culprit? The outbreaks flared abruptly, always taking out kin. This strongly suggested transmission within households. Although household spread of malaria, like typhoid, was common enough, the unknown killer struck adults and teens more often than small children, malaria's chief victims; tests for malaria were usually negative among those stricken. When seven of nine new patients in Guéckédou tested positive for cholera—likely false positives—most Guinean health officials put their faith in these results.

It's not that deadly viruses weren't considered. The clinical course and high mortality, and the apparent nature of spread, were consistent with what are classed as "hemorrhagic fevers." Ebola and Marburg, the filoviruses, are considered two of these. ("Filovirus" was the name given to what would grow into a family of viruses that appeared filamentary, or stringlike, when viewed through an electron microscope.) Marburg, the first named filovirus, was identified after a lethal and unknown affliction in lab monkeys imported from Uganda caused human outbreaks in Germany and Yugoslavia in 1967.[8] Less than a decade later, in the course of a spectacularly lethal outbreak of acute febrile illness near Zaire's Ebola River, a related virus was given the name Ebola and added to the filovirus family.

The virus that causes another sometimes-hemorrhagic disease, Lassa, leaps to humans from a species of rat common in the neighborhood. That alone, in the view of critics of West African health authorities, should have brought Ebola to mind. But few of those afflicted during the expanding outbreak showed signs of hemorrhage, which was alleged to be typical of Ebola but isn't (one reason infectious disease doctors avoid the rubric of hemorrhagic fever). Some local authorities who missed the diagnosis later claimed to have been steered away from it by international health authorities and bona fide Ebola experts, who continued to insist that the virus was unknown in West Africa. This was false: a handful of medical studies from previous decades had suggested that the Ebola virus was already present in the region.[9]

It's hard to fault beleaguered West African health professionals for missing these clues. Few—even those who'd helped conduct these studies—had access to the expensive scientific journals in which these surveys were published. Nor had local facilities been left with improved lab capacity for diagnosing the varied causes of febrile illness after expatriate researchers had returned to Europe.

When Ebola was recently loosed among humans living in Guinea, whenever and wherever that may have been, its rapid and accurate diagnosis wasn't possible even in Conakry, where neither public nor private institutions boasted the sort of labs that led to the initial 1976 identification of Ebola. Four decades after this discovery, Sierra Leone and Liberia also lacked the bulky and expensive tools of mid-twentieth-century virology that had permitted the identification of many new pathogens. Many villages and towns in the Kissi Triangle still lacked even the point-of-care tests used to distinguish one cause of febrile illness from a dozen others.

Bureaucratic obstacles also impeded a coordinated Ebola response. In mid-March, for example, a team assembled by Guinea's health ministry and the local offices of the World Health Organization left Conakry for the increasingly deforested forest region in order to investigate what was happening there. On the fifth day of its mission, the delegation interviewed the family of a thirty-seven-year-old woman who'd fallen ill in late February with fever, diarrhea, and vomiting, and who may have shown hemorrhagic signs as well. The woman died in southeastern Guinea on March 3, but the team learned that she had been visiting from Kailahun District—the Sierra Leonean patch of the Kissi Triangle. The team also learned that the deceased woman's daughter was sick and had fallen ill *within* Sierra Leone's borders. She would survive, but one of her own children had died in Kailahun a few days before the team arrived.

Throughout late February and March, relatives of these women and their sundry caregivers fell ill, and at least one of them died in a hospital in Kailahun. (In some retrospective reports, this was on March 19; in others, ten days later.) This was all vital information. But nobody communicated it effectively across national borders and in local languages, jobs that many deemed the responsibility of the World Health Organization. The team did write a seventeen-page report upon returning to Conakry and insisted they'd sent it on to authorities in Freetown. But officials at Sierra's Leone health ministry—and the country's WHO representative—later claimed they never saw it.

So how and where *was* Ebola identified as the culprit shortly after the investigations in southeastern Guinea? In Europe, and from samples shipped north from the medical desert. This story, too, begins in the Kissi Triangle.

In the early months of 2014, Doctors Without Borders, the world's largest medical humanitarian organization and its most Ebola-savvy one, had a small brigade in Guéckédou, where they were working to rein in malaria. Members of the MSF team—the organization is better known by its French acronym, for Médecins Sans Frontières—were as perplexed as others by the mysterious affliction spreading right in front of them, so they sought clues about its etiology by reviewing the signs and symptoms of the stricken. On March 14, they sent a summary of their findings to an MSF epidemiologist in Brussels. Paradoxically, the identification of Ebola as the culprit was based on two of its less common but best-known signs: when he noted that a number of the afflicted had hiccups and a few had signs of a bleeding disorder, the epidemiologist worried that they might be stricken by a filovirus. He sounded the alarm.

In response, one MSF team in Brussels packed for Guinea, and another was summoned from Sierra Leone to Guéckédou, where its members joined logistics experts hired to pack up blood samples from the sick and from survivors. The samples were sent north from Conakry on Air France's overnight flight to Paris, and from there to a lab in Lyon.[10] A team of virologists and lab technicians in full biosafety gear got to work at once. A few minutes after 7:00 p.m. on March 21, the MSF epidemiologist's hunch was confirmed: the samples teemed with the Zaire Ebola virus—the species identified as the cause of the 1976 outbreak, which had centered around a Belgian mission hospital, where almost 90 percent of those sickened had died. A day later, and along with the World Health Organization, health authorities in Guinea announced that their country was home to what was in all likelihood already a large and geographically diffuse Ebola outbreak.

These authorities acknowledged its spread to Conakry and expressed fears that the virus had already crossed Guinea's borders. Many outbreak watchers assumed the borders in question were those with Liberia, because the Sierra Leonean pieces of the puzzle hadn't yet been put together or communicated effectively. A week later, the Liberian health ministry confirmed cases of fatal Ebola in Lofa County, just south of the country's border with Guinea. That's when one high-ranking UN official based in Monrovia began pressing for a more aggressive response from the World Health Organization and the alphabet soup of humanitarian agencies associated with the United Nations. I knew this official and had clearance to read her dispatches, which make clear some of what happened—and didn't happen—within those institutions as Ebola continued to spread. In essence, she felt stonewalled by headquarters, and reached out to MSF and other nongovernmental agencies with experience in Ebola response. There weren't many of those, as MSF stalwarts often noted.

Bureaucratic sluggishness, infighting, and miscommunication—much discussed in subsequent studies and commentaries about what went wrong with the international Ebola response—were the subject of heated debate in the midst of it. There were many open conflicts among various protagonists. On March 31, for example, MSF leaders correctly declared the epidemic to be "unprecedented" in scale and ample cause for an unprecedented and concerted response; they demanded the world pay attention. This demand was made, in typical MSF fashion, in a press release. (The organization issues an average of one press release per day.) The next day, the World Health Organization, in typical WHO fashion, cautioned against overreacting: the outbreak was not unprecedented, its chief spokesperson claimed from Geneva; it was quite similar to previous ones. An Ebola Twitter war ensued, the first of many.

At one level, a strong similarity between present and past did exist. As in previously documented Ebola outbreaks, the contagion pattern suggested human-to-human transmission in the course of caregiving and burying the dead. The West African epidemic had, however, reached the region's capital cities; this level of urban spread was new and should have worried the World Health Organization more than it did. There was, by then, a real risk of an Ebola surge overwhelming hospitals and health-care professionals, and abundant evidence that social distancing and other mitigation strategies might be materially impossible in these cities. During the civil conflicts that had recently ravaged the region, rural refugees had flooded into all three cities, trebling or quadrupling the size of their populations. They continued to grow after the conflicts ended.

The region's political and economic elites, most of them city dwellers, quickly developed concerns about the stigma associated with Ebola and the effect it might have on trade. (Tourism hadn't yet rebounded after civil war.) But the authorities didn't turn down early offers to help, either. Within two days of its announcement, the World Health Organization, not in the habit of issuing errata, dispatched an outbreak SWAT team to Guinea. In late March and early April, public-health agencies from around the affluent world followed suit. Among them was the largest of the lot, the U.S. Centers for Disease Control and Prevention (CDC). But the job at hand wasn't only disease control and prevention. Nor was it solely the study of transmission chains, contact tracing, the counting of the dead, or confirmation of cause of death. The people of the trizone region, and soon many others, were looking for something else: if Ebola has always been a caregivers' disease, it's because people always seek care when they're sick.

There's little evidence that stricken villagers and their urban kin, regardless of their own diverse notions of disease causation, were unwilling to seek care from doctors and nurses, even though national and international authorities and journalists soon made claims along the lines of a *New York Times* headline, "Fear of Ebola Breeds a Terror of Physicians."[11] The sick may have consulted traditional healers of all stripes, but they also sought care from doctors and nurses in public hospitals and private clinics, and in towns and cities; there just weren't a lot of physicians in the medical desert. What drove Ebola sufferers underground, and sparked or fanned conspiracy theories and overt resistance to health authorities, was not the arrival of doctors, nurses, and other professional caregivers. It was, rather, the arrival of a vast machinery of disease containment: once the global alarm sounded in late March, the control-over-care paradigm was officially ascendant.

To be clear, effective containment in the spring of 2014 would have prevented much of the suffering and death described in the pages that follow. The question raised in these pages is whether effective containment is possible without safe and effective care. From the start of the West African Ebola epidemic, the order of priorities advanced by international health officials was in view: the first order of business was to stop transmission, the second was to protect health professionals, and the third was to save the lives of those already afflicted. This was crystal-clear from the outset.

The SWAT teams dispatched by various national and international organizations, and soon enough by military forces from all over, counted fewer nurses than epidemiologists, researchers, managers, health educators, communication specialists, and soldiers. This April influx also included a slew of short-term consultants focused on safe burials, health promotion, health security, infection control, the elaboration and enforcement of building and safety codes, the proper conduct of what's termed "incident management," and the cultivation of something else called "cultural resilience." These consultants began training thousands of locals (underpaid, of course) to be contact tracers tasked with identifying and surveilling all those in contact with each person confirmed to have Ebola. They trained a similarly numerous contingent of sprayers of chlorine, crowd controllers, town criers, and "burial boys." This last term may not have been introduced by Ebola SWAT teams, but it was of European origin.

So, too, was the colonial-style inversion of clinical priorities. Even those with clinical training were often directed to nonclinical tasks. The inversion of medicine's idealized social contract, with saving the sick the highest priority, required such redirection.

The tasks assumed by these teams, homegrown and expatriate, were of critical importance. But the personnel of the international disease-control machinery soon learned that the majority of locals, whether in villages or cities or moving between them, didn't wish to be contained, instructed, traced, controlled, managed, monitored, sprayed, isolated, quarantined, or buried safely—even in a culturally resilient manner. Nor did many desire to be guinea pigs. They did, however, want proper medical and nursing care and pragmatic assistance with food, water, and social services, especially when ordered to remain in place or formally quarantined.

People at risk of Ebola could also, surely, have used some reassurance regarding their chances, as opposed to lectures on the perils of bushmeat and brief workshops on faddish concepts like cultural resilience. The messages initially disseminated in 2014 by health-promotion and communication consultants—who relied on cues from the sort of scientific authority previously described—didn't help lessen the control-versus-care conflict, nor did they lessen growing fear. Radio spots, commissioned songs, and billboards showcased a confusing set of troubling, punitive, or contradictory messages and commands: Ebola is real, not caused by witchcraft or curses. It kills 90 percent of those afflicted. Don't eat bushmeat. Don't eat bats. Don't eat plums (which few West Africans seemed to fancy) gnawed on by bats. Don't play with or eat baboons (a species largely absent from the region in which the spillover event was held to occur) or monkeys of any sort. Don't touch your sick or bury your dead, or you'll be punished. Don't shake hands. Don't touch anyone at all, ever. Stay at home, or shelter in place. Go to a hospital. Don't go to a hospital, as there's no known treatment for Ebola. Go to an isolation center. Isolate yourself if you can't get to one of those because of travel bans. Practice social distancing.

Ham-fisted hectoring was not unfamiliar to the people of the forest districts, who like people everywhere had their own complex and discrepant notions of what caused the very real affliction spreading in their midst. Nor were the *forestiers*—as they've been termed from Conakry since it became the capital of French Guinea in 1904—unfamiliar with the inversion of medicine's social contract, with care replaced by containment as the sanctioned priority. They were, on the other hand, unaccustomed to a benevolent and effective health system able to care for them when ill or injured, regardless of the nature of affliction or of perceived etiologies.

In both Guéckédou and Macenta Districts, there was by early April evidence of what francophone Guineans called *réticence*—overt resistance to quarantine and isolation and hostility to powerful outsiders. In previous decades, influential outsiders had been associated with disease containment, the restriction of free movement, calls to abandon polytheism and other superstitions, and heavy-handed efforts to prevent the *forestiers* from cultivating forest gardens while industrial logging flourished. (In 1976, Conakry decreed felling a tree a capital crime, if it was those living among the trees doing the felling.) As efforts to ban funerals were followed by others forbidding home-based care in the absence of trusted alternatives, conflict erupted across the forest districts.

It's easy enough to understand both the mixed messages and the motivation behind these bans. Funerals and caregiving are the two main sources of contagion in Ebola outbreaks. But last rites and caregiving are deemed social obligations as least as important in the medical desert as anywhere else. Across Guinea, people fled disease-control campaigns or responded to them with violence. Contact tracing, and many contact tracers, were often met with open hostility. On April 4, a newly opened MSF isolation unit in Macenta was looted and shut down by an angry and fearful crowd. Ebola got real, all right.

As "Ebola is real" began trending as an official and expert response to fearful and distrustful local responses, ongoing spread was missed by seasoned Ebola hands. This was in part because, across the region, the machinery of containment was largely untethered from the delivery of effective care. Such was the conclusion, if not the language, of a two-month-long investigation of what transpired during April and May by medical reporters from *The New York Times*:

> Although conditions were ideal for the virus to go underground, some of the world's most experienced Ebola fighters convinced themselves that the sharp decline in newly reported cases in April and May was real. Tracing those exposed to Ebola and checking them for symptoms, the key to containing any outbreak, had been lacking in many areas. Health workers had been chased out of fearful neighborhoods. Ebola treatment centers had gained such reputations as deathtraps that even desperately ill patients devoted their waning strength to avoiding them.[12]

"Health workers" is, of course, an expansive rubric. It didn't include, during those early months, many nurses and doctors with expertise in caring for critically ill patients. Guinea's clinical desert remained arid as the control-over-care paradigm blossomed.

The same process unfolded in Liberia. By April 9, having isolated what they believed to be the last of twelve Ebola cases, Liberian authorities began counting the days without report of new ones. According to the World Health Organization, if Liberia reached forty-two consecutive days in their countdown without any new cases, the country could declare an end to its outbreak. Emergency responders from MSF and Samaritan's Purse, the missionary organization that had converted its Monrovia chapel into an ETU, declared an end to their Ebola work in Liberia, with the former pulling its team back to Guinea for the mopping-up phase. The disease-control and Ebola experts who'd shown up in late March also began winding down operations.

Meanwhile, officials and international authorities were still making the improbable claim that the epidemic had spared Sierra Leone entirely, even though the Guinean villages and towns hit early in the outbreak were a lot closer to Sierra Leone's Kailahun and Kono Districts than to Conakry. Given the region's porous borders and the nature of Ebola's human-to-human spread, the international teams dispatched to West Africa had ample reason to suspect the virus had already spread there.

And then there was the seventeen-page report that officials in Conakry had produced in March, which had revealed a number of cross-border Ebola introductions and the death in a Sierra Leonean hospital of a woman with ties to Guinea's epidemic. The authors of that report had linked the deceased woman to a friend described, in an unflattering and misleading epidemiological epithet, as a "superspreader." This was a locally famous traditional healer and diviner who for decades had helped diagnose and respond to diverse afflictions on both sides of the border. (Thrown cowries were this woman's medium, but she was also known to converse with the dead.) The alleged superspreader had visited her sick friend at home and in the hospital. By month's end, she herself was suffering from nausea, vomiting, diarrhea, and severe headaches. She soon died, sometime around April 8.

Hundreds attended the healer's funeral in Kailahun District. Within weeks her husband and a grandson had fallen ill. But there's little doubt that more than close family prepared her for burial and helped to inter her: impoverished homes and understocked and understaffed clinics and hospitals were, along with an absence of well-provisioned undertakers or burial teams, the real Ebola superspreaders in the region. By the end of April, others who'd tended to her, including fellow healers, began to fall ill, and through their own caregiving (or receipt of it) helped forge new links in the chain of transmission. One of these was the healer's sister-in-law, whose blood sample—carried by a health-surveillance officer over rough roads between Kailahun and Kenema, a center of the diamond trade and capital of the district of the same name—yielded the first laboratory-confirmed case of Ebola in Sierra Leone on May 25.

The sample was logged shortly after many Ebola experts had returned to whatever tasks they'd been previously assigned, or had simply packed up and flown home to Geneva, Brussels, or Atlanta.

Hard as it might be to believe, there were fewer health professionals in Sierra Leone than in Guinea. But one of the former was already knowledgeable about Ebola: Dr. Humarr Khan, the director of Kenema Government Hospital. Khan was born to a large family in the town of Lungi, home to Sierra Leone's international airport. He was among the first generation of Sierra Leoneans to graduate from the country's only medical school, which was opened well after the end of colonial rule in the 1960s.

By the time I met him, Humarr Khan was known as a collegial and hardworking physician-researcher with a particular interest in Lassa fever. He was compact, jovial, and an ardent soccer buff. As Ebola spread from nearby Meliandou to Conakry and Liberia, Khan was monitoring developments from the hospital and lab. Although the hospital was a decrepit mess, the lab was not. Khan and his American colleagues, including several from Tulane and Harvard, had long dreamed of creating a network of laboratories in West Africa that, using new diagnostic technologies and the tools of genomics, would help unravel the mysteries of Lassa's epidemiology and how it caused human disease. A few years prior to the outbreak in Meliandou, Khan had teamed up with Pardis Sabeti, who'd been a student of mine at Harvard Medical School and was now a colleague. He had the patients, she had the supercomputers, and together their teams sequenced the Lassa genome.

This work was supported by the American government, which, panicked by the homegrown anthrax attacks that had followed 9/11, had pumped up investments in research on pathogens that might conceivably be weaponized. As part of that effort, Lassa had been put on a new list of "Category A bioterrorism agents," in part because Soviet scientists and defense authorities had previously included filoviruses on their roster of bioweapons.[13] After this new classification, a group of Sierra Leoneans, working with American colleagues and funding, was able to build a modern laboratory to study the virus on the war-battered campus of Kenema's district hospital. The U.S. Centers for Disease Control had pledged to help build and sustain another lab in N'Zérékoré, southern Guinea's regional capital. But armed conflict, dwindling enthusiasm, and bureaucratic Balkanization between multiple agencies from several nations ended that dream well before the Ebola nightmare began.[14]

When the boy branded Patient Zero fell ill, in other terms, Kenema was pretty much a clinical desert, but not a diagnostic one. Its hospital, where Khan directed the Lassa ward, was the only place in Upper West Africa that had the capacity to diagnose any kind of hemorrhagic fever. But Kenema's clinicians, who were mostly nurses, knew that no laboratory network could slow Ebola's spread unless it was embedded in a health system strong enough to deliver high-quality care—and that was lacking from the Kissi Triangle to the coast.

Unlike some of their colleagues in the world of disease control, Dr. Khan and his colleagues were seeking the causes of febrile illness not just to identify and contain them but also to treat them. They knew that diagnosis alone does not a health system make, so in doing his work Khan regularly called for investments in Sierra Leone's entire care-delivery system, including its hospital infrastructure and network of nurse-run public clinics. All of them, Khan complained, lacked staff, stuff, and safe space in which to deliver care. Well after the war ended, the rebuilt Kenema Government Hospital and its

Lassa ward were poorly supplied and worse than dilapidated, and remained so even after Kenema's shimmering new lab arose from the sands of the clinical desert. But, as would become tragically clear during the Ebola epidemic, even that lab lacked the meticulous infection-control practices required to handle dangerous infectious pathogens.

One of these was Ebola, supposedly new to Upper West Africa. Over the years, Khan and his coworkers had demonstrated that a substantial percentage of patients with signs and symptoms suggestive of Lassa fever, but without laboratory evidence of it, did show evidence of recent Ebola infection. One study put the number at more than 8 percent.[15] That meant the virus wasn't only present in eastern Sierra Leone; it wasn't rare. These findings had been presented in scientific meetings and in a manuscript submitted for publication in an academic journal months before Patient Zero fell ill. Improbably, the article was rejected, with at least one reviewer arguing he just didn't believe Ebola occurred in West Africa. It didn't appear in print until shortly before the Kenema facility's director and many of his nursing colleagues were dead of Ebola.

On May 23, for the first time, Ebola reached the Kenema Government Hospital in a living human host. She was a twenty-year-old pregnant woman who hailed from a town in Kailahun District—from the same neighborhood, in fact, as the traditional healer tarred by epidemiologists as a "superspreader." The young woman arrived with a fever and was later found to have attended the superspreading funeral that took place in Kailahun in early April.[16] But all that she and others knew when she arrived at the hospital was that she had miscarried and was bleeding. The team in Kenema took her to the OR in an effort to save her.

Most physicians and nurse-midwives working in the region might have assumed the young woman's fever and miscarriage to be due to a peripartum infection caused by bacteria, or to a case of malaria. But lab tests did not support these diagnoses, and so Khan and his colleagues also tested her for Lassa. When it came back negative, they worried she had Ebola and requested that the lab perform the test the next day. By the time a blood sample from the alleged superspreader's sister-in-law arrived from a small health center in Kailahun. And so it came to pass that, on May 25, both the twenty-year-old and the healer's sister-in-law tested positive for Ebola. Both women would ultimately survive. Once within the hospital, the virus spread rapidly through its cramped and crowded wards, including the Lassa unit. The staff was overwhelmed and frightened, but the sick kept on coming.

At first, they came mostly from Kailahun District, with many linked one way or another to the nexus of healers and kin mentioned above. (As in Meliandou, the birth attendant looking after the pregnant woman from this nexus was among the first to die.) Then they came from Kenema and, after that, from across the country. As the crisis widened in June, Kenema Government Hospital was named the national Ebola referral center. Humarr Khan was suddenly Sierra Leone's Ebola czar. By the end of that month, with more than a hundred confirmed Ebola diagnoses, Khan and his team began admitting patients to a makeshift ETU erected on the campus. In the words of the Irish ambassador to Sierra Leone, a young diplomat who'd visited the hospital a dozen times before Ebola hit and was to become something of an Ebola czar herself, the unit was soon "operating very much on a wing and a prayer."[17]

Prayers did not suffice to conjure the staff, stuff, space, and systems needed in Kenema. On July 8, with fifty-three confirmed cases in the ETU, the campus ran out of chlorine. Stockouts of gloves and other PPE were also reported. Infection control was, in the word of a WHO physician dispatched to the hospital, "catastrophic."[18] International disease controllers called for the hospital's closure, even though there was no obvious alternative in the more heavily populated west, where cases were mounting rapidly. Facilities in Freetown and Port Loko—a large town not far from the Atlantic coast and not far from Humarr Khan's hometown of Lungi—were already transferring critically ill patients east to the hospital in Kenema. Many didn't survive the jolting six-hour drive, especially patients with nausea and vomiting. Their lost fluids went unreplaced, a depletion worsened by the oppressive heat of a suffocating, fouled jeep. Since the rainy season was only half over, some vehicles didn't make it through the mud. It's not difficult to imagine what became of their passengers.

It wasn't difficult, in any case, for me to imagine, since I happened to be in Freetown just then. Before the outbreak began, I'd helped organize a medical conference on surgical care there in late June; it was my first time in the country. When we made plans to gather in Freetown for the conference, I knew only four Sierra Leoneans. One was Humarr Khan; the second and third, surgeons involved in the conference; the fourth, a student of mine at Harvard Medical School, who began telling me about the dread moving west over my first meal in Freetown. By November of that year, Khan and one of the surgeons were dead of Ebola, my student had taken a leave to work full-time on efforts to halt it, and the other surgeon was struggling to keep the nation's chief referral hospital from collapsing under the weight of Ebola's assault on Freetown.

Kenema's collapse, and Humarr Khan's, was not prevented by these or any other efforts. Over the course of June and July, Ebola picked off the hospital's brave but poorly provisioned nurses and other caregivers like a hidden sniper. Fear bordering on panic rippled through the staff, including its Lassa stalwarts; rumors and conspiracy theories and protests swirled around outside the hospital gates; some nursing aides and ancillary staff refused to show up for work. Khan watched as several of his closest friends died. Then, on July 19, after a day or so of weakness and malaise, he, too, mounted a fever. Like just about every other clinician feeling feverish at that time and in that place, Khan hoped it was "only malaria," a leading killer across the region. A couple of days later, when he learned it was Ebola, he asked to be driven east to Kailahun, where MSF had just opened a fifty-bed ETU.

Humarr Khan knew from begging for chlorine and other supplies that the MSF unit was better stocked than his facility in Kenema—and staffed by doctors and nurses who'd signed up for the job. He also worried that staying put might mean he'd die as a patient in his own hospital, which he feared would force its closure. Khan wasn't the only one who didn't want to see Kenema shut down, even though surviving staff were clearly unable to deliver care safely. The Lassa ward was, along with the new unit in Kailahun, the only place in the nation trying to pull these patients through. A purpose-built ETU had been promised for Kenema by the Red Cross but was delayed by controversy and bureaucratic haggling; a functioning unit in Freetown was still months away. Neither would come online quickly enough to prevent Kenema's ignominious downfall.

As one of a fairly small number of Sierra Leonean physicians with an international reputation, Dr. Khan was urged by friends and family to seek care elsewhere. He of course knew that his chances of survival would be better outside the country, but no one sick with Ebola in Upper West Africa had yet been allowed to leave the clinical desert. When he arrived in Kailahun, Khan still had reason for hope: he was young, only thirty-nine, and otherwise healthy. Cared for in an American hospital, say, most people Khan's age survive serious viral ailments, even those for which there are no specific therapies and that may cause death primarily through mechanisms other than fluid loss leading to shock. But Ebola is exceptionally virulent, and Kailahun was about as far from an intensive care unit (ICU) or emergency room as Khan could get.

There was one other ray of hope, called ZMapp, an experimental Ebola therapy developed by a Canadian research lab. Like promising Ebola vaccine candidates, ZMapp had gathered dust on the shelf for years, because few in the pharmaceutical industry had shown much interest in developing preventives or therapies for Ebola. The costs of developing them were high, and (in the common calculus) the potential rewards too low. But, improbably, the only ZMapp doses on the continent were in three vials stored in a refrigerator at the MSF unit in Kailahun, a few hundred yards away from where Khan lay dying. The staff there debated whether or not to administer it to him.

The Khan-ZMapp debates played out during three days of international conference calls. These palavers, to use the term common in this part of West Africa, included a handful of Ebola experts from MSF headquarters in Paris and Brussels, WHO officials in Geneva, and health authorities representing Sierra Leone, the United States, and Canada. The calls became public and contentious. Every new incident of nosocomial transmission—Khan's was likely one, of course—pushed influential voices to argue that all patients should receive an oral solution of rehydration salts and, for most, nothing more, including ZMapp. MSF was calling the shots, and several of its physicians in Kailahun threatened to resign if a "medical VIP" were to receive treatment unavailable to all. But the real debate was less about favoritism or administering an experimental therapy than about what therapies would be administered within the Kailahun unit.

The government of Sierra Leone and others made emergency efforts to get

Humarr Khan flown to Switzerland or Germany, engaging a medevac plane to await him in Lungi. But when pilots and crew learned that he was vomiting and had diarrhea, they refused to take him. Khan died in Kailahun on July 29.

After Humarr Khan died, his friends, family, colleagues, and fellow citizens—and various pundits—argued about whether he had received adequate care in Kailahun and (if not) why he hadn't been flown to a safe haven. Newspaper and radio reports, as well as commentary on social media, made much of the fact that Khan had died without receiving ZMapp. But more tragically than dying without ZMapp, Khan died without receiving adequate—and nonexperimental—treatment for significant losses of fluids and electrolytes. An epidemic of mistrust had already been mounting. Now, in a climate of angry disagreement sparked by Khan's death, it took hold among the ranks of frightened and often disgruntled health-care workers.

The drama I would later witness in Monrovia in mid-October, when two young brothers with "wet" Ebola collapsed within the world's largest ETU, had by then been playing out for months. Not all Ebola patients die from, or with, dehydration, but prolonged vomiting, diarrhea, and fever were prominent early symptoms among many who fell ill in 2014. If a substantial proportion of the afflicted caregivers were dying of hypovolemic shock triggered in part by lost fluids and electrolytes, wasn't that a paradoxically reassuring detail for clinicians willing to replace them on the front lines? After all, there's therapy for that, and *someone* had to take care of wet patients, as families and traditional healers—Upper West Africa's primary caregivers—had already demonstrated. But by July it was being argued, usually by outside experts, that infection control within hospitals was so ineffective that the primary goal of an Ebola *treatment* unit was to isolate patients suspected or known to have Ebola and to encourage them to try to rehydrate themselves with oral rehydration salts—a goal met, in Khan's case.

What patients critically ill with Ebola needed was *supportive* and *critical* care, which is delivered primarily by skilled nurses. Supportive care doesn't mean handholding. It means fluid resuscitation together with the prompt treatment of intercurrent or secondary infections, many resulting from Ebola's attack on the immune system or from damage to the gastrointestinal tract. It means treatment of the malnutrition, anemia, and wasting that accompany serious illness. It might also mean transfusions of whole blood, plasma, or platelets, or administering drugs called vasopressors, which elevate blood pressure. Critical care requires more gadgetry—a breathing machine for ventilatory support, a dialysis unit for renal failure, various monitors—but it's not rocket science, either. Both supportive and critical care are considered routine in any American hospital with an intensive care unit.

Critical care was perhaps out of reach in Sierra Leone—in the summer of 2014, there were no ICUs to speak of in Sierra Leone, not even in Freetown's chief referral hospital—but many hospitals and clinics still had the ability to offer supportive care. During the West African Ebola epidemic, however, such care was discouraged because the slightest breach of contact precautions could and did result in nosocomial spread. Even those in full protective gear (gowns, gloves, masks, and goggles) were often called to observe a "no-touch policy," meaning no physical contact at all. This approach was unlikely to save those unable to keep down orally administered therapies but was safer than anything that might involve needle sticks. Messy procedures like emergency cesarean sections, and even assisted vaginal deliveries, were of course casualties of this view and of the dread that underpinned it. Since most Sierra Leonean women delivered at home, they'd long endured a de facto no-touch policy from skilled professionals. But that didn't help the traditional birth attendants who were left holding the babies.

Medical personnel had ample cause for fear when the Ebola outbreak occurred. Ninety-two health professionals in the district of Kenema were stricken with the virus during the epidemic, of whom sixty-six were employees at the hospital. This was about a third of its clinical staff, and most died.[19] Many of these workers had been infected while providing care outside of the facility, sometimes within patients' homes, as part of a parallel fee-for-service health system that sprouts when and where nurses and nursing assistants are underpaid—or not salaried at all. The dangers were real, in other words. But many West Africans, including frightened clinicians, disliked having their fates decided by those advocating a standard of care that in many cases didn't resemble care at all.

The fraught debates fanned by Humarr Khan's death unfurled just as two American missionaries contracted Ebola in Liberia and were flown to the biocontainment unit at Emory University Hospital in Atlanta. They weren't medevacked to receive ZMapp or some other experimental therapy; they shared three vials of ZMapp, flown in for them from Kailahun, while still in Monrovia. No, the missionaries were evacuated so that they could receive supportive and (if necessary) critical care. Many involved in such triage believed that Humarr Khan and the nurses and allied health professionals in Kenema would have survived if they'd had similar access to such care.

When health workers across Sierra Leone went on strike after Khan's death, it was in part to protest work conditions and the failure to afford occupationally exposed West Africans the same sort of medical attention received by Americans and Europeans stricken with Ebola. But it was the debate about ZMapp, not the one about the quality of basic medical care, that went viral. Remonstrations about the Khan case—and about differential exposure to risk of Ebola and differential access to things that might save one from it—spread quickly. By mid-August, they were a staple of mainstream news across Africa and beyond. *The Onion*, a satirical weekly published in the United States, ran a story about Khan's death under the headline "Experts: Ebola Vaccine at Least 50 White People Away."[20]

International experts may have debated the question of access to experimental therapies, vaccines, and better-equipped isolation units, but they did so in the narrow terms of quandary ethics. Notably, should Humarr Khan, Sierra Leone's top expert on hemorrhagic fevers, have been given "special treatment"? One critical question, of course, was whether enough was being done to make basic supportive and critical care—nonspecial treatment—possible in Sierra Leone, Liberia, and Guinea. Many West African clinicians, especially those who were unable to charter a plane or count on their governments or sponsors to bring them to safety if need be, thought not. The no-touch policy didn't help, deepening anguish among clinicians and deepening resentment among patients and their families.

With international attention focused on containment, and in the absence of prompt and massive efforts to safely introduce supportive and clinical care, local clinicians began to fear that they and their patients were, to use the scholarly term, screwed.

Roiling debates about the quality of care proceeded as if West African clinical deserts were somehow immutably arid and suddenly and forever cut off from the rest of the globe. This hermetic fiction was jarring when the international response, and much public discussion, focused largely on spread across national borders. But it was downright surreal from a historical point of view. The rest of the world has been connected to West Africa for centuries—and is still connected, as diamonds from Koidu and Kenema, and the weapons that more recently leveled those towns, attest.

The myth of hard borders became more difficult to sustain in the face of pressing need to break that seal. It didn't take long for Ebola to be exported beyond Upper West Africa. In late July, a sick Liberian-American businessman sought medical care in Lagos, the largest city in Africa. The patient and one of his doctors died in the attempt, along with six others, prompting Nigeria's president to call the doomed Liberian a "madman." But he hadn't been crazy at all. He'd gone to Nigeria because he knew that as an Ebola patient he could expect to receive better care, in better conditions—air-conditioning surely helped those in biosafety gear tend to patients without the minor distraction of drowning in sweat—than elsewhere in West Africa.

In the weeks that followed, a total of nineteen people were infected with Ebola in Lagos, and most survived. Global public-health authorities breathed a sigh of relief, but not because of the lower mortality: A major Ebola outbreak in Africa's largest city had been prevented—without hospital closures or hospital bans. This was not because Nigeria had invested its oil wealth in its public care-delivery system, but because Nigeria at the time was conducting a massive polio-eradication campaign. Once Ebola turned up in Lagos, the health authorities diverted the resources and know-how of this campaign, which calls for meticulous contact tracing, toward containing the new threat.[21] Caregivers then helped avert disaster by bravely providing supportive care to patients once they were in isolation.

By the time Ebola reached Nigeria, however, any notion that the West African epidemic was under control had long been dispelled. On August 8, the World Health Organization took the rare step of declaring Ebola in West Africa a "public health emergency of international concern." (COVID-19 was the next declared one, in January 2020.) But health authorities didn't use this announcement as an opportunity to radically and rapidly improve the quality of care offered to those ill with the disease. In the tyranny of the either-or, and as deaths mounted, officials remained focused on containment, as if prevention and care were competing tasks rather than complementary ones. Such views were common even after quarantine, travel bans, border closures, and martial law had already failed to control the epidemic, and even after it became clear that patients who received better supportive care, as they did in Lagos and Atlanta, had good odds of survival.

Réticence about the control-over-care paradigm among the general population remained fierce in Guinea. In mid-September, villagers in the south of the country killed eight members of a national "awareness team" trained by "social-mobilization experts" (to invoke two of the unwieldy neologisms of the international disease-control apparatus) and dumped their bodies in a latrine.[22] Such teams, referred to as "health workers" by many reporters, had been trained by the consultants who descended upon all three countries to lecture the locals about the reality of Ebola and the risks associated with caregiving, burials, and bushmeat. The Guinean Red Cross and its international partners would later report an average of ten attacks per month on its burial and infection-control teams.

The story was similar in Liberia, and not only in rural areas. On July 23, a man called (truly) Edward Delay set fire to a conference room in the Ministry of Health. The day before, and in the same room, Delay informed Liberia's president, Ellen Johnson Sirleaf, that he was distraught over the recent death from Ebola of his teenage brother, who had been turned away from a Monrovia hospital. Sirleaf responded to this act of arson and to other developments by seeking to seal national borders and calling the army into the fray. When these measures proved ineffective, she requested, on September 9, assistance from the U.S. armed forces. Several other West African leaders, and some humanitarian organizations, also called for rich-world militaries to contribute to the Ebola response.

Within days of his Liberian peer's request, President Barack Obama committed to sending three thousand troops to Liberia. "If we move fast," he told the world, "even if imperfectly, that could mean the difference between 10,000, 20,000, 30,000 deaths versus hundreds of thousands or even a million deaths."[23] Donald Trump, not yet a presidential candidate but already with a Twitter following that exceeded that of many pop stars, responded with this tweet:

Obama won't send troops to fight jihadists, yet sends them to Liberia to contract Ebola. He is a delusional failure.[24]

The American troops sent to Liberia actually stood little risk of contracting Ebola, because they weren't being sent to staff mobile army surgical hospital (MASH) units. Instead, their job (with the help of slow-motion civilian subcontractors) was to erect new Ebola treatment units, help coordinate logistics, and assist with transport—of disease controllers, clinicians, and other healthy personnel. U.S. troops weren't even permitted to transport properly packed blood samples.

American soldiers were also there to back up the Liberian army, a role they'd played during much of the twentieth century. Liberian armed forces certainly needed mentoring on crowd control: on August 20, they fired live ammunition into a crowd protesting the quarantine of West Point, a Monrovia slum that was home to some seventy-five thousand people. A teenager bled out on the spot. Some of the protesters then attacked and pillaged an Ebola isolation facility that had been recently erected in the neighborhood. Many in the crowd loudly dismissed Ebola as a fabrication or a plot, and the international media were soon reporting with alarm (and sometimes a mix of consternation and bemusement) that looters at the facility had carted off the center's soiled mattresses and linens.

Sirleaf called off the West Point quarantine after ten days.

The control-over-care paradigm clearly had scant popular appeal. It also had limited effectiveness. By September, the Ebola outbreak in West Africa was already ten times larger than any previously recorded, with no end in sight. Sierra Leone was then registering more than two hundred cases each week, leading even sober U.S. health authorities to issue doomsday scenarios.

The most notorious of these, which in September bore the august imprimatur of the U.S. Centers for Disease Control, predicted over a million cases by January if current trends were to continue.[25] Prior to 2014, the largest documented Ebola outbreak had been registered in 2000, in the war-torn clinical desert of northern Uganda, where an estimated 425 fell ill from a Sudan strain and 224 died. Now, predictions of worldwide spread from West Africa whipped up a parallel epidemic of journalistic and public hysteria that had already gone global. This emerging social pandemic was heightened at the close of September when Thomas Eric Duncan, a Liberian visiting his Liberia-born fiancée and their son in Dallas, became the first person ever diagnosed with Ebola in the United States.

Like others stricken with the disease, Duncan—who went by Eric— was a caregiver of sorts. He'd shared a taxi with a pregnant nineteen-year-old in distress as her family frantically sought care in Monrovia. Ominously wracked with convulsions, the young woman was referred to an ETU, where treatment for her condition, likely eclampsia, would be available—had she been admitted. The staff there turned her away, as the unit was already filled to capacity. Duncan then helped carry her from the taxi back into her house, where she died a few hours later. This occurred at the time of our own team's first trip to Monrovia, when we'd seen a couple of sick people lying in its streets. Passersby gave them a wide berth, awaiting emergency personnel in hazmat suits. With some shame, we'd done the same.

Shortly after trying to help the dying teenager, Eric Duncan headed to Texas on a commercial airline. On September 25, a few days after his arrival, he went to the emergency room of a major Dallas hospital, complaining of a low-grade fever, headache, and abdominal pain. He was sent home with a typical emergency-room diagnosis—"sinusitis and abdominal pain"—even though he forthrightly stated that he'd just come from Liberia, then the most Ebola-affected country on earth.[26] Three days later, critically ill, Duncan returned to the same hospital in an ambulance, and on September 30, after reviewing test results, the Centers for Disease Control declared him an Ebola sufferer. Because of tardy diagnosis and inadequate infection-control measures within the hospital, two nurses caring for Duncan subsequently fell ill with the disease. These were the first cases of Ebola transmission ever recorded in the United States.

Print, television, and social media blew up, and little of its content reflected kindness or concern. Twitter, in particular, became a superspreader of Ebola hysteria and of meanness. On October 4, Donald Trump, leading the charge, demanded that Duncan be punished:

This Ebola patient Thomas Duncan, who fraudulently entered the
U.S. by signing false papers, is causing havoc. If he lives, prosecute![27]

Even Liberia's mild-mannered president invoked the possibility of legal action against Eric Duncan and offered her apologies to the American people for his care seeking. Although he and his family were tried in the Twitter court of popular opinion, there would be no legal action against him, even if he had committed a crime: Duncan died on October 8. The Texas shitshow was, however, echoed across the globe.

More countries declared travel bans and the like, just as Mr. Trump was recommending on Twitter and in other free forums granted him. In October, the Australian health minister imposed a travel ban on all visitors from the three most affected countries, suggesting that traditional funeral rites there made their welcome "an unacceptable risk."[28] The anthropologist Paul Richards, who'd worked in Sierra Leone for decades and had done more

empirical research on the matter than the authorities Down Under, offered
a tart reply:

> If it is stubborn to wash the dead then it is stubborn to nurse the
> sick. To insist otherwise blames the victim. Courageous refusal
> to abandon loved ones normally elicits admiration, not blame.
> So commentators on the Ebola epidemic, whether in Australia or
> elsewhere, ought to avoid stigmatizing West Africans for no other
> reason than that they care for their loved ones.[29]

Xenophobic and punitive reactions, terrifying to Eric Duncan's family and disturbing to many traveling West Africans, were dispiriting to the expatriate clinicians who'd responded to the call to serve in West Africa. To nurse the sick and
to introduce supportive and critical care was what led us there in the first place.

We had begun to suspect we wouldn't always be welcomed home well before October 24, when Kaci Hickox, an American nurse volunteering in Sierra
Leone, was detained in a holding unit near Newark's international airport on
the orders of the governor of New Jersey. This happened just as Craig Spencer, an American emergency-room physician, fell ill with Ebola in New York
City shortly after returning from a stint in Guinea with MSF. By then, Ebola
hysteria—fanned by the hot air of the upcoming American election season—
had reached its peak in the (again) Ebola-free United States. We'd continue
to feel its sting in the months to follow, but poor Spencer got a hornet's nest
full of venom just when he most needed support. Rather than being praised
for his service, he was pilloried in the tabloid press and on social media for
trying to take his mind off what he'd just witnessed by going bowling—even
though he promptly reported to Bellevue Hospital when he mounted a fever.

Bowlers and balls were unharmed, but Donald Trump didn't miss the
chance to disparage Spencer's irrational wish to return home after his tour of
duty in the clinical desert, and Obama's obvious lunacy in letting him do so.
Just prior to the midterm elections, the future leader of the United States (if
not the free world) leveled his Twitter guns at both the sick physician and the
sitting president:

> If this doctor, who so recklessly flew into New York from West
> Africa, has Ebola, then Obama should apologize to the American
> people & resign!

Trump, a self-described germophobe, now used Twitter to shower disparagement on his allegedly Kenyan-born rival, on black and brown immigrants,
and on returning clinicians. Dr. Spencer, Trump wrote with strangely poetic
inaccuracy, had "touched many, bedlam!" Obama, on the other hand, was a
"stubborn dope."

> I have been saying for weeks for President Obama to stop the
> flights from West Africa. So simple, but he refused. A TOTAL
> incompetent![30]

The surgeon Martin Salia, a native of Humarr Khan's adoptive city of Kenema, was the second of my Sierra Leonean acquaintances to die of Ebola. He,
too, was the target of opprobrium during the madhouse season of American
elections.

Humarr Khan and Martin Salia were friends with much in common.
Both had the misfortune to begin their medical studies as war broke out in
eastern Sierra Leone, and both became refugees when war reached Freetown.
Upon his return, Salia took a junior position at the country's main teaching hospital—a battered colonial relic named Connaught—and later went
on to graduate from the Pan-African Academy of Christian Surgeons after extensive training in Cameroon and Kenya. During the war, Salia's
wife, a nurse, and two sons emigrated to Maryland, where they would
eventually become U.S. citizens. Salia kept a green card. But like Khan,
he wanted to focus his attentions on the medically underserved of Sierra
Leone. This eventually led him to Kissy, a poor neighborhood in Freetown,
where he served as chief medical officer of the United Methodist Hospital.
As one of only a handful of surgeons practicing in a country of over seven
million people, Salia also performed surgeries at Connaught, serving as the

director of its emergency department. That's how I came to meet Salia a few months before he died.

Passionate about extending emergency surgical services to those who'd never known a safety net, which would have included almost all his fellow citizens when he finished medical school, Martin Salia attended the Freetown conference we helped organize in June. Although soft-spoken, he vigorously supported notions of progressive universalism (health care for all) and of social protection (health insurance for all), since these would in principle help remove barriers to life-saving surgical care. Shortly after the conference ended—and as Ebola brought most surgery to a halt within Sierra Leone—Salia went to Maryland for a brief respite with his family. His wife and sons hadn't wanted him to return to Sierra Leone. But Salia was a devout Catholic who felt it was his calling and his duty, and Humarr Khan's death had shaken him deeply. In August, after promising to return to the States if he fell ill, Salia flew back to Freetown.

Martin Salia surely knew the coming-home part would be easier said than done—harder, in any case, than tending to Connaught's trauma patients and performing emergency cesarean sections without coming in contact with Ebola. That said, it's not clear exactly how or where Salia contracted the disease. His hospital in Kissy had simply halted surgical services, and efforts to muster the staff, stuff, space, and systems necessary for treating surgical disease had largely petered out elsewhere by late October, by which time Freetown had supplanted Monrovia as the most Ebola-affected city on the face of the earth. All we know is that in the first days of November, he felt the onset of fever, muscle aches, and fatigue, at which point Salia called his wife to say he hadn't "knowingly made contact with an Ebola patient," but promised to get tested just in case.[31] He was probably soft-pedaling his fears, because the first place he sought care was a newly established British facility dedicated to the care of Ebola-stricken health professionals.

The British facility promised some real T in its ETU, but Martin Salia never received it. After some debate, the unit's gatekeepers turned him away. It had been set up to serve only those Sierra Leonean health professionals who were "directly involved in delivery of Ebola response programmes in U.K.-funded treatment facilities."[32] (Also ineligible for admission were Sierra

Leonean caregivers stricken with Ebola in the course of working in what were termed community-care centers, most of them short on the middle *C*.) An initial discussion of Salia's merits as a patient meeting such admission criteria concluded with a no—even though, as director of Connaught's emergency services, he played a key role in U.K.-funded Ebola programs.

Martin Salia next went to the suburb of Hastings, where the national police academy had been converted into an Ebola treatment unit at the close of September. He was by then pretty sure he had Ebola, but an initial test came back negative. So he was sent home from there, too. This led to relief in Maryland—and to premature celebration among colleagues in Kissy and at Connaught. But Salia's fever persisted, and soon he was losing fluids to vomiting and diarrhea. The surgeon turned next to Connaught, where the doctor tasked with leading the hospital's Ebola response had recently perished, as had several nurses, a couple of them during the brutal overland transfer to Kenema. On or around November 10, about eight days after the onset of his symptoms, he finally got confirmation that Ebola was the cause of his rapidly worsening signs and symptoms.

At that point, Martin Salia's friends at Connaught, several of whom had attended our June surgical conference and at least two of whom were British, pressed him to return to the U.K. facility that had turned him away. Its medical director already had designated a bed for him. By then, however, the surgeon was critically ill: he was showing evidence of renal failure. This might have been caused by a viral attack on his kidneys, but it also might have been caused—or worsened—by the drop in blood pressure that accompanies severe dehydration. Salia returned to Hastings, knowing he needed fluids urgently.

For days, Martin Salia had been taking oral rehydration salts, which several international organizations continued to insist was the best care they could offer in such circumstances. A few even still touted oral rehydration as the standard of care for all patients. But, as every surgeon knows, intravenous replacement is the mainstay of therapy for hypovolemia in the face of inability to take fluids by mouth, and the doctors at Hastings put an IV in Salia in order to administer fluids and antibody-rich blood from an Ebola survivor. He also received antibiotics and antimalarials. But by then, only critical care, of the kind available in any operational ICU, was likely to be able to take the measures likely required for him to survive long enough for his own immune system to rein in the virus. Critical care remained unavailable in Sierra Leone, however, even in the British ETU.

Hoping he might receive the kind of care that had allowed other American victims of Ebola to survive, Salia's friends and family made heroic efforts to airlift him to the United States. Quickly—through the generosity of their local Catholic church, the Methodists who employed Salia, and, it was rumored, the tech titan Paul Allen—they raised the promise of $200,000 in order to charter a biosecure plane to fly the surgeon to Omaha, where the University of Nebraska's biocontainment unit had agreed to take him in. Salia left for Nebraska on November 15, having boarded the plane on his own two feet, more than ten days after his symptoms had first appeared. By the time he reached the biocontainment unit, however, his kidneys had failed, he was agitated and in respiratory distress, and he had evidence of marked hypovolemia and liver dysfunction.[33] The clinicians running the unit did their best, initiating dialysis and mechanical ventilation shortly after his arrival. But it was too late. On November 17, Martin Salia, forty-four years old, was pronounced dead.

Several days later, Salia's wife returned home with his ashes, which had been sealed in a rubber box. She placed it on his side of the bed. She then organized a funeral mass in Hyattsville, Maryland, which was attended by hundreds, including Ron Klain, President Obama's Ebola czar. Months later, after another mass in her home parish, she placed the rubber box inside a wooden urn and then buried what remained of her husband.

Two questions in the tradition of social medicine: Why did Ebola spread so rapidly in some places and not in others? Why did it kill some of the afflicted while sparing others?

Conspiracy theorists raised these same questions throughout the epidemic, of course. But so did many local and national health authorities, who knew—in spite of the guesswork, hyperbole, and error that followed in the wake of Ebola—that the three countries heavily afflicted have some of the world's weakest health systems. Had they been more robust, it might have been possible for an acutely ill child like poor Émile from Meliandou, whether he was Patient Zero or not, to be seen by a well-trained village health worker. That worker, recognizing the urgency of the situation, might in turn have been able to summon a safe means of transporting the child to a hospital or clinic with proper infection-control capabilities and a clinical laboratory. Once at a decent hospital, a child like Émile might have received the care he needed to survive.

That kind of care requires emergency rooms, intensive care units, and operating rooms waiting at the end of an ambulance ride or referral—resources that rarely figure in the recommendations made by international health authorities and aid organizations promoting "health systems strengthening" in medical deserts like Upper West Africa. These systems, go the arguments, don't need such frills—the very ones we argued were essential investments during the Freetown surgery conference in June. Even after September 2014, when aid money began to trickle in to Guinea, Sierra Leone, and Liberia, there was never much evidence of the staff, stuff, or space that might have stopped the spread of the disease and saved those afflicted by it: Émile and his caregivers in Meliandou; Humarr Khan and the Kenema and Connaught nurses; Martin Salia; the convulsing pregnant teenager aided by Eric Duncan; and so many of the other victims whose names one never hears.

As for the second question—Why did some die while others were spared?—it's one always front and center in social medicine, which looks around (at social context) and back in time (at social history) in order to answer it. But the default explanation for significant differences in rates of mortality has long been a simple idea: different variants of Ebola kill differentially, with Zaire being the worst. Research such as that conducted by Pardis Sabeti and Humarr Khan may ultimately help reveal if specific mutations confer increased transmissibility and virulence. But the idea is simplistic as well as simple: many exclusively biological hypotheses about the variable virulence of pathogens are pretty quickly swamped by the variable virulence of the world we inhabit. Giving all the credit to the virus is dubious when we humans have been the architects of the stunning inequalities that characterize our shared world.

It's been the task of social medicine to sort out how multiple factors—ranging from nutritional status, age, comorbid disease, route of inoculation, relative lack (or absence) of the staff and stuff required to deliver supportive and critical care—contribute to differential mortality among those sickened by Ebola. The Americans and Europeans who fell ill were infected, after all, by the same Zaire strain that killed 70 percent of their West African peers. The great majority of stricken expatriates survived because they were flown back to the United States or Europe for the kind of care that can only be delivered safely in a modern hospital with rigorous infection control. These survivors had the luck to be diagnosed earlier than Martin Salia and, with a few exceptions, evacuated more promptly. Others, like Craig Spencer, survived because they fell ill shortly after returning from service in West Africa and went straight to a well-equipped medical center. The nurses infected while caring for Eric Duncan also recovered promptly. It was a similar story for most European health professionals.

Most sickened Americans and Europeans had the fortune, it must be added, to be nursing or doctoring while white. Unless we believe (as some clearly do) that Africans, and those of African descent, are innately more susceptible to Ebola than others, it's difficult not to believe that more of our African colleagues might have survived with proper care. Humarr Khan and the Kenema nurses didn't die of blood loss. Nor did Martin Salia, although he suffered, at the end and along with renal failure and possibly a bowel perforation, hemorrhagic manifestations of the disease. There is a widespread belief that Ebola and other viral hemorrhagic fevers cause profuse and irreversible bleeding in the humans they afflict. This is only rarely the case. So why has this belief taken hold?

Here we leave the domain of medical science for that of fantasy. Ebola may have caused only a couple dozen documented outbreaks prior to 2013, but it had already starred in movies, novels, and at least one nonfiction bestseller: *The Hot Zone*, by Richard Preston. His book, which reconstructed episodes of illness characterized by massive bleeding, drew more from an outbreak among lab monkeys housed near Washington, D.C., than from outbreaks among actual people in Africa. (A lab colony in Reston, Virginia, was invaded by an Ebola strain now held to be avirulent among humans.) In Preston's account of the disease in humans, blood weeps, seeps, or gushes from every orifice, or oozes from the eyes. Clinicians called up during the West African epidemic have, alas, seen people die this way, but the endgame was usually much different. In the most thorough reviews of Ebola's chief signs and symptoms, uncontrolled bleeding doesn't even make the top ten. In the West African outbreak, the most common signs and symptoms were fever, intense fatigue, loss of appetite, headache, nausea, vomiting, and diarrhea.[34] These signs and symptoms—especially when accompanied by delirium or disorientation—can all lead to dehydration and, when persistent and untreated, to hypovolemic shock: a more common mode of exit than the massive blood loss implied both by the term "hemorrhagic fever" and by many journalists' descriptions of Ebola.

At any rate, solely biological factors cannot account for why some die and some do not, or for why almost none of the Ebola caregivers in the United States—whether of the nearest-and-dearest variety, meaning family, or the professional ones, meaning nurses, physicians, and others in contact with patients, samples, or infected waste—were infected in the course of providing care. If you want to explain wildly varying fatality rates among those infected with the same strains of a virus, you have to understand the social context in which care is given. The same is true of transmission: the setting determines what kind of care is available *and* how safely care is delivered. Similar points have been made regarding most communicable pathogens for well over a century. That century has also taught us that medical impoverishment and high fatality rates and untrammeled contagion can be radically and rapidly reduced by vigorous human countermeasures. This point was not made, alas, during the first months of the West African Ebola epidemic.

The disparate fates of professional caregivers afflicted in the course of the West African epidemic reflect the grotesque disparities seen among our nations, bound together and yet held apart for centuries. Unequal bonds of the sort evident during the colonial period, but also before and well after it, have linked the home countries of the researchers, clinicians, and sundry others whose reports and studies are cited in this book. Even as those credited with authorship of studies in academic journals have tended to reflect a tardy (if now de rigueur) interest in reciprocity, the health systems on either end of these bonds have become more disastrously disparate. One sad reminder of this growing inequality appeared in an article published at the height of the Ebola epidemic in *Science*, perhaps the world's premier scientific journal. The article, which was based on work conducted in Pardis Sabeti's lab, analyzed the genomes of the Ebola variants circulating at the time. By the time the article appeared in print, five of the study's fifty-eight authors were dead, killed by Ebola.[35] One of them was Humarr Khan.

Understanding how Ebola and related pathogens spread, and how they kill, allows us to learn from the West African outbreak and make a broader case for what our priorities should be. So does COVID-19. But to do that, and to understand social context, we need to retrieve more than a little history from the dustbin. We also need to pay closer attention to the lived experience of the afflicted, which requires social proximity. For me, that proximity did not begin in late June 2014, at the surgery conference we held in Freetown; it began in September of that year. But social proximity was nonetheless the unexpected result of that chance meeting.

2.

Tough Calls

The division of responsibility, authority, and power between public health and medicine has been a continuing source of concern and conflict. Although representatives of both fields have traditionally voiced strong commitments to health and social betterment, the relationship between public health and medicine has been characterized by critical tensions, covert hostilities, and, at times, open warfare.

—Allan Brandt and Martha Gardner, "Antagonism and Accommodation," *American Journal of Public Health*, 2000

I FIRST LAID EYES ON FREETOWN IN MID-JUNE 2014, WHEN A GROUP OF US traveling from Rwanda flew there for a medical conference. The topic at hand was surgical care—or the lack thereof—in what are these days inelegantly termed "resource-poor settings."

None of us who'd helped organize the meeting had then been thinking about Ebola, even though post-conflict Sierra Leone would prove fertile ground for the virus. In May, as some planning to attend the meeting questioned whether or not Freetown was a safe venue, the World Health Organization had announced that the outbreaks in Liberia and Guinea were soon to be contained. When the question was raised again, and when that announcement was rescinded, I reassured a couple of surgical colleagues that no, Ebola wasn't spread by attending medical conferences. But there was no cause to be glib.

As reports of new cases climbed in those countries, we worried that our presence might be an added burden on our Sierra Leonean hosts. Since they didn't want to cancel the conference, I continued to hope for the best. A couple of weeks before a contingent of us headed west from Kigali, Rwanda's capital, it was clear these hopes, too, had been misplaced: eastern Sierra Leone was by then the theater of a major Ebola outbreak. When our hosts again insisted we come, we boarded a regional jetliner not knowing what we'd find on the ground. Now, as our delegation approached the continent's west coast, the virus and international disease-control experts alike began to invest Freetown.

Our plane made its descent toward Freetown in the early evening. It was a clear day, and the view was spectacular. Before us: the great dull green Atlantic, dappled with orange under a westering sun; the shoreline, a brighter green and fissured by innumerable rivers, streams, and estuaries also reflecting the orange light, their banks lined by a darker green margin of meandering mangroves; and imposing headlands that reared over the western edge of the continent. Freetown surrounded those hills, reaching up steep inclines and sprawling across every valley. But if the city looked lovely from the air, there were signs that it might look less so on the ground. We saw neighborhoods perched in the wrong places, gashed red hillsides that suggested recent landslides, plumes of smoke coming from sources clearly larger than cookfires, the leaching of reddish topsoil all along the seaboard. It didn't look much like pristine (and landlocked) Kigali. But my friends who lived in Freetown loved the place and I was pretty sure I would, too.

Our plane touched down at Lungi International Airport at about 6:00 p.m. We assumed we'd be able to enjoy the best time of day to see a west coast city this close to the equator—as the sun sets and the heat wanes. I was looking forward to meeting up with a handful of Sierra Leonean friends for dinner. Their number included one of my favorite students. He was a busy doctor, and I'd insisted he not bother meeting us at the airport. In truth, I wanted to take in the initial sights in silence, or something close to it. That hope evaporated as soon as we stepped onto the tarmac and were greeted by a blast of damp heat unfamiliar in Kigali.

Also unlike Rwanda, the airport was dilapidated and congested, a cacophonous mess. The same might of course be said of LaGuardia, but the Lungi airfield still bore scars of war, even though the conflict that had inflicted them had ended a decade earlier. Some of the buildings were pocked with bullet holes, and others were missing bowl-size chunks of plaster. Some had been covered by paint, but other structures near the terminal looked to be abandoned husks. And, if conditions out on the tarmac were scorchingly hot and humid, they didn't get much better inside the terminal, which was tiny, and where the odor of jet fuel gave way to pungent smells of salt water, cook smoke, diesel exhaust, and sweat; the power twice flickered off as our luggage was being unloaded.

The scene reminded me of Haiti, which was oddly comforting, but not everyone converging on Freetown that evening viewed the surroundings with equanimity. We were joined in the terminal by others arriving for the conference from elsewhere in Africa, and we somehow arrived shortly before several colleagues arriving from or via Europe. Gradually, this jet-lagged collective was herded onto a bus headed, we were told, to "the next terminal." Those herding us (and at least some of our bags) gestured vigorously, smiled readily, and barked orders at us in a language that sounded a bit like English to me. I understood almost none of it.

Off we went to that next terminal. The heat inside the bus was suffocating, and those who could leaned out the windows. We bounced down a short and mostly unpaved road, raising an orange dust that coated everything in our vicinity: people (including us passengers), houses, little shops, and the garbage that lined the roads. We made a sharp turn and headed down a steep decline, at which point, through a sparse collection of leaning coconut palms, we saw the terminal in question—a long, narrow, rickety wooden dock that reached out into the choppy dun water. Several small boats and one large ferry bobbed up and down on dauntingly large swells. The sun was growing redder as it sank, and lights began to appear across the water. *That must be Free-town*, I thought, but didn't want to reveal my ignorance by asking. I couldn't see any tall buildings on the far shore, but by then the light was fading. I'd forgotten that getting from Lungi to Freetown meant crossing a giant estuary.

The prospect was less than inviting. The estuary's near shoreline was littered with debris. I saw plastic, foam food containers, bobbing coconuts, a few palm trunks, shards of painted wood that bore a troubling resemblance to what might have once been bits of boats. There were also a couple of drowned kapok trees, replete with shredded leaves and propelled before us at a mysterious clip by some unseen current not far offshore. As we gathered under a large open gazebo to await the crossing, thin young men began hoisting our bags onto the ferry from the jetty, which wobbled precariously. They were cheerful and confident, and soon began helping the first of our lot to board. The rest of us nursed lukewarm beers as the dark enveloped the landing; it took three trips to get us all to the other side. Our passage, across twenty kilometers of open water, was punctuated by sudden decelerations for unseen masses of seaweed and plastic flotsam.

That evening, in Freetown, we had dinner with my student and several others, most of them physicians. The Ebola outbreak, we soon learned, had everybody on edge. I hadn't ever felt such an undercurrent of shared anxiety during the decade I'd practiced medicine in Rwanda, and knew our dinner companions were right to worry: Ebola aside, the country was becoming a medical no-man's-land that steadily swallowed people with far more common ailments or injuries. To the east, we heard, health professionals were fleeing their posts as the epidemic moved west toward the city from Kailahun and Kenema. Surgical care, and even basic first aid, was evaporating. Roadside trauma was a ranking killer. More women were dying in childbirth, as were their infants—and their malnourished, unvaccinated, older, and now often motherless children. For many citizens of Guinea, Liberia, and Sierra Leone, it was as if an ambush waited around every corner.

And that was in mid-June. By September, when we returned to Freetown to tackle Ebola, western Sierra Leone was ground zero of the epidemic, and

Upper West Africa was just about the worst place in the world to be critically ill or injured.

More than just the Ebola outbreak convinced us at Partners In Health to establish a presence in Upper West Africa, which was, along with the eastern Congo, perhaps the most arid patch of Africa's clinical desert. To explain what drove us, let me turn to the backstory, which I'll relate from my own point of view—that of an infectious-disease physician trained in the late eighties and early nineties and who since has battled several epidemics in the medical desert.

In the past century or so, especially since the advent of vaccines, the story of humankind's struggle against infectious disease has been one of steady progress, at least in the affluent world. Some infections still kill, of course, even in medical oases like Boston, but the general trend is positive. Thanks to a mix of specific therapies (antibacterial, antiparasitic, antifungal, antiviral) and nonspecific therapies (supportive and critical care), we have made most formerly fatal microbial diseases eminently survivable. I've been fortunate to witness this process several times over the past three decades.

One obvious example is AIDS—a disease with disputed (but likely zoonotic) origins that emerged in force in the 1980s, made headlines, and triggered numerous social epidemics. During that era, AIDS surged across the United States to become the leading infectious killer of young adults and, through transmission from mother to unborn or nursing infants, a ranking cause of death among children. The same was true in Haiti, where I spent the year between college and medical school, and part of every year in the ensuing decades. This was why I came to specialize in infectious disease, and it was how I met Dr. Anthony Fauci, the director of National Institute of Allergy and Infectious Diseases, or NIAID for short. The institute is the nation's primary sponsor of research on infectious pathogens—even those, like Ebola, that are unknown in the United States.

When Tony Fauci took over as NIAID's director, in 1984, HIV—the human immunodeficiency virus, which causes AIDS—had only just been discovered. He directed the attention of researchers, clinicians, policy makers, and political leaders to AIDS, winning a massive increase in federal funding for basic and clinical research on the affliction and the virus that caused it. Such investments bore fruit rapidly. Fauci also helped break down barriers between researchers and the afflicted. During the worst years of the American epidemic, he listened to the voices of AIDS activists and came to be a voice for people affected by HIV. Under his charismatic and effective direction, an unlikely coalition of scientists, clinicians, and activists moved forward the discovery, development, and delivery of new drugs and diagnostics that, even in the absence of a vaccine, saved millions of lives across the United States, as was Fauci's duty, and across the world, which was not.

AIDS established Dr. Fauci as the nation's premier infectious-disease doctor and an indefatigable bridge builder. It also made him uncommonly aware of obscure zoonoses that jump out of forested obscurity and into towns and cities, and from there across continents and oceans. NIAID became, during his happily long tenure, the chief institution tasked with identifying new or resurgent microbial threats around the world. He argued that the full force of science, and the sprawling network of NIAID-supported researchers and clinicians, be brought to bear on allegedly exotic and far-off problems like Ebola and Marburg. Bighearted, physically compact, curious, hard-driving, compassionate, inclusive—Tony Fauci was a rock. During the West African Ebola crisis, just hearing his robust Brooklyn accent on the phone reliably dropped my blood pressure by twenty points.

As we've seen, one reason Dr. Fauci was able to draw attention and financial resources to obscure pathogens that had never been seen in the United States was a post-9/11 concern about the threat of bioterrorism. Because of their lethality, filoviruses such as Marburg and Ebola were included on NIAID's list of pathogens that might be used as weapons. The research conducted more recently on the Lassa and Ebola genomes by such researchers as Pardis Sabeti and Humarr Khan was also supported by NIAID and by other branches of the U.S. government.

But knowledge of genetic codes does not always inform an understanding of where these viruses lurk or how they come to infect humans. By the time of Khan's death, in July 2014, more was known about the Ebola genome than about where and in what natural host the virus lived. Several species of bats common across Africa were invoked as reservoirs, but so were organisms as varied as fungi, certain plants, and pigs.

The epidemiology of human infection was also sketchy. There was evidence that filoviruses could live on in testes and in breast tissue, which raised, among the tiny number of researchers studying such matters prior to 2014, the specter of spread through sexual contact and transmission from mother to child. Knowledge of the clinical course and optimal treatment of Ebola and Marburg was even more limited. In Africa, at least, the Zaire species of Ebola seemed to kill the great majority of those infected. But what fraction of those infected in the desert was ever diagnosed? What fraction received even rudimentary medical care?

The work that Humarr Khan did sorting out the etiologies of febrile illness in Sierra Leone suggested that many Ebola victims, during both recognized and unrecognized epidemics, hadn't received a diagnosis, much less anything approaching adequate medical care. At the time of Khan's death, in other words, the encounter between Ebola the *virus* and modern science was confined largely to a handful of research laboratories deemed able to handle highly contagious and lethal pathogens, while the encounter between Ebola the *disease* and modern medicine was glancing, at best. Little was known about clinical management of Ebola because so few had taken up the fight to save the afflicted, who were largely people from rural parts of central and eastern Africa. The small number of brave and undersupplied health professionals who'd taken up that cause were also mostly Africans.

In the decade prior to Ebola's rapid spread across Upper West Africa, I'd been lucky enough to learn from and train hundreds of health professionals from rural areas in Rwanda, Malawi, and Lesotho, and, thanks to Partners In Health, had been able to help them be better supplied. These doctors, nurses, social workers, and community health workers were drawn to their work by an idealism that often gets beaten out of young health professionals dispatched to rural backwaters. But when they had the tools of the trade, and similarly inspired coworkers, we saw in rural Rwanda, Malawi, and Lesotho what we'd seen in Haiti: high rates of staff retention and a keen interest in advanced training.

So there we were, in Freetown, to discuss the obvious. We knew that safe surgery requires highly trained staff, clean and well-maintained operating rooms (safe space), an uninterrupted flow of supplies (lots of stuff, including instruments, anesthetics, and blood products), and ongoing attention to infection control (systems). Needless to say, most such ingredients are missing in most settings of poverty, and without them, surgical care and anesthesia—even for such straight-forward procedures as an appendectomy or removal of blinding cataracts—are ineffective, painful, and morbid. But can't the missing ingredients be found?

That's the problem we flew to Freetown to talk about. As we converged on the capital city, the borders of Sierra Leone, Guinea, and Liberia were officially closed. This meant little to the Ebola virus, which continued to spread as those afflicted with it continued to move back and forth within and between these countries along countless unmonitored footpaths and across the region's rivers. Nonetheless, we stuck with our plans for the conference. It hadn't been easy to find a hotel and conference space able to accommodate close to a hundred surgeons, anesthesiologists, obstetricians, surgical nurses, sympathetic economists, and policy makers. And those of us who were short-term visitors to Sierra Leone knew we wouldn't be sickened with Ebola: none of us planned to attend any funerals, even though the conference participants who were our hosts were increasingly obliged to do so.

One our hosts was T. B. Kamara, a urologist who also served as the chief medical officer of Connaught Hospital. He had a lot to say about access to safe and affordable surgical care. Not long before our conference and years after the end of Sierra Leone's civil war, Dr. Kamara had co-authored an ar-ticle in the *World Journal of Surgery* that had made the alarming case that the Sierra Leonean surgical teams working in the district hospitals in Port Loko and Kenema, among others, were working with resources that were equivalent or inferior to the resources available to the surgical teams that had worked with the Union Army during the American Civil War.[1] This was both a warning and a plea, and it was especially ominous now that Ebola imperiled Sierra Leone's shaky medical progress since the cease-fires of 2002.

Sierra Leone's lack of surgical services was not, however, rare. Just prior to the conference, colleagues of mine at Harvard had suggested that two billion of the world's population lacked access to safe surgical care. That might strike you as a high number, but to those of us on the clinical teams at Partners In Health, it seemed suspiciously low. That's because of how rarely, in the course of our work in Haiti and parts of Africa, we'd seen functioning and affordable surgical services in rural areas unless we put them in place and removed economic barriers to them. In these backwaters, clinics and hospitals often lacked electricity and running water. The polite euphemism that described these as being in short supply or "limited" in Sierra Leone made it sound as if the country were a temporarily understocked Sweden.

Referral and transportation posed huge problems for the rural poor of Africa, especially those needing surgical care. Steady urbanization across the world had brought sick people closer to well-provisioned hospitals, but it hadn't always made it easier for the poor to obtain quality care. That matters: even in cities blessed with staff and facilities, safe surgical care often remained unavailable to the poor, because the fee-for-service scourge and its twin— the lack of health insurance—remained global pandemics. In most countries surveyed, catastrophic health expenditures ranked as the number one trigger pushing poor and near-poor families into abject destitution.[2] During our time in Freetown, some of us calculated the number of people lacking ready access to safe and affordable surgical care as closer to five billion.

The difference between two and five billion is a pretty big one; and the capital of a clinical desert proved to be a good place in which to draft a report on the dimensions of this problem and to propose remedies. T. B. Kamara and Martin Salia helped us see the big picture by outlining the challenges faced in postwar Sierra Leone. By and large, its small towns and provincial cities lacked even a single formally trained surgical team. In most of these places, clinical officers (a term used to describe providers with four years of general medical training) lacked the wherewithal to perform even cesarean sections and to transfuse blood safely, which meant that mothers and babies were dying needlessly. Even before the Ebola outbreak, Sierra Leone had the world's highest maternal-mortality ratio, with many of these deaths due to obstructed labor or hemorrhage: surgical deaths.

There was ample cause for concern that things could get worse by the time our workshop ended, on Saturday night, June 21. That evening, during our last supper in Freetown, my student Bailor Barrie gripped my arm and pulled me aside. He told me that although he had planned to conduct his thesis research on tuberculosis in Sierra Leone, as I had encouraged him to do, he now felt it was his duty to focus on Ebola instead. Barrie's anxiety had little to do with the mundane matter of choosing a thesis topic. He was desperate to draw Partners In Health into the struggle against Ebola. Given our existing commitments and resources, I didn't think there was much chance of our staff and board agreeing to that, and told him so. Besides, I added while extracting myself from Dr. Barrie's grip, larger groups with deeper experience were already responding to the epidemic.

These were unsatisfactory responses, and we both knew it.

My wife, Didi, a community-health specialist and advocate for women and girls, also attended the Freetown meeting. We were returning to Rwanda the next evening but during the day visited two very different health facilities stood up by two sets of acquaintances. The first was an Ebola unit that a team from London's King's College was hastily setting up with staff at Connaught; the second was a new surgical center built by friends from Emergency, an Italian nongovernmental organization focused on trauma care.

Clinicians from both organizations had participated in our conference, and we were pleased by the invitations. But neither visit was reassuring. At Connaught, we found a tiny new "holding unit" with six beds, separated by grimy sheets of plastic. Once diagnosed, Marta Lado and Oliver Johnson explained, Ebola patients would be "transferred" out of it. Infection control and clinical care would be assured in the unit by three European physicians—including Johnson, a young but composed British doctor, who led the King's College team, and Lado, a sunny and knowledgeable infectious-disease specialist from Spain—along with three stoic Sierra Leonean nurses. Nobody on the team looked to be over thirty; a couple of the nurses appeared to be barely out of their teens.

As they showed us around, I struggled to keep my game face on. The unit was a dank place, already cramped and stifling even without a single patient yet in its care. What would it be like when its beds were full of patients, its linens soiled, its buckets overflowing with vomit and diarrhea, and everyone's eyes were stinging from chlorine? And where and how would those patients be transferred once they had been diagnosed with Ebola? There were, in late June, no treatment units in the city or anywhere near it; there was only the beleaguered Lassa ward in Kenema and the Ebola unit in Kailahun soon to be opened by MSF. These were hundreds of miles to the east. How would desperately ill patients survive the jolting, overland transit to these places?

And what about the hundreds of administrators, nurses, doctors, aides, cleaners, and future chlorine sprayers who staffed the hospital? Even the most careful and well-protected of them would be in grave danger once Ebola breached its defenses—if it hadn't already. Didi, a veteran visitor of horrible hospitals, was soon feeling nauseated. So she excused herself early and headed to an open courtyard littered with the rusting skeletons of hospital beds. As she headed out, she pointed to two sheets of paper tacked crookedly to the wall with surgical tape. They were funeral announcements for two nurses who'd died of unspecified causes in the previous week. *Li gen tan la*, she said in Haitian Creole. *It's already here.*

We were led on a tour of the rest of the hospital, which did nothing to ease our anxiety. Right across from this isolation ward was what our guides called "Casualty," a pitifully small and poorly staffed emergency room under the direction of Martin Salia, to whom we had said goodbye earlier that morning. (It would be the last time we saw him.) The two wards shared an entrance. Everybody on the team must have known as well as we did that this was not a safe space in which to care for someone with Ebola, or even to hold them for transfer to some as yet unidentified place. I had visions, right then and there, of piled-up bodies and sickened health workers.

From Connaught, we drove to the trauma center built by Emergency. Its founder was an Italian transplant surgeon who had dedicated himself for years to banning land mines and caring for their victims.[3] In the aftermath of civil war, which had left land mines and other ordnance across the country, these still killed civilians, many of them children. The new center had been built to address the need for trauma care in Freetown as motorcycle accidents quickly eclipsed wounds of war as the ranking cause of trauma deaths. Emergency's leadership was divided (it seemed to me) as to whether or not providing care for those injured in road accidents was central to their mission. That's one reason the local staff had attended our conference, but it wasn't clear they were much interested, just then, in Ebola.

Living through the aftermath of Haiti's 2010 earthquake had left us with strong opinions on the need for trauma care, regardless of the cause of trauma. But on that day, I could think only about the coming plague. What we saw at the Italians' center differed dramatically from what we had just seen at Connaught's holding unit. The unit was spotless, air-conditioned, and well laid out; its staff were gloved and gowned; and, in general, it had more of the staff and stuff required to prevent nosocomial spread. Even so, it only had nine beds. If Ebola reached Freetown in force, and even if the staff chose not to convert the center into an Ebola treatment unit—something those leading the tour told us they didn't plan to do—they would nonetheless be endangered by the rapid advance of the disease. Our unplanned discussion of the matter was interrupted by Oliver Johnson. "It's time to go," he said. "You're going to miss the ferry."

It was hard to hear over the engine of the smaller boat that took us back to Lungi. As we lurched our way noisily across the debris-filled estuary to the airport, I quickly lost myself in thought. Some of the staff we'd just met at the holding unit and the trauma center were sure to fall ill with Ebola. What would happen when they did? The Europeans would probably be medevacked home, but getting them to the absurdly sited Lungi airfield, which was in Port Loko District, would be a logistical nightmare. The Sierra Leoneans we'd just met wouldn't likely have the option of being airlifted to safety. Would Emergency end up offering them intensive care if they needed it? In the face of an epidemic, would that even matter? What difference could nine beds, or ten times that, really make?

As the boat neared Lungi, I didn't have to close my eyes to call to mind the faces of the people with whom I'd spent the past few days: the Sierra Leonean nurses, doctors, orderlies, ambulance attendants, lab workers, and sundry staff, many of whom would soon be working on the front lines of a new battle; Marta Lado and Oliver Johnson and the embryonic Ebola team at Connaught; the staff at the Emergency center; and, of course, Humarr Khan, Martin Salia, T. B. Kamara, and Bailor Barrie. If past Ebola outbreaks were any guide, it was only a matter of time before some of these people would begin to sicken and die.

Nor did I have to close my eyes to survey the faces of the conference attendees with whom we were leaving Sierra Leone that night. In the departure lounge, at least, they looked more troubled than relieved. I imagine all of us felt roughly the same way: as though we were running away from people trapped in a burning building.

These impressions, reflections, and worries accompanied me as I made my way back to Rwanda. On or between flights—it took more than twenty-four hours to cross the continent, in part because airlines had already started to cancel stopovers in Freetown, Conakry, and Monrovia—I ruminated about the chances of convincing my friends and colleagues at Partners In Health to work in West Africa.

I must have looked terrible as I worried about all of this. I hadn't slept well on my final night in Freetown, and my eyes were red, which almost led an anxious Kenyan flight attendant to eject me from the second leg of our flight. The Ebola hysteria was already that bad. Bailor Barrie's plea had moved me more than I'd let on, but the odds felt long. To be of use in the mounting crisis, we'd need to mobilize a huge team, as in hundreds and perhaps thousands of people. We'd need the resources to launch and sustain a far broader endeavor than one narrowly defined to stop Ebola. Sierra Leone needed a health system like Rwanda's, which had taken years to build.

I was still brooding when we reached East African airspace. Maybe those of us who had attended the conference could return to help out as clinician-teachers and researchers? No. I knew a research mandate, even a well-funded one, would not suffice in the midst of such a crisis. And what good would another book or a bunch of articles about Ebola do if their insights weren't linked to improving the delivery of care? How would research and teaching alone improve the space in which care was delivered? How would they prevent stockouts of personal protective gear, medications, and the lab reagents needed for clinical services? What could be done to address the lack of local clinicians on hand to care for the sick?

These were the sorts of questions posed to me more than thirty years earlier by rural Haitians, who had nothing against research, writing, or teaching. These questions had been echoed in pretty much all of the places I've been lucky enough to work in the decades since, and it was in response to such questions that we'd founded Partners In Health. It was why many of us kept trying to grow it. But after mulling these matters over during those flights back to Rwanda, I couldn't see how I'd be able to convince friends on our board that we had the bandwidth necessary to expand to West Africa. That board counted the most generous people I knew, many of them inspired by Tom White, a Boston construction magnate who'd helped us build or rebuild dozens of health facilities in Haiti, Peru, and beyond. But our resources were always stretched thin. Our existing clinical operations cost tens of millions of dollars each year, and we were already struggling to raise the money to fund them.

During the last leg of the trip home—a short one from Arusha, Tanzania, to Kigali—I thought of several other reasons to justify our inaction. We had no experience with Ebola and little appetite for short-term engagement in disaster response. After the 2010 Haiti earthquake, we'd seen how badly that could go.[4] Once in West Africa, we'd be there for years. Training doctors and nurses was central to our mission, and this takes time in a clinical desert, especially one without functioning teaching hospitals. Many factors argued against our direct engagement in West Africa. I understood them well, but even so, ultimately it didn't matter. None of them convinced me.

In the days and weeks after we got back to Rwanda, peaceful and on the upswing after hitting rock bottom in 1994, my dread mounted. Grisly and disheartening images of the epidemic began coursing across the world. One by one, members of Humarr Khan's team fell to the plague sweeping through Kenema. And then so did he. Khan's death, on July 29, was the tipping point for me. I had been more of an admirer of his than a friend, but I had hoped to change that. Had fate been kinder, Khan would have spent the upcoming academic year at Harvard, in Pardis Sabeti's lab.

I began lobbying everybody I could think of to leap into the fray. Just a couple of weeks after Khan's death, with Ebola now on the front page of U.S. papers, I was begging and haranguing not just the leadership of Partners In Health but also every influential figure I could: Dr. Jim Kim, a cofounder of Partners In Health and now the president of the World Bank; Hillary and Bill Clinton; Dr. Tony Fauci; Dr. Raj Shah, the head of USAID; sundry UN leaders; and a handful of philanthropists who I knew were willing to make quick decisions in the face of the unanticipated, among them George Soros, Paul Allen, Bill and Melinda Gates, and several supporters who'd quietly served as angel investors for Partners In Health in Haiti after the 2010 earthquake.

Several of these people ran organizations and bureaucracies that could be frustratingly slow to spring into action. In the case of Ebola, however, they had sound institutional reasons to act quickly. The foundations headed by Soros and Clinton had been supporting medical and recovery efforts in Liberia since the end of the war a decade earlier. Bill and Melinda Gates, in a class by themselves, had invested billions in polio eradication and were helping fund a vast machinery of surveillance and vaccination in Nigeria—the continent's most populous nation and one of the world's last known settings of polio transmission. Given Nigeria's long and costly engagement in Sierra Leone's and Liberia's recent civil wars—and its sheer size—it stood to reason that Ebola in Upper West Africa was likely to spread there, too.

It was obvious from the outset that the entire neighborhood was at risk of contagion. The World Bank is a bank for development, and Ebola was already stalling it. As country after country shut down air travel to the region and closed borders, trade was dwindling. As markets were upended, and as food and fuel shipments ceased, hunger and unrest spiked.[5] The United Nations had thousands of peacekeepers in the region, some of whom would surely be exposed to Ebola, even if their numbers included few professional caregivers. And on August 8, the lead UN health agency had declared Ebola to be a "public health emergency of international concern," a declaration that had been made only a couple of times previously in the history of the World Health Organization. That same week, Liberia's government—having already shut down its schools and universities, banned soccer matches, and threatened to quarantine entire neighborhoods—declared a state of emergency. Sierra Leone had done the same a week previously, hours after Humarr Khan's death.

In spite of all this local hubbub, the initial response from the so-called international community was tepid at best. No army of nurses and other professional caregivers was mobilized in the wake of these declarations and pleas. The World Health Organization, weakened over the years by political feuds and funding shortfalls, had little operational capacity and was unable to act promptly or effectively. Eventually, many regulatory bodies, development banks, governments, and private foundations—spurred on by leaders who belatedly recognized the threat to their national and international interests—did mobilize resources and attention. But few of them had the hands-on capacity to care for the sick or injured in operations conducted simultaneously around the world. MSF, the world's largest medically focused humanitarian organization, did have that capacity, but it wasn't nearly enough to contend with the crisis unfolding in Upper West Africa.

Given the scale of the problem, it was no surprise that the staff and board at Partners In Health might feel we didn't have the resources to help in a meaningful way. We certainly didn't have the operational capacity of MSF, nor did we have a roster of on-call clinicians and other first responders. And then there was the bigger question of finances: in 2014, far more Americans sent contributions to MSF, a charity founded in Europe and funded largely by Europeans, than they did to Partners In Health. Our list of donors was tiny. After the Haiti earthquake, we'd opened Partners In Health–Canada with a staff of two, but we had no significant capacity to raise funds in Europe or Asia. MSF has close to thirty offices on those continents alone—and more on others.

Partners In Health had received a welcome influx of unsolicited donations after the quake, which had permitted us to build and open Haiti's first modern academic medical center, just to the north of the quake zone. But now our reserves were depleted. The Sisyphean task of raising operational funds each year blunted appetites for further expansion, and some at our headquarters, in Boston, longed for its opposite. With long-term efforts in ten countries and close to fifteen thousand employees—most of them community health workers working in or near the places they'd been born and raised— many of the Partners In Health staff based in Boston felt we were already trying to do too much, while those stranded in medical deserts naturally enough felt like we were doing too little.

This wasn't a new tension. But that summer I couldn't shake the feeling that Ebola was a fire that we had an ethical obligation to fight. Saving lives is, after all, what doctors and nurses take oaths to do. Even after tardy WHO warnings and appeals for assistance, however, a familiar and unambitious logic proliferated in public-health circles around the world: the priority was containment, not delivery of clinical services. This was clinical nihilism: the tools and funding required to improve supportive and critical care, we heard every damn day, were not in the budget.

But if Ebola wasn't in the budget, didn't that mean that the budget, not the virus, was wrong?

Saying we weren't experienced in responding to Ebola also seemed like a cop-out. Even if we weren't trained to tackle the disease specifically, we could learn on the job. The most important contribution I could make, I realized, was to press our executives and board to sign on. For more than a month, I stewed over the best way to make the case. One thing we'd learned in our work—from Haiti to Peru, Russia to Rwanda—was that improving the quality of care during major outbreaks of infectious diseases had improved efforts to control them as well. That's certainly what had happened with AIDS in Rwanda and in much of Africa.

By late summer 2014, when I was back in Rwanda, the Ebola outbreak and its threat to major urban areas in West Africa and beyond meant that the control-versus-care debate had finally spilled into the mainstream press. This seemed to me to be a moment of opportunity. Shouldn't we use it to *integrate* prevention and care? Here's our chance, I wanted to shout, to link an emergency response to Ebola to efforts to build a proper health system! We (the collective Rwandan we) had done it before, for ten million people! Here's our chance to admit that low-ball treatment protocols would not save the majority with serious complications of Ebola infection any more than they'd saved Humarr Khan and his colleagues! Here's our chance to admit we're afraid for nursing and medical staff but to keep pressing for more and safer supportive and critical care in West Africa!

The exclamation points kept piling on. Most clinicians in Guinea, Liberia, and Sierra Leone seemed to feel similarly emphatic. (Their lives depended on it.) Well before the summer ended, they were joined in that sentiment by many public-health authorities. (Their families' and neighbors' lives depended on it.) The focus, a growing number of people agreed, had to be on improving the quality of care. If we wanted to improve that, we would need clinicians with expertise delivering supportive and critical care, especially nurses, along with safer spaces in which to provide them.

By late August, many of the world's disease-control gurus had also connected the dots between poor-quality care and the failure of containment. One influential figure on the scene, an American physician who had been working for years in the region using the smallpox-control playbook, laid out the debate in stark terms in a private conversation as I was pushing our own team (and others) to act. "In previous Ebola outbreaks," he confided in conspiratorial tones, trying to help me hone the message, "the public-health people didn't much care if mortality approached a hundred percent, as long as they could make sure everyone was accounted for on a contact list. But now that Ebola is in the cities, they"—his fellow disease-control experts—"recognize the need for us to improve the quality of care in order to bring people into the system."

Global public-health authorities were forced to concede that they were losing the battle. The measures that had been taken during the spring and summer, isolation without proper care, had backfired. Citizens of the three most affected nations were frightened of those measures, and the result by September was so much resistance and obstruction that it had become difficult—impossible in many communities—to isolate the sick and keep track of the contacts of confirmed cases. Contact tracing was hard.

It was a similar story when it came to the unsafe burials that were contributing to the spread of Ebola. There have always been cultural differences in last rites and the preparation of the body for them, but always and everywhere families honor the remains of their dead.[6] Helping the bereaved make burials safe, dignified, and respectful of local traditions was the ethical way to slow funeral-related Ebola transmission. Instead, Sierra Leonean officials passed laws banning "traditional" funerals and imposed stiff fines for infractions—before they were able to provide safer and acceptable alternatives. Liberia began a cremation campaign and also threatened to criminalize burials.[7] In both countries, as in Guinea, these moves were widely resisted.

That cycle needed to be broken. If families were allowed to participate in some meaningful, safe way in last rites and interment, we suspected, there would be less household spread, and fewer attacks on burial and public-health teams.

By September, international calls for engagement with the mounting Ebola crisis were growing louder. Speaking before a specially convened forum at the UN General Assembly, President Barack Obama made the case resonantly:

> I want us to be clear: We are not moving fast enough. We are not doing enough. Right now, everybody has the best of intentions, but people are not putting in the kinds of resources that are necessary to put a stop to this epidemic. There is still a significant gap between where we are and where we need to be. We know from experience that the response to an outbreak of this magnitude has to be fast and

it has to be sustained. It's a marathon, but you have to run it like a sprint. And that's only possible if everybody chips in, if every nation and every organization takes this seriously. Everybody here has to do more.[8]

Others at the forum voiced mounting frustration at the lack of a rapid and coordinated international response. There was more than one "high-level meeting" on Ebola convened by the United Nations that month. The international president of MSF, Dr. Joanne Liu, a Canadian pediatrician and emergency-room doctor, repeated a warning she'd been making for weeks: that the international institutions and governments that might have helped combat the epidemic had formed little more than "a global coalition of inaction."[9]

Sitting next to me as Dr. Liu spoke at one of them was Ophelia Dahl, the longtime director of Partners In Health and one of its cofounders. We agreed with Liu. We both wanted to be in West Africa, doing our part, and Dahl prepared to voice her opinions to our board, a group of thoughtful, compassionate, generous people, each of whom had pledged significant fractions of their personal resources whenever we'd insisted in the past on the need for action, whether it was in Haiti or Russia or Rwanda. They weren't billionaires, and each had been dragged into years-long, ongoing commitments in a dozen countries. So they had reason to feel that as an organization we were "trying to do too much" or "trying to move too fast." These arguments were psychologically plausible but not empirically correct regarding any humanitarian organization, charity, funding agency, or government concerning itself with Ebola.

Ophelia Dahl assembled a group to help her prepare a plan. It included Jon Lascher, a member of our team in Haiti. He had cut his teeth in Togo a decade earlier as a Peace Corps volunteer, and flew back to Boston to help a small team, led by Sheila Davis, our chief nursing officer, cobble together an Ebola-response proposal for the next Partners In Health board meeting, the first since Humarr Khan's death; it was scheduled for September 10. By then, we'd received formal invitations from all three of the most affected nations, and the head of USAID had exhorted us and other American medical and relief organizations not yet working on Ebola to do so, promising financial support. But invitations and promises did not guarantee prompt or sustained action. The only pledges that had materialized at the meeting of the UN General Assembly, for example, had been for a short-term emergency response.

In their proposal, Jon Lascher, Sheila Davis, and the rest of the team laid out the broad outlines of what they called the "PIH Ebola Response." Partners In Health, they wrote, would need to provide clinical care *and* help get shuttered hospitals and clinics up and running, and then keep them running. This would be hard to do, and even harder to fund, once the emergency was declared over. As of September 9, we had no funding or formal pledges. To break through this impasse, we proposed to form a coalition with two smaller organizations founded by Partners In Health protégés.

One of the outfits was in Sierra Leone, the other in Liberia, but there was no question that we would be asking our board to assume the lion's share of the responsibility. They had every right to exercise due diligence before making long-term commitments, especially since we'd never worked in West Africa before. Some of them later complained we didn't give them time to do that. But that was time that a growing number in West Africa simply didn't have. Would our small group of overburdened trustees trust us on this one? On the day of the meeting, we made our case, and the board unanimously approved our appeal. Not only did its members grant their approval of the effort, they also personally pledged a million dollars to kick-start it. "Up until this point," Jon Lascher remembers, "there was still uncertainty whether or not Partners In Health would establish itself in two new countries in the midst of an emergency. 'Green Light Day' removed any lingering doubt." I felt like weeping for joy.

Wheels now quickly started to turn. Within a record ninety hours, George Soros and his Open Society Foundations approved a proposal short on details; less than a day later they transferred money to Partners In Health. Paul Allen's foundation soon followed suit, and the gears of USAID and the international disaster-relief machinery began to grind. But there were plenty of hurdles still to clear once we had the cash to launch operations. We needed short-term clinician and logistician volunteers, for one thing, but we didn't have a list of those ready to be called up for duty. We'd had good luck when we made a plea for volunteers after the Haiti earthquake, but the situation in West Africa was very different.

Several of the first expatriates to pitch in during the Ebola crisis had been stricken, and this was shaping world opinion. When a French nurse volunteering with MSF in Liberia had fallen ill, it had taken a fraught fifty hours to arrange her repatriation. She survived, but an elderly Spanish priest—a missionary physician airlifted from Monrovia to Madrid—didn't make it. A second priest fell ill, as did a British nurse and a Senegalese epidemiologist. All three were medevacked and two survived. A Massachusetts doctor, the third American stricken, was evacuated from Monrovia to Omaha, Nebraska. He recovered fairly quickly.

Then there was Ian Crozier, American Patient Four, who fell ill in Sierra Leone in early September. All we knew about Crozier, whose name wasn't revealed, was that he was an infectious-disease doctor who'd been sent to Kenema by the World Health Organization after Humarr Khan's death. In spite of dozens of front-page stories in the world's most influential newspapers about Kenema's ordeal, the city's hospital was still an understaffed and undersupplied shithole. That's not a term to be used in describing countries or continents, but it was the mot juste for the hospital in Kenema, which was receiving a growing number of transfers from holding units like the one we'd visited at Connaught. These makeshift centers didn't even have enough personal protective gear or body bags to cope with the crisis.

Mechanical ventilation and renal dialysis—which would soon save Ian Crozier's life—weren't even part of the discussion.

Not long before Crozier fell ill, he had opened up an ambulance sent from the Connaught holding unit, in which he found the dead bodies of two young nurses afflicted with Ebola. One of them was the twenty-two-year-old nurse we had met during our visit in June. Unable to work out which woman was which, the burial team had decided to inter them both in graves labeled "anonymous Freetown cases."[10] (Oliver Johnson and Marta Lado, and no doubt many others struggling within the confines of Connaught, had been heartbroken.) Now, on the day of the Partners In Health board meeting, I learned that Crozier had just been airlifted to Emory's biocontainment unit.

Because I have friends and former trainees at Emory, I heard through the infectious-disease grapevine that Ian Crozier was critically ill. But he also received critical care. He had respiratory failure and was mechanically ventilated; he had renal failure and was dialyzed. Ultimately, the staff at Emory saved Crozier's life. But even as his life hung in the balance, an undertow of censorious opinion from the international control-over-care crowd swelled. Imagine if the resources invested in the care of these expatriates, I heard more than once, had been invested instead in prevention efforts!

This was a radically different critique from that offered by West African clinicians. *They* were asking us to imagine if the resources invested in the care of people like Crozier had also been invested in the care of their sickened peers.

Despite the climate of fear and the very real dangers, several staff members from across the Partners In Health archipelago—nurses, physicians, logisticians, researchers—dropped what they were doing to sign up; others volunteered to assume extra duties while they were gone. And many from beyond that archipelago did, too. Soon Sheila Davis, having launched the PIH Ebola Response, was able to announce that hundreds of experienced clinicians were offering to serve via the Partners In Health website.

As this collective turned its attention to Liberia and Sierra Leone, I felt my dread abate for the first time since I'd left Freetown, almost three months earlier. In spite of persistent anxiety and much sadness, it would not recur while we were fighting back. In *The Plague*, Albert Camus describes the same action-impelled shift in sentiment, attributing it (in proper French fashion) to sound logic. "The essential thing," he wrote, "was to save the greatest possible number of persons from dying and being doomed to unending separation.

And to do this there was only one resource: to fight the plague. There was nothing admirable about this attitude; it was merely logical."[11]

We couldn't fight Ebola with logic alone, of course. In the absence of material resources, the kind of logical attitude that Camus described—along with admirable courage—was what killed Humarr Khan, the Kenema nurses, and several of the nursing students subsequently sent into the breach. It's what claimed the life of that twenty-two-year-old nurse from Connaught, enthusiastic and brave, who had the misfortune to begin her career in 2014. It's what led American Patient Four, Ian Crozier, to fall ill at the height of Kenema's crisis. What these people lacked were not logical attitudes or sterling personal qualities. They lacked the staff, stuff, safe space, and systems needed to do their jobs. How would we get them in place?

Dread gone, a new anxiety accompanied us to new destinations. Much of it concerned gathering the required resources and getting them to West Africa. Simply reaching Freetown and Monrovia was a major challenge. Only a couple of commercial airlines still served Ebola-affected regions, and—in contrast to what occurred after the earthquake in Haiti—few offered to put private aircraft at the disposal of humanitarians headed to and from West Africa. (None, to my knowledge, offered to transport the afflicted.) But Tony Banbury, an American with long experience in conflict zones, including Cambodia, was one of the UN officials I'd been nagging from Rwanda. He had just been tapped by headquarters to lead its first-ever emergency-response mission dispatched to quell an epidemic. Banbury let me know, in the run-up to our board meeting, that the United Nations could provide logistic support to teams like ours.

Tony Banbury had been deeply involved in the response to the 2010 earthquake in Haiti. The quake had destroyed UN headquarters in Port-au-Prince, taking out almost all of the organization's leadership team—his friends and long-term colleagues. Banbury and I came to know each other well during that terrible aftermath. His Ebola mission now faced an undertow of resentment from established UN bureaucracies, their staffers grumbling about workarounds and parallel efforts. But he was determined to help. Minutes

after Partners In Health's board approved our involvement in the Ebola crisis, I walked along a leafy Boston side street to call him in private. Banbury
instructed our team—which included me, Sheila Davis, and Joia Mukherjee,
along with a couple of fellow infectious-disease clinicians—to fly to Ghana,
where we'd board a jet bound for Monrovia.

This team left Boston almost immediately, and soon saw hints that the
world's largest public-health endeavor remained clinically paltry. Shortly after touchdown in Accra, we were led to a sleek white jet marked with a large
black "UN" on the fuselage. We expected it to be full of relief workers, including fellow clinicians. But on that first trip, it was just us, along with a couple of
folks from Last Mile Health, a nongovernmental organization based in eastern Liberia that had been founded by a young physician born in Liberia and
trained at Harvard. Last Mile Health was one of the two groups with which
we would form a coalition to fight Ebola. The second was Wellbody Alliance,
launched by Bailor Barrie and based in eastern Sierra Leone.

Few of the humanitarians we saw on subsequent runs looked like they
were headed there to put in intravenous lines or to offer supportive care to the
sick, and it was soon apparent that the alliance we'd formed with Last Mile
Health and Wellbody Alliance would not be able to make much of a difference without rethinking our collective commitment solely to rural regions in
eastern Liberia and Sierra Leone: Ebola had become a heavily urban (and
thus western) epidemic, and our new sister organizations were much smaller
than we'd understood. We had to rethink our approach and couldn't do this
at a remove, from Boston. So we turned for help to Corrado Cancedda, who
had volunteered to lead our efforts in Sierra Leone.

Dr. Cancedda, who hails from Genoa, is the Partners In Health clinician introduced in the first pages of this book, in which I described a visit I made
with him to an ETU in Monrovia. He did much of his training, including a
fellowship in infectious disease and a doctoral degree in immunology, in the
United States. We were colleagues at Boston's Brigham and Women's Hospital and at Harvard Medical School. More significantly, we'd worked together
in the mountains of Lesotho, a small country surrounded by South Africa,
and then for years in rural Rwanda. Cancedda had made his mark in Rwanda

through clinical teaching in the midst of epidemic malaria, tuberculosis, and HIV disease. This part of West Africa, Ebola crisis or not, would prove a quite different posting.

Rwanda is compact and densely populated and boasts a decent network of paved roads. It also had, for well over a decade, a government strongly committed to investing public dollars in efforts to strengthen the national health system. Rwandan political authorities were and are strongly committed to rooting out corruption. Such efforts had failed in postconflict West Africa, as those from beyond its borders rarely failed to note. The levels of material and social investment made in Rwanda after the genocide had not been made after the end of civil war in either Sierra Leone or Liberia, even though from afar they looked (at least to myopic development economists) to reliably outperform tiny and landlocked Rwanda.

The illusion is shattered within minutes of touchdown at the strangely sited international airports serving Freetown and Monrovia. As soon as we landed, we realized the enormity of the tasks ahead of us. The first was to set up offices, recruit local staff, and open bank accounts, but these were relatively straightforward chores. We also had to manage large teams of clinicians, logisticians, and accountants and find places to house them. Beyond logistics, getting started required more than just passion and commitment and good leaders, and more than just mastery of infection control; it required surviving what seemed like endless meetings. We didn't always like them but recognized their necessity and took part respectfully.

We'd learned over the years not to go rushing off during emergencies without the approval and direction of local health authorities, who in this instance were overwhelmed by well-intentioned but unvetted teams offering varied and not always helpful forms of assistance. It had been the same story after a barrage of hurricanes hit Haiti in 2008 and was followed by the 2010 earthquake. (A few days after the quake leveled much of the neighborhood around Haiti's primary referral hospital, I was tasked with explaining to its weary and suddenly homeless medical director that no, the Scientologists in the casualty-strewn courtyard were not "volunteer scientists.") Those who signed up to serve in Haiti were also required to spend time in regular coordination meetings, most held in capital cities. In UN and disaster-relief argot, these were the dreaded "cluster meetings," which went by a more colorful term whenever confusion, backbiting, and complaint dominated.

We'd seen a lot of this in Haiti and were aware that health officials in Liberia and Sierra Leone, as in Guinea, were beyond beleaguered. But we hoped official invitations and personal connections would expedite our assignments. We'd already met some of the top health officials; our friends from Last Mile Health and Wellbody Alliance knew many of them well. The health minister of Liberia, a genial surgeon, was still hanging in there, but the young minister we'd met in Freetown in June had been sacked after the Humarr Khan debacle. As we awaited instructions from the authorities, who were flat-out as they tried to cope, it was already clear that no purpose-built Ebola treatment units would be completed in the immediate future.

To manage, the authorities had therefore begun to requisition public buildings—including schools, army barracks, and police headquarters—and to patch up temporary structures erected during the long, stuttering close of civil war. Like other public assets, health professionals themselves were also being requisitioned and repurposed. Nonetheless, the central governments of all three countries were still short-handed—and that was before all sorts of dismissals, defections, and deaths bedeviled their ranks. Even though we offered to start work without awaiting purpose-built ETUs, it took time for the authorities in Liberia and Sierra Leone to assign us to our posts. To them, we probably (and understandably) seemed just to be one group among many.

MSF, the only organization that might reasonably claim to be moving fast or doing enough, continued to expand its efforts; Cuban authorities had announced a willingness to send clinical brigades, as did a number of African nations, including Rwanda and South Africa. While we were still awaiting official instructions, a Ugandan physician who'd previously worked straight through an Ebola outbreak in strife-torn northern Uganda managed to outfit an abandoned building in Monrovia as an Ebola treatment unit, with help from a team of experts and volunteers under her direction.[12] At the same time that we'd visited the ETU described in the first pages of this book, we also inspected this ersatz one not far away. It was cavernous, with unfinished cement walls stained black by fire or mildew, but it had a hundred beds, and that was a start. I insisted on buying flowering plants for the Monrovia unit, which some of my coworkers found strange, but the Ugandan physician appreciated the gesture. I wanted to hug her. By then even shaking hands was officially discouraged. I hugged her anyway, and she hugged back.

A lot happened in the weeks that followed. As the new Monrovia treatment center opened its metaphorical doors—it didn't really have doors—we headed back to Ghana on UN transport. From there, Corrado Cancedda, Sheila Davis, and Joia Mukherjee traveled to Alabama to join others from Partners In Health attending a CDC-sponsored training for U.S. clinicians headed to West Africa to fight Ebola, the first of its kind. Partners In Health had the largest number of clinicians present for the training. This made us proud but also made us worried.

By the first week of October, with the epidemic moving full speed ahead, we'd established beachheads in both Freetown and Monrovia, met with two heads of state, attended numerous briefings, and met with just about every one of the UN-affiliated agencies. But we still hadn't been assigned to particular towns or cities. In Sierra Leone, being posted required meeting the new health minister. After sacking his old one in August, the president of Sierra Leone, Ernest Bai Koroma, had turned to the diaspora to recruit a new one: Dr. Abu Bakarr Fofanah, a mild-mannered tropical-disease expert who'd been based in England. Fofanah had returned to a country in crisis, and to ongoing deaths among the already thin ranks of health-care professionals. Since we'd been invited into the country by President Koroma, arranging a meeting with Fofanah was easy; the assignment he gave us, not so much.

Dr. Fofanah and other government officials, all of whom were surely sicker of meetings than we were, received us on October 9. Their chief worry was what they termed "Ebola's western surge." "We're making gains in the east," Fofanah said. "Occasionally, we have a few days of zero cases reported. But the epidemic has now shifted to the west and north of the country." He argued that we shouldn't be based only in Kono, the diamond district where Bailor Barrie (also present that day) and Wellbody Alliance had long labored. The minister insisted that we needed to work to save lives in the more heavily populated parts of Sierra Leone. Periodically consulting notes on a piece of paper that read "Partners In Health" at the top, Fofanah mentioned Port Loko several times. We weren't surprised; he was echoing Koroma, who'd spoken to us of the same district a couple of days earlier. Both knew of our work in Rwanda.

As we sat listening to Dr. Fofanah in his conference room, we began to understand for first time that we were going to be sent to Port Loko. As newcomers, we had no idea where it was; we weren't even sure if it was a town, a district, or both. But he wasn't yet through with the details of his proposal. With laser-like focus, Fofanah asked us to "help complete the conversion of an abandoned vocational school in the chiefdom of Maforki" into an Ebola treatment unit and to staff it with clinicians trained to observe strict infection-control procedures. "I understand several of you are specialists in infectious disease," he said with a look around the table, letting his gaze fall briefly on a couple of us. There were few of us left in the country, he said, and infection control would be weak. If we were genuinely interested in strengthening the health system, as we had done in Rwanda, we should work not only in Maforki but also in Port Loko's district hospital. The hospital, he said, had ceased most clinical operations. We should do all this, he added, while also initiating our proposed work in Kono District.

At this, Bailor Barrie smiled; he was getting what he had asked for back in June. The minister added that Partners In Health would report directly to the District Ebola Response Centre, or DERC. He didn't seem to doubt our willingness to accept these assignments and mentioned a couple of others for consideration after complaining of a lack of volunteer clinicians willing to work in Freetown's grotesquely understaffed referral hospitals. Fofanah was especially troubled by the example of the national maternity hospital, where laboring mothers without Ebola were now being left unattended.[13] Ophelia Dahl, who was leading our delegation, had insisted we visit the facility the previous day with precisely these fears in mind.

The health minister did offer one scrap of good news: the Cubans were coming, and they, too, might be assigned to help in Maforki, which would likely become "very busy, very quickly." Having worked for years with Cuban clinicians and laboratory technicians in Haiti and elsewhere, we felt like cheering. We in turn proposed to engage, hire, and train Ebola survivors to work with us. Fofanah, although not an ebullient type, applauded the idea, and two other officials present at the meeting promised us a list of survivors and their contact information. We knew, as did the minister, that many of them would need follow-up care.

Before we left his conference room, Dr. Fofanah warned us that Ebola was rapidly undoing the progress his country had made in the decade since the end of the war. "Can you imagine what will happen?" he asked us as he considered the possible side effects of the epidemic. "Children not coming for vaccinations? Expectant mothers not coming for antenatal care? Even when the Ebola epidemic is over, this is another time bomb. Can you imagine?" Yes, we could imagine. Dahl said as much in just the right tone. "We are eager to get started," she said. "We're aware that this has been going on for a long time. We do have experience moving fast. With your permission and encouragement, we're ready to do that."

Abu Bakarr Fofanah did not mince words or smile in responding to this pledge. "We needed this help yesterday," he said. "Today, it's still not here. Please, let's not let tomorrow pass us by."

Bright sunlight and acrid chlorine fumes assaulted us as we left the Ministry of Health that day. As we got in the car, we wondered what exactly we had just signed up for. We knew Maforki would be bad—after all, what kind of school, or any building for that matter, is abandoned in provincial Sierra Leone? We didn't even know in which direction we were headed. Where was Maforki and what was a chiefdom? Where or what was Port Loko? A city? A port? A district?

Bailor Barrie had answers for us. The Maforki chiefdom and the town of Port Loko were a couple of hours north of Freetown, and both were within

Port Loko District. Barrie mumbled something about the airport but didn't add much more. By that point in my travels, I was lugging around articles about Ebola and books about West Africa, and as soon as I got back to my room, I began combing through them all to learn something about where we were going. The books were mostly ethnographic, including a couple of new volumes written by colleagues (such as the anthropologist Adia Benton), as well as colonial accounts. The older volumes had maps, and the town of Port Loko, with various spellings, was on every one.

Like many other enduring settlements from previous centuries, Port Loko was established on a major estuary. The surrounding district of the same name lay squarely in Temne country, suggesting the area would have been predominantly Muslim by the time English-language accounts began to appear in the seventeenth century. I didn't have any of those handy, but did have *A View of Sierra Leone*, published in 1926 by a retired British colonial officer who'd spent six months in the colony almost a century before Ebola was recognized in Port Loko. His description of this part of Sierra Leone, and of the Temne tribe, began with a seven-hour boat ride from Freetown to Port Loko, some of it along or through mangrove swamps thinned in order to plant rice. "The native town of Port Lokko," wrote the official, "clusters on a steep hillside with two tumbling streams, one of large size, dividing it."[14] From the British emplacement, a hundred feet above the rivers, one had "fine views" of a nearby town and, sometimes, the elevations around Freetown and (to the northwest) Conakry.

That didn't sound all bad. The British officer was unimpressed, however, by Port Loko's infrastructure. Although it had been "a prosperous town for a hundred and fifty years, there seems never to have been a market place, sales of food taking place along the streets." I found no mention in my fervid reading of clinics or hospitals. In the end, the Briton wasn't convinced that Port Loko had much of a future. "For four hundred years," he wrote, "Europeans have traded up and down this estuary, yet at the present day very few of the European residents of Freetown have been up it. Its day is over."[15] Leaving aside whether or not the absence of the Europeans was bane or boon—the British had wrought havoc in and around Port Loko in the decades prior to the author's visit—this was chilling to read a few hours after our session with the health minister.

We may not have known where to find Port Loko on a map, but we'd been hearing about it on the radio and in weekly Ebola reports from national and international authorities. By the time of our meeting with Dr. Fofanah, Port Loko town had reported the sharpest rise in new cases in the country—which meant, just then, the sharpest rise in the world. Between June and October, Ebola had taken hundreds of lives in the surrounding district, and the number of cases kept going up as new chains of transmission spread through families and their caregivers.

Since Ebola had emerged from the forest still covering parts of the tri-zone region, Port Loko's rising caseload was part of its "western surge," the term used by Dr. Fofonah and by epidemiologists in the weeks prior to our setting up operations there. Those new to Sierra Leone didn't know that the same language had been used to describe rebel incursions during the civil war, which had followed a similar east-to-west trajectory. The country's eastern reaches—comprised of Kenema, Kono, and Kailahun Districts—had fallen, and now Freetown and the coastal region, including Port Loko, had to be defended against invasion. War metaphors are too often used in discussions of public health, but what we learned about Port Loko District after we were asked to provide clinical services there did make it seem like a combat zone. When we finally set up camp, in October, we learned that the government facilities we'd been tasked with supporting in Port Loko were death traps.

Maforki was the worst. On paper and in official reports, the abandoned vocational school was primly listed as a 108-bed Ebola treatment unit. But like many other structures newly converted to care for the stricken, it was unsafe by any standard. It had no walls and seemed more like a bunch of decaying sheds than a permanent structure. Maforki had no running water or electricity. It lacked proper drainage, an incinerator or other waste disposal, chlorine-production capacity, a triage area in which to sort the sick, and a morgue. Fofanah had informed us its infection-control measures would be "weak," but he was wrong: there were none at all. Unfortunately,

Port Loko's health authorities, now clustered in the DERC, had no other options within the district. The days of transferring moribund patients across the country were over, and not because of concerns with the safety of transport. Now there were simply too many dying patients to transfer cross-country.

Those sickened by Ebola within Port Loko District were referred to Maforki. The ETU had opened a week before our team got there and was filled to capacity within a single weekend. On the day our team arrived, Bailor Barrie and Jon Lascher counted 167 patients in the 108-bed facility. Bodies were lying in the courtyard, and at least two employees had contracted Ebola within the first week of government-run operations. Not that it was clear how many of the dead and dying in the area were sick or dead from Ebola. Laboratory capacity was also absent in Port Loko District, making it impossible to distinguish Ebola from other prevalent causes of fever, headache, fatigue, diarrhea, and vomiting. One driver, a young Sierra Leonean man, was as horrified as his new American colleagues upon visiting Maforki in the third week of October. He quit the next day.

Neither Bailor Barrie nor Jon Lascher, veterans both of some awful conditions, liked the idea of working in Maforki. But they'd already unsuccessfully scouted other potential sites. Lascher later recalled that trip in sobering detail:

> There was little if any care being delivered in Port Loko district in October. Before we went to Maforki, Bailor and I went to see the district medical officer, who was alone in his office, sweating. He looked like he was about to have a stroke and later did. He sent us with a British military officer to scout an alternative location in a village not far away. When we got there, we saw three nurses sitting on a bench. One of them didn't have a shirt on, which should have made it clear they weren't on duty. They were awaiting the results of their own Ebola tests, which then took days to get back . . . The British officer pointed to a nearby soccer field and said maybe they could build an ETU there, but that it would take time. It was hard to

imagine that even the best military engineers could stand up ETUs in time to save even a minority of those already sick or about to be. Sick people were piling up in that village and across the district and in the hospital . . . When we inspected Maforki, it was difficult to know who was dead and who was alive. The smell was awful, and the first thing I thought of was the General Hospital in Port-au-Prince right after the earthquake . . . The trip back to Freetown that night took a long time because of all the roadblocks, which made Bailor think of the war. But I kept having a different thought: Here it was, almost November. How is it possible that the government had no partners to help provide care or to speed up diagnosis in the most affected district?

As far as skilled nursing went, Maforki was so short-staffed (we heard from nurses there) that many patients were checked on only once a day. The Cubans, still undergoing training, had yet to arrive. We'd heard the agreement had been to send a couple hundred clinicians to Sierra Leone, but we had no clue how many might end up in Port Loko.

Several Port Loko caregivers, including surviving medical and nursing staff in the hospital, begged us to sign up for service there. So did the overwhelmed and stroke-bound district medical officer. And Partners In Health, it transpired, wasn't the first international nongovernmental organization to have been assigned clinical duties at Maforki. Others with greater experience in disaster relief, and even prior Ebola stints, had declined the assignment. Our fellow humanitarians, whether working with nongovernmental organizations or UN agencies, had reason to be afraid. We were afraid, too, and it would have been easy just then to say that such working conditions were intolerable. We could have refused to work there and insisted on building a well-laid-out and safer space from scratch. The problem with such prudence was reality: Port Loko District didn't have a purpose-built ETU, and the sick and dying were already piling up in Maforki, in the district hospital, and in shabby health centers and homes across the region. Maforki may have been a hellhole, but we'd promised to go there.

In the days that followed, we had intense, extensive debates about what to do.

Meanwhile, on October 24, the American nurse Kaci Hickox, upon returning to the United States from Sierra Leone, was detained against her will in Newark and, even though she was asymptomatic, put in an isolation facility not much better than those planned for West Africa. At the time, I was in Morocco for a conference on Ebola and had plans to make a quick trip to Boston to celebrate my birthday with friends. But the climate of fear taking hold in the United States made me worry about being detained if I returned, so instead of traveling I spent two unplanned days in Marrakesh.

This gave me time to think, and to read. I hadn't known that Donald Trump was then doing his best to inflame sentiments by tweeting disparagingly about President Obama (who could fend for himself) and Dr. Craig Spencer (who'd been fending for the destitute sick in Guinea at his own peril and had just been admitted to New York's Bellevue Hospital with Ebola):

> With all that is happening with Ebola, including the doctor who
> so easily came back to New York, Obama still refuses to stop the
> flights![16]

While I was stuck in Marrakesh, Corrado Cancedda called me to rehash our debate about Maforki. He launched into a monologue about the parlous conditions there and wondered out loud if we might have a better chance of delivering care safely in Port Loko Government Hospital.

Dr. Cancedda already knew my thoughts on the question. The situation in Port Loko town wasn't much better than at the facility in Maforki. The hospital had largely been shut down, although, despite the risks, its medical director and surviving nursing staff continued to see pregnant women and sick children. The campus was now home to a sixty-bed holding center—basically a large, open ward to which Ebola "suspects" were sent while awaiting lab results sent from Freetown—where nosocomial transmission was surely taking place: by the time some suspects had tested negative for Ebola, or positive for malaria or some other cause of acute febrile syndromes, they had been housed next to Ebola patients and exposed to the virus. (Of twenty health workers in the district who'd died in the previous two weeks, eighteen had been on its payroll. As in Kenema, it wasn't clear that they had been infected at the hospital, because many of them had also been caring for the sick at home.)

One point of ETUs—and of community-based diagnosis, isolation, and referral to them—was to prevent district hospitals from suffering the fate of Kenema's, which had finally been shut down after a majority of its senior clinicians had been sickened. So if we were to reopen Port Loko's hospital, we'd need to make sure that the facility in Maforki functioned as an ETU, as Minister Fofanah and his staff had concluded. Cancedda, Lascher, and their team ultimately reached the same conclusion.

At the tail end of October, Partners In Health planted its flag in both Maforki and Port Loko Government Hospital. By then many flags had been planted across the district, and several sigils hung. But with the exception of the government's emblems, these did not announce the direct care of the sick. Instead, they announced the construction of Ebola treatment units (a long time coming), the installation of solar panels able to light them during the night, rudimentary waste-management systems, the recruitment and training of sprayers of chlorine solution, the care and feeding of short-term volunteers, and the safe burial of the dead.

The first week the Partners In Health team spent in Port Loko District was grim. Ibrahim Bah, recruited as a driver to replace the young man who'd fled upon seeing Maforki, described his first two days on the job:

> I was in Freetown. Then I came to Port Loko as a driver to work with
> Partners In Health because the driver who had been hired ran away
> because of fright of Ebola. I received a call that I should come to
> replace him. My first day in Maforki, on October 26, I saw the burial
> team carrying nine corpses. That made me very, very, very sad. I
> nearly ran away too. But because of the love I have for my country,

I wanted to save sick people. On the next day, October 27, I saw 14
corpses removed.

In early November 2014, we deployed our first short-term volunteers to Sierra
Leone and Liberia. These recruits, mostly American clinicians, were to work
with scores of Partners In Health staff from the United States and Haiti.
They'd been vetted to ensure they'd be able to deliver supportive care safely
in unsafe places and to handle the stress that inevitably comes with time in
an Ebola treatment unit. Many West African clinicians, mostly nurses and
nursing aides, volunteered to join the effort, creating a legion of ancillary
staff—many of them Ebola survivors—who took charge of logistics, record
keeping, infection control, and a host of other nonclinical activities. Partners
In Health was suddenly sponsoring a substantial fraction of professional
caregivers in Sierra Leone and Liberia, and scores of survivors.

In Sierra Leone, our collective set up shop in Maforki, Port Loko town,
and Koidu—the capital of Kono District and a bustling diamond-trading town
that had been trashed by war. Because of the diamond trade, the town had
been partially rebuilt, but in a ramshackle way. Its public hospital looked as
if a neutron bomb had gone off within it—the kind of bomb, that is, that kills
the living but leaves buildings intact. There were few staff left to run it, even
though the booms and thuds of the mines would be audible throughout the
epidemic.

In Liberia, we were dispatched to two district hospitals in the most underserved regions of a grotesquely arid medical desert. One was in Zwedru,
where Last Mile Health was working with a group of community health workers; the other was in Harper, a small city that served as the seat of Maryland
County, in the southeastern corner of the country. Like Koidu, Harper had
been half leveled by a war that ended a decade previously. But unlike Koidu,
parts of Harper looked as if the cease-fire had just been declared. Abandoned
and gutted buildings still lined its main drag, which is where we established
our headquarters in (yes) an abandoned house. Trees and vines were growing

within and on it. There was precisely one physician providing regular clinical care in all of Maryland County when we were sent there. The region's nursing school had been shut down.

In the aftermath of war, which had spared no part of the region and laid low the health systems of Sierra Leone and Liberia, it was clear to the newly arrived that scant resources had been invested in rebuilding these systems, or in training those needed to run them. The peace had cost billions, we knew, but the budget for UN troops alone dwarfed that allocated to the kind of peacemaking that involved health care, education, and helping ex-combatants find gainful employment. The abandoned vocational school in Maforki now full of the dead and dying had been part of one such effort; we later found on the premises a sign that declared part of it a bakery. It was hard to know, and didn't seem to be a good time to ask, if these efforts had really led to the transfer of new skills or the social reintegration of newly skilled former combatants. But at least the war had ended.

Most of our expatriate volunteers knew no more about this troubled history than I did. Learning about social and historical context was not part of our remit or our purpose. Our growing army was assigned two primary tasks: the first, in concert with scores of poorly coordinated teams, was to halt the advance of Ebola in these districts while trying to save those already sick from it. The second was to reestablish basic health services in hospitals, clinics, and rural health posts. A small but valiant team was also dispatched to Freetown's maternity hospital. In Maryland County, we were also asked by Liberia's president, Ellen Johnson Sirleaf, to help reopen its nursing school and to tutor its almost-graduating class through national board exams.

Accomplishing these tasks simultaneously posed all sorts of logistical and security challenges. Liberia, which hadn't conducted a robust truth-and-reconciliation process to reckon with the legacy of war, was notoriously fragile. A number of its warlords still served in public office, while others jockeyed for power from the sidelines. Sierra Leone was riven by deep division and mistrust, in spite of efforts to work through its recent bloodletting. The week before we arrived in Koidu, a clash between security forces and the family and neighbors of a ninety-year-old woman thought to have Ebola left two dead. Contact tracers had insisted on taking a sample of her blood, even though there was then little offered in the way of care. As proof of that, nine out of nine nurses working in Koidu Government Hospital's holding unit would be infected by January 2015; seven of them died.[17]

We encountered few security problems, however, because it was pretty clear we'd arrived to provide medical care. We never had trouble drawing blood—even when we screened close to two hundred seemingly healthy residents of a village near Koidu in an effort to see if symptom-based screening had missed folks with Ebola. (It had.)[18] The problem for us wasn't hostility to professional caregivers, foreign or homegrown. It was simply the lack of them, and of the required stuff. This was especially true within government health facilities outside of the capital cities. We believed in strengthening these institutions as a public good. That's why, from November on, so many of us—eventually including forty-one Cubans—spent so much time in Port Loko Government Hospital and within the blue plastic walls of Maforki.

As the new year began, the number of cases in the western reaches of Upper West Africa finally began to decline. But conditions on the ground remained challenging. Those of us providing clinical services had more resources to buy stuff and pay staff than at the outset of the surge. Even counting the Cuban brigade, however, the number of available clinicians per patient in Port Loko would have been laughable in a U.S. emergency room or intensive care unit.[19] There had been movement on few of the Ebola commitments made at the United Nations—and by "movement" I simply mean the transfer of money out of one general bank account into another designated for aid to the region.[20] Resources in the hands of care-delivery teams on the ground remained paltry and sharply focused on Ebola, to the exclusion of the vast array of suffering we saw in district hospitals, in health centers as they slowly reopened, in homes, and in the streets of towns and cities.

As regards systems and space, the situation in Port Loko District remained parlous. Systems that increased the chances of local staff being paid for their labor were far more popular than infection-control protocols linked to resupply of gloves, gowns, and face shields. The space in Maforki had been radically improved since the end of October, but that was true because intermittent electricity was better than none; because a triage area, even if outside under a mango tree, was better than none; because rented houses for short-term volunteers were better than tents; because water from a hundred-gallon tank, though inferior to running water, was better than water from a bucket; and because a roof patched together with plastic tarpaulins was better than no roof at all.

Who on earth wouldn't have preferred a purpose-built (and thus well designed) Ebola treatment unit? The problem, of course, was timing. Most safe ETUs built for the crisis took months to open, and when they finally did, it was too late. The British unit at Kerry Town, where Martin Salia unsuccessfully sought care, cost an estimated £80 million, but it saw few patients. Nine of the eleven facilities built by U.S. military contractors in Liberia, at a cost of hundreds of millions of dollars, never cared for a single patient and weren't much use for anything else.[21] We refurbished Maforki with less than a hundred thousand dollars, and close to 8 percent of Sierra Leone's Ebola survivors walked or were carried out of its doors. As rickety as the facility was, it nonetheless represented a solid monument to cost-effectiveness.[22]

The question of clinical effectiveness, however, remained a sore point in Maforki. We never managed to drive mortality down to anywhere near 10 percent, as we'd wished. That was simply impossible without the staff and stuff available in American hospitals. The trend was positive while we were there, but as the epidemic and interest in it began to shrink, so did the chance of strengthening the care-delivery system by acquiring needed equipment and training local providers to use it. In Guinea, Liberia, and Sierra Leone, the care-delivery system in the first weeks of 2015 was as weak or weaker than it had been a year previously.

By then Ebola had killed nearly ten thousand people, including hundreds of nurses, nursing aides, doctors, and other health workers. Even at that stage the odds of surviving an Ebola diagnosis were barely even, unless you happened to be American or European or had some other ticket out of the West African clinical desert. And that's not even mentioning all of the other causes of medical concern in the region. In general, the chances of sick

West Africans remained poor at the end of the epidemic—a state of affairs not mentioned when, in December 2014, *Time* magazine named "the Ebola Fighters" as its "Person of the Year."[23]

By February 2015, new cases of Ebola were becoming rare in parts of Sierra Leone and Guinea. Liberia was itching to declare victory. Many emergency-response organizations were scanning horizons for the next crisis. On the ground, however, our teams knew to be wary of Ebola triumphalism.

On March 10, in between trips to Sierra Leone and Liberia, I kept a long-standing promise to give a lecture at a Colorado university. At that point, new Ebola diagnoses in those countries were declining rapidly, and national and international health authorities again were predicting impending victory. Several of the big funders were chafing to pull back and manifested scant interest in health-systems strengthening or in medical education, both necessary to address the deadly dearth of professional caregivers well before Ebola, like war, further thinned their ranks. Now, as funders and humanitarians alike spoke of moving on, new transmission chains continued to link urban households and rural villages across Upper West Africa. Guinea would register more cases in March than in either January or February.

This dilemma—Ebola wasn't over, deficiencies in the health systems hadn't been addressed, the three affected countries were now bereft of hundreds of health professionals, and relief workers scrambled for the exit—gave us more reasons to seek supporters in places like Colorado. I struggled to lay out the dimensions of the dilemma to my audience. In addition to the losses caused by the virus, thousands were dying not of Ebola but because of it; those still stuck in Upper West Africa faced an impending crisis as short-term volunteers packed their bags. It was a difficult message to share outside of the clinical desert. Some in that audience surely felt that the massive global Ebola response, belated though it was, had addressed that dilemma.

Even as I tried to undermine Ebola triumphalism from the lectern, a flurry of messages appeared in rapid succession on my phone, which I was using as a stopwatch for my talk. This inrush made me anxious, in a familiar way that tended toward dread, but reading these messages would have to wait. The Q-and-A session, usually the most enjoyable part of any lecture, seemed to drag on. Afterward, I was ushered to a reception hosted by a group of eager and earnest students planning careers in global health. Before talking to them, I apologized and retreated to a corner with a young colleague from Partners In Health. He'd received the same messages I had and already knew what they said.

The messages contained news that we'd been fearing for months: an American clinician volunteering with us in Sierra Leone had just been diagnosed with Ebola. I quickly scrolled through my e-mails. The stricken volunteer, whose identity wasn't yet revealed to me, had been tending to the sick in Port Loko, which I'd just left. One message, sent at 10:31 p.m., about an hour earlier, came from Tony Fauci.

Paul:
See below. I will be taking care of one of your people.
Best regards,
Tony

What followed were exchanges about the events of that day, including an e-mail to Fauci under the subject heading "AMCIT in Sierra Leone EVD Positive." AMCIT, I guessed, was State Department jargon for an American citizen; EVD, I knew all too well, was shorthand among infectious-disease doctors for "Ebola virus disease," which in our circles was preferred to "Ebola hemorrhagic fever." Plans were already being made to transport the volunteer to a biocontainment unit in Bethesda, Maryland, where Fauci and his army conducted their own research and clinical practice. The other e-mails didn't provide much more information.

This was bad news. But because our sickened colleague was American, we had some confidence about his fate. Fauci's message meant he would be quickly evacuated to a clinical facility able to provide supportive and critical care. In the summer and fall of 2014, we'd learned that even the sickest Ebola patients could be saved with aggressive and carefully monitored intensive care. Not only that, we'd learned a lot about the complexities and variations of Ebola's clinical course from the well-documented hospital stays of each of the previously repatriated victims—far more than we'd learned in decades of epidemiological reports from Africa's clinical deserts.

My colleagues in Lungi and Freetown prepared to evacuate the volunteer to Dulles International Airport on *The Phoenix*, a biocontainment plane that had been doing brisk business in recent months. I was tasked with calling his family, but first I needed to consult with Tony Fauci in Bethesda and with Corrado Cancedda in Port Loko. What was the volunteer's clinical status? Was he stable for transport? Did we have any lab data? How had he fallen ill? Had others been exposed? What would happen next? These were the kinds of questions family members ask, and I didn't yet know the answers to any of them, much less the most pressing one: What were his chances of survival?

I reached Cancedda as the sun was rising in Colorado. Within half an hour, I had the basics down. Like other Partners In Health volunteers, the young man—whose name we never disclosed—had gone through training on how to don and doff personal protective equipment. He'd been in Sierra Leone for sixteen days and had worked for a week or so in Maforki before being assigned to Port Loko's hospital. Four days before his diagnosis, he had suddenly "felt weak" and then had spiked a fever. The day after that, Cancedda told me, he'd "passed out during rounds." For any physician or nurse, the word "rounds" conjures an image of a crowd of clinicians moving from bed to bed. Although bedside rounds, like doctors, had been rare in Port Loko prior to the fall of 2014, they'd become more routine after the arrival of teams from Partners In Health and Cuba.

That meant the American volunteer would have been surrounded by fellow clinicians when he collapsed. They would have rushed to his aid, naturally. In the cramped and crowded hospital, as opposed to the ETU in nearby Maforki, they wouldn't have been wearing much in the way of personal protective gear. It was unlikely that all of them would have been sporting even gloves: a fresh pair was worn to examine each patient, but not all those rounding examined each patient. Since the man's symptoms had not yet included vomiting or diarrhea—he was still, in the jargon, a dry patient—the likelihood of Ebola transmission to those helping him to his feet was low. But in the algorithmic logic of epidemiology, all those who came to his aid, even those with the presence of mind to glove up, would be classified as "exposed" once his symptoms were attributed to the virus.

Corrado Cancedda had been up all night, but he read my thoughts. "Exposure in this sense means they will be quarantined for observation," he added. Quarantined where? "The CDC thinks they should be quarantined in the States," he told me. Like me, Cancedda was probably already imagining harsh public debates about whether potentially exposed but asymptomatic returnees should be allowed out in public during three long weeks of the intrusive observation that even lax or mild versions of quarantine generally require. In the United States at least, such monitoring had never once worked to diagnose Ebola before simple self-report had. It had, however, cost millions of dollars and engendered no small amount of umbrage.[24] "The CDC will want them near one of the designated treatment centers," Cancedda continued. That meant the biosecure units in Atlanta, Bethesda, and Omaha. It seemed unlikely that any of those classed as exposed would be natives of these cities. "How many came to his aid?" I asked. Cancedda paused, then replied, "We're up to a dozen already."

We now had a new logistical nightmare, an American one, on our hands. And there was more: the volunteer clinician, whom I'd never met, hailed from Dallas. My heart sank. The only cases of Ebola transmission in the United States had been to two Dallas nurses involved in the care of Eric Duncan. One had been treated by Tony Fauci and his team, the other by colleagues at Emory. Both of the Dallas nurses had recovered promptly, but their experience had sparked a veritable frenzy in the press and on social media.

Even before Duncan was diagnosed, much of the world was falling prey to an outbreak of Ebola fear and loathing, as anthropologist Adia Benton and a colleague had noted back in September in *The Washington Post*. "Amidst irrational fears of infection through air travel," they wrote,

> multiple international airlines have ceased flights to West Africa. Fear has even halted travel to unaffected regions, revealing the spillover

effects in our "map-challenged" world: there are reports of airlines canceling flights to East Africa—where there are fewer people infected with Ebola (zero) than in America (two). There is also evidence that Ebola-fueled racism is on the rise in Europe. In the U.S., over a quarter of Americans think they or their families are at risk.[25]

After Duncan became the first person diagnosed with Ebola in the United States, and then died, his fiancée and their son suffered not only his loss but also enough rejection and stigma that they had felt compelled to seek shelter at an undisclosed address afforded them by the Catholic Church.

The media circus that had surrounded all previous American cases, and many more non-cases, had been debilitating to volunteers from across the country, as I knew from personal experience. It wasn't much better in Europe, where the low-water mark may have been reached when a Spanish nurse, infected while caring for one of the priests serving in Liberia, was obliged by the authorities to have her dog euthanized.

After talking to Corrado Cancedda, my next step was to call Tony Fauci. He'd remained a voice of reason throughout the first Texas drama, reminding a fearful U.S. public avid for news that the real problem lay in West Africa, which needed and deserved U.S. assistance and support.

Several members of Fauci's team had gone to Liberia to help clinically, among them a sharp young doctor named Dan Chertow, who was trained in both infectious disease and critical care. Others from the National Institutes of Health (NIH) had helped design or fund studies of therapeutic agents and vaccines protective against Ebola in nonhuman primates. These were as yet unproven in humans, in large part because of what one pundit termed "Ebolanomics": there was scant interest in testing, developing, and marketing therapies for a disease afflicting mostly rural Africans.[26] During the decade prior to the West Africa epidemic, a Canadian vaccine able to protect 100 percent of experimentally infected macaques just sat on the shelf.[27] So did promising therapies like ZMapp.

I got through to Fauci on the first try, and it was not a tough call. As usual, he was upbeat and encouraging. But he suggested that it might be best if the family avoided speaking to journalists or even to close friends about the diagnosis. Others at Partners In Health would give the same advice. But before I called the family, I wanted to talk to the new CEO of Partners In Health. Gary Gottlieb, a Harvard psychiatrist, had served for close to a decade on the board of Partners In Health and been among the most supportive of the lot when we made the decision to go to West Africa. I wanted his counsel and maybe a bit of his clinical expertise. I was, to put it clearly, more than a bit anxious.

At dawn on March 11, headed back to a Colorado airport, I still hadn't called Dallas. But rumors were already circulating on the Internet that a clinician working with Partners In Health had fallen ill with Ebola. Meanwhile, I knew that *The Phoenix* was scheduled to reach the Lungi airfield at 11:45 the next morning. That would be day seven of the Texan's illness, which had come to include profound muscular weakness and diarrhea; he also had laboratory evidence of both hepatitis and abnormal blood clotting. But he had no bleeding. His blood pressure was fine, perhaps because his fluid losses had been replaced. Intravenously, of course.

When I finally dialed the home number of our volunteer, after the sun came up over both Colorado and Texas, I was shamefully relieved to hear an answering machine on the end of the line. But before I could hang up, one of his younger brothers, a nursing student himself, picked up. Those first conversations are a bit of a blur in my memory, but it was possible to convey a positive message: still lucid and clinically stable, his brother was headed from the epicenter of the epidemic to an epicenter of knowledge about how best to care for those critically ill from all manner of infections. He would receive attention from the team of doctors and nurses who'd cared for a fellow Texan, the Dallas nurse Nina Pham. They were top-of-the-line clinicians, I told him, and wonderful people, too. The young man connected me to his parents, with whom I shared the same opinion and several more. They made plans to head immediately to Bethesda.

Their son reached Dulles International Airport in discomfort due to diarrhea, fever, and persistent neuromuscular weakness, but his blood pressure remained normal. Dan Chertow, the NIH doctor who'd likely seen the most cases of Ebola after traveling to Monrovia at the height of Liberia's surge, was waiting for him on the tarmac. I wanted to be there, too. While the volunteer had been flying across the Atlantic, however, I'd flown from Colorado to Peru, for reasons that had little to do with Ebola—Partners In Health had been working there for years on drug-resistant tuberculosis, and there were finally a couple of new drugs to offer these patients. I promised Tony Fauci and his new patient's parents that I'd head to Bethesda as soon as possible.

Tony Fauci and the volunteer's father kept me abreast of developments while I was in Peru, letting me know he took a turn for the worse shortly after arriving. Although his viral load had plateaued, he was displaying the signs of one kind of Ebola sepsis syndrome: fluids were leaking into his lungs and other places they shouldn't go, and the team in Bethesda worried he'd need help breathing. And even though he'd been protected from hypovolemia, his kidneys weren't doing their job, his profound weakness didn't let up after his diarrhea did, and he was starting to display changes in mental status—all evidence of direct viral attack on his kidneys, gut, lungs, and brain.[28] (Evidence of its attack on his liver, for which Ebola displays a marked affinity, was evident prior to his arrival.) But the irrepressible Fauci remained optimistic. Five days later, when I was boarding a flight in Lima and on my way to Bethesda, he offered me reassurance. "We're going to pull him through," Fauci said.

When I reached Bethesda, Tony Fauci himself drove me over to the NIH biocontainment unit. On the way there, he told me that his patient was intubated. The unit, I soon learned, was tiny. Then again, it had only one patient at the time. He was in a private room, of course, hooked up to all sorts of gadgets. I found these familiar and reassuring: they were the kinds of gadgets used in every ICU in which I'd worked. The staff were sympathetic, encouraging, and kind to the patient and his family. His mother, who looked about ten years younger than I'd expected, often sat in the nursing station, which looked like the control tower of a small airport. Monitors were everywhere, and thick panes of glass separated us from her son. It was staggering to count the number of doctors, nurses, social workers, lab technicians, respiratory therapists, and others who were dedicated to the care of a single patient.

I spent a week in Bethesda. During rounds, which occurred promptly at four in the afternoon, a dozen physicians—Fauci always in blue scrubs—were routinely present to discuss the developments of the day. It was hard not to think about Humarr Khan, Martin Salia, and all the patients I'd been seeing in Maforki and Port Loko. More than once, I thought about those two young nurses who had died somewhere between Connaught and Kenema and been buried with the help of Ian Crozier shortly before he became Patient Four. I thought about others I'd never met but whose dreadful ends I'd heard about and was now haunted by: the pregnant teenager who had seized in front of her family and Eric Duncan after she was turned away from medical assistance, the nurses of Kenema, and the dead family members of the survivors to whom I'd become close over the previous few months. I'd heard so much about their kids, siblings, spouses, and parents—all lost—that I thought of them, too.

Another hard part of visiting the NIH unit was that I couldn't enter the patient's room or converse with him. Even in full gear, that wouldn't have been possible when I arrived, since he was on a ventilator and sedated. But he didn't stay on the vent for long, and I was grateful to be around when he was extubated. His mother and her sister were there that day and the team was excited and optimistic. Minutes after the breathing tube came out, we could hear the young man talking garrulously—"the drugs talking," he later joked, although it's not clear it was so—even if he couldn't hear or see us. The same phone that had delivered the barrage of e-mails a couple weeks earlier was replete with the wonder of FaceTime, and my first conversations with the sick man, and his with his mother and aunt, were on that marvelous invention called the iPhone.

The volunteer got worse before he got better. His renal function worsened throughout the second week of his illness; then, the NIH team was on the verge of initiating dialysis when his kidneys began to recover. Although it was difficult to assess his mental and neurological status while he was intubated, the Bethesda team was able to determine that he'd developed meningoencephalitis, as had Ian Crozier—and as had probably thousands of those who had fallen ill in West Africa. Because we were in Bethesda rather than Port Loko, we were able to see from daily blood tests that his deterioration occurred after an innate, or nonspecific, immune response began to clear the virus. In week three of his illness, an adaptive and specific anti-Ebola immune response revved up, his viral load dwindled to nothing, and his meningoencephalitis slowly resolved. His life saved, the young Texan would go on to make a full physical recovery, although, not surprisingly, he suffered lingering psychological and emotional distress.

Not long after he fell ill, Partners In Health and I showed up on the front page of *The New York Times*. We didn't get a flattering treatment. The article quoted people who felt that because we had chosen to put our volunteers to work before new purpose-built Ebola treatment units were ready, we were to blame for nosocomial transmission that occurred in the Ministry of Health's designated unit in Maforki. Some took that criticism to heart, but the family was having none of it, and neither were Fauci, Chertow, and others on the NIH team. I often wondered what the volunteer himself felt, but then, on June 8, he sent me a beautiful letter that dispelled that anxiety. I cite part of it here with his blessing:

> Dear Dr. Farmer,
>
> I've been meaning to write this letter since my hospital discharge— but I'm just now getting around to it. Though I have never met you in person (unless you count iPhone's "FaceTime" while one party is coming off of powerful sedative drugs), I feel like I know you, and even more so after talking to you the other day via phone. This whole journey has been a whirlwind, though now it has slowed down a bit and I am just biding my time until I am able to work again. I'll never forget March 10, 2015, the day I was informed that my Ebola PCR test was positive. It was a day that started me down a path that never in my wildest imagination would I have gone down. It also introduced me to a wonderful group of people, some with PIH and some with NIH, whose kindness I can never repay.

Once the volunteer made it through this episode, Ian Crozier stepped in to walk him through the tough process of survivorship. He was one of those whose survivorship has been harnessed to the well-being of others.

After his own recovery, Ian Crozier became deeply engaged in work with survivors across West Africa and something of a folk hero (and walking Ebola encyclopedia) to many of us at Partners In Health. Inspired by Crozier's example, the Texan made a pledge to return to West Africa—and kept it. Within a year of his diagnosis, he, Tony Fauci, and I would find ourselves in Liberia together. Dan Chertow and Crozier were working there, too, seeking to understand late complications of acute Ebola, which continued to affect a substantial minority of survivors in West Africa.

It's to their lived experience of the epidemic that we turn next.

3.

Ibrahim's Second Chance

All those who have thought about the bad state of things refuse to appeal to the compassion of one group of people for another. But the compassion of the oppressed for the oppressed is indispensable. It is the world's one hope.

—Bertolt Brecht, "The World's One Hope," circa 1938

IBRAHIM KAMARA, WHO BY THE AGE OF TWENTY-SIX HAD SURVIVED EBOLA and the loss of more than twenty members of his family to it, isn't good with secular calendar dates. The night we met, in Freetown, he told me, "The worst month of my life began at the close of Ramadan." This period of fasting and reflection is announced by the Islamic lunar calendar, where a year is ten days shorter than the solar year. I had to look up the dates: in 2014, Ramadan started at sundown on June 28 and ended on July 28, when the sun dipped below the ocean that has shaped the history of this westernmost tip of Africa.

Ibrahim and I met in November, more than three months after Ramadan's close, in the restaurant of the Mammy Yoko, a seven-story hotel that promoted itself as a "luxury beachfront resort." By then Ebola, raging through the city, had ended what little tourism Sierra Leone had known. But you wouldn't have known it inside the restaurant. The place was plush, sleek, and busy. In the background, we could hear the dull boom of the nearby surf. Ibrahim was dressed in what might be called generic hip-hop style: baseball cap cocked at just the right angle, sunglasses perched on his forehead, a polo shirt, and jeans hanging low by some miracle of suspension on a slim frame. Most young men in Freetown, whatever their creed, dress in similar fashion—one that would make them look at home in cities on either side of the Atlantic. Except on Fridays, that is, when many of them wear brocaded shirts and matching trousers, a traditional outfit seen across West and North Africa.

The Mammy Yoko's dining room, which had a vaguely European vibe, had been gutted during the 1997 battle for Freetown. More than a thousand civilians from two dozen nations had taken refuge in the hotel in the days just after the Sierra Leonean army's high command had joined rebel forces to overthrow the country's first elected civilian government. After those forces had swept in from the east, and as Nigerian warships steamed west to stop them, the hotel's top floors had been struck by mortars and grenades; fires broke out on several floors, and hundreds scurried to the sweltering basement. A U.S. aircraft carrier churned north from the shores of the Congo to deliver the AMCITs, journalists, Lebanese business folk and their families, and sundry expatriates deemed worthy of rescue besieged in the hotel, which was defended by a doomed contingent of Nigerian peacekeepers.

Of course, I knew none of this the night I first broke bread with Ibrahim, even though the scars of civil war were then evident in and around the refurbished restaurant. Like most adult Ebola survivors, however, Ibrahim had a grim familiarity with both sickness and war. For them, the rebel attacks had barely faded from memory before the viral one had begun. The foreigners present in the Mammy Yoko the night I met Ibrahim weren't refugees or war correspondents; they were the worn and worried officers of the international anti-Ebola brigade. That night's diners included several Ebola experts and public-health functionaries from Atlanta, Washington, and Geneva, some in the company of a handful of tired-looking Sierra Leonean officials.

Ibrahim and I met for a dinner gathering of some of the city's first Ebola survivors. The event was intended to bolster morale among the bereaved survivors, and among my weary colleagues. Since I also knew a few of the Ebola and public-health experts at the other tables, I worried they—or the hotel's staff—might not approve of our timing. By late November, Freetown and its environs were reporting hundreds of new cases each week. No city on the face of the earth had ever been so Ebola-afflicted, and it wasn't clear that December would be any better.

A visual survey of the dining room suggested we were separated from one another by a lot more than having survived an Ebola diagnosis or not. The Partners In Health team, including its Sierra Leonean leaders, were the beneficiaries of university educations. We had jobs and prestige, and the only Ebola stigma we AMCITs endured was when we returned to our home country, which had adopted a defensive and corrosive posture. Of the survivors present that night, none were professionals, most were less than half my age, and all were poor or downright destitute after trying to save family members from a virulent affliction that seemed to come out of the blue.

One of the guests seemed to be known and admired by pretty much everyone gathered, regardless of nationality or medical history: Dr. Marta Lado. She was the Spanish infectious-disease doctor—"the Spanish Angel," as one of her former patients called her that night—who in late June had shown me the newly assembled isolation unit at Connaught Hospital. Between July and late November, she'd lost patients, colleagues, and friends—including the surgeon Martin Salia and a couple of young nurses to whom she introduced me. The Mammy Yoko dinner had to be the first time that Ibrahim and several of the others had seen Lado out of a hazmat suit, but they recognized her and her ready smile, and more than one of them embraced her warmly, in hugs that she gladly returned—violating the tenets of the city's ABC campaign. (Although public-health acronyms change rapidly, this one still meant "Avoid Body Contact.") Lado sat across from me but didn't stay long. During our dinner, the blare of sirens led her to look anxiously at the cell phone sitting near her plate, which she barely touched.

Ibrahim, who was seated next to me, was among those who recognized Lado. It didn't take him long to let me know he'd gone through hell that summer. The most grievous of his losses, I'd later learn, was the death of his mother. It was outside the doors of Connaught that he last saw her, when he turned her over, limp, to a group of masked, unknown clinicians dressed in full bioprotective gear. Among those clinicians had been Lado and her young British colleague Oliver Johnson, who'd also shown me around the unit at Connaught in June. He was at the dinner, too. Almost all the survivors present that night knew both of them, and the hospital, for the same reasons that Ibrahim did. The Mammy Yoko, on the other hand, was foreign territory.

Few of those who a month or two previously had been at death's door, and seen their loved ones trip over its lintel, had ever been in a hotel dining room. They were unsure of how—or what—to order from the menu. Most settled on traditional fare, a mush of cassava, palm oil, and potato leaves, which the expatriates skipped in favor of pizza or pasta or fish. Any awkwardness quickly evaporated, however, replaced by a welcome air of levity. Soon most of the noise in the restaurant came from our three tables, pushed together to form a T. Once in a while, other patrons would look up from their computers or handheld devices to see where all the noise was coming from. A few, drawn to the unexpected merriment, joined us.

Most of the survivors were chatting in Krio, an English creole that is the lingua franca of Sierra Leone. But at a certain point in the evening, one of the survivors stood up at the clinking of a glass and made some remarks in the Queen's English. The young man's name was Mohamed, but he was known to everybody in the room simply as the Chairman for the efforts he'd made on behalf of fellow Ebola sufferers. "We don't think we should be called 'Ebola survivors,'" he told us, "although we're proud to have survived. We should be called 'Ebola conquerors'!" At that, Ibrahim raised his glass and cried, "To the conquerors!"—a response that provoked cheers and peals of laughter.

No one had forgotten—could forget—Ebola, but the evening offered us all a bit of respite, camaraderie, and encouragement. The moment reminded me of similar celebrations of survival that I'd been lucky enough to be part of, in Peru, Russia, Rwanda, Malawi, Boston, and Haiti. Most of all, I was reminded of rural Haiti, where, even in the darkest of times, the survivors of deadly disease and injury I'd cared for as a physician consistently sustained themselves with similar confidence, humor, and ebullient conversation. It was a wonderful dinner that stretched well into the night.

Looking around the tables, I couldn't identify a single Sierra Leonean who'd received care that might reasonably be termed modern—and, with the exception of Ibrahim, I knew their medical histories pretty well.

A couple of them were Maforki survivors, but most were the folks on a list we received the day after our October meeting with the health minister, Dr. Fofanah. We'd promised him to keep an eye on their medical progress and to remain alert for signs of relapse or complications. This group had conquered Ebola in large part by virtue of being young and previously healthy and willing to fight back by gagging down liter after liter of oral rehydration salts, or by begging for "drips" to replace the fluids and electrolytes they'd lost to vomiting, diarrhea, and fever. They then forced themselves to eat and drink even when, because of grief and despair and sickness, they didn't feel much like fighting back. Yet all of them credited nurses and doctors with saving their lives—thanking us, in essence, far more than we deserved.

Ibrahim was one of the fighters, for sure. He's naturally wiry and compact, and at the time considerably diminished by illness, but even so he came across as larger than he is. He certainly wasn't shy, at least not one-on-one. Soon after the Chairman's toast we were again deep in conversation, even though my lack of Krio and our divergent versions of English (and Ibrahim's enthusiasm that night) led to a lot of sign language and emphatic gestures. He told me two things during our conversation that have stuck with me.

The first concerned the ABC campaign, which rankled Ibrahim. "So you're telling me," he said, more or less, "that my mother, who carried and birthed and bathed and fed me, has just fallen down on the floor in her own vomit, and I'm not supposed to go and help her up and clean her? That I'm supposed to call some emergency number that never works and not help her myself? That pisses me off!"

The second involved the number twenty-three. That's how many members of Ibrahim's family had died from Ebola, among them his mother and grand-parents, along with aunts, uncles, and cousins. His mother's side of the family tree had been cut down, root and branch, in a single month. Ibrahim repeated just the number, twenty-three, and waited for a response. I didn't have one at hand. By then, I'd met, worked with, or taken care of scores of Ebola patients. But I didn't recall meeting or hearing of anyone whose family had been so devastated by the disease, nor was I familiar with any pathogen that could take out an entire family. (Later, we'd meet survivors with similar stories of bereavement, and we were already hearing accounts of wiped-out villages.) It took me a couple of years, and a lot of help, to sort out Ibrahim's calculus.

Family networks are famously fluid and complex in West Africa. In most parts of Sierra Leone, you can find "co-wives"; twins who turn out to have been born at different times; and siblings who didn't share a parent but had been taken in as wards. Sometimes husbands and wives are not married, at least in any formal or local sense; sometimes they have secret spouses whom they don't mention. Sometimes "brothers" are either half brothers, adopted, or members of the same cohort going through the ubiquitous rites of passage that outsiders, at least, have long called "secret societies." "Uncles" are older cousins and "grannies" are elderly aunts; godparents and other sponsors (in-cluding nonnative ones) are often also introduced as mothers, fathers, aunts, and uncles. The massive dislocations of the war that the country had just lived through had scrambled things further. At one point during the conflict, half the country's citizens were refugees or displaced.

Whatever Ibrahim actually meant when he referred to his family, it was hard to imagine a more apocalyptic fate for kin, however defined, than the one he described. I think I finally said as much. "Well," he said in response, "I'd like you to interview me about that terrible month." The directness of his request surprised me. I'd already conducted more than a handful of cursory interviews with the Ebola survivors around the table and knew how painful their stories could be.[1] But I viewed Ibrahim's invitation as an opportunity. I was in Sierra Leone, after all, in part to advocate for the development of a proper health-care system, and to help overturn the nihilistic control-over-care paradigm that still reigned—and learning from the stories of Ebola survivors was an important part of that work. So I took Ibrahim up on his offer, agreeing that night that we'd meet in short order so that he could tell me his story, or as much of it as he wished to share.

As it turned out, Ibrahim had so much to say, and I had so much to learn, that we would end up talking for a couple of years. In the process he would inspire me to write this book.

Although uneasy with the secular calendar, Ibrahim sometimes speaks with a strange precision. When I asked him, a day or two after his toast to Ebola conquerors, to start at the beginning of his story, he offered the following: "I was born on a Saturday, at twelve o'clock, in March 1988, at Connaught."

Of Ibrahim's earliest years, there remains little in the way of testimony, and little chance of ever obtaining it. Most of those who might have supplied it—parents, grandparents, uncles, aunts—have been claimed by Ebola or other acute afflictions and injuries. This account of Ibrahim's youth is therefore based solely on his own recollection of it, with a bit of help from an older half brother, Mamoud. The two often lived apart during their childhoods but would look out for each other, and their other kin, when their family came under attack by Ebola.

Ibrahim was the first son of Hawanatu and Abdullai Kamara. The young man told me that his mother, Hawanatu, came from "upline," a reference to the rural reaches of Sierra Leone.[2] She hailed from the village of Mabanta, in Port Loko District, and identified as Temne, the country's largest northern tribe. Her father was a local chief, but certainly not of the paramount variety, to use the title bestowed upon British-backed leaders; Ibrahim's maternal grandparents were smallholder farmers and poor.

Abdullai was a Susu (also spelled Soso)—one of the smaller ethnic groups in Sierra Leone, with deep, mostly Muslim, roots in Guinea. Born in the Guinean village of Geva, which I could never locate on a map, Abdullai worked as a minor dockside functionary in eastern Freetown, sometimes said to be the third-largest deepwater port in the world. Much of the country's mineral wealth—diamonds, of course, but also gold, titanium, rutile, and bauxite—passes through Freetown, as does rice, containers full of electronics, gadgets, used clothing, you name it. Although most diamonds are now shipped legally from the port or shipped by air, some are smuggled out through the same overland channels of trade that smuggled in Ebola and weapons of war before it.

Ibrahim considered colonial rule remote history. But it influenced his life in the contingent ways that historic precedent always does. Before and after independence in 1961, most young men and women in Sierra Leone were shut out of secondary education and the formal economy. The likes of Abdullai and the stevedores he monitored have rarely enjoyed the benefits of what passes, legally or illegally, through Freetown's port. He and his brother (who offloaded imported sacks of rice for a living) were part of Sierra Leone's urban proletariat, a class that had grown extensively during the twentieth century, when Britain had marshaled its subjects and their resources in support of its efforts to fight two world wars. After Sierra Leone declared its independence from Britain, Freetown continued to grow. Although Ibrahim was born there, he spent part of his childhood in the small villages of his parents, where much of his family practiced subsistence agriculture, along with a small-scale trade in palm oil, cocoa, groundnuts, kola nuts, and such staples as rice, cassava, bananas, and millet.

Ibrahim's rural kin—especially those in the north, where most of his cousins and his grandparents lived—remained mired in want. Sierra Leone is verdant, but its soil is poorer than a visitor might believe, and the north has less rainfall than the coast or the richer agricultural land to the east and south. As a result of this (and of land grabs on top of a lack of access to fertilizer, decent agricultural implements, and credit), harvests in Port Loko District didn't often provide much surplus. As under British rule, the residents of the district's smaller hamlets received almost nothing in the way of assistance beyond that from their own kin. Ibrahim described to me what the conditions were like in Mabanta, his mother's village, when he was young. "There was nothing at all," he said. "No proper primary school, no secondary school, and no hospital or clinic unless you walked for hours or could get someone to take you on a bike."

This was the life Ibrahim's family had sought to spare him and Mamoud by moving to Freetown, and to some extent it did. But even the most hardworking parents could not shield their children from the former colony's warped political economy and the structural violence it perpetuated. The nation's economy could be summed up (in rather grim terms) as based largely on poorly managed trade in diamonds and minerals, on faltering subsistence agriculture, and on risky markets for cash crops and rice, their prices prone to wild fluctuation thanks to the actions of speculators, hoarders, or international financial institutions.

Abdullai and Hawanatu moved to Freetown in search of not only jobs but also a formal education for their children—something they themselves never received. Both Ibrahim and Mamoud attended a large Christian school, which, as Ibrahim put it to me, was "full of Muslims." (Most accounts of Sierra Leone over the last couple of centuries agree that Christians and Muslims got along well, even when feuding tribes and colonizers did not.)[3] Ibrahim made it his goal at school to learn to speak English well. "Without proper English," he told me, "you can never get a job with the government or in administration. You can't even study what you want."[4] By the time Ibrahim was in school, however, even good English and a devout application to study were unlikely to get one far. That's because he was born just before Sierra Leone's civil war, which made the term "blood diamond" famous.

If you read the history of the region backward, that war seems inevitable. After independence, the country's new leadership had created a Westminster-style parliamentary government, but ethnic regionalism, created through decades of British divide-and-conquer rule, rose significantly in the 1960s. This strife often peaked during political contests, which had less to do with tribal affiliations than with control of the country's mineral wealth. The price and supply of its staple food was similarly marked by sudden peaks and troughs. Whether locally grown or imported, rice became scarce during Ibrahim's youth. It was a scarcity that recurred reliably (and usually worsened) with political upheaval. That, on the other hand, had been anything but scarce in Sierra Leone. "By the time I was old enough to think," Ibrahim said, "I saw that a man like my father could work and work and get nowhere. The country had riches, it's true, but corrupt politicians took them all, leaving us to get by on scraps fit for dogs." Sierra Leone had become, he said, little more than "a corrupt one-party state that gave some things to a few, and not much to everyone else."

The party in question was named the All People's Congress (APC). Across Sierra Leone, as the APC tightened its grip, the gap between reality and the aspirations of the urban poor continued to grow. This divergence was hastened in the late eighties by policies of international financial institutions widely termed "structural adjustment." As the anthropologist Paul Richards has put it:

> The APC regime hoped to fend off political trouble by paying attention to the food needs of the urban poor (especially Freetown youth). But in recent years, with structural adjustment forcing the price of rice upwards, and reducing prospects of a government job, many young people in Sierra Leone have seen themselves locked out of the urban areas, perhaps permanently. Life is a stressful shuttle between bouts of digging in a rural diamond-mining slum and bouts of even harder labour digging in the farm.[5]

The growth of Freetown led to the shrinking of agricultural aspirations among those, like Ibrahim, who came of age during the war, by which time the "dreams of the village," another anthropologist has noted, were "no longer their dreams."[6]

No wonder. In 1990, when the United Nations ranked 130 nations on its Human Development Index, it put Sierra Leone in 127th place. It would soon fall to dead last.

In 1991, the Revolutionary United Front (RUF), with a helping hand from Liberia's Charles Taylor and Libya's Muammar Gaddafi, invaded Sierra Leone from the forest around Kailahun. Early on, RUF "rebels" took their greatest direct toll on those outside Freetown, whose residents initially considered the conflict a far-off border war. But the influx of refugees from the war—five hundred thousand of them during the course of one violent year, mostly from rural areas—sped the city's growth considerably. Many of the country's villages were destroyed or abandoned during the conflict and remained empty shells afterward, while Freetown and larger regional towns grew.

The causes of the war were and are much disputed. Young Sierra Leoneans often cite corruption among post-independence government officials as the leading cause—corruption not just in Freetown but also, thanks to politically indebted paramount chiefs, across the nation. Dashed expectations regarding development, and the lack of it in rural areas, were often blamed on Siaka Stevens, who ruled the APC and the country from 1967 to 1985. The fight for control of mineral resources, including the diamonds that helped finance war on both sides of the Mano River, is another factor often cited by scholars and young people alike. "But it wasn't just diamonds," Ibrahim told me. "It was everything: land and rice and all the minerals under the earth. They sold it off, and out it went in ships and planes, while they got richer and we got poorer." (Ibrahim used "they" in this way to refer indistinctly to several groups of people: the wealthy, the warlords and politicians of his teenage years, government officials, and military leaders. They were, he said, the same cast of characters.)

Sierra Leone's civil war lasted more than a decade, killed an estimated fifty thousand, created millions of refugees, and left a bitter cup for Ibrahim's generation to sip. Many of his peers had been forced to fight. Had he been born in a village or town, rather than in the nation's capital, Ibrahim might himself have had to fight on one side or the other of the war as a child soldier. "I was lucky," he reflected. "Although we were poor, we lived in Freetown. Even if I wasn't able to finish school, I did not have to do evil things." He would see plenty of evil things, however, when the war reached the city. War gave Ibrahim his first experiences of hunger and fear, he told me. It disrupted his education. And, he said, it killed his father.

Ibrahim was nine when Abdullai died. Initially, all he told me was that his father had "got a blockage." That's not the most descriptive term, medically speaking, so I asked Ibrahim to elaborate. "My father could not urinate or defecate," he replied. "He was in great pain after an accident"— one that he had suffered, Ibrahim continued, "after the war hit us directly, where we lived and worked." When Ibrahim and I had this conversation, we were once again in the Mammy Yoko restaurant. Bailor Barrie was with us, listening quietly and ready to step in at any moment to clarify and help translate between our discrepant versions of English.

By this time in our friendship, Ibrahim assumed I'd understand the barrage of place names he evoked, especially parts of Freetown. Because I did not, I laid a map of the city on the table and asked Ibrahim to walk me through what had happened to his father, and where. He first located his neighborhood and tapped his finger on it, as if sending Morse code. "Lumley," he said without looking up. It wasn't far from where we sat. A long pause ensued. "The army soldiers got together with the rebels and invaded the city," he said. "We didn't know what was happening until it was upon us."

I wasn't sure, just then, which invasion, but I knew the invaders were sobels. Sierra Leoneans, I knew, referred to allied soldiers and rebels as sobels, a combination of the first letters of "soldier" and the last letters of "rebel." Bailor fidgeted a bit—he clearly had his own sobel stories—but he remained silent, his gaze fixed on the map to which Ibrahim had returned. "This was just after May," he said, and the doctor nodded. Invoking the month alone was supposed to mean something obvious, I could tell. When I didn't get the point, Ibrahim finally stopped studying the map to say, by way of explanation, "May 1997." Bailor added that this was when the first big assault on Freetown occurred. That sobel project marked the end of Freetown's insularity—and much of Freetown.

In May 1997, Freetown and a recently elected civilian government were ostensibly protected from rebel incursions by Nigerian peacekeepers, but once the Sierra Leonean army's high command had merged forces with the rebels, the peacekeepers could do little to stop their advance on the city. Ibrahim's eyes and hands were back on the map. "I was in Lumley," he said, pointing again to the neighborhood. "My father was working at Water Quay." He moved his finger north and east, toward the port. So what had happened to

Abdullai? I asked. Had he been injured in an attack in Lumley? Or at the port, which the sobels sought to seize? Ibrahim answered no to these questions. "The rebels didn't get to Lumley," he said, tapping somewhere in between the neighborhood and the quay. "So we survived. But it was because of the war that my father died."

Ibrahim's explanation unfurled slowly. For weeks during that period, he said, it was impossible to move freely in Freetown. His family wanted to escape but found themselves trapped. Where Abdullai worked, at the docks, turned out to be close to some of the fiercest fighting. "Because the rebels were in the east where he worked," Ibrahim continued, "he had to bike there, and the guys tried to stop him, but he sped through a roadblock, and that's how he had his accident." By "guys," Ibrahim meant a frightening mix of sobels and teenagers armed with machetes, bush rifles, and the occasional automatic weapon. By "accident," he meant that his father lost control of his bike just after careening through the roadblock.

Abdullai knew he'd injured his ankle badly. But, scared of what these guys might do to him, Ibrahim's father picked himself up, righted his bike, and fled toward Lumley. His ankle hurt so much he had trouble pedaling and barely made it home. En route, Abdullai developed symptoms that suggested he had suffered an injury to not just his ankle but also his spinal cord. By the time he got home, he was having difficulty passing urine. This was the "blockage" Ibrahim had mentioned, and it panicked Abdullai's wife and children.

Although there was never a good time to be sick in Sierra Leone, the sobel attack on Freetown made it one of the worst times and places in recent African memory to fall ill or sustain an injury. Many health professionals had already fled the country by then, and others had been killed. Nonetheless, in a pattern to be repeated during the Ebola epidemic, the family turned first to the formal medical system, or what was left of it. Abdullai and Hawanatu risked their lives three days in a row to see a doctor and obtain relief for his worsening pain, which was mostly from urinary obstruction, and because Abdullai could no longer walk. On the fourth day, with Abdullai now in deep distress, they decided to try their luck with an herbalist in Waterloo, a town not far to the southeast of Freetown.

This would be an even riskier journey. The marauding sobels had already invaded part of Waterloo, and their positions were being bombarded by Nigerian jets. But the couple felt they had no alternative, so Abdullai's brother and Hawanatu loaded him into a crowded van known locally as a *poda poda* to make the journey. The van managed to evade any fighting, but Abdullai died in agony along the way. Ibrahim got the news later that day. "I didn't understand what had happened," he told me. "I was at school, in class, and my brother and mother came to school to collect me for the burial." He paused before adding, "My father was a Muslim."

That meant (in Ibrahim's telling) that Abdullai should have then been buried in his hometown in Guinea. But with Sierra Leone in chaos, and much of it in rebel hands, this wasn't possible. Abdullai was buried hastily in a Muslim ceremony in the Quay Port area of Freetown. These last rites weren't up to standards, and not in what he had wanted as a final resting place. This was the fate of many during war, but the failure caused the family grief, anxiety, and even dread, "for a long, long time," Ibrahim added, his deep voice dropping to a whisper.

Perhaps it was his father's sudden death that led Ibrahim to the peripatetic fate known by many who lose a parent; perhaps it was the growing penury of the war-wracked nation to which he was born. His generation knew little but conflict.

These were years of open war and failed military coups, their alleged perpetrators sent to Pademba Road Prison, where many were hanged or executed by firing squad. Civilians routinely were shot by vengeful partisans and looters—at home, on the beach, or on the bridge linking the city's western peninsula (and Lumley Beach) to the business district. By the time Abdullai died, families fleeing violence and political instability in the east were pouring into Freetown, where Nigerian and other West African peacekeepers sought to keep rebels and sobels from taking the city. Some already there, however, sought to escape the coups and executions by heading back to farms and families in the countryside. The war had cut off rural areas to the east and south, toward and beyond the Liberian border, but many with origins in or closer to Guinea—then the only neighbor not consumed by civil strife—sought refuge to the north.

That's what Hawanatu, Ibrahim's mother, did. She moved her family back to Mabanta, where they packed into her parents' tiny compound. There and then, Ibrahim became close to his maternal grandmother, Mary, who became an important influence on the suddenly fatherless boy. "When I was near her," Ibrahim told me, "I always behaved better, quieted down." But he received no formal schooling in Mabanta. His family, including his grandmother, still longed for him to attend school. At thirteen, Ibrahim went north to Guinea, to his father's home village of Geva, to live with his uncle and paternal grandmother.

In doing so, Ibrahim was far from alone. Close to a third of the population of Sierra Leone sought refuge away from their homes before its civil war ended, in 2002, tracing routes throughout the region from the bush to the big cities and back again, from villages and towns in Sierra Leone to the Ivory Coast, Nigeria, and, especially, Guinea and Liberia.[7] These routes, determined by family and economic ties, would later constitute the social pathways of many Ebola transmission chains.

Ibrahim never ended up attending school in Geva, because, as he put it, "the fees were too high." Instead, he became a motorcycle taxi driver, known in much of West Africa as an *okada* rider. (The word was borrowed from the name of a defunct Nigerian airline once famous for skirting air-traffic delays.) "I liked to ride," he said, "and was good at it." During his teenage years, Ibrahim helped both sides of his family as an *okada* rider, and also regularly crossed the porous border with sacks of rice for his mother and favorite granny. Sometime after a cease-fire held in 2002, Ibrahim returned to Mabanta, but that meant another year far from any secondary school.

Finally, in 2004, when Ibrahim was seventeen years old, Hawanatu's elder brother Ousman—who by cultural convention owed them favor and protection—invited her and the children to live with him in postwar Freetown, where he worked as a petty trader. This was in part so that Ibrahim could finally attend secondary school and partly so that he might "help with his business." Uncle Ousman's trade proved petty indeed: he lived on a busy street, selling jugs of black-market diesel and soft drinks from a table outside his front door. Soon he had Ibrahim hawking items from the stall, and, when possible, working as an *okada* rider with a rented bike. Ibrahim did, however, enroll in Islamic College, a secondary school in western Freetown. Although boys and girls attended classes in different shifts, Islamic College was a far cry from the madrassas depicted in U.S. news reports. Even during the worst years of the war, the country retained its reputation for religious tolerance.

Sierra Leone was also a place of religious syncretism. In much of the country, as across West Africa, this syncretism plays a role in the way many people respond to serious illness. That was the case, for example, when Ousman became paralyzed, suddenly and mysteriously during the time Ibrahim lived with him. Not long before, Ousman had fallen in love with a married woman, and much of his family considered his paralysis to be some kind of supernatural retribution—as Ibrahim and many other Sierra Leoneans put it, "native business." Ousman nevertheless first sought care in a hospital, where the staff attributed his paralysis to a stroke. Unsatisfied with this diagnosis, or merely covering his bases, Ousman went upline (in his nephew's word) in search of alternative therapies.

Through smartphones and the Internet, young people in cities were well acquainted with the pull of global youth culture, but that didn't mean they were cut off from their rural roots or from the complex cosmologies and traditions of their parents, rural kin, and ancestors. Most of the patients we got to know well in 2014 and after—whether in Freetown or in rural districts, whether young or old—proved capable of sifting through multiple explanatory paradigms when confronted by serious illness. In such circumstances, most of them did what Ousman did: they sought help from the country's formal health infrastructure *and* from upline practitioners deemed expert in the arts of taking care of native business.

In Ousman's case, such syncretism proved costly and ineffective. He survived his stroke (if that's what it was), but his business collapsed, a turn of events that threatened Ibrahim's chances of finishing high school—and the family's chances of simply getting by. Ibrahim, his mother, and his half brother were now in desperate need of a breadwinner or a patron. According to the received wisdom of colonial anthropology, the tradition in rural Temne households in such circumstances is for the widow to marry her husband's younger brother. But Hawanatu didn't want that, and her parents didn't suggest it. Instead, she married a man without roots in Port Loko, and the family regrouped anew in Lumley.

After the war, Lumley became a commercial hub of markets and nightlife, a place where poverty and wealth existed cheek by jowl. The family was joined there by Mary, Ibrahim's beloved grandmother—and soon, Ibrahim recalls, "two little ones." These weren't easy times. They suffered chronic financial problems. Ibrahim struggled at times to get along with his stepfather, which only worsened his chances of remaining in school.[8] But some of the problems he had in the house, Ibrahim told me, were of his own making. He preferred playing soccer and working as an *okada* rider to focusing on his studies, and was prone to altercations with others his age. "I was the cause of complaints," he told me, "because I was running with wild friends."

Tired of struggling to pay fees and buy books, Ibrahim dropped out of school in the tenth grade. He told himself he would go back, but he was twenty years old and felt it was time not only to fend for himself but also, as he put it, to "help my mom and granny." In this part of West Africa, at least, kinship networks and related patronage have almost always been the means by which young people like Ibrahim make the transition from student to worker, usually far too early for their own good. Patronage networks are also the way young adults find places to live—a room in a crowded house or a bed or mat in a crowded room. Ibrahim turned to one of his father's brothers, who worked as a vendor in a stall, trying to cash in on the exploding market for mobile phones.

If there's been any recent boom among West Africa's street merchants, it's been cell and smartphones, the main means by which poor urban families remain connected to their rural kin and increasingly important as a means of requesting and transferring cash. Almost everybody in Freetown has a mobile phone. They're sold in street stalls, but also hawked, as are SIM cards and credit, by mobile vendors. Ibrahim's job was "selling in the street." He became a whirling dervish of a street vendor, working the neighborhoods from Kissy to central Freetown, the area including the larger markets and federal buildings and banks rebuilt after the war. But no matter how industrious he was, Ibrahim didn't earn enough to help his mother and grandmother. So he also continued his work as an *okada* rider.

Ibrahim spent the next year living between eastern Freetown, with his uncle, and Lumley, with his mother and half-siblings. The two sides of the city, east and west, are divided by Tower Hill, which rises six hundred feet above the floor of a narrow valley between the Sierra Leone River and the higher hills to the east and south. His father long gone, Ibrahim was now the tenuous link between the two families. His everyday life was a "stressful rush," and it was in this period that he had his only brush with the law. On his rented motorcycle one day, he collided with a car. The collision destroyed his headlamp but did no damage to the other vehicle. Unfortunately for him, however, it was a police car. Ibrahim got down on his knees and begged for forgiveness, but the officer had him sent to Pademba Road Prison, where political prisoners and the instigators of the country's recent military coups and war had been tortured, hanged, or shot.

Ibrahim would spend three nights in Pademba, during which time, he told me, he became a more observant Muslim. "If you get into an accident on the bike," he told me, "only God can save you. While in prison, I really turned to prayer." His were answered after his third night, when a judge threw out his case. After that, Ibrahim went home, but his reprieve was short-lived. This was the summer of 2014. Ramadan was upon him, and the real horror was about to begin.

The unraveling began on a Wednesday, Ibrahim told me, just after Ramadan had ended, when an uncle of his arrived in Lumley. If Ibrahim's recollection is correct, the date would have been June 30.

As Ibrahim would later clarify for me, the "uncle" was actually Ibrahim's mother's older sister's first son. The man was an imam at one of northern Freetown's tiny mosques and came to Lumley "because he wasn't feeling well." His muscles ached, he felt tired and weak, and he had no appetite, but, Ibrahim said, neither he nor anybody else knew why. The imam doubled as a taxi driver, so maybe he was just suffering the ill effects of the fast and a busy month for a cleric with a side job? But when vomiting followed nausea, and diarrhea followed abdominal pain, Hawanatu and Ibrahim had to be aware of the possibility that the imam had been stricken with Ebola. The disease was already rampant in the city, and everybody in town was talking about it.

Just a few days before the imam's arrival—on the day after Humarr Khan's death—Sierra Leone's president had declared Ebola a national emergency. A dozen vehicles equipped with loudspeakers that day had crisscrossed Freetown to alert the population, as had scores of *okada* riders hired for this purpose. Stories about the spreading epidemic were leading the news—not only in Freetown but all over the world. Earlier in the month, MSF had declared Ebola "totally out of control." Airlines had canceled flights to the city, and several international nongovernmental organizations, ubiquitous in the region since the end of the war, had pulled expatriate staff out of the country. As it would turn out, more cases of Ebola would be reported in Freetown that week than had been reported in a city ever, anywhere.

Adding to the family's concern was the fact that the imam had recently helped to bury a couple of young congregation members. But "my uncle didn't say how they died," Ibrahim recalled months later. By this point in the story, I was getting confused about which uncle was where, which ones were on which side of the family, and which ones were uncles in the sense of being a parent's sibling. I kept thinking of the number twenty-three—as in twenty-three dead—and was determined to grasp Ibrahim's accounting. But this wasn't the time for clarifications. He was, in that particular session, fully caught up in his narrative; it was better not to interrupt when he was on a roll.

The morning after the imam reached Lumley, Ibrahim had to leave before sunrise for work. He did so with regret, because he didn't like the idea of leaving his mother to care for his uncle without his help. Ibrahim told me, in this long session, that he sensed that something bad was going to happen, and indeed it did: that morning, the imam's symptoms worsened dramatically. Hawanatu took him to a neighborhood pharmacy, where she bought medicine recommended for him by a "pharmacist"—probably a shop assistant with no formal training. She kept Ibrahim up to date on the situation by phone, and soon called with bad news. The imam was vomiting uncontrollably, Hawanatu told her son. "Anything he ate came right back up," Ibrahim paraphrased, "including the medicines."

With her concerns mounting, Hawanatu called a newly established Ebola hotline for an ambulance, as the city's inhabitants had been instructed to do in such cases—a service that had never before been made available to poor Sierra Leoneans. But none arrived, and the imam grew sicker. By midday, his vomiting and diarrhea were uncontrollable, and he was unable to sit up, much less stand. "It was so bad," Ibrahim told me, "that my younger brother called me, as did about five other members of my family, including my granny, asking me to come back to help." But that day Ibrahim's phone-selling uncle had gone to Guinea and told Ibrahim to mind his stall, so now Ibrahim was stuck across town, unable to do anything other than worry. And worry he did. A feeling of dread descended on him, he said, "like some crushing weight."

At home, surely invaded by the same dread as Ibrahim's, Hawanatu and others, duty bound to nurse their ailing relative, mopped his fevered brow and tried to keep him clean. Again they called the Ebola hotline for an ambulance, again without success. By the time Ibrahim returned home that night, shortly before ten, the imam was dead. "Everyone was crying," he remembered. Not long afterward, people from the imam's mosque, fulfilling their obligations to the dead, came to help prepare him for burial. "They used a cream to rub and clean him," Ibrahim explained, "and then took him straight to the cemetery." There he was buried by his family and members of his faith community. Most were surely aware of the peril they faced in doing so. An estimated 120 new cases of Ebola were reported the week the imam died, and the government had declared it a crime to "harbor an Ebola suspect."

The hours just after death are probably when the Ebola virus is most infectious to those who touch the bodies of the deceased. Why would anybody court such risks? Decades earlier, the anthropologist Michael Jackson had provided an answer. "Death is not denied," he wrote about attitudes toward death and burial in Sierra Leone. "Nor do people react to suffering with the outrage and impatience so familiar in our own society—the tormented sense that one has been hard done by, that one deserves better, that permanent health, unalloyed happiness, even immortality, might one day be guaranteed as a civil right." In Sierra Leone, he continued, what's considered terrible is not death itself but "to die alone, to be refused decent burial, to have one's lineage die out."[9]

New laws, enacted that summer, banned the preparation of bodies for burial and interment itself. Families throughout the country agonized about whether to obey them, given what they understood to be their obligations to the dead. During the westward march of Ebola, the choice to continue honoring these obligations was viewed by the international media and many outside observers as evidence of cultural obstructionism and an uninformed devotion to "traditional" or "exotic" funeral practices. But there's a much more mundane and meaningful explanation: families took care of the dead and the dying because for generations they had received little help in these tasks from either governments or from civil-society institutions beyond mosques and churches. In Sierra Leone's cities and towns, the costs of caregiving and its final act were borne almost wholly by families without insurance.

Across West Africa, many knew by then the risks they ran. They ran them because they felt they had to—because so few others were willing to help in that last act of caregiving. Even after Ramadan, with Ebola nonstop news, victims and those who cared for them were offered little help with nursing, infection control, or prompt and dignified burials. What had happened to the imam was a case in point. "We called the number we were supposed to call," Ibrahim recalled bitterly, "but no one ever came, not even after he was dead and gone." This abandonment—by health authorities and by the mortuary industry—was far worse in rural regions. It was complete in villages beyond the reach of paved roads.

Caught between social imperatives and growing awareness of how Ebola was transmitted, and new and punitive laws, thousands of families in Sierra Leone that summer were torn apart trying to meet these obligations; others were torn apart by failure to do so. In October 2014, when we interviewed two dozen survivors, every one of them told us that when they fell ill, they had suspected the cause might be the care they had given to other victims, or their help preparing them for burial. This was true regardless of what they might have said to health authorities or to the clinicians who evaluated them hastily and often fearfully; it was true even when the afflicted and their families entertained multiple and discrepant hypotheses about what was happening.

Desperate for any alternative diagnosis, members of Ebola-stricken households were also awash in confusing information. Across the region, airwaves and billboards were still dominated by public-service announcements insisting "Ebola is real" and "Don't eat bushmeat," but offered little, in those days after Ramadan, in the way of pragmatic assistance. The survivors I came to know understood the dangers they faced in providing the care they did. But what choice did they have?

Events unspooled quickly after that, as did Ibrahim's account of them. The imam's teenage son, who'd accompanied his father to Lumley, didn't eat for days, a bad sign after breaking the Ramadan fast, and began to feel profoundly weak. (He was, in Ibrahim's words, "not feeling bright.") The boy and his family attributed these symptoms to grief, but Ebola was the cause, and he, too, soon fell to the virus. This time the family did not attempt to prepare the body for burial. "We took him to the morgue," Ibrahim said, "and they washed him there." But they still wrapped the youth in a shroud and laid him in his grave themselves.

Other caregivers in Hawanatu's family—those who tried to keep the sick clean, transported them to hospitals, or prepared the deceased for burial—continued to sicken and die. The imam's oldest daughter died three days later, and the next day his wife—both in a makeshift isolation unit cobbled together north of the city. In almost every instance, they sought care from the medical system, including the overwhelmed Connaught, where several nurses and the physician leading its Ebola response died shortly after Ramadan. (Marta Lado and other friends there, taking every precaution, were devastated by these developments.) "Then," Ibrahim told me, after a long pause, "we lost my granny, and my mother's older sister died the same day." That was Thursday, August 7. Both had died at Connaught.

Hawanatu and her sons tried to retrieve the bodies for burial. This was now illegal not only for any person dead of Ebola but also for those dead of anything that *might* be Ebola. But Ibrahim told me that a "corrupt doctor" working at Connaught said that his grandmother Mary, unlike his aunt, had not succumbed to the disease. For a fee he could get the family a certificate stating as much, so she might be buried according to her wishes. Ibrahim then believed (and still does) that Mary, like the rest of her family, was felled by Ebola, but his family paid the doctor and retrieved her body. "I think he was a bad doctor," Ibrahim told me. Then he paused and shrugged. "But a few days later he was dead, too."

The doctor at Connaught, Ibrahim added quickly, wasn't representative of those he later met there. By then, Sierra Leonean health workers were enduring risks of Ebola infection that have been estimated to be one hundred times greater than those faced by the general population. August and September were the peak months of such losses, when deaths among doctors, nurses, ambulance drivers, hospital cleaners, and burial-team members accounted for almost 10 percent of all Ebola deaths. In Kenema District, where Humarr Khan and his nursing colleagues worked, 15 percent of those sickened were health professionals.

The body of Ibrahim's grandmother, once retrieved from Connaught, was placed in a morgue—Freetown had several, all of them profitable fee-for-service business ventures—while the family, certificate in hand, discussed Mary's dying wish to be buried in her home village along with her ancestors. "My mother and some of my aunties argued about it," he said. "Some advised us not to take her body to the village. But our granny had told us many times that she did not wish to be buried in Freetown, but in her Mabanta." Ibrahim stopped for a moment, and when he continued, his voice broke. "My granny, who loved me so much, told *me* to do this."

What remained of the Freetown branch of Hawanatu's family struggled mightily to reach a tenuous consensus. She and her children decided that the right thing to do was to bring Mary back to the village for a traditional burial, which, as Ibrahim put it to me, involved buying "some kola, water, and whites" and calling the imam "to pray for the dead." Kola nuts, a ritually significant stimulant throughout the region, are given as gifts in times of trouble and of celebration; clean water is used to bathe the dead, who are wrapped in white linen and interred.[10] The family at last had a plan—but it wasn't at all clear that they could carry it out.

By this point in the epidemic, such traditional burial practices, common among both Christians and Muslims in West Africa for centuries, were now formally and expressly forbidden. And the authorities' approach to preventing them had become increasingly militarized, a move supported by some of the disease-control experts who had arrived in the region. Travel to certain districts now required an official pass, which had to be shown at police checkpoints, where everybody passing through would have their temperature checked before being waved on. Several such roadblocks had been set up between Freetown and Mabanta, which meant that getting Mary back there would be next to impossible. There was widespread fear of repatriation in rural areas, too. Some villagers began to invoke laws and bans with a regret that masked a growing relief about *not* having to nurse the sick and bury the dead. "People in the village told us not to come back," Ibrahim recalled. "We started sitting down and thinking: What is going on right now? We couldn't go back there."

So Mary was buried in Freetown.

The tragedies continued. Within a week, Hawanatu learned that three of her sisters' young children had died in Mabanta. Two other relatives, both young women living in Port Loko District, perished at about the same time, as did the newborn of one of them.

Overwhelmed by grief, and by a sense of having failed her family, Hawanatu resolved to go home to be with her father. Ibrahim and his older brother, Mamoud, pleaded with her not to go, but she wouldn't budge. "I'm the only one left now," she told them. Her father needed help, she said, with his religious and social obligations. The family might not have enough money to offer up a sheep or a goat, as was traditional, but at least she could cook rice to honor ancestors and feed what remained of her shrinking family. In mid-August, over her sons' strenuous objections, Hawanatu set off for Mabanta in a *poda poda*. These were mostly packed even at the height of the Avoid Body Contact campaign.

Ibrahim and Mamoud already feared something was wrong with their mother, but they couldn't tell if she was sick or just grief-stricken and exhausted. They got their answer just a couple of days later, when Ibrahim got a call from the village. "Your mother," said one of his cousins, "is not feeling so bright." This everyday Sierra Leonean expression has many meanings, but in this context it had only one. They needed to get Hawanatu back to Freetown, and early the next morning, Ibrahim hired a car to bring his mother to Connaught. When they arrived in the village that afternoon, the driver saw that Hawanatu was sick—at which point he threatened to leave Ibrahim and his mother stranded in Mabanta. The implacable Ibrahim offered to double the fare and begged the driver to take him and his mother back to Freetown.

By then, the sky was darkening and it began to rain; Hawanatu was vomiting. After much public palaver, the driver acceded. Ibrahim and Hawanatu sat in the back seat, her head on his lap. Somehow they managed to pass through the checkpoints and made it back to town. "I took her straight to Connaught," Ibrahim recalled, "but they said it was too late, come back early in the morning. So we went home." It was pitch-black when they arrived: there was no electricity in the house.

Retching and incontinent, Hawanatu was so weak she couldn't stand. Ibrahim carried her to her tiny room and laid her on her bed after covering it with towels and whatever clean clothing was handy. It was a sleepless night. "We gave her coconut water," Ibrahim said, "and tried to keep her clean." He next had to find another driver to return to Connaught. By dawn, desperate and bone-tired, he found a taxi, who, for another exorbitant fee, took him and his dying mother to hospital—where he found a long line of desperately ill people already waiting to be tested for Ebola. "By then," he said, "I was carrying my mother in my arms. She had Ebola, and I knew it. And I knew we were all dead anyway. Her children, everybody."

The despairing young man, carrying his limp and barely responsive mother, took his place in line. Liquid stool covered his jeans and shirtfront. Ibrahim, feeling exhausted and weak himself, didn't know how long he could keep holding his mother. He began to tremble and sweat. Just as he felt he was about to collapse, a triage nurse came out and gave them a yellow band to mark Hawanatu as needing urgent attention, and then staff in full protective garb took her away. "I waited outside, not knowing what to do," Ibrahim told me. "It was Friday, so I went for prayer at the big market mosque."

Ibrahim returned to the hospital immediately after prayers and began searching the wards of chaotic Connaught for Hawanatu: "I starting shouting 'Where is my mother?' I was angry I couldn't find her, even if the worst had happened. Then I saw many other people crying, and I started crying, too. I finally went home." He returned to the hospital the next morning to receive the news: Hawanatu had died on Friday, at about 8:00 p.m. Ibrahim, grieving, returned home to wait for the inevitable. "I knew," he said with a shrug, "I would soon be sick."

He was right. Three days later, Ibrahim continued, "I started not feeling really nice." His muscles ached, but he didn't bother to consider this a possible consequence of holding his mother aloft in Connaught's dreadful queue. His head throbbed. He had no appetite and felt too weak to eat anyway. Then came abdominal pain, followed in short order by vomiting and diarrhea, which worsened the pain. Soon he could barely stand, but he didn't really know whom in his family to call. On his mother's side, so many had perished. He hadn't been in touch with Abdullai's relatives since before Ramadan; his stepfather had left at about the time the imam fell ill. As for his neighbors, they were fully aware of the sickness in the tiny house in Lumley and considered it a contaminated deathtrap: everyone gave it a wide berth. "I had no one to talk to." Ibrahim didn't want to frighten "the only one left"—Mamoud, his half brother—but realized he had no choice. Mamoud took Ibrahim to Connaught, where he tested positive for Ebola. He shrugged again, as if to add "of course."

It was then that Ibrahim met Dr. Marta Lado. Several Connaught staff had already perished by then, even though it wasn't likely they'd been infected within her holding unit—it may have been the safest place in the hospital. The recent death of the physician Ibrahim named corrupt had shaken the

Europeans who'd led us on a tour of Connaught in June, but they remained at their posts. They were, in my view, torn between fealty to the idea of deferring to Sierra Leonean nationals and an awareness that rigorous leadership was needed in the midst of crisis. They ended up in leadership roles themselves. This—again, in my view—saved many lives.

Dr. Lado admitted Ibrahim to Connaught, where he was given intravenous fluids ("a bagful, one time, every day"). After three days, as he recalls it, "people in suits" took him by ambulance to the national police academy in Hastings, which just that week had been precipitously converted into the country's largest Ebola treatment unit. That unit would do remarkable work in the months ahead, but Ibrahim may be forgiven for believing that "almost everyone admitted died." In fact, slightly more than half of those admitted to the Hastings unit in its first months survived; at the end of 2014, more than three-quarters did.[11] He was one of the unit's first patients, and, given his month of hell, he had ample reason to be terrified. The ride there didn't ease his fears. "There were four of us in the ambulance," he told me. "A woman eight months pregnant died on the way." The two others were also young men who'd been caring for sick family members. Neither survived.

Ibrahim didn't willingly provide much detail about his initial days at Hastings, but he had arrived when mortality was highest, and at a time when stockouts of medical supplies, power outages, and shortages of food were all frequent. The few details he did share were plenty telling. "I could not sleep, not sleep, not sleep," he said. "Someone dying every day. Seeing small children dead. Mothers dead. I heard people saying 'I need water' or 'Help me,' but no one came, especially at night. And I couldn't help anyone, either. I was on a drip."

Despite the conditions, and in his view because of that drip, Ibrahim began to improve physically after a week in Hastings. But this didn't lift his spirits. Grief washed over him in immense and regular waves.

During the course of our discussions in late 2014 and early 2015, Ibrahim repeatedly mentioned wanting to help those sick with Ebola. "Maybe I could be a nurse's aide," he said, "or just help people know they have a chance to get better? At least I could talk to them."

It wasn't entirely clear back then what someone like Ibrahim—who wasn't alone among survivors wishing to help the afflicted—might do to help. By then we knew more about what Ebola sufferers needed than we did in October 2014, when assigned to the overrun ETU in Maforki and to help out at Port Loko Government Hospital. The hospital, which was only a couple of miles from Maforki, had then been practically empty, although its chief medical and nursing officers were still struggling to provide prenatal care and a handful of other services. As in previous Ebola outbreaks, many hospitals had been formally closed; others simply ground to a halt by fear, attrition, and loss. This wasn't the sort of place to send idealistic young folks, no matter how hale.

Even eager-to-help Ibrahim might have been dismayed by the conditions at Port Loko's hospital in October. It sits in the shadow of a large ochre mosque, the only thing of note in the eyes of the British officer surveying the unpromising town ninety years earlier.[12] When I first visited, just before meeting Ibrahim, a half dozen cars had been abandoned in the roundabout inside the hospital gates. The only shiny-looking item on display outside the hospital was a new incinerator from England, but it wasn't working. A huge mound of medical waste abutted it.

There were early calls to allow Ebola survivors to serve in such settings because they were likely immune to reinfection by the same strain of the virus. But there were obvious reasons to spare survivors the trauma of being anywhere near these facilities. At the height of the western surge, many who reached Port Loko facilities were dead on arrival. During the course of a single hour in late November, Maforki received in transfer four patients who'd died en route. On that date, we watched as Port Loko District edged out Freetown—its population three times as large as Port Loko's—with the highest number of new confirmed cases in a single day: 13. The report issued daily by the National Ebola Response Centre showed that this wasn't anomalous. Of the country's 5,441 confirmed cases at that point, Port Loko had reported 792 of them, most registered in the previous few weeks. Only the district including Freetown had reported more.

There were plenty of reasons to believe that conditions were generally worse in rural ETUs than in urban ones, or that patients in rural areas were sicker than their urban counterparts. That's one reason Ibrahim was so keen to get his sick mother back to Freetown. Many patients from the north of Port Loko District—from places like Mabanta—were carried in on death's door after finding rural facilities abandoned and going home to await an ambulance. As they waited for professional assistance, their kin did what kin do: they looked out for one another. This sped up household transmission. During the days before Ibrahim first asked me if he could help Ebola patients, we saw whole families reach Maforki from hard-to-reach villages. Often the sickest victims would be put on a stretcher, but then the younger and stronger ones would be left to sit in chairs in the hot sun in the triage area, or holding the hand of a nurse or aide in full protective gear. They would then stagger and weave across the chlorine-parched courtyard of the red zone. We'd seen this unsteady gait and dazed, disoriented look in every Ebola treatment unit, but it was our impression that diagnoses of patients who exhibited them were made more quickly in Freetown.

Neither Maforki nor Port Loko's hospital seemed safe places for Ibrahim to help out in even a nonclinical role. It was hard to argue that he or other young survivors would have much to offer in the midst of a dangerous health emergency, especially considering their losses and persistent or new symptoms. In late November, not everyone who reached Maforki received intravenous fluids and adequate electrolyte replacement. When the most dehydrated did, it was far short of what would have passed for adequate fluid resuscitation in the home countries of the short-term volunteers. What these patients needed was skilled nursing care and careful medical follow-up. Many of the survivors we now counted as coworkers also still needed follow-up.

During the last weeks of 2014, some disease-control experts were still calling into question the very notion of providing even basic supportive care within Ebola treatment units—Plan A, as some people called it. These experts instead argued for a focus on preventing further spread by shifting funding toward Plan B, which involved home-based care for those stricken with Ebola. Plan B made some sense, especially in rural areas, where delays in response from professional caregivers made the idea of home-based care potentially life-saving, as long as afflicted households could be supplied with protective gear and oral rehydration salts while awaiting safe passage to a staffed and stocked ETU.[13] But Plan B was clinically inadequate. In both Mabanta and Freetown, Ibrahim's family had in a sense been wiped out by a poorly implemented version of Plan B.

In a devastating story published on November 28 in *The New York Times*, the veteran reporter Jeffrey Gettleman brought the nature of the debate into sharp focus. (Gettleman was then East Africa's bureau chief for *The Times* and had reported on a 2007 Ebola outbreak in the Congo. He headed west as the virus did.) He organized his piece about Plans A and B around a teenage girl named Isatu. It's a story not unlike the one Ibrahim told me about what happened after his imam-uncle fell ill. Isatu lived in Kissi Town, about an hour's drive south of Freetown. When she fell ill, Gettleman wrote, her family had called the government's Ebola hotline for help, but got no response. He quoted a community volunteer whom he found pacing around in front of Isatu's house. "I've called 10 times myself," he said as the drama was unfolding. "No response."[14] According to Gettleman, Isatu's family and neighbors made more than thirty-five calls for help, but the only team that ever actually turned up was the burial brigade.

Such failure in the face of mounting Ebola incidence led to less clinical ambition rather than more. By this point, according to the reporter, overwhelmed "health officials"—some of them European and American expatriates advising local officials—were making an explicit case behind closed doors for Plan B over Plan A, with grave consequences for Isatu and patients like her. Gettleman wrote,

> The health officials admitted Plan B was a major defeat, but said the approach would only be temporary and promised to supply basics like protective gloves, painkillers and rehydration salts. Even that did not happen in Isatu's case. Nobody brought her food. Nobody brought her any rehydration salts or Tylenol. No health workers ever talked to her about whom she might have touched, which means

anyone directly connected to her could now be walking through
Freetown's teeming streets, where—despite the government's ABC
campaign, Avoid Body Contact—people continue to give high fives,
hug and kiss in public. Community volunteers said Isatu's case was
the norm, not the exception.[15]

It was worse in rural areas to the east. One anthropologist and his coworkers
described in grisly detail the fates of those living in the villages around the
Gola Forest, where no one showed up for weeks after Ebola outbreaks—even
though officials threatened the villagers with punishment if they tried to bury
the bodies themselves.[16]

I was tending to patients in Port Loko when Gettleman's report was
published, but Jon Lascher somehow procured a hard copy of *The New York
Times* in Freetown, just before my first formal interview with Ibrahim. I read
part of the article aloud to him and then looked for a reaction. After a long silence, which led me to wonder if I'd been reading too quickly, he said, "This
is what we all experienced in August. But it shouldn't be happening now." He
then asked once again if he might help us provide care for the sick. "Am I not
immune to Ebola now? Can't I work in an ETU?" Having heard the question
from many quarters, I told him I didn't know for sure, and that in any case
he still needed time to recover from his own illness. This response deflated
Ibrahim visibly.

Ibrahim's reaction made me wonder: How had I come to be the decider?
His offer was not one to be dismissed lightly, and I promised to reconsider
it when I returned in a month. It was one of the first times I'd seen Ibrahim
smile.

Late November proved to be the peak of the Sierra Leonean epidemic. Cham-
pions of both Plan A and Plan B claimed credit for the turnaround, which occurred in Sierra Leone as it had in Liberia and Guinea: when Ebola reached
the coast. The roaring Atlantic remained mute on the subject.

Trying to implement Plan A took a lot of resources, human and otherwise.

By the end of December, the size of the Partners In Health team in Port Loko had grown to close to eighty people, mostly nurses and doctors, but also logisticians and record keepers. Scores of sprayers and cleaners, most from around Port Loko and including several survivors, tried to keep the place clean and supervised the donning and doffing of personal protective gear. A Cuban contingent of about forty finally reached Maforki. This meant that individual clinicians spent less time in sweltering protective gear. But even with their help, and with what we hoped was a declining caseload, the Ebola victims who made long and punishing journeys to Maforki were sicker, and for longer, than those transferred by ambulances over short distances to Hastings from holding units in Freetown.

Throughout the rest of the year, and into the next one, as the number of new cases at last began to fall, patients continued to reach Port Loko in terrible condition, often referred from far-off clinics or health posts and often after having walked or been carried even to those. Ease and time of transportation explained some urban-rural disparities of outcome, but so did fear and confusion. Sick villagers had been instructed to avoid clinics and hospitals, but at the same time to report to them. Debate over Plans A and B—and about the control-over-care paradigm—reflected a similar ambivalence.

That said, there were always patients well on their way to recovery in Maforki and other units, and they cheered the clinicians and sicker patients. If there was anything that got us through the western surge—and by "us" I mean clinicians in general, regardless of country of origin or affiliation—it was the encouragement offered by patients who were doing well, and by survivors who were deemed out of the woods. And by the new year, mercifully, Ibrahim was one of them. When I saw him in early January, he'd put on a couple of pounds and seemed less depressed. His brother Mamoud had found a job in the city of Bo, to the east, and Ibrahim was mostly living alone, an almost unheard-of arrangement in Freetown.

Then again, Ibrahim was by then spending most of his time with survivors who worked with Partners In Health, including the always ebullient Chairman, and a young taxi driver named Momoh. That is, Momoh had been a taxi driver before falling ill. When we first met him, in September 2014, he had a frail, shaky look, and his skin was sloughing. This was just days after he'd been declared Ebola-free; Momoh had a laminated certificate from the Ministry of Health to prove it. But no one, it seemed, wanted to get in his cab, which is how he came to be a driver for Partners In Health. When I saw him in January, at another dinner at the Mammy Yoko, he looked like a new man—a "regular linebacker," according to one of the nurses. (The reference was lost on the survivors around the tables.) Our dinners were becoming a tradition, one welcomed by both attendees and hotel staff. They were certainly uplifting to me, and so was seeing most survivors look like they'd truly conquered the disease.

At least physically. It was during the new year that Ibrahim unleashed the full story of his family's demise to me. We saw each other almost every day I was in Freetown. Still eager to work with us, Ibrahim kept up his charm offensive, often complemented by guilt trips. Both had their intended effect. I'd not stopped thinking about either him or his offer, but he just didn't seem to have the set of skills we needed at the ETU I knew best, the one in Maforki. We had three urgent needs there, and all of them required increased nursing capacity. First, we needed to improve the triage process, and to begin a more aggressive and standardized initial treatment regimen for each patient, one that would include rehydration with oral and IV fluids.

Second, we needed to improve the quality of care within the facilities to which Partners In Health had been assigned. Many patients—maybe most—arrived looking malnourished and anemic. But how could we know without checking hemoglobin levels and weights? And some with Ebola were surely afflicted with other infections: blood-sapping parasites beyond malaria, such as hookworm; pneumonia and other bacterial infections; perhaps other viral infections, including HIV disease but also Lassa fever, which may have killed more Sierra Leoneans than Ebola did in 2014; tuberculosis; and a host of other diseases, from leptospirosis (like Lassa, spread by rats) to tick-transmitted pathogens endemic to the region. In addition to infections known to be prevalent in West Africa, Ebola's attack on the immune system and gut also made patients vulnerable to what are termed intercurrent infections. The most common of these were probably caused by the invasion of the bloodstream by gut bacteria due either to Ebola's direct damage or to that sustained during days of vomiting and diarrhea. Failure to treat them with the right antibiotics was likely one of the reasons Ebola patients were still dying within Ebola treatment units in West Africa, while those lucky few who reached Europe or the United States survived.

Third, there was still the matter of electrolyte losses and imbalances. Most patients we saw with severe gastrointestinal symptoms had low levels of potassium, sodium, and magnesium. But some presented with high serum levels of sodium, and there was no way to tell the difference simply by examining them in a mango-shaded triage area. That meant that even in cases of severe dehydration, the type of intravenous solution called for varied from patient to patient and over the course of a single patient's illness, especially when Ebola hit the kidneys. Some sudden deaths were likely due to losses of potassium, calcium, or magnesium, which were not likely to be replenished by either oral rehydration formulations, coconut water, or commercial sports drinks (some of which worsen low levels of potassium). Addressing such challenges required increased lab capacity and, again, better nursing care.

The volunteers we were looking for to help out there were nurses and physicians accustomed to working in ICUs, surgical suites, and emergency rooms. Ibrahim certainly had hard-won experience nursing sick family members, and as a survivor he probably was (as he suspected) immune to reinfection by the same Ebola strain. Those factors, along with his eagerness to help, made him an appealing prospect as a volunteer. But they didn't magically confer advanced nursing skills on Ibrahim. And his having survived the disease didn't actually ensure that he was no longer able to transmit the virus. Even months after blood tests become negative, live virus can often still be isolated from urine, semen, and breastmilk. Not only that, being declared Ebola-negative didn't mean that a patient was on the way to recovery. A few of those who left the ETU as survivors did a little happy dance, but most staggered or were carried out as malnourished and weak as when they came in, or more so. They would be convalescent for months.

Several of the American and European survivors, who benefited from evacuation and intensive care, still ended up gravely ill for long periods. Ebola had not only acute but also chronic effects. In Sierra Leone, its sequelae may have been overlooked within overwhelmed ETUs, but they were a ranking topic of discussion among survivors discharged to home or to the nearby public hospitals. Some Port Loko survivors had already developed seizure disorders, blindness, and other visual problems; others had disabling joint pain; and all suffered from the sort of trauma that accompanies the loss of family. Previously, in those rare circumstances in which Ebola or Marburg had been countered with modern medicine, these complications had been addressed by effective therapies. But in West Africa in 2014, the containment-over-care paradigm left little time or resources to study or attend to sequelae.

As I considered Ibrahim's offer, all of this gave me pause. At the same time, we couldn't shake the feeling that we needed to do much more for patients who were out of the ETU but not out of the woods. Maybe this was where Ibrahim and others might make a difference.

During January, mortal dramas and debates were still playing out across Upper West Africa. Everyone in Port Loko Government Hospital had heard about a baby named Jariatu, one of the charges in the hospital's pediatric unit. She'd been found by a burial team, barely alive in a houseful of dead family members, and taken to Maforki.

Jariatu was, on arrival, too unresponsive to drink, and the nurses and physicians there had been unable to find a vein for an IV. So colleagues from Partners In Health did what they would do in Boston (or in central Haiti): they inserted a needle into a bone in her leg—an intraosseous needle, as it's called—and began resuscitating her through her bone and marrow. Shortly thereafter, Chuck Callahan, the Baltimore physician who'd performed the procedure, went to check on her, fearing the worst. Here's how he described the moment in his diary:

25 December
A Christmas miracle. Went ahead of everyone because if little Jariatu was dead I wanted to see her alone. She wasn't. Her little eyes opened. I picked her up and picked up a cup of ORS—she reached

for it with both hands and started drinking it and formula. I walked her over to Susie to see her—we both cried—me under my suit.

The nurses in Maforki returned her gold earrings, which they had removed and plunked in chlorine solution on the off chance that she might survive, knowing that they were likely to be the only memento of the parents who'd once loved her. Well before she was discharged to Government Hospital a couple of weeks later, Jariatu was dubbed the "Miracle Baby."

By then, often propped up between stuffed toys, Jariatu had developed a magnetically cute aura, and had become the star of the ward. Nurses were ever popping by to see her. But her recovery wasn't really miraculous. What made the difference was not some new technology or treatment. The reason that she and many others would survive that month was simple: they got rudimentary medical services of a sort that had been unavailable to others living in the medical desert. If any miracle was involved, it was the miracle of equity.

At about the time Jariatu was transferred from Maforki to Port Loko Government Hospital, a nine-year-old girl named Mariatu made the same trip. But the clinical course of her disease was quite different. On December 28, 2014, the day Mariatu was admitted to Maforki, she had a fever, was vomiting, and suffered with severe diarrhea. She'd seen her mother and sister die of Ebola but was saved from that fate by fluid resuscitation. On or about January 10, a blood test showed no evidence of the virus in Mariatu's bloodstream, a sign that her own immune system had kicked in to clear the virus. Unlike the Miracle Baby, however, Mariatu didn't then bounce back. At that point, she still hadn't spoken or eaten, and was of course losing weight. By no means beyond a blood test had she recovered, but her bed was needed. Mariatu was transferred to Government Hospital.

Mariatu weighed twenty-nine pounds when she arrived—a nine-year-old wraith. Having survived acute Ebola, she now lay dying of malnutrition, just a few beds down from the lively Jariatu. A physician volunteer at the hospital tried feeding her through the nose, using what's known as a nasogastric tube, but the girl, still mute, pulled it out. One of the survivor-volunteers, a woman roughly in her fifties who'd been assigned to sit with Mariatu, tried to get the

girl to eat a high-protein, high-calorie peanut paste that usually worked wonders with younger malnourished children, but she refused that, too.

Some of the clinicians who were monitoring Mariatu's case, shocked by
her emaciation, suspected a second and undiagnosed infection, something
other than the bacterial ones sometimes seen in the course of Ebola, and
asked me to evaluate her. The teams in and out of Port Loko had already
nursed patients through the acute phase of Ebola only to discover the patients
also had tuberculosis, AIDS, malaria, or (in one memorable case) disfiguring
Buruli ulcers of the legs. But Bec Rollins, one of my nonmedical colleagues,
a close friend and a wise one, would advance a different diagnosis for Mariatu. Bec led our communications team in Boston but traveled often to Sierra
Leone. I'd already been asked to see Mariatu and a couple of others recently
discharged from Maforki. Corrado Cancedda and I had planned to head
there the day before but got tied up in the ETU, only five minutes away. Bec
met Mariatu, Jariatu, and others at Government Hospital the day before I did.

Upon returning to Freetown, Bec Rollins found me having dinner with
Ibrahim in the Mammy Yoko, where she reported to us what she had seen. She
showed us photos, too. Based on what I saw in those pictures, I thought Mariatu might be suffering from a wasting, consumptive disease like tuberculosis—
perhaps a quiescent or latent infection reactivated by Ebola and anemia
and malnutrition. But Bec's diagnosis was simpler: the nurses and Mariatu's
assigned companion (whom Bec termed a "grumpy grandma") were avoiding the skeletal Mariatu while lavishing attention on Jariatu and some of
the other kids.

Ibrahim listened with rapt attention as Bec was talking. After seeing
the photographs, he asked both of us, "Can't I help this girl?" Bec and
I had plans to meet the next day at Maforki, bearing bougainvillea plants
we hoped to place around what everyone called the survivors' tree: a mango
festooned with colorful scraps of cloth, one for every patient who made it
out alive. But I was pretty sure both of us worried about the idea of Ibrahim
returning to an ETU. He'd seen enough Ebola to last several lifetimes. His
wasn't an offer to be spurned, either, and I figured I could first go to Port
Loko town to evaluate Mariatu and get the lay of the land.

I hadn't been to the hospital since early December, and when I got there the next day I was struck by the changes. The rusting hulks of cars still littered the courtyard, but the hospital itself, now bustling with clinicians and patients, had been repainted, repaired, and (in places) reroofed. Most of the clinicians were Sierra Leonean, but many were Americans and affiliated with Partners In Health. The hospital also had lots more of the supplies necessary to properly care for Ebola patients, most of them donated by the same handful of countries and international nongovernmental organizations that had dominated previously declared humanitarian disasters. The clinicians appreciated the largesse but at the same time feared (correctly, alas) that it was self-interested and would be short-lived. Not only that, but they all were painfully aware that the physical improvements at Port Loko Government Hospital had outpaced clinical improvement among a substantial subset of Ebola patients.

Mariatu was proof positive of that. I didn't need help identifying her, since she was the sickest-looking child in the ward. I found her just a few beds away from Jariatu, in a bed that had been jammed against the wall, which seemed to have Mariatu's full attention. Sitting next to her was the middle-aged survivor who'd been assigned to look after her. She didn't look especially grumpy, but she didn't say anything, either. The girl's father, who had brought her to Maforki, was (I'd heard) nowhere to be seen.

"Mariatu," I said, and then placed a gloved hand on her shoulder. She looked away from the wall when I repeated her name, but that was it. "We think she's also suffered brain damage," one of the nurses said to me, in English. "She almost never speaks, and makes no sense when she does." Busy with patients deemed more likely to survive, she left the ward after handing over Mariatu's thin medical dossier.

With the exception of Jariatu, all of the other kids on the ward were suffering the sequelae of Ebola. A six-year-old boy named Ibrahim, his bed directly across from Mariatu's, had no evidence of persistent infection. But he couldn't see. This seemed to surprise our new and hard-pressed colleagues at the hospital, but in fact Ebola and Marburg had long been associated with visual loss. I thought of this boy as Little Ibrahim, and could guess what he needed: nursing care, physical therapy, and the attention of an ophthalmologist, since there was still a chance his vision could be improved by a brief course of steroids and some eyedrops. And, of course, some TLC. Little Ibrahim was quiet when the charge nurse introduced me, but he had a great smile. Once he grew accustomed to my presence, he showed himself to be affectionate and chatty.

A couple of beds down from Ibrahim was Isatu, the six-year-old girl I'd already met in Maforki. Her mother, and probably others in her family, had died of Ebola. After a rough first week, Isatu had seemed to be doing well, her signs and symptoms of Ebola diminishing steadily. But midway through her ETU stay, she'd suffered seizures, from which she hadn't fully recovered, and the staff at Maforki had been heartbroken. I'd tried to reassure them, saying that maybe Isatu was still all there but just needed antiseizure medications and more time. She had been transferred to Government Hospital a day previously, and looked fine. I'd assumed she was receiving the recommended medications.

With the nurses busy elsewhere in the hospital, the grumpy grandma and I were soon the only adults on the ward. Mindful of the purpose of my visit, I sat on Mariatu's bed, with my back against the wall so I could keep an eye on Ibrahim, Isatu, and the others. Every time I spoke to Mariatu, she looked at me with what seemed like fear followed by disinterest, and then turned her eyes back to the wall. Finding no documentation of a recent fever, and no evidence that she'd been weighed since admission, I did a fairly extensive clinical evaluation, which led me to conclude that she didn't have tuberculosis or any other undiagnosed infection, or cancer. Reinserting a feeding tube was my only and wholly unoriginal suggestion, along with obtaining a few basic lab tests, measuring her weight and height, and stopping her antibiotics. She'd lost a couple more pounds since her transfer, and was starving to death by any measure. I promised those taking care of her that when I got back to Freetown I would call Harvard colleagues of mine (an expert on eating disorders and a pediatric surgeon accustomed to feeding kids unable to eat) to discuss Mariatu's case and return the next day.

On the ride back to Freetown that night, I thought long and hard about "Big" Ibrahim's request, and shared some thoughts with the two colleagues

I was traveling with, Jon Lascher and the driver, Alex Jalloh. Mostly we were quiet. I thought about Ibrahim's story, and how often he returned to the importance of talking to patients, offering them a kind word, listening to what they had to say. That was why we had assigned Mariatu her companion, but I saw little more evidence of tenderness and warmth in her than Bec Rollins had. Then again, who knew what the grumpy grandma had been through, what losses she'd incurred, what uncertainties she now faced? As it happened, a phone call interrupted this reverie.

It was Ibrahim. He'd been thinking about Mariatu, he told me, ever since he saw Bec's photos. He desperately wanted to accompany us back to Port Loko the next morning to see her. "Sure," I said, feeling anything but sure, and stalling for time by promising to call him back with a plan after getting back to Freetown. In the end, I couldn't come up with a compelling reason to keep Ibrahim from helping out directly, and was able to muster several justifications for allowing him to do so. Most of all, I was aware of my bizarre fortune, being in charge of such a decision. I owned it, as the Americans say.

When we got back to Freetown, we made our way to the Mammy Yoko, of course. I called Ibrahim from there. Alex Jalloh would pick him up early the next morning, I told him, and we'd all head to Port Loko. After that, I could almost see him beaming as we talked.

Three of us left for Port Loko early the next morning: Alex at the wheel; Ibrahim behind him, the seat and floor next to him piled high with supplies; and me riding shotgun. Our conversation, in English, was stilted and intermittent. Ibrahim leaned forward to answer any questions, and would often ask me to repeat them. Since the two of us got along well, and since this was clearly not the best time to continue the tale he'd been telling me, we soon slipped into companionable silence.

On the outskirts of Freetown, Ibrahim lowered his sunglasses and promptly fell asleep. Sleepiness, he'd told me in late November, was one of the enduring symptoms of his bout with Ebola. This wasn't unusual. Many who survive Ebola suffer significant neurological sequelae. Most of the kids

I'd seen in the pediatric ward the day before had suffered from them: Little Ibrahim with his blindness, for example, and Isatu with her seizures. Blindness could often be reversed with simple steroid therapy, and seizures could be prevented with medications. But insomnia was harder to parse. How much of it could be attributed to Ebola, and how much, say, to the grief and loss they'd experienced?

As we bumped along on our way to Port Loko, getting stopped at checkpoints periodically to have our temperatures taken, I made mental rounds on the ten children in the ward, bed by bed. Who knew what was going on in Mariatu's, Little Ibrahim's, and Isatu's minds? They were young, but they weren't oblivious to the magnitude of the catastrophes they'd just endured—and were still enduring. Those catastrophes, it seemed to me, weren't unlike those many children experienced during Sierra Leone's civil war. Many children had been conscripted as combatants, lost their families, or both. Almost every adult Ebola survivor in Sierra Leone had also lived through the catastrophe of that war and were still suffering material, social, and psychological aftereffects.

As far as I could tell, the people sent to West Africa during the Ebola crisis knew very little, if anything, about the war and its devastating effects on the population, even though these had been documented amply by humanitarians, psychologists, anthropologists, journalists, and others. My American colleagues and I certainly didn't, but at one level this wasn't a problem. At the peak of the crisis, we didn't need our staff and volunteers to be deeply versed in local history, or to have strong opinions about how best to resurrect the health system of a nation ravaged by war. As in similarly devastated Liberia, and surely in Guinea, we just needed them to tend to the sick. But now, with the epidemic subsiding, the problems that survivors of Ebola would have to deal with were becoming increasingly apparent, and we needed to figure out how to address them. As we drove, I found myself wondering: What if Ibrahim had PTSD—a category of fairly recent confection—as a result of the trauma he had just lived through?

Was it really advisable to bring Ibrahim back to Port Loko and Maforki, settings like those where he had witnessed such awful things and had lost so much? I pulled down the sun visor in the car and angled its mirror to get a surreptitious look at him. Ibrahim was still asleep, or seemed to be: shades down, head tipped back, unusually still. He was wearing a plaid short-sleeve shirt, open at the collar, jeans made to look acid-washed, and bright red-and-white Adidas sneakers. A big fake-gold watch was on his left wrist, which rested open-handed on his knee, as if in prayer. Hair shaved tight in a fade, Ibrahim looked fitter than he was when we'd met, a couple of months earlier. Somehow he also looked smaller and more vulnerable.

"Let's go directly to the hospital," I said to Alex Jalloh. "Then we'll see about Maforki."

Although Port Loko Government Hospital was far and away a more cheerful-appearing place than an ETU, most patients there were gravely ill. Regardless of diagnosis or age, they were malnourished and anemic. But the most emaciated of the lot was Mariatu, who, when we arrived, still had her face turned to the wall and didn't seem to have budged since I'd seen her last.

The feeding tube we'd placed the day before dangled from her nose, fixed in place with surgical tape. Mariatu now weighed less than when she was admitted to the hospital, just as she'd weighed less when transferred to the hospital than when admitted to Maforki. Even from the door, she looked beyond recall, and—seeing her in person for the first time—Ibrahim was visibly distressed. "Poor *pikin*," he said to no one in particular. Instead of beating a hasty retreat, however, he sat down on her bed, leaned over her, and started to talk to her softly in Krio, his hand resting gently on her bony right shoulder. I'd tried the same the previous day, to no effect. She'd scarcely looked up. But a minute later, while thumbing through her chart for new lab results, I saw something I won't soon forget.

Mariatu turned away from the wall and toward Ibrahim, and then, trembling, sat up, leaned her tiny frame against him, and began whispering in his ear. None of the staff at the hospital, American or Sierra Leonean, had even known she could still speak, but Ibrahim seemed to have no trouble coaxing her into conversation. I had no doubt that she was telling Ibrahim something important. I watched, mesmerized, and might have stayed that way for a long time, but then, suddenly, a few beds away, Isatu had a seizure and fell to the floor.

At that moment, no nurse or other doctor was present, nor was there a supply of gowns or other protective gear beyond gloves, which I was already wearing. Cursing, I yelled for help while signaling Ibrahim to stay put. It was obvious enough what needed to be done, and I did it: picked Isatu up, called for an injectable antiseizure medicine, jabbed it into her thigh, disposed of the syringe, and helped an anxious nurse wipe up the mess: Isatu had become incontinent, as patients do when they have seizures. It was after she stopped seizing that I noticed that my pants were soaked with her urine. This made me anxious. Viable virus, as noted, can often be found in urine well after it's cleared from the bloodstream. There wasn't anything I could do right then and there, beyond washing up, looking surreptitiously for any nicks about my wrists or under my dampened pants, and calling for one of our logistics volunteers to install bed rails.

Besides, I was overwhelmed by curiosity about what Mariatu had told Ibrahim, so I asked him. "She said, 'I want some juice,'" he replied. "And a certain type of cookies."

Right there, in the children's ward of Port Loko Government Hospital, Ibrahim had been transformed into a man with a mission. His job now, he felt, was to find precisely the type of juice and cookies that Mariatu wanted. So armed with petty cash from Jon Lascher, who had arrived in another car, Ibrahim and Alex went on their errand of mercy, hoping to find the juice and cookies in a shop they'd been told was "right around the corner." They were gone for what seemed like hours. Meanwhile, having proceeded to Maforki, I tried not to think about whether or not lifting a damp, seizing six-year-old constituted an Ebola exposure. By epidemiological algorithms maybe it did, but not by the clinical ones I understood well and could observe firsthand.

While waiting for Ibrahim and Alex, Jon and I sat down for lunch. The "dining room" at Maforki consisted of a folding table and a dozen chairs, sheltered by a tent pitched not far from the tree where we'd planted bougainvilleas the day before. The atmosphere was much more relaxed than it had been in early December, when I'd eaten there last. Then, almost everyone had seemed too harried—or too revolted by the smell of death and chlorine—to stop for lunch, but now a number of volunteers came in and out. A couple of expatriate nurses greeted me and asked for updates about the patients they'd discharged to Government Hospital. Ibrahim and Alex didn't show up until long after Jon and I finished eating.

As Jon had guessed, they'd gone first to the hospital. Ibrahim launched right away into a report of what had happened. "Mariatu was so happy to see me back," he said, speaking uncharacteristically fast. "We got her the kind of cookies and juice she wanted." Surprising everybody, including her father, who had reappeared, she'd polished off a sizable package of the cookies, washing them down with two bottles of fruit juice. Mariatu had then taken Ibrahim's hand and had asked if at some point Ibrahim could take her for a walk—this from a girl with bedsores who, the nurses had told us, *couldn't* walk. She'd told Ibrahim she wanted to go home. "You need to stay for a while so you can stand on your own two feet," he told us he'd responded. "Eat all this reserve food, and you will soon be able to go home."

Ibrahim said he'd also spent time with Mariatu's father, a forlorn-looking, weathered fellow who we'd seen sitting alone outside the ward. Ibrahim introduced himself, explained that he was a survivor, and insisted that Mariatu would recover. This boosted the man's spirits—as did seeing Mariatu talk to Ibrahim. She hadn't uttered a word to him since her mother and sister had died of Ebola, he told Ibrahim. Nobody at the hospital had talked to him, either. Ibrahim felt that the father, confronting the prospect that another daughter might also die of Ebola, was terrified. "No one has explained to him that it's not Ebola that's killing her now," he told me. "It's *sadness* and a refusal to eat and talk."

The two of them also talked about what he, Ibrahim, termed "stigmatization," a term with broad currency in Sierra Leone. We'd heard the word invoked in every meeting with survivors, and from health authorities, paramount chiefs, and caregivers. "Psychosocial" has similarly broad currency in this part of West Africa, and likely a similar source—the humanitarian organizations that had flooded Sierra Leone and Liberia after the end of civil war. But Ibrahim described the effects of stigma on Mariatu's father in sharply materialist terms: after Mariatu's mother and sister had died, he had been laid off from his job as a carpenter in a workshop, Ibrahim explained—because of fears that he, too, might harbor the virus. So he had turned to his younger brother for help, but he, fearing contagion, had also kept his distance. Now, at the hospital, Mariatu's father felt helpless as he watched his daughter decline. "He didn't have money to buy her the things she liked to eat," Ibrahim explained, "because he has no money. And no money to get back and forth from home."

Ibrahim clearly had much to tell us. But I'd made plans that afternoon to visit the Cuban brigade working in the ETU, and had to cut him off. One of the Cuban doctors had just returned from Switzerland, where he had been treated for Ebola, and I wanted to congratulate him on his recovery. I also wanted to discreetly ask a friend, an Ebola-experienced French nurse, what she thought of my potential exposure. (Not much, it turned out, to my relief.) I explained the situation to Ibrahim and got up to go to the inner sheds, where the afflicted lay. "No need to come inside," I told him. But Ibrahim jumped to his feet, began walking with me, and without missing a beat kept talking about Mariatu as we entered the green zone. "I really sat and talked to her," he said. "The problem is that the nurses are so worried and busy."

Ibrahim had to pause his account as people greeted me, but he always picked up right where he had left off. "The lady hasn't been trained properly," he told me, referring to the grumpy grandma. "But she *could* be trained, I think." The red zone came into view, separated from the green zone merely by waist-high barriers. We halted some thirty yards from it and took in a now-familiar scene: suited-up clinicians stooping over very sick, prone patients. "You've had enough of ETUs," I said, putting my hand on Ibrahim's shoulder. "No need to continue." But seeing the patients and their gowned-up caregivers didn't deter him in the least. "I want to go to talk to other survivors," he said, "and, across these barriers, to those still sick." We didn't enter the red zone that day, but everywhere we did go in the ETU, Ibrahim seemed at ease, just as he had in the hospital.

That was our next stop. When we returned to the pediatric ward after a few hours at Maforki, we found that Mariatu's "reserve food" was gone. She needed much more than juice and cookies if she was to recover, of course, but her new interest in such treats was a sign that we would be able to coax her to eat the protein-rich supplements she desperately needed. We noticed another promising sign: when we arrived, Mariatu was sitting up, leaning against the wall, and listening to Little Ibrahim. He couldn't have been completely sightless, because he gave us a merry greeting as soon as we walked in. We soon learned that Mariatu had shared her juice and cookies with him. Free of her feeding tube, she may have even given us a smile.

On the way back to Freetown late that night, Ibrahim was on fire. Still ebullient, if not quite manic, he pleaded with us to let him work with Mariatu and her father, and told us how good our day had made him feel. "I was able to meet my goal," he said. "To talk to the survivors, but also to remind the nurses how the patients feel, and to ask them to be more gentle with them. I want to go back and work with them more." He didn't pause even when we stopped at checkpoints to have our temperatures checked.

Jon Lascher, who rode back with us to the city, asked Ibrahim to compare Maforki, where staff outnumbered patients, to the big ETU at Hastings. "What I liked most about Maforki," he replied, "was how many doctors and nurses go inside. That didn't often happen in Hastings." Ibrahim told us that the makeshift facility in Maforki was cleaner and better maintained, with more toilet facilities, than what he'd seen in his time at Hastings. (Still riding shotgun, I turned to look at Jon, having just complained of the *lack* of toilets at Maforki. It was too dark to make out his face.) "But the main difference," Ibrahim continued, "is the human contact with the doctors and nurses and other staff." Jon asked him why he thought Maforki was better in this regard. Were there simply too few staff at Hastings? "This was early," he replied. "We were the first patients there. The epidemic was just starting in the city, and so many people were dying. There were dead people everywhere. The nurses and doctors were so afraid. That's what I think."

It was close to midnight by the time we reached Freetown and parted ways. Exhausted, I collapsed into bed—only to be jolted awake just a few hours later by a phone call. It was Ibrahim, of course, eager to know what time we were heading back to Port Loko. Any irritation I felt at being awakened before dawn melted away as Ibrahim once again began talking about the day we'd just spent together. "Yesterday was a great day for me," he said. "That's the first center I visited since my family died. In fact, it was the greatest day of my life." I held the cell phone to my ear, unable to say anything. I knew, from the time I'd already spent interviewing Ibrahim, that he wasn't given to hyperbole.

Jesus, I thought. *The greatest day of his life?*

I was grateful to be alone as my voice caught in my throat. After a few long seconds, Ibrahim asked if I was still on the line and reiterated his plea that we allow him to go work with Mariatu and her father. "Sure," I said finally, "you can come back tomorrow."

A few days later, Ibrahim moved to Port Loko. "I will stay until Mariatu is better," he told me. I didn't even know where Ibrahim was to eat and sleep—or if he would sleep—but I was confident that Jon and his team would look after him.

Mostly confident, that is: there was something about Ibrahim, something that struck me even before he accorded me the painful gift of his story, that made me feel protective and anxious. A few days later, I had to leave for Liberia, an hour away by plane, and these sentiments made my departure even harder than usual. But Ibrahim called me a few hours after I reached Monrovia. "Mariatu is doing better," he told me, his voice still booming and assertive. "I promise you she will make it. She is eating more every day."

I wasn't the only one to notice Ibrahim's newfound zest for a life of service. Just after I left for Liberia, one of our young American colleagues, who'd helped to run the survivors' program for Partners In Health, wrote me the following:

> You have no idea the joy it brings watching the directness of a
> hiphoppin' Ibrahim as he advocates for health and solidarity.
> One moment that stands out is when we walked into Government
> Hospital late one night and a startled security guard shouted, "Halt,
> who goes there!" With no hesitation, Ibrahim yelled "PIH!" as he
> strode off to check on his patients.[17]

Bec Rollins called me the night I reached Liberia, which she'd just left for Boston. I filled her in on the story of Ibrahim and Mariatu. She was happy that Ibrahim seemed to have found new purpose, but my story made her worry about how he'd fastened his hope, fervor, and passion on Mariatu. "What would it do to him if she, too, were to die?" Bec asked. "It's as if she's all he has left. It could break him. I know it would break me."

Bec had put my own anxiety into words. But Mariatu did not die. A few days later, Ibrahim called again to tell me she had gained five pounds. And at the close of February, when Mariatu went home, she was, by Ibrahim's report, "as human as ever." When I saw her again, a couple of weeks later, I found her almost unrecognizable: her face and frame had filled out and her smile had returned. Not only that, she was affectionate, grateful, and anxious to return to school. A few months later, in August, she did just that. But I heard from Mariatu herself well before her wish was granted.

It was Ramadan again, and I was back in Rwanda, working at the hospital where I'd been helping out for a decade. And one day, toward the end of the fast, I got an international call during rounds. The country code was 232—Sierra Leone. I answered thinking it might be Ibrahim, but heard nothing on the line. A few minutes later I received a text from Mariatu. Her English was imperfect, so I paraphrase: "May God reward you all," she wrote, "for taking care of me."

I forwarded the note to Ibrahim.

4.

The Two Ordeals of Yabom

A staunchly, resolutely unalone
existence is a windfall, I'm aware.
My mother, widowed young, was on her own.
She sliced a single life out of a shared
one almost overnight. She'd been one thing
at dinner but by dawn was something new,
something that no one envied. Friends would bring
us things to heat up, casseroles and stews,
and whisper thanks to Jesus for their luck
as they drove home. Our quiet, giant house
was stuffed with silence. We watched TV, stuck
our fingers in the cakes. Without a spouse,
with grieving children eating on the floor,
my mother put a brick beside her door.
—Mary Block, "Crown for a Young Marriage," 2014

History rounds off skeletons to the nearest zero.
A thousand and one is still only a thousand.
That one seems never to have existed.
—Wisława Szymborska, "Starvation Camp Near Jaslo," 1962

I FIRST LAID EYES ON YABOM KOROMA ON A MORNING IN EARLY OCTOBER 2014. The newly bereaved woman, thirty-eight years old, was sitting on a concrete ledge a few dozen yards from her house, a tin-roofed shanty nestled into a steep hill in a part of Freetown called Foulah Town. While the city had been christened in the late eighteenth century by British abolitionists, Yabom's neighborhood was named after Fula-speaking refugees who settled there in the early nineteenth century.

The Fula, who hailed predominantly from the north and east, were among many fleeing the violence of the slave trades. In Freetown, they joined captives plucked from the high seas by British antislavery patrols. If the ties of these "recaptives" to their ancestral lands had been severed, their religious affiliations, languages, and cultures were not so readily erased. Many had been born and raised Muslim, and their numbers grew. On the morning we first sat with Yabom, I counted four picturesque mosques. One of them, the Foulah Town Mosque, looked more like a Bible Belt church, with stumpy minarets and a Greek-appearing façade, but elegant Kufic verses spanned the cornice.

Yabom was sitting next to a teenage boy. Both had just been discharged from an ETU, and both had compelling stories to tell. But while the teen was downright cheerful in recounting his, Yabom was soon in tears. A busy intersection didn't seem the best place for an interview about her ordeal, but passersby didn't stare. All of us knew that Ebola was on everyone's mind. As the second call to prayer spiraled mournfully heavenward from the many minarets rising from the ramshackle quarter, it was hard to believe that the disease was spiraling out of control. Mountain Cut, the town's potholed thoroughfare, was packed with purposeful pedestrians and creeping vehicles. Both kinds of traffic seemed to slow and eddy between the largest mosque and the alleyway below Yabom's house. Most were heading downhill, and it didn't take long to see that this part of Foulah Town tilted toward the Big Wharf down below.

Up high on the hill, Mountain Cut began as a corridor of roadside stalls, where retail merchandise (small tins of evaporated milk, sliced bread replete with pats of butter, a bowl of cooked rice smothered with palm oil and cassava or potato leaves, a bar of soap, a single cigarette or a pack of them) could be had from before dawn to well after the Ebola curfew supposedly then in effect. Closer to the dock, the stalls gave way to stores selling used clothing, new and refurbished electronics, pirated DVDs, and wholesale soap, rice, and palm oil. When we climbed up to Yabom's tiny courtyard and looked back down at the city, we could see the taller buildings of Freetown's business district spread out in an impressive panorama, their bases obscured by the smoke of the daily ritual of burning trash. A tang of salt and the smell of fish hung in the air, heavy but not unpleasant.

We soon learned more about Yabom in the relative calm of her yard. She'd just returned from a miserable but life-saving stay at the commandeered police academy in Hastings, but there was no joy in her homecoming. Colorful laundry was drying all over the house, but it did nothing to relieve the sense of absence that enveloped the space like a shroud. Prior to her time in the ETU, she had lost her husband, two of their five children, and close to a dozen more relatives to Ebola. Yabom had cared for or helped bury most of them before falling ill herself. Upon returning from Hastings, just a few days prior to our visit, she discovered that, during her isolation, Ebola had taken her mother.

It took many visits to learn all of this, but some details of Yabom's life before Ebola came into view shortly after that first glimpse of Mountain Cut and its descent toward the docks. Before the virus invaded, Yabom and her husband had been supporting their family across this economic gradient. She had plied a trade in new and used clothing, mostly shipped by container from China via Guinea; her husband, Saidu, sold unfinished lumber—really just stakes, hewn from what was locally termed a plum tree, and used to frame the informal dwellings that had sprouted across the poorer parts of the city during and after the war. Yabom, Saidu, and their children lived in one of these houses, a tin-roofed and partially tin-walled structure with neither electricity nor running water. The couple struggled to send their kids to school, and the household was often short of food, but Yabom told us that day that the family had been happy nonetheless.

Bailor Barrie was with us at our first meeting with Yabom, and on many subsequent ones, too. She spoke little English and he served as my interpreter during most of the difficult exchanges I'd have over the years that followed that first meeting. That day, when he began talking in Krio to Yabom, they soon realized that they were neighbors. Bailor told her during that first roadside exchange that he lived just on the other side of Mountain Cut, in a five-story apartment building erected over the foundations of wooden buildings that had been razed during the war. He pointed to the building as we talked. Already weathered-looking, it was a concrete box that lacked the elegance of even the more modest mosques in the neighborhood and seemed out of place among the dilapidated houses that leaned into or away from the street. Watching the two of them—the stout doctor and the rail-thin widow who were neighbors and contemporaries—made me think hard about my protégé.

By then, it was already hard for me to imagine going anywhere in Sierra Leone without Bailor. He was dearer to me than most of my students. We'd broken bread many times during my first trip to Freetown in June, which already seemed like remote history. Yet before that visit to Foulah Town, I'd never asked him where exactly he and his family lived. Then again, if I was there only to attend a brief medical conference, why should I have needed to learn anything about its neighborhoods and its history? Everything was different now that I was back to stay, and a bond between the three of us—Bailor, Yabom, and me—was cemented over the course of the next few years. We would get together often, and gradually I would learn their stories, as they learned each other's.

The process was anything but linear; it was often halting, sometimes painful, and full of twists and revisions. This was of course to be expected when the topic was the mortal peril that Yabom and (as I discovered) Bailor had survived. Such uncertainty faces anyone seeking to understand their significance, but this deciphering was often interrupted. We were all caught up in the epidemic still unfolding around us, and even straightforward matters took time. It took me weeks, for example, to learn that Yabom (like Ibrahim's parents) identified as Temne, and years had gone by before I learned that Bailor identified as Fula. You might wonder why it took me so long—all I had to do was ask, after all—but such matters recede into the background during a medical emergency. What's more, a decade in Rwanda had made me reluctant to ask impertinent (if not irrelevant) questions about anything to do with tribes or tribalism. Never mind the checkered past of Africanist anthropology. I did know that Bailor was Muslim, but only because I'd seen his first name, Mohamed, on his application to a graduate program at Harvard Medical School.

As Bailor and I got to know Yabom, I learned that many of my initial impressions of her were incorrect. Although forthcoming about her experience of Ebola, she'd seemed shy and not much given to small talk. The reason was grief, of course—a subject obliterated from much expert discourse during the first months of the epidemic, when many pontificated about "local beliefs" about sickness, death, burial, funerary ritual, and the afterlife. Yabom's own stated views on these matters were as subject to revision as anyone else's, and she was still making sense of her losses as life went on.

By the beginning of 2015, although her vision was failing acutely, her depression seemed to lift. Nothing seemed to please her more than chatting with new friends, among them Ibrahim, the Chairman, other survivors, and some of us who'd taken care of them. She opened up her house as a meeting place for survivors, and during their gatherings I often saw a radiant smile light up her face. Despite what she'd been through, Yabom was somehow able still to see most matters in a positive light, a trait that lifted my spirits like nothing else. And when I was with her my spirits often needed lifting, because the stories she told were grim.

Even Bailor was at times struck dumb as Yabom told us about the extraordinary extent of her losses as a daughter, a sister, a mother, and a wife. But those stories are vital for us to hear, because they can provide a powerful understanding of Ebola, and the structural forces that made it so deadly. Since every Sierra Leonean her age who survived Ebola had also survived brutal civil war, Yabom's story offers an insight into the role armed conflict played in setting the stage for the epidemic. Hearing it brought into view the lives of those who split their time between village and city.

Finally, Yabom's story was told from the point of view of a woman.

Yabom was born on January 30, 1976, in the hamlet of Bantoro. The village, which sits in a small chiefdom of Port Loko District, was situated about a dozen miles from Port Loko town. Bantoro abuts the Little Scarcies River, which, like others crossing this part of West Africa, has its origins in the highlands of Guinea. Port Loko District may have long been Temne terrain, but people of diverse backgrounds and means inhabit its chief towns and trading posts. Bantoro, on the other hand, was tiny and homogenous, inhabited by a half dozen families related by blood or marriage, and usually both.

Yabom described her parents as "humble and peaceful," but "poverty-stricken" would have been closer to the mark. Like others, they grew rice, corn, millet, cassava, potatoes, and palm products in small gardens cleared from bush and woodlands on the southern shore of the river. Her father, Amadu Mohamed Koroma, didn't own his land in the legal sense of having a deed, but his family had tilled it for generations by the time she was born. He had two wives: Fatmata, Yabom's mother, bore him seven children; her stepmother, five. There were a couple of other kids in the mix, but I never quite got the genealogy straight. I did learn that Yabom was her mother's fourth living child and her father's ninth, and that Fatmata's first four children, three boys and a girl, were from a previous marriage. All of them perished before Yabom was born. The oldest, the girl, died in the course of Yabom's older sister's naming ceremony. She was bitten by a venomous snake during the festivities.

Yabom didn't share this detail with a shrug any more than Bailor or I received it with one. Nor did she gloss over the fact that five other siblings and half siblings were lost to unknown childhood illnesses—unknown, in any case, to her. This towering mortality and an absence of medical care, to say nothing of antivenom, serves as a grim report card on the health-care system of Sierra Leone in the 1970s. The penury endured by its largely illiterate peasant farmers at the time of Yabom's birth serves most of all as a report card on colonial rule. The British legacy of rural neglect—and the control-over-care approach it adopted with the natives—would have taken even the most visionary and well-resourced leaders decades to overcome. By the time Yabom was born, however, it was clear that the nation's rulers envisioned something other than sharing its resources.

In principle, Sierra Leone's first independent leaders had access to diamonds and mineral wealth. But they didn't share this bounty with the rural, poor majority: if profit margins were slim in the city, they were razor-thin in rural communities like Bantoro. Yabom told us that her family regularly experienced hunger at the outset of the rainy season, before the rice and cassava ripened. Though the harvest was often insufficient for household needs, her mother sold some of it (especially cassava) in the market to buy essentials: matches, soap, candles, kerosene, salt, spices, shoes, and clothing. During the dry season, which usually runs from November to April, Fatmata refined oil from wild palm fruits (a favorite food of bats, according to Ebola billboards) she harvested in the forest. She produced around six hundred liters a year, selling the oil in Foulah Town for, Yabom thought, about $150. Like Bantoro's other families, hers supplemented its income by mining sand from the banks of the Little Scarcies.

None of Yabom's older siblings—including Kadiatu, whose naming ceremony had been cursed by a snakebite—had been able to attend school. There wasn't one in Bantoro, and paying for fees, food, school supplies, and safe lodging for children in a town with a school was out of the question. Yabom considered herself fortunate, because when she was five or six years old, one of her father's sisters had come back to the village from Foulah Town and invited Yabom and Kadiatu to live with her in order to attend school. Yabom described that day to us as one of the happiest of her life: she'd heard a lot about the city and was excited to see it; school would be an added bonus.

With independence and an easing of colonial efforts to keep the rural poor in place, Foulah Town had become Bantoro's gateway to the capital and the world beyond. When Yabom and Kadiatu first passed through that portal, their aunt was a single parent already responsible for seven children, four grandchildren, and a couple of other relatives. She lived in a two-bedroom house on Grant Street, another narrow alley off Mountain Cut, not far from where Yabom lived when Ebola struck. The house was without modern amenities, including running water. The aunt tried to make ends meet by selling foo-foo, a fluffy paste made of pounded cassava that would remind Americans of mashed potatoes. She sold it from an awning-covered table planted on the edge of a street running along the Big Wharf.

Yabom's aunt managed to send a couple of her younger kids, Yabom, and Kadiatu to Freetown Baptist Primary School, not far from the house. But she couldn't feed, clothe, and school her dependents through the foo-foo trade alone; Yabom's father supplemented his sister's meager income by sending some of each harvest from Bantoro to Freetown. And, as in the village and most poorer urban households, children were expected to contribute directly to the budget. Each day after school, Yabom, Kadiatu, and three of their cousins sold cups of chilled water for a penny each, from buckets perched on their heads. The girls walked up and down Sani Abacha Street, Freetown's busiest, until they'd met their quota. Yabom understood that this daily grind was the only way to contribute her share, but she often longed to be home.

Bantoro was only a few hours away by *poda poda*. But it wasn't until Yabom was in the fifth grade that she and Kadiatu finally managed to return. "I was so happy to be back," Yabom later exulted of that first trip home, "that part of me wanted to stay there." Her parents discouraged such sentimentality: most girls of Yabom's age in Sierra Leone didn't get the chance to be students. She and her sister were soon back in Foulah Town, but staying enrolled in school there would prove to be difficult, because the country's embryonic educational system was threatened before it was even born.

National politics was a big factor in this stillbirth. For seventeen years, Sierra Leone was led by Siaka Stevens, a corrupt, self-serving autocrat who'd revised the country's constitution to keep himself in power, transforming what started out as a British-style parliamentary democracy into a one-party state that derived most of its income from the extractive industries. Diamonds were far and away the largest source of foreign exchange during Yabom's early years, and Stevens controlled that trade. As his reign neared its end, and as she began school, the price of diamonds and other minerals dropped sharply. When Stevens retired, in 1985, he again overrode the constitution and appointed a new president himself: Major-General Joseph Saidu Momoh, the commander of the armed forces. A couple of years later, with rumors of an insurgency trickling in from strife-torn Liberia, Momoh introduced a new and harsh "austerity program."

This was another term for structural adjustment. Already, international financial institutions had made aid to Sierra Leone dependent upon the government's adopting policies that discouraged public investments in education, health care, and other social services. As a result of this "conditionality," as it's termed in development economics, the government had slashed public expenditures in the years just prior to the war.[1] This imperiled even modest support for teachers' salaries, school supplies, and the administration of national exams. The costs were passed down to families like Yabom's, who were expected to buy school uniforms, shoes, and supplies. Exam fees became prohibitive, as did the cost of rice, previously subsidized.

Teachers and others in the educational sector, even those who didn't lose their jobs, were among those hit hardest by these measures. "By the time I was in fifth grade," Yabom told us, "the teachers began a go-slow"—that is, a strike. The country's teachers would strike on and off during the brief remainder of Yabom's schooling, which came to an end in 1988, when her aunt ran out of money and couldn't pay for Yabom, then twelve, to sit for exams at the end of the seventh grade. Kadiatu suffered the same fate, as did a cousin then in the fourth grade. These were supposed to be temporary hindrances, but the following year was even worse. As a couple of her cousins donned new or refurbished uniforms, Yabom, Kadiatu, and their out-of-school cousins were forced to sell water, austerely and all day long, and to help their aunt in the foo-foo business.

After a year or so as full-time street peddlers, with their hopes of resuming school fading, the sisters began shuttling—as Ibrahim Kamara, too, would do—between village and city. This back-and-forth didn't last long, though, because Yabom and Kadiatu were soon to pass through the portal of adulthood.

Yabom and Kadiatu returned to Bantoro—for good, they thought—in the first months of 1990. "At first," Yabom told me and Bailor, "being back was strange and different. My mom had twins while we were gone, and one had died. Life was always hard for her, but she didn't complain. It was always work, work, work, and she was glad to have us back." Being home, Yabom said, also allowed her to "join society."

Yabom was referring to the rites of passage known as initiation. By this time, she was living in a small house in the village with her father, her mother, her grandmother, her stepmother, four initiated sisters, and two initiated half sisters, along with several babies, toddlers, and young kids who hadn't yet gone through initiation. All girls in Bantoro and its environs joined what's known in the Krio and Temne languages as Bundu, the allegedly secret society for girls. (In other languages, its either Bondo or Sande.) The girls just back from Freetown knew they were different from the others in their Bundu cohort. "People had respect for us, as we had lived in the city," Yabom added, "but they sometimes called us *oporto*." This was, Bailor Barrie added with a smile directed my way, the Temne term for whites.

Although initiation into these sodalities, as they're termed by social scientists, was initially more awkward for the Freetown girls, there was no question that Yabom and her sister would be included. Integration into village and family life, which in Bantoro was hard on everyone but especially on girls and young women, is the primary function of Bundu initiation. "These sodalities," anthropologist Carol MacCormack has written about the process, "initiate virtually all pubescent children into the first grade of adulthood, designating them 'those who may procreate.' They also sustain individuals in reproductive and economically productive activities throughout life."[2] Yabom described the process a bit more simply. "Among women," she told us, "if you don't join the Bundu, the others talk about you."

Yabom didn't mind talking about her initiation with us, and smiled at times as she recalled those first months back home. Initiation takes place in what are widely termed "bush schools." A ritual specialist, or *sowei*, led the process, which involved seclusion in the bush school for the transmission of life lessons and for ritual circumcision. "They make a cage," Yabom added, "fenced in under a mango tree, and in the enclosure they teach the women how to become wives, how to take care of their husbands." (Bailor, who by then had finished a year of coursework at Harvard, at one point translated the entire process of initiation as "female genital mutilation," which elicited a puzzled look from Yabom.) Initiation in Bantoro, she told us, was a family affair. Of the eight others initiated in Yabom's cohort, five were her sisters—if you included, as she did, stepsisters and a distant relative given as a ward to her mother. The group was rounded out by a couple of cousins. The *sowei* was Yabom's grandmother, who was also Bantoro's midwife.

The size of a Bundu cohort and variations in perception of how old girls need to be to enroll in the bush school are in part a function of the size of a village; small ones like Bantoro don't have annual initiations. The youngest initiate in Yabom's group was five, which is very young compared to anthropologists' accounts; Kadiatu, then fifteen, was the oldest. "Members of the same cohort," Yabom said, "are like sisters from the same mother." Time spent in this sacred grove was one of the ways the girls learned how "to make a peaceful household." The precise amount of time was shorter than described in classic texts. According to Yabom, "It normally takes three weeks to one month."

Perhaps in keeping with her oaths, Yabom told us little about what went on in bush school other than to describe the instruction as "mostly singing and dancing and girls talking to each other." But MacCormack, who did her fieldwork in the 1970s and in a larger town, has described what the process was probably like for Yabom and her cohort:

> There are pleasures to be enjoyed as well as ordeals, and the girls go gladly into the initiation grove. Food is plentiful since the initiation season occurs in the post-harvest dry season and each girl's family is obliged to send large quantities of rather special food into the initiation grove on her behalf. There are also special Bundu songs, dances and stories to be enjoyed around the fire in the evening. The stories usually end with an instructive moral linked to Bundu laws given to the living by ancestresses of the secret society.[3]

Yabom described her initiation to us as a welcome and necessary step toward full inclusion in her extended family. "I wasn't happy at first," she said. "I was scared until we were all alone together for a while, and then again before they took us out. Then I was happy."

Happiness was generally in short supply in Bantoro; just getting by was increasingly difficult. Yabom's second rainy season there began after a poor harvest, and Kadiatu had several new obligations: Soon after initiation she was married, had a baby, and got pregnant with another. Yabom was sent back to her aunt in Freetown, where she went right back to selling water and helping her aunt peddle cassava. "That was pretty much all I was doing," she said, "when the rebels invaded."

The year was 1991 and the place was Kailahun District. At first, the residents of Freetown considered the RUF invasion a far-off affair. For Yabom, the daily grind in Bantoro, and on Grant Street, was struggle enough. But she nonetheless recalls clearly the day she first heard of the rebels:

> There was a man I knew from Freetown who was doing business in Koindu, in the east. He was on his way there when the rebels attacked the town, and he escaped back to the city. There were already people coming from Liberia as refugees. We saw them arrive, of course, but that conflict didn't seem to concern us. Before the rebels came to Freetown, the Krios were saying, "Who are these rebels? Are they human beings, or do they have tails? Are they specters or just thieves?"

Yabom had plenty of her own concerns by then, and they had little to do with the war or its specters. When she was fifteen, she met a man named James Kanu, a twenty-nine-year-old who hailed from the northern district of Tonkolili, which borders Port Loko District.

Like Ibrahim's father, James Kanu worked as a day laborer at the port. "I met him as I was going to sell water," she said. "He asked a friend of mine if she knew how old I was." Since Yabom already was initiated and there was then no Facebook, it wasn't considered incorrect for him to inquire about her status. (Back then, most Temne girls were married or spoken for by age fifteen.) James plied Yabom with gifts, and they began dating. Two years later they were still dating, and Yabom was visibly with child. Her aunt pressed James to make it official, but he pleaded being too poor to marry. Even though her grandmother was the village midwife, Yabom stayed in Freetown to have the baby, a girl she named Kadiatu after her favorite sister.

A year later—unmarried, without James, still in her teens, still nursing the baby—Yabom moved back to Bantoro. This time, the adjustment was harder. She had grown unfamiliar with the rhythms of the farm and was new to juggling work and caring for a newborn. Still, she was with her family and loved living with Kadiatu, who had young children herself. Despite the rigors of rural life, especially for young women, Yabom described this period to us as one of simple pleasures. "We used to have one of those big boom boxes," she said, "which we played in the evening. The kids were always dancing."

Yabom knew, too, that the capital was then in turmoil. There were strikes, riots over the price of rice, and demonstrations in the streets by angry students and foot soldiers. In April 1992, junior officers and disgruntled rank-and-file who'd been fighting in the east marched into the palace and deposed President Momoh in a bloodless coup. The folks in Bantoro, Yabom said, didn't worry much about the coup or the steady westward creep of the rebels. War remained a problem in the east, not in the city or elsewhere in the west, and not in the northwest. "There had been coups when my parents were young," she told us, "and many stories about political conflict. What worried us was the price of rice."

Yabom was further distracted by a budding romance. After two years back home, she took up with Saidu Turay, a young man helping her father with the rude tasks of clearing brush, plowing, planting, and harvesting. As Yabom first recounted the story to us, Saidu "was helping my parents to farm, and my father liked him, so they gave me to him," adding that he was an orphan who'd been raised by an elder cousin resident in the village. There was more to the story, which emerged in dribs and drabs. Yabom used the term "orphan" loosely; Saidu's father was alive and well in Freetown, but he wasn't sending money back to the village, which was then one of the chief reasons for villagers to go to the city. She would later explain that in fact she and Saidu were related; he was the grandson of her grandfather's brother—by an American reckoning, her second cousin. She also added that the two of them wanted to marry. But Saidu's family was even poorer than hers, and he didn't have the money to pay her bride price, so their relationship was never official. Yabom always referred to Saidu as "my husband," and soon enough everybody in her family accepted the arrangement.

A few years passed, and Yabom remembers them as happy ones. She was deeply disappointed by a couple of miscarriages, including a stillbirth. But early in 1996 the couple became the parents of a baby girl. Kadiatu and their mother helped her with new duties, and soon even little Kadiatu did, too—and she soon knew how to fetch wood and water. Not long after Yabom gave birth to her second child, a nationwide ordeal began that for years would ravage Yabom's life, and the lives of so many in Sierra Leone, from Freetown to forest. As she put it to us, "The war met me in the village." The story of that tragic ordeal is rarely told from the perspective of those who lived through it. And it *needs* telling.

If you want to understand the Ebola crisis in West Africa—what it was like to live through it, and why so many rural Sierra Leoneans responded as they did—you first have to understand what it was like to live through civil war. Nobody I've met has made that clearer to me than Yabom, even though she spoke unwillingly of the conflict.

By the time Yabom and Saidu and their girls settled into family life, a growing fraction of the army was clearly complicit with the insurgents, who fought to control the diamond districts in the east.

Freetown and the northwest hadn't yet been overrun by the RUF, but sobels had clearly infiltrated the high command. From top to bottom, Sierra Leone's armed forces—bolstered by Liberian rebels—were hostile to elections. As long as the conflict continued, the ruling junta and the rebels knew that wealth from diamonds and minerals, and rice, would flow their way, while a strong civilian government would upset their gravy train. But in February 1996, amazingly enough, elections happened anyway. A lawyer turned UN bureaucrat named Ahmad Tejan Kabbah was elected president in what were held to be fair elections, although much of the citizenry couldn't safely cast ballots. His mandate was to end the war.

Kabbah knew the Freetown sobels were as great a threat to him and his government as the RUF, so he surrounded himself with a Praetorian guard of Nigerian soldiers. Nigerian troops were also the mainstay of a regional peacekeeping contingent of the Economic Community of West African States (ECOWAS) known as the ECOWAS Monitoring Group (ECOMOG). The force would grow dramatically in the period that followed and would shape the destinies of both Yabom and Bailor Barrie. Before the 1996 elections, though, it was heavily concentrated in Liberia, which had disintegrated during a civil war launched a couple of years before Sierra Leone's began. With the insurgency moving west, ECOMOG established bases in Port Loko and other large towns in the north, but by that point neither those forces nor the newly elected president seemed to have much chance of speedily bringing the conflict to an end.

In May 1997, the rebels made their first big western surge, crossing through Port Loko District. With spectacular violence, they entered Freetown and overthrew the government, forcing Kabbah to flee in exile to Guinea. "I was living in the village and listening to the radio," Yabom recounted. "We saw refugees coming from Freetown, and alpha jets flying overhead and heard them bombing the rebels who came into the area." The alpha jets belonged to Nigeria, which had purchased them from Germany; they'd been a fixture of West African skies for years. But neither the jets nor ECOMOG ground forces were able to hold back the rebels. They spared Bantoro during this first western surge, but their advance spelled the end of any sense of security in the village.

The families of Bantoro had few weapons beyond the tools they used to farm; they knew these were useless against the rebels' weapons of war even before the rebels gained access to those of the sobels. Anticipating attack, the villagers made plans for flight and secretly stocked refuges in the bush with food and farm tools. The villagers felt secrecy was essential, Yabom told us, because they believed the 1997 coup was an inside job. When she mentioned this, Bailor Barrie stepped out of his role as translator and interjected, "It certainly was!" Since Bailor had been in Freetown during the events of May 1997, Yabom let him share his recollection of events.

Bailor's life was improbably full of promise before the coup. The son of an itinerant tailor, he'd grown up in a village not far from Makeni, a big trading town a couple of hours east of Port Loko. As a boy, he had loved school and decided early that he wanted to become a doctor. So he dedicated himself to preparing for his medical exams, which he then aced, leading to his acceptance to Sierra Leone's only medical school—a triumph for a young man in his circumstances. Bailor moved to Freetown, where he became the ward of an unrelated "auntie" married to an army general opposed to the rebels and their allies within the armed forces. On the day of the coup, Bailor and his host family hid in the basement of their house while the rebels raged through the city and President Kabbah fled. Reinforcements were soon dispatched to Freetown from ECOMOG bases in Liberia and from Nigeria. They eventually beat back the rebels, also with spectacular violence. Before any semblance of peace was restored to Freetown, however, much of the city was looted and parts of it were burned. Even after things settled down, the conflict was far from over, because the capital remained in the hands of uniformed sobels.

The situation, Bailor knew, was worse to the east. His hometown of Makeni had been one of the rebels' targets well before the first western surge. Before the war, his father had traveled regularly between Makeni, his wife's nearby home village, and Guinea, where he, like many Fula, had roots. Once the fighting started, Bailor's father abandoned his trade as a tailor and headed to Tonkolili District to mine gold. He had all of his money and gold stolen there, Bailor told us, which precipitated a psychotic break. Then, as now, there was only one psychiatric facility in the country. (Founded in 1820 as Kissy Lunatic Asylum, it is West Africa's oldest.) There would have been no sure way for Bailor's father to get there during these events, nor much reason to: the asylum was without medications. He then took to shuttling between Makeni, his home village in Guinea, and Bailor's mother's village, an hour or so from Makeni.

After the rebels' western surge and the coup in Freetown, Bailor tried to get news of his parents but heard nothing. He assumed the worst, in large part because of what he'd seen happening in Freetown. At a protest a few days after the rebels had entered the city, he'd seen a friend of his shot dead as he stood right next to him. He'd also seen fellow students arrested and taken to prison, where some were killed. By that point, many students were making contingency plans for flight: aspirants to the middle class, unlike the folks in Bantoro, tended to think first about fleeing to other nations rather than other districts, and there was clearly no point in heading south to Liberia. Violence and repression continued throughout the summer, and by the end of August, Bailor informed his auntie that he had decided to seek refuge in Guinea. Since his family had roots there, he hoped to find news of his parents. On August 28, he packed a few things in a backpack, including his school records and certificates, and headed north.

Bailor had limited options. The overland road had been closed by clashing armies, leaving two ways to head north to Conakry. One was a helicopter ferry from the Lungi airfield, which cost $400; the other was a ride north in a boat, which cost $40. He had about $60, so naturally he chose the boat. Bailor reckoned he passed through a dozen checkpoints to get to the docks. When at last he reached them, what he saw terrified him. The boats on offer resembled huge wooden canoes with outboard motors, and none of them looked seaworthy. He continued:

> I was worried about the boats and the risk I was about to take, and decided to take a short walk to decide if it was worth it. Then I heard gunshots, and people started to panic. I ran toward the boats, as did hundreds of others . . . I got to one of them, pushing my way through the crowd. The boat, which had a capacity of maybe sixty, had two hundred people in it. The captain was yelling at people to get off when soldiers starting shooting us. I fell to the deck, and people fell on top of me. The captain asked everyone to pray.

Remarkably, the overladen vessel made it to Conakry, on a pail and many prayers, as passengers scooped out waves washing over the gunwales. By the time they arrived, Bailor was sick and almost unable to stand. By then, Sierra Leonean refugees were streaming into Guinea by air, land, and sea. Bailor and most of his fellow passengers knew to head to their country's embassy in Conakry, where they joined hundreds camped on its grounds.

When Bailor Barrie couldn't find his parents, the medical student was referred to a camp. He was now formally a refugee, allotted "a bucket, a towel, soap, and some toiletries" and a daily ration of bulgur wheat, cornmeal, beans, sugar, and cooking oil. Hearing this, Yabom nodded silently. As we would learn when she told us more of her story, she had deep experience in such matters. Bailor found his father's brother in short order, and two months later the two of them located his mother and other relatives from Makeni in a refugee camp. It was there that he learned his father had been shot during a rebel attack on his wife's home village. He initially survived his wound, but his mental illness flared. Bailor would later learn that he died not long afterward, "alone in his room."

It took ECOMOG the better part of a year, and a unilateral Nigerian blitz on the junta in Freetown, to restore constitutional rule. When President Kabbah returned from his exile in Guinea, in early 1998, he had no small number of army officers hanged or shot for treason. Bailor returned that May and began focusing on his studies again—no small feat, given the atmosphere in the city and the ongoing menace to the east.

Meanwhile, Yabom and her family in Bantoro—spared during the first western surge—were increasingly worried about the conflict. With good reason: by then, thousands had perished in the war, and the rebels, strengthened by army defections, and armed by Liberian factions and by profits from blood diamonds, were again pushing west. In the latter months of 1998, many of Port Loko's neighboring districts were coming under fire, as were ECOMOG-controlled corridors stretching from Freetown to the Lungi airfield, across Port Loko District, and on to the border with Guinea. Nonetheless, Kabbah and Nigerian commanders maintained in announcements to a frightened populace that the western part of the country, including Port Loko District, was safe from rebel attacks. But they weren't, especially not after the sobels launched a second assault on Freetown and again began moving through Port Loko on their way to the city.

The people of Bantoro knew they were in peril, and many made preparations to flee into the bush. They were wise to do so, because this time, in October 1998, the rebels did attack. Yabom and her family first realized what was happening on a Wednesday morning, about half an hour after returning from morning prayers in the village mosque. "We heard gunfire," she told us, "but far away. People started arguing. Some said we were under attack; some said we weren't." The imam called them all back to the mosque to confer. The consensus was that the rebels had attacked the town of Mange, the seat of the chiefdom in which Bantoro lay. It was only about five miles away, so a number of young men from the village—including Saidu, two of Yabom's brothers, and one of the imam's sons, their cousin—sneaked along hidden paths to the town to reconnoiter. When the scouts confirmed that Mange was indeed under attack, they rushed home to alert those still sheltered in the mosque or in their homes.

Panic now seized the families of Bantoro. "People were running left and right," Yabom told us. "Some of the men hid close to the village. We fled to our farm in the bush, about a mile away from the house, that same Wednesday morning." Yabom and her relatives knew their refuge was dangerously close to both Mange and Bantoro, but they were faced with a dilemma. "We wanted to flee farther," Yabom said, "but knew we had to eat. There were about fifteen people hiding there. We had rice and other stuff on the farm, but no cooking oil, only unprocessed palm oil. I was cooking alone. We were so scared we didn't even sit together. The old men, older women, and young men went to keep watch."

Chaos now spread across the chiefdom. A substantial contingent of Nigerians was billeted in Port Loko, not much more than ten miles from Mange. When the Nigerians got word of the attack on the town, they rushed to defend it. But by the time they reached Mange, rebel forces had launched an assault on Bantoro. The young men watching from the bush ran to Mange to alert the Nigerians, who then followed them back to the village. The soldiers and scouts ran into trouble on the way. "There were three footpaths to the village," Yabom recounted, "and the boys showed them each trail. The rebels had laid an ambush on the one taken by the imam's son, and he died when he was hit by an RPG. The Nigerians captured the one who fired it, but the others fled. They took him away, but he escaped later, taking one of the girls from our village." It's not clear the imam ever learned of his son's death, since he and his family were killed, the mosque looted and set on fire.

The rebels, who now included openly mutinous soldiers, attacked scores of defenseless villages during that campaign, and for a shifting set of reasons. These included forced recruitment, especially of girls and boys, and looting of cash, food, and what few portable valuables were to be found in such settings. "For our own village," Yabom told us grimly, "they said the purpose was to kill people." They carried through on that threat and then put Bantoro to the torch. By the end of the day, the village was destroyed, and the rebels had either captured or gruesomely murdered many of its inhabitants, including several members of Yabom's and Saidu's extended family.

As smoke rose above Bantoro, survivors of the attack scattered. Some headed west, but Yabom's immediate family—her father, his wives, Kadiatu and her husband, Saidu, one of Yabom's younger brothers, and a passel of kids—headed for a village south of the shifting front lines. Or, as Yabom put it to us, "We ran deeper into the bush."

The first night was a terror. Yabom and her family stumbled through thick undergrowth and trackless fens for much of the night. They tried to sleep for what remained of it, but only the youngest ones managed to do so. At dawn, afraid for their lives, they decided to make their way to Freetown. Because they avoided roads, the journey took them several days. Reaching the capital alive was one thing; finding safe haven there was another. The sobel advance continued, but so did official reassurances that the city was protected. Tens of thousands from Port Loko and other disputed districts had taken President Kabbah and the Nigerians at their word, and Freetown was flooded with refugees, many with stories not unlike Yabom's. She and her family sought news of those who had fled Bantoro by different paths and looked for shelter with kin or friends, trying to avoid the despair of refugee camps already packed with the ill, hungry, and injured.

Even the Bantoro survivors who made it to Freetown together were forced to split up. Yabom and her daughters stayed briefly in Foulah Town with her aunt, who had indeed escaped the first sobel assault. The tiny house on Grant Street was packed to the rafters, so Saidu and a couple of others stayed with relatives in the eastern part of the capital. He'd finally located his father, who—unlike many in Freetown—still had a job. But Saidu didn't feel he could move Yabom and the kids into a house full of people he hardly knew, so he ended up bunking with an uncle who was also related to Yabom. In December, Saidu managed to reunite his family under this kinsman's tin roof.

By that point, roughly a quarter of the Nigerian army, and more than a thousand troops from other West African nations, had been deployed to Sierra Leone. Their remit was to protect civilians and enforce the latest of several broken peace accords; they were scattered across the western districts and the rest of the country. In December the RUF and its sobel helpers launched another assault on the refugee-swollen city. They began by attacking Hastings, which Yabom, Ibrahim, the Chairman, and many others would come to know years later when the national police academy was converted into the country's largest ETU. These attacks continued during the last week of the year, by which time many regretted their choice of refuge. As December gave way to January, some decided to seek safety elsewhere.

Saidu was unsure of what to do next. Six ECOMOG battalions were deployed on the outskirts of the city, but there were gaps in their perimeter, and an attack seemed imminent. His sister suggested that Yabom and her children flee to Wallah, which she described as "an island-like area, almost surrounded by water." (Wallah, known as Tombo Wallah on the map, was in Kambia District, north of Port Loko town and close to Guinea.) It was a wise suggestion, but Yabom was reluctant to split up the family. So she put off making a decision—and then it was too late. Near dawn on January 6, the rebels and sobels launched a major assault on Freetown. They called it Operation No Living Thing, a name that accurately described their plans for the civilians sheltering in the city.

By some estimates, some fifteen thousand rebel and sobel forces poured into the city during Operation No Living Thing. They were met with a counterattack by a similar number of Nigerian troops, and much of eastern Freetown was destroyed. Over the course of more than a year, in many conversations with me and Bailor, Yabom would reveal bits and pieces of her experience of armed conflict—the first of two ordeals she would live through, the second being Ebola in 2014. Hearing about the sack of Bantoro took a toll on Bailor, but he translated dutifully. When Yabom spoke of Operation No Living Thing, however, he would shift uneasily, having lived through it himself. In one session, over an almost untouched meal at the Mammy Yoko, Yabom paused her account and asked him to launch his.

On the night of the attack, Bailor began, he had stayed up late studying anatomy. At about 3:00 a.m., a friend called to let him know that the rebels had reached town. An hour or two later, Bailor began hearing automatic gunfire. "We turned on the radio," he said, "and heard reassurance from the minister of information, saying everyone should remain calm." Meanwhile, a battle was under way not far from where a Nigerian battalion was headquartered. Bailor soon heard alpha jets overhead, scrambled into action by the Nigerians. "They were bombing rebel positions," he said. Yabom broke in to correct him: "They were bombing *everywhere*."

Yabom lived closer to the action during the early days of the assault, so Bailor let her resume the story. "When the rebels entered the city," she said, "they were firing from afar." Saidu woke her up to show her the arcs of tracers. The rebels, they learned, were closing in on a neighborhood close to the wharf and using civilians as human shields. The alpha jets, for their part, "were looking for crowds and bombing them." Much of that neighborhood was destroyed. (Among the material losses were the stall and stock that belonged to their host and uncle.) The besieged government imposed a curfew not long afterward. According to news reports, the minister of information informed those listening to the national radio (or the BBC) that "anyone found on the streets after dark would be shot."[4]

The beleaguered government and its demoralized Nigerian protectors retained the ability to threaten civilians—including those alleged to be RUF sympathizers—but not to protect them. They lacked the means (or the will) to distribute food or water to the civilian population, to say nothing of medical care for the ill or injured. Many deaths occurred when civilians, foraging for food and water, were caught in the cross fire or, as Yabom remembers it, targeted by the rebels. "They would kill people over minor arguments," she told us. The fighting in Freetown raged for three weeks, until at last the attackers ran out of ammunition. When they were finally expelled from the city, they inflicted more death and disfiguration on the way out. "They burned houses and cut off limbs," Yabom told us. "They didn't have enough ammo, so they used machetes and kerosene."

Saidu's father met an awful end during this period, at the hands of a child soldier. He'd been working as a pharmacy assistant and had no work after his shop was looted early in the course of Operation No Living Thing. Like most trapped in the city, he spent days hiding at home. But when a group of rebels turned up in his neighborhood and began demanding money from neighbors who he knew were already destitute, Saidu's father pleaded on their behalf. Whether irritated by his pleas or high or terrified, "a *pikin* no older than twelve shot him, point blank." Yabom told us this part of the story a couple of years after I met her. I hadn't seen her cry in a long time, even during her recounting of the destruction of Bantoro. But she did then. Bailor, who'd witnessed similar scenes, put his face in his hands.

After a long pause, Yabom said, "It made me sick to see kids dragging guns bigger than they were. I love kids. Seeing them used in this way made me cry then, and still does now. It's because the rebels threatened and drugged those kids that they could make them do anything. I don't blame the kids, but the rebels were wicked people."

Operation No Living Thing was beaten back, but it achieved some of its objectives. In Freetown, citizens and refugees alike lived in fear of the sobels' return and in uneasy symbiosis with their demoralized Nigerian protectors. Reports of pitched battles farther east, some of them between sobels and militias loyal to the government, suggested that the RUF had sustained heavy losses. And allegiances break down quickly during a dirty war.

Few in Freetown believed they were safe after the second sack of the city; rumors of an imminent attack circulated incessantly. Like many others, Yabom and her family ended up fleeing to Guinea. But they first sought refuge in island-like Wallah. To make money there, Yabom sold water, and Saidu sold cigarettes and candy, but they found themselves unable to earn enough to feed the family. Then tragedy struck again. Zainab, their younger daughter—unvaccinated, newly weaned, and malnourished—died after a bout of diarrhea. (With no access to medicine or professional health care, untold numbers of other children displaced by the sobels suffered a similar fate during this awful period.) In mourning and still struggling to feed their surviving children, Yabom and Saidu worried that the whole family would starve.

In May, along with a few other young adults, including Kadiatu the elder, they left their children in the care of other family members and returned to Bantoro to see if it was safe to resettle. They found its dwellings deserted, its mosque looted and mostly razed, and their plots of land overgrown. But the land was still arable, so they set up makeshift shelters on the bank of the river and began clearing it by hand. Burning the overgrowth would have been easier, but with bands of rebels were still marauding, they didn't want to send up any telltale signals of smoke. The strategy worked. Without attracting notice, they planted rice and cassava and prepared for the return of the extended family—although they almost starved as they waited for the crops to grow. "We barely survived," Yabom told us. But survive they did.

Eventually, when the rice was almost ready, they summoned the family back to Bantoro. Reunited at last, the survivors struggled to rebuild their homes and their lives. Yabom was soon pregnant again, and she and Saidu decided that the village simply wasn't a safe place for a baby and a nursing mother. So once again she, Saidu, and their children traveled north to Kambia District, near the Guinean border, in search of a safer haven. But Kambia, too, was soon under threat from the rebels. At that point, Yabom and Saidu—like hundreds of thousands of their fellow citizens during this period—decided it was time to flee Sierra Leone altogether. With Yabom heavily pregnant and three children in tow, they crossed the border and made their way to Kalako, a grim refugee camp not far into Guinea. Saidu helped get the family installed there and then headed back to Freetown, hoping to earn some money and return. Yabom gave birth to a baby boy on May 29, 2000.

Another cease-fire was declared, this one to be enforced by UN peacekeepers. Six months later, now with four young children in her care, but without Saidu or her sister to help her, Yabom crossed back into Sierra Leone and made her way to her aunt's place in Foulah Town. She reunited with Saidu soon afterward, and the two of them began pounding what was left of Freetown's pavement, selling new and used clothing, bags, and shoes. After a year or so, as the new peace accords took hold, the couple started growing their own tiny trade network. Life wasn't easy, but they made ends meet. By the end of 2001—with blue-helmeted peacekeepers all over Freetown, and as the dazed residents of the city began to think of work, school, and other matters beyond survival—they managed to rent a place near Yabom's aunt's. It was right above Mountain Cut and offered a bit more space for their children, who now included another boy. There they were often joined by relatives, mostly fellow war refugees from Bantoro and including Yabom's younger brother. Their hillside house was soon as crowded as any other.

The family had its ups and downs in the years that followed. Saidu lost his job and for several years had trouble finding steady work. Yabom continued trading in used clothing and other wares. They welcomed two more children, a boy and a girl. In 2010, Saidu landed a job on a fishing boat and shipped out to sea for months; when he returned, he had enough capital to start working in the brush-stick business. Another baby, a boy, arrived in 2011. During the next three years, and for the first time, the couple had enough money to feed their growing family and to send their children to school. At last, Yabom concluded, the war and their long ordeal was over. Thinking back on that period, she again recalls feeling happy.

Whenever possible, she and Saidu sent money back to the family in Bantoro, who they knew would remember them at harvest time.

Ebola, like the war, met Yabom in the village, even though she and Saidu were in Freetown. The beginning of her second ordeal occurred in July 2014, when Saidu's uncle—the one who had raised him in Bantoro—fell ill with fever, muscle aches, diarrhea, and vomiting. Unable to help as his condition worsened, the family turned to Bantoro's sole surviving traditional healer, but her efforts proved ineffective. Saidu headed to Bantoro in order to take his adoptive father to St. John of God Hospital, in Lunsar. The hospital sits about halfway between Freetown and Makeni, where Bailor Barrie's shattered family was trying to put things back together.

Saidu's uncle at first seemed to get better, an improvement Saidu associated with "a drip" and antibiotics. But he soon went into decline again, and the bills were piling up. In a temporizing measure, Saidu took his uncle to his sister's home in Freetown, where the family did their best to keep him clean and scrambled to find enough money to take him to Connaught or another Freetown hospital. Saidu chipped in for medical fees and helped to nurse him. ("Just like he later did with the children," Yabom added.) But to no avail: his uncle died, prostrate on a soiled mattress, on his third day in Freetown. Before he died, he made his nephew promise that he would take him to Bantoro to be buried with his ancestors.

Saidu and his family now faced the same dilemma that Ibrahim's had, and at about the same time: In the midst of the epidemic, should they honor those wishes? New laws banned such repatriation; formal and informal checkpoints designed to prevent the transport of Ebola victims were springing up along the roads and paths between cities, towns, and hamlets. Some worried villagers were calling to suspend traditional burials to help avoid the spread of the disease or out of fear of the authorities. "But Saidu had promised," Yabom recalled, "and I agreed with him that such promises should be honored." Saidu and his sister and Yabom brought his uncle home on August 6, a few days after the end of Ramadan. He helped to wash and shroud the body, carried it with two relatives to the cemetery, and lowered it into a grave. A new imam from the village's half-rebuilt mosque presided over the ceremony and prayed for the dead.

Saidu and his family returned to Freetown in the days following the funeral; one by one they soon began to fall ill themselves. It started with Saidu's sister, who was taken to Connaught. The hospital was in crisis as Ebola surged through the city. It's not clear why she would not have been tested for Ebola, or, if she was, why her test would have been negative. She'd been sick for days and was not referred, Yabom told us, to a holding center. (The police academy had yet to be transformed into an ETU.) A few days later, Saidu—who nursed his sister, too—started complaining of generalized body pain and a headache;

he had no appetite. "He took some tablets and felt a bit better," Yabom recalled, "so we thought maybe we were okay." But during this period, eight other family members fell ill. Six went on to die, most in hospitals or newly designated holding centers. But Saidu and his sister clung to life.

Something had to be done, and the nature and origins of the siblings' illness would determine what was needed next. Ebola seemed to some members of the family to be the culprit, but not everybody agreed and some entertained more than one explanation for this disastrous unraveling. Several family elders insisted Saidu and his sister suffered from a bad case of "native business." Yabom explained: "One of Saidu's uncles insisted, 'This is not a hospital sickness. The family is cursed, especially the lineage of the old man who died first, so we must get everyone, including Saidu and his sister, back to the village.'"

Yabom's views on this matter seemed to change over time. During many of my interviews with her, I'd had Bailor Barrie with me as a translator. But the first time Yabom told me this part of her story, the two of us were on our own; Bailor had resumed his studies, put on hold by Ebola. By then I could understand a bit of Krio, and Yabom could speak some basic English. In that moment, when the subject of curses came up, she recognized that I was struggling to understand but eager to learn more, so she slowed down to explain, as if to a child. By then, I'd been reading about divination and secret societies for months and had questions of my own.

I started with the obvious. "How do these curses work?" I asked. "Who pronounces them? Why would Saidu's uncle be cursed?"

Yabom responded slowly in English mixed with Krio. "Say, for example," she said, "that someone has lost a fowl to thieves. They could easily go to people to find the name of the thief and others, to punish his family. There is a society they can go to, called *gbom*"—this sounded like "bomp" to me—"in order to answer questions and take revenge."

"Are these *mori* men?" I asked, dropping recently acquired knowledge.

But Yabom was unimpressed. "No," she said. "*Mori* men are diviners. They find out things. The *gbom* people, they don't find out so much as punish. They have a place they go to do the *sweh*."

Generously, she waited until she was confident that I'd grasped that *sweh* was a variant of "swear."

I had. Swears were much discussed in the ethnographic literature on West Africa—an obscure branch of scholarship that had taken on sudden prominence during the Ebola epidemic, after perplexed and frustrated international disease-control authorities began seeking background on "traditions," "superstitions," and "beliefs" new to them.[5] The same terms, it should be added, were used by Sierra Leonean health authorities, some of whom seemed embarrassed by the entire notion of native business. All of us had trouble recalling the contingency of the moment, the weight of the war, and the degree to which rural families had been obliged to cope with illness and death on their own.

Yabom wasn't done with her lesson. Masters of the *gbom* society, she continued, can throw curses and reverse them. "I don't know the words they say exactly," she said, "but something along the lines of, 'This person came to me and said so-and-so has stolen our fowl. If so, I want this *sweh* to go and affect the thief's household.' There are different *sweh*. Some are for the whole family, and some they do for the person who did the act. They do the first type to punish someone dear to the person who took the fowl." In the evolving view of some in Saidu's extended family, the sickness and deaths that had afflicted their kin were the result of a *sweh*, and the person behind it must have cursed Saidu's whole lineage.

Yabom shrugged as she laid out the logic she attributed to family elders. "Sometimes," she said, "those who are victims aren't even aware of the reason for the curse. This is how it's been." Most of Saidu's family, she continued, eventually decided that they were the victims not of a *sweh* but of Ebola, an "ordinary sickness that had come to the village."

I asked Yabom what *she* believed.

"If it was a *sweh*," she said, a year or so after these events, "I don't think it worked, because my own family kept dying."

Why, I persisted, couldn't a curse have caused an ordinary sickness? "Ordinary sickness means it's not caused by man," she said. "Besides, a *sweh* afflicts one family line, but this was two."

I would revisit these questions with Yabom in future conversations. The last time we discussed them, at the Mammy Yoko in the summer of 2016, she made it clear that she was still struggling to account for the great misfortunes that afflicted her family. "I don't know what it was all about," she said. Maybe Ebola had just found them on its own, as ordinary sicknesses do, but Yabom still hadn't ruled out the possibility that she and her extended family were the victims of a vengeful curse. "There's too much wickedness in the world," she said with a shrug.

I never brought the subject up with her again.

During that summer, again at the Mammy Yoko and again during Ramadan, Yabom had finally described to me the most difficult part of her ordeal: the death of Saidu and her children. By that point, we had been meeting on and off for almost two years and had covered much of her story, but she'd never been able to venture into that terrible terrain. It was exceedingly painful for her to talk about, and for me to hear. Bailor Barrie hadn't wanted to hear that story, either. Yabom began it with a sigh.

In August 2014, after several of his relatives had fallen sick and died, Saidu's temporary reprieve came to an end. His symptoms returned, this time accompanied by fever, nausea, and copious diarrhea. Soon he was as sick as his sister. Those of the family left standing, still concerned about the possibility of a curse, decided that they should return to Bantoro to make a last-ditch effort to take care of native business. On Thursday, August 21, Yabom and her siblings found a driver willing to take them home, and made the difficult journey that evening. It was all for naught: gentle, reliable Saidu and his sister both died the next day. "It was then," Yabom said, "that I decided that, yes, we were cursed." Whatever the cause of the sickness, her grief did not drown a deep sense of foreboding. "I knew it was coming for me and the children," she told us.

Yabom was right. A few days after Saidu's death, still in Bantoro, two of their sons fell ill almost simultaneously with much the same symptoms. Once vomiting and diarrhea hit, the boys declined rapidly. Yabom's mother tended to them as Yabom, wracked by muscle pain and nausea, felt her own temperature rise. Her youngest, Hassan, died on September 2; Alpha, born a couple years earlier, died three days later. Nor were others in her extended family spared: during the same week, a niece and a nephew died in Bantoro. (They were also related to Saidu, and number among the eight of his relatives lost that month.) Yabom was despondent and sick and sure that if she didn't leave the village, she would be next. She called her sister Kadiatu—back in Freetown with their younger brother—and begged her to find a way to get her back to the city.

On September 8, Kadiatu and their brother engaged a taxi to collect Yabom in Bantoro. On the return journey, as they neared the outskirts of Freetown, they got caught in the public-health dragnet. Yabom, visibly ill but still able to walk, was ordered to get out of the taxi and wait for an ambulance. Inside a tent by the side of the road, she was offered oral rehydration salts but was unable to keep them down. Kadiatu stayed at the roadblock, outside the tent, while their brother went home to scrounge cash. Only if they could offer it to those manning the roadblock, they were sure, would anybody move Yabom anywhere. Sure enough, no ambulance had yet arrived when her brother returned almost thirteen hours later, in yet another rented vehicle.

Yabom was no longer vomiting and didn't have a fever. Angrily, her brother demanded he be allowed to take Yabom home. "This is unacceptable," he'd said with some heat. "You can't hold her here without anything to offer her!" The authorities at the roadblock gave in, on the condition that Yabom's brother leave them his address in Freetown. If she were indeed sick with Ebola, all of them would be counted as contacts and isolated. At seven the next morning, an official of some sort showed up at the house looking for Yabom and her contacts. Kadiatu and her brother chose not to tell him that she was there, at which point the contact tracer began announcing loudly to everyone in the crowded household, and anyone else within earshot beyond it, that Yabom had Ebola. This was an educated guess, since she hadn't been tested. But it put fear into the hearts of the neighbors, who soon ringed the house and started yelling at Kadiatu and her brother—an example of contact tracing as it was often practiced in Sierra Leone in 2014.

Yabom's siblings had already decided to take her to Connaught. Unnerved by the hostility of their neighbors, they left with her for the hospital as soon as they shook the official. After two days on the women's ward, Yabom, now confirmed to have a fever and once again vomiting, was seen by a harried Marta Lado, who wore full protective gear while examining her. Lado, whose kindness Yabom recalled well, had her transferred to the in-house holding center I'd visited in late June—a place of terrible suffering but one that, thanks to Lado and her dedicated colleagues, saved many lives and prevented many new infections.

Yabom's ordeal, however, was far from over. The staff at the holding center soon confirmed that she had Ebola and decided to transfer her, along with three others newly diagnosed with the disease, to Hastings. "By the time we arrived," Yabom recalled, "it was night. There was no one there to attend to us." The four of them then had to wait for more than an hour inside a vehicle reeking of vomit and liquid stool. When at last they were admitted, they discovered that the electricity had gone out in the ward. None of the patients received any therapy or nursing care that night; an aide instructed them to self-administer oral rehydration salts. The following morning, the newly admitted patients were finally seen by staff, including a physician who prescribed intravenous fluids and a cocktail of antibiotics and antimalarial medication. At the time, Yabom had no appetite at all and turned down all offers of food. "It was the drip," she believed, "that kept me alive during those first days."

As protocol dictated, the staff confiscated her phone and dropped it in chlorine solution. From that point on, she was in isolation, the primary and sometimes sole purpose of most ETUs in Africa. During her stay, Yabom had no contact whatsoever with her family or anyone else. Instead, on her own and still gravely ill, she often lay awake, torn between grief and disbelief. Were her beloved boys and steadfast Saidu really gone? Had this really happened? How? Why? She felt as if she had nothing left to lose. Gradually, as she received a bit more of the care she needed, and as her immune system cleared the virus, her symptoms subsided. With her improvement came a new and gnawing anxiety. What had become of the rest of her family?

Yabom found out on October 5, when, after testing negative for Ebola, she was discharged and sent home. Her jewelry was returned, but her chlorine-marinated phone was useless. Upon reaching Mountain Cut, she found her sister

Kadiatu and her younger brother alive and well, but they had awful news to report. While Yabom had been at Hastings, Ebola had taken their mother.

When Bailor and I first met her on Mountain Cut, just days after her release from Hastings, Yabom was gaunt and felt dizzy upon standing. Although fever, nausea, and diarrhea were behind her, she had headaches and felt "sore all over." These symptoms lasted for another week or so, and a generalized weakness persisted for well over a month. During this period, as she came back to life only to have to reckon with the enormity of her losses, depression took hold. She didn't feel like talking and ventured no farther than her stoop. Her eldest, Kadiatu, begged to come home and cook for her. But she was expecting a child of her own, and Yabom forbade it.

Things started to turn around in January. By then, Yabom had put on some weight, and her depression was lifting. She attributed her improvement to the work she'd started to do with children orphaned by Ebola—work that had been arranged for her through the expanding survivors' program started by Partners In Health, which was at this point increasingly run by the ex-patients themselves. Whether at work or at home, Yabom always seemed to be surrounded by a clutch of small kids, one or two of them clinging to the hem of her dress. Some of the younger Ebola survivors she met in Hastings— among them the cheerful teenager at her side on the day we met her, but also Ibrahim and the Chairman, who was then only twenty-two—were also drawn to her den-mother vibe.

Yabom's daughter gave birth to a baby in late January, and she brought the baby to Foulah Town for an extended stay. This cheered her, she said, as much as anything else. But Yabom's trials weren't yet over. Ever since December, it turned out, Yabom had been experiencing clouded vision in her right eye—or, as she put it to me, in language that even I could understand, "Me begin see smoke wit mi eye." By February, she could barely see out of the eye and it turned out that she already had extremely limited vision in the other, because of a cataract problem that surgery had failed to correct. Now Yabom was at risk of blindness. How had we missed this? In part, because we were all still focused on the immediate symptoms of Ebola rather than its sequelae. But as the epidemic died down and survivors began to contend with the disease's aftermath, we saw an epidemic of blindness sweep through their ranks and knew we'd been slow to address it.

Thanks in no small measure to the efforts of Ian Crozier—who, in the fall, as American Patient Four, had almost gone blind himself—Partners In Health already had volunteer clinicians screening and treating patients for visual loss in Lunsar, the town where Yabom's Ebola ordeal began. So in mid-March, partly to assuage a guilty conscience, I took Yabom there myself. After examining her carefully, the staff prescribed a regimen of steroid and atropine eye drops and a short course of oral steroids—a regimen that, using generic medications, cost just a couple of dollars. Yabom rapidly regained sight in her right eye and continued her return to good health. Soon the survivors' program found her a job as caretaker at the Observational Interim Care Center, where she was able to mother eighty-four kids orphaned by Ebola. Since "interim" means what it does, Bailor Barrie and those running the survivors' program subsequently helped her find related work in a center that provided care to runaways and abandoned children, up to seventy of them at a time.

Working at the center became a passion for Yabom—so much so that, a few months after starting that job, she opened her own home up to a thirteen-year-old runaway. Still hopeful about the future even after surviving her two ordeals, Yabom invited her to stay.

DOWN THE RABBIT HOLE

We can only understand the present by continually recurring to and studying that past; when any one of the intricate phenomena of our daily life puzzles us; when there arise religious problems, political problems, race problems, we must always remember that while their solution lies in the present, their cause and their explanation lie in the past.

—W.E.B. Du Bois, "The Beginning of Slavery," *The Voice of the Negro*, 1905

THREE MONTHS AFTER MY FIRST STEPS ON SIERRA LEONEAN SOIL, AFTER A tardy return with reinforcements, I was shuttling between Boston and places like Port Loko, Maforki, Freetown, Koidu, Monrovia, and Harper. Each of these places—like every village and household, and each person who belongs to one of those—has a history.

These are usually unknown to the newly arrived and were to me. Yet it wasn't possible to sit still long enough to become familiar with people or places in the manner congenial to anthropologists and physicians. While many coworkers stayed put to join new colleagues from Sierra Leone and Liberia in order to care for the sick, it was my charge to beat the bushes for the staff and stuff required for safer and more effective clinical care, and to sound the alarm in places with a relative surplus of these ingredients. But as airlines shut down routes to the region, and as the logic of containment hardened, getting in and out of this part of West Africa was easier said than done.

By the fall of 2014, Americans were largely restricted to reentry via a handful of East Coast airports; fear and unfriendly public opinion greeted clinicians and others upon return. (If Donald Trump had had his way, American Ebola responders wouldn't have been allowed back home at all.) Quarantine and reporting requirements shaped by the whims of state governors, and by a surge of politically stoked fears of contagion, were heaviest at the height of Ebola's real surge, which occurred only in Guinea, Liberia, and Sierra Leone. Despite any inconvenience we experienced, we knew that West African passengers had it much worse, lessening any appetite for public complaint among our ranks. Privately, we fumed.

This tumult and conflict waxed during the last months of 2014. In mid-November, on the day of Martin Salia's death—announced to me on television screens throughout Boston's Logan International Airport—I headed back to Sierra Leone, where the real peril lay. The number of new Ebola cases there continued to rise, but so had, finally, the number of clinicians seeking to save the sick. One Partners In Health volunteer on the scene was a French nurse based in Seattle. I'd last seen her in early October, in the eastern Liberian town of Zwedru, as Ebola headed west to Monrovia. (Zwedru had been termed "Ebola-free" by local authorities, but it was also lab-free. So who was to know?) My friend was in high demand in French-speaking Guinea, but we were glad she came and stayed put in Port Loko, where everyone called her Frenchie. "Do you remember?" she asked by e-mail exactly a year later. "Bodies dumped in the triage zone, half-dead, dead. By the ambulance-load."

Of course I remembered. We were surely both thinking of one awful day at Maforki, where we stood in the scant shade of a mango tree as the stricken reached the triage area she and others had organized in the ruins of a bakery, once part of a vocational school for demobilized combatants. A month earlier, the school's disintegrating remains had been designated as an Ebola treatment unit. But the sick and dying arrived before the staff and stuff did, and Maforki reeked like a battlefield. By late November, it stank of chlorine, imperfectly masking the smell of death. This was progress, as was a new whiteboard in the bakery-turned-triage unit—a rare sign of optimism in part because it recorded the names and ages of the patients ready for discharge home or to Port Loko Government Hospital. An on-call schedule was laid out on the board, which further proclaimed the staff "the most awesome team." If the sting of chlorine meant more dead virus, the schedule meant there was now electricity at night and that Maforki's awesome team included short-term volunteer clinicians, most of them expatriates, who'd joined dozens of chlorine sprayers, cleaners, and nursing assistants, all Sierra Leonean.

Any elation over improvements was fleeting. Within an hour of my arrival, several members of that team stood at rigid attention as an ambulance pulled up. Its back doors slowly opened from inside, revealing two dead passengers. Watching a twelve- or thirteen-year-old girl extract herself from the vehicle and wobble across the chlorine-scorched courtyard was enough to break anyone's heart. An elderly man made it out to collapse into a wheelchair but didn't stir again; I wondered if he might be related to the girl, who didn't look back as she stumbled toward a cot inside the ETU. Those tasked with running the unit witnessed such dramas several times a week during the following month.

The scene at Port Loko's hospital, where another nursing assistant had just been diagnosed with Ebola, wasn't much more heartening. Many of the sickest in Maforki had been diagnosed and referred from the hospital, a late stop on a long or last pilgrimage if the afflicted hailed from rural areas far from the town. That they'd reached it at all was a miracle, if too rarely the one they needed: dessicated by days of fever, vomiting, and diarrhea, they came to resemble one another in their extremity. The professional caregivers, who hailed from a half dozen countries, also looked alike in their standard-issue light-blue or yellow masks and gowns, rubber boots, and plastic face shields. Their tasks resembled those required in any other makeshift structure full of the sick and dying in any other medical desert. A heady stench of sickness, chlorine, and an intravenous solution called lactated Ringer's—which triggered in many of us involuntary memories of Haiti's runaway cholera epidemic—was familiar and everywhere.

The one unexpected comic moment in Port Loko came during a Thanksgiving meal, when the ceiling over an impressive spread started to collapse with a loud crack. About the only thing I could give thanks for just then was the chance of working with people like my French colleague and the Sierra Leoneans, Haitians, and Americans holding down the decrepit fort of Maforki and helping to keep the hospital open.

Meanwhile, the people of Port Loko were living their own particular hell. Three incidents that week—the week during which I met Ibrahim Kamara and six weeks after I'd met Yabom Koroma, both of them from that district— stiffened my resolve to learn more about the region's history. All three incidents were unremarkable, but they stuck with me.

The first occurred on November 19 in the small village of Matweng, not far from the town of Port Loko. Relatives of an Ebola casualty attacked one of the District Ebola Response Centre's burial teams during a dispute regarding whether they could pray over their kinsman at home, where he still lay hours after his last breath. The young man's nearest relatives hadn't yet arrived because of roadblocks and travel restrictions, and those keeping vigil at the house refused to hand him over to the cloaked and masked burial team until all had gathered. The family voiced suspicions of plots to abscond with the body to some "imaginary place" for nefarious purposes. I heard these details a couple of days later during a daily briefing at the DERC, which had been hastily organized in the offices of Port Loko's health department. The story was reported as an aside, with weary shrugs from the authorities present about "native business."

There were, in the half-mast eyes of those gathered that morning, far graver problems to consider. Sunk into sofas covered with frayed fabric of leopard-skin design, most of the Ebola responders were too tired to muster visible concern. Perhaps they knew no one had been harmed. The bereaved in Matweng had contented themselves with throwing rocks at the burial vehicle, which had (by the standards of the day) arrived fairly promptly. The matter had been referred to the paramount chief and to local police. Similar incidents had occurred across the region since the start of the outbreak, and that would have been my last consideration of the Matweng matter if we hadn't listened to the news on the way back to Freetown late that night.[1]

The newscast and the long drive furnished the second incident. As during the war, getting from Port Loko to the capital entailed negotiating roadblocks and checkpoints; once again, these were manned by people in uniform and by young helpers. Guns were in evidence, though less numerous than the omnipresent thermometer: those at the barricades were now searching for fevers, rather than weapons, loot, or signs of partisan affiliation. Still, it was a tense drive in the dark, and I imagined coworkers present during the war must have experienced it as a flashback. About half the passengers in our two-jeep convoy had known the war; most (with the exception of Jon Lascher) had been refugees.

For varied reasons, none of us was in the mood for small talk. To forestall it, I turned on the radio. After a bit of fiddling with the dial for something in English or French, I happened upon a local news program. It was all Ebola, all the time. The announcer reported that, across the nation, more than five hundred new cases had been confirmed during the previous week, surpassing all previous records. What's more, the district of Port Loko had reported more cases than any other outside of Freetown—just then the most Ebola-stricken city on the planet, having edged out Monrovia by mid-October.

This news didn't improve the mood in the jeep, where silence reigned as the announcer went on. As during the DERC meeting that morning, national officials and international health authorities continued to complain of being hampered by "native superstition," including the attribution of Ebola to witchcraft, which the newsreader equated with the belief that "Ebola is not real." Across West Africa, significant resources had been invested in erecting billboards declaring as much: "Ebola is real" was second only to the exhortation to abstain from bushmeat (and any congress with monkeys or bats) in public-service announcements, billboards, and murals conceived by consultants and paid for largely by international donors.

Granted, such notions may have been more widespread than American beliefs that vaccines cause autism, and it would be hard to point to a single named and sanctioned Ebola outbreak during which similar commentary wasn't registered.[2] But after what I'd just seen, heard, and smelled, it was hard to believe that these messages merited, just then, such lavish investment.

None of the dead or dying I'd seen that week had contracted Ebola because they doubted its reality or ate bushmeat. What Ebola-afflicted families then doubted most was the availability of real medical care—or of help burying their dead in keeping with cherished traditions.

I turned to the man at the wheel, Alex Jalloh. We'd shared many private conversations since, unlike fellow passengers other than the Haiti-hand Jon Lascher, we both spoke French. I pointed to the radio dial. "What do you make of that?" Jalloh knew what I meant and why I'd asked in that language. He'd been at the DERC that morning, but I wasn't sure if he'd heard about the Matweng matter. (He had.) "It's true that people are superstitious," he replied cautiously. "That's why they didn't want to put the body in the burial car." Suddenly, "the burial car" seemed more sinister than a vehicle sent to help bereaved families by safely burying their highly infectious dead. Another pause as Jalloh gauged my response. "Then they disappear the body," he continued, "and you don't know where to, maybe a city far away. No one can recognize them behind their masks." He then added, "It is like witchcraft." Jalloh hesitated once more before adding, with a sidelong glance my way, "In *their* minds."

This second "their" was in sympathetic reference to the bereaved. I decided not to pursue the matter, since Jalloh seemed mildly embarrassed, but I hoped to read more about such understandings upon reaching the privacy of the Mammy Yoko. The hotel was where the third incident occurred, a predawn phone call. It was the front desk calling to say that someone was awaiting me in the lobby. Groggy, I asked if the caller was an American coworker from Partners In Health or a Liberian. "I'm not sure," came the polite Sierra Leonean reply. "I didn't ask to see a passport." The rehabbed Mammy Yoko looked nothing like my previous lodgings in Monrovia, and my disorientated assumption that I was in Liberia must have been evident to the receptionist. But the blurring of national identity was due less to sleep deprivation than to growing appreciation of the historical antecedents common across this part of West Africa.

The Mammy Yoko Hotel was where I'd first read about the connections between Kono's diamond mines and civil war in both Liberia and Sierra

Leone. It's where I read about war's impact on Guinea, and about the co-lonial occupation of West Africa and the rise of Islam across the region well before the Europeans' arrival. The hotel was one of the places where I read about hemorrhagic fevers elsewhere in Africa, but not so far away, as the bat flies, from the rain forest that still cloaked part of all three nations—including the Upper Guinean forest, where Ebola's spillover event from animals to hu-mans was held to have occurred. This forest once subsumed the Gola Forest, where diamonds erupted from the earth and from which the recent war was launched. The more I read, the more I was overwhelmed by stories of violent conflict, recurrent epidemic disease, and rapacious extraction of rubber latex, timber, minerals, gold, and diamonds—not to mention human chattel. These stories were integral to the process of Upper West Africa's becoming a clinical desert. Liberia and Sierra Leone and Guinea were in this regard as similar as the gaunt and drawn patients—"almost skeletal" is one way of saying "almost the same"—we'd seen that week in Maforki and in Port Loko's hospital.

Of course, every generalization risks washing away the messy details of social life and social history, and should be corrected by the specificity of historical and ethnographic accounts and informed by the lived experience and clinical condition of the sick. But with Ebola, even the standardized and tidied data were being curtailed: openly and unselfconsciously qual-ified, in weekly updates from national and international health authorities, as "cleaned," "scrubbed," or "censored." (Much of this process of sanitation was performed by professionals once termed sanitarians.) As it dawned on me, telephone receiver in hand, that I'd confused Sierra Leone with Liberia in the pitch dark, it was clear I wasn't trying hard enough to link clinical knowledge, so often standard and standardized, to the personally and cul-turally specific.

Part of my personal penance for inaction between July and September, by which time Humarr Khan and thousands of others in need of reinforce-ments were dead and buried, was to learn more about the personal histories of the Ebola dead, of survivors, and of their caregivers. We sometimes speak of history from below.[3] But what I needed was more like history from next door—more information about what had brought the entire region to this pass. The next four chapters are meant to make amends for my ignorance. Even at four in the morning, it's not right to mix up Liberia and Sierra Leone.

On the face of it, the three most Ebola-affected nations are countries with markedly different (if equally dark) histories. Former colonies of France and Britain shouldn't be confused with one another, or with Africa's oldest independent republic, even if all three are home to the same blended "tribes"— Mende, Temne, Sherbro, Kuranko, Kpelle, Mandingo, Gola, Grebo, Fula, Susu, Krahn, Kru, Vai, and many others—and smaller, influential populations of coastal Creoles and Lebanese.

Or should we say Guinea and Sierra Leone are predominantly Muslim countries and Liberia a largely Christian one? Two countries rent by civil war and one ostensibly spared such strife? Two third-world countries long integrated into the mercantilist-then-capitalist world (exporting unpaid labor, as well as precious metals and raw materials) and one later integrated, at least in principle, into what was not long ago termed a second world, shielded by an Iron Curtain but engaged in similar traffic? Or might we better consider them as lands similar in being rich in the same kinds of natural resources and inhabited by people who rarely enjoy the vast profits derived from them?

Each of these formulations is too pat. Any stab at understanding what shapes epidemics and social responses to them leads back to a vast range of contributing causes. No one could argue with the assertion of the anthropologist Paul Richards and colleagues about Ebola in this part of West Africa: "If human-to-human contact is the main mode of transmission, attention needs to be paid to underlying social factors."[4] These factors include, as the experiences of Ibrahim and Yabom suggest, extreme economic and physical insecurity and the absence of anything resembling an effective health-care system, capped by the effects of civil war. Assaults on survival began well before that conflict, which flooded Guinea with refugees and shredded its fragile safety net.

Across West Africa, weak health systems are a legacy of colonial rule, which, promises and propaganda aside, knew few successes in public health—

and almost none in providing medical care for the natives. The dominant development and humanitarian paradigms now generating endless acronyms, and buzzwords like "resilience" and "sustainability," have similar origins. So does the near-exclusive focus on disease control rather than care, evident throughout the Ebola epidemic. In the West African nations that were once European colonies, attention to underlying social factors takes us back before independence in the mid-twentieth century—back at least to 1884, when European powers formalized their scramble for Africa by carving it into pieces.

In Liberia, never a European colony but suddenly hemmed in by them, Ebola's spread was hastened by the same social factors. Fevers, feuds, and diamonds moved freely across its borders, and its civil war sparked Sierra Leone's. But even before the latter began, Liberian refugees streamed into Guinea's forest districts, where they sometimes outnumbered citizens. Weapons from across the world poured into Liberia, as did armed factions from Guinea and, later, Sierra Leone. Some of them consisted largely of resentful "Mandingo traders" denied Liberian nationality on the grounds that they weren't native to Liberia, even though they'd lived there and athwart its borders for generations.

Nor can it be honestly argued that Liberia was spared the taint of colonialism. The chief reason for long U.S. dominance in Liberia is that seaboard settlements like Monrovia and Buchanan and Harper were, as their names suggest, founded by Americans. Liberia's American settlers may have been of African descent, but they shared many of the views and tactics of European colonists, including those who settled North America. The Americo-Liberians, famously anti-indigenous, were as hostile to imperial Britain as George Washington et al. When European powers squeezed Liberia a century before Ebola did, Monrovia sought U.S. protection against expansionist Britain and France—all the while continuing to subdue the unruly natives who dared to resist its civilizing mission. Like its neighboring countries, Liberia was drawn into two world wars, since the combatants needed labor, timber, coal, iron ore and other minerals, and rubber latex.

Especially latex. In 1926, in an effort to break Britain's rubber monopoly, the Firestone Tire and Rubber Company—Ford Motor Company's chief source of tires—negotiated a ninety-nine-year, million-acre concession in Liberia at six cents an acre. By World War II, there was probably a little bit of Liberian forest in many, if not most, American automobiles. If there weren't a lot of U.S. dollars in the pockets of those who planted, tended, or tapped rubber trees, the dominant Americo-Liberians did not view this as a problem: their pockets were lined, they weren't the ones doing the work, and prevalent conditions meant that Firestone's pittance was more than what had been available to most of the natives, who were forced to pay British-style "hut taxes" in cash. Thus was independent Liberia shaped by far-away colonial capitals, and even more so by the United States—for close to two centuries its ambivalent midwife and inconstant patron.

A similar ambivalence marked Britain's ties to Sierra Leone. At the start of the industrial revolution, when slavery in the Americas was first challenged by activists not themselves in fetters, Freetown and Monrovia were established as experiments, indeed as formal arguments against slavery, the transatlantic slave trade, and—for a while and in theory—white rule over black subjects. Both outposts claimed to promote "legitimate trade." As palm oil lubricated the gears of European industry, Palmolive and other soaps of West African origin kept its workers clean. Meanwhile, as in French Guinea, colonial authorities pushed farmers to plant groundnuts, coffee, cacao, cotton, and other export-ready tropical produce. But the slave trades, Atlantic and local, did not end with European declarations of abolition. Throughout the twentieth century, and until civil wars ended in this one, allegedly legitimate commodity production in West Africa often relied on serfdom or outright slavery.

Armed conflict and forced labor are among the causes of the causes that rolled out the red carpet for rapid human-to-human spread of Ebola in Upper West Africa. These wars weren't fought, nor labor forced, for strictly local gain. An understanding of today's West African epidemics, and social responses to them, requires consideration of the region's integration into an economic web spanning the Atlantic Ocean and linking four continents in a suffocating and interminable embrace. The narrative history that follows seeks to chart West Africa's thorough integration into a global economy of extraction, highlighting—in the interest of illuminating developments of relevance to its Ebola epidemic—regular outbreaks of epidemic disease, the extractive trades, conflict, and outright war.

If you want to understand the magnitude and dynamics of this Ebola epidemic, in other words, think in terms of fevers, feuds, and diamonds.

PART II

FEVERS, FEUDS, AND DIAMONDS

Until the very recent penetration by Europe the greater part of the continent was without the wheel, the plough or the transport-animal; almost without stone houses or clothes, except for skins; without writing and so without history.

—Margery Perham, "The British Problem in Africa," *Foreign Affairs*, 1951

If you should penetrate the campus of an American Ivy League college and, challenging a Senior, ask what, in his opinion, was the influence of Africa on the French Revolution, he would answer in surprise if not pity, "None." If, after due apology, you ventured to approach his teacher of "historiography," provided such sacrilege were possible, you would be told that between African slavery in America and the greatest revolution of Europe, there was of course some connection, since both took place on the same earth; but nothing causal, nothing of real importance, since Africans have no history.

—W.E.B. Du Bois, "Africa and the French Revolution," *Freedomways*, 1961

The legacies of the trans-Atlantic slave trade, colonialism and structural adjustment programs have helped to shape the political, social and economic environment in which Ebola thrives as much as they shape the response to the crisis itself.

—Adia Benton and Kim Yi Dionne, *The Washington Post*, 2015

5.

The Upper Guinea Coast and the World the Slaves Made

Historians cannot speak of the history of modern slavery and emancipation without recognizing the complexity and centrality of Sierra Leone and Liberia.

—Nemata Amelia Blyden, "'Back to Africa': The Migration of New World Blacks to Sierra Leone and Liberia," *OAH Magazine of History,* 2004

Stolen bodies working stolen land. It was an engine that did not stop, its hungry boiler fed with blood.

—Colson Whitehead, *The Underground Railroad,* 2016

HOW DID WEST AFRICA BECOME A CLINICAL DESERT—A PLACE IN WHICH the rapid human-to-human spread of Ebola was not just possible but almost inevitable? The answer begins centuries ago, when pathogens and pathogenic forces were linked to a worldwide web of maritime commerce that bound expansionist European economies to the Americas and Africa. This web began to take shape in the mid-fifteenth century, when Portuguese explorers and traders gave Port Loko, and indeed Sierra Leone and much of the Upper Guinea Coast, their names. The result would be violent conflict, recurrent disease, and rapacious extraction—of rubber latex, timber, minerals, gold, diamonds, and human chattel.

European sovereigns first sponsored maritime explorers of the African coast in order to dominate intercontinental trade, which continued to grow as new Atlantic networks complemented trans-Saharan trade. Trade routes spanned that sea of sand, as the widespread use of cowrie currency—the shells were from the Maldives, in the Indian Ocean—suggests. In the estuary that would later berth the port of Freetown, Iberian mariners found a deep harbor and a readily accessible source of fresh water. But they didn't discover, as they claimed to in Brazil, vast and thinly settled regions: West Africa, and especially its northern interior, was long settled when the Europeans arrived. Along the Niger River, which cuts across West Africa in a mighty arc, large towns and far-reaching trade networks had flourished for centuries by the time the Portuguese came calling. By the fourteenth century, the Niger Bend boasted several cities—Timbuktu, Gao, Niani, and Djenné—that were likely larger and more prosperous than Lisbon was at the time.

Most towns and cities along the Niger were then under Muslim rule. Medieval Islam was at least as technologically and militarily advanced as the avowedly Christian and ever-feuding states of Europe. In coastal West Africa south of the Muslim strongholds, the Iberians found metallurgy and textiles that could more than rival theirs. (Some wondered if the exquisite bronzes from Benin and the Ivory Coast might have been the work of the master craftsmen of ancient Greece.) Because they stretched along an inland delta, towns and cities along the Niger Bend were initially shielded from European attention, but they were further shielded because many West African sovereigns of the era had big armies. For example, the Songhai empire—which at its height stretched across much of the Niger's 2,500-mile course—had a standing force of up to 200,000 men by the time the Portuguese began trading along the coast. These garrisons guarded the towns and trade networks under their sway, exacting tribute within and beyond shifting borders.

Although horses and camels never flourished in the tropics, in part because of pestilence carried by tsetse flies, imperial forces from the Sahel and the savannah also turned south toward West Africa. The most significant of these southward population movements have been termed the "Mane invasions," which Portuguese sources date to about 1540.[1] They led to a gradual process of conquest and integration through marriage, acquisition of new languages and customs, and the spread of Islam. This process was slower where forests were drenched with up to two hundred inches of rainfall a year. It was in such hostile environments that the residents of littoral and inland regions had long carved rice paddies out of mangrove swamps, fields, and forests—a formidable technical achievement relying on farming techniques different from those common in Asia.

Unlike the African invaders from the north, the Europeans who traveled to West Africa weren't out to assimilate, win converts, or grow rice. They were after a perch on the region then supplying the majority of the world's gold, and they knew that a foothold on the Gold Coast might enable them to break a Muslim monopoly on supplies of the metals that were then the basis of many European trading currencies. And there were many other treasures to covet. A Portuguese official, writing in the late 1530s, compared his native land with societies he encountered inland of the Upper Guinea Coast:

> I do not know in this Kingdom any yoke of land, toll, tithe, excise or
> any other royal tax which is more certain in each yearly return than
> is the revenue of the commerce of Guiné . . . It is, besides, so peaceful
> a property, quiet and obedient, that—without our having to stand at
> the touch-hole of the bombard with lighted match in one hand, and
> lance in the other—it yields us gold, ivory, wax, hides, sugar, pepper,
> and it would produce other returns if we sought to explore it further.[2]

They did seek to explore it further. Thanks in part to reports home from merchant-traders who ventured inland, the gears of covetous European expansionism were set in motion.

Once established along the coast, the Portuguese, and soon Europeans from other coastal nations, looked north and east toward the great mud-walled cities and giant mosques of the Niger Bend. Commerce and taxes—and surpluses of rice, sorghum, and millet—had permitted the emergence of powerful chiefdoms across this part of West Africa. They contested each other from the stockaded towns and walled cities in which crops, trade goods, and treasures could be stored and citizens and subjects shielded from marauders. Europeans who wished only to trade didn't fall under this category. But it didn't take West African sovereigns long to detect gold-lust among the new-comers, and to learn that many of them were also after free labor. Within a few decades of the 1471 arrival of Portuguese ships on the Gold Coast, writes one of its best historians, "the basic nature of the next three hundred years of contact between West Africa and Europe had been established: commerce in gold and slaves."[3]

By the good offices or acquiescence of the Atlantic, this traffic quickly bound together four continents. In Africa, these binds remained largely coastal. Hardy Iberian agents of maritime commerce dominated African shipping lanes for over a century, until they were contested by French and British traders, who fought them—and each other—for hegemony over the Atlantic trade with Africa and in Africans. The Dutch, Swedes, and Danes also joined the contest, which dragged in its wake all manner of private and state-backed profiteers. Inland incursion was resisted by political and religious leaders, overlapping groups in West Africa as in Europe. But would-be invaders found themselves repulsed by unseen forces more deadly than anything the Africans might design. "West Africa's most effective defense against Europeans was disease," explains another eminent chronicler of the era: "blackwater fever, yellow fever, breakbone fever, bloody flux, and a whole zoo of helminthic parasites."[4]

Growing rice, then as now Upper West Africa's staple, required water, much of it slow-moving, stagnant, or rolled by brackish tides into estuaries and lagoons. Europeans entered these swamps and forests, dotted with hidden fens and marshes, at their peril. It didn't take them long to learn it, as the words of the previously cited sixteenth-century Portuguese official suggest:

It seems that for our sins, or for some inscrutable judgment of God, in all the entrances of this great Ethiopia that we navigate along, He has placed a striking angel with a flaming sword of deadly fevers, who prevents us from penetrating into the interior to the springs of this garden, whence proceed these rivers of gold that flow to the sea in so many parts of our conquest.[5]

The flaming sword of deadly fevers, regardless of who or what wielded it, would prove important across a world now linked, rather than divided, by the Atlantic. But events following the rise of transatlantic trade transpired differently on either side of the ocean.

Within a century of first contact, the empires of Central America and the Andes, like the indigenous people of the Caribbean before them, had fallen or were falling. Indigenous populations had been reduced by as much as 90 percent; Haiti's natives, some of Columbus's earliest and most welcoming hosts, were completely obliterated by the mid-seventeenth century. How this happened has been the subject of brisk, centuries-long debate. A series of "virgin-soil hypotheses" attribute the great American die-off largely or solely to a lack of immunity to Old World pathogens, including smallpox, measles, yellow fever, influenza, and leptospirosis.[6] But much more than susceptibility to unfamiliar pestilence was at play. Europeans introduced steel weapons, armor, and guns to the equation. Although disease, warfare, siege, and famine abounded before European arrival, the newcomers intensified them by appropriating land, conscripting native inhabitants to work farms and mines on that land, and then making off with the wealth extracted from those places.

Epidemic disease sometimes preceded the colonists, setting the stage for such improbable events as those reported from the heart of the Incan empire, whose rulers were as warlike as any Iberian conquistador. Shaken by civil strife after smallpox felled the emperor just prior to the arrival of Francisco Pizarro, a newly deified replacement saw his vast army routed by the conquistadors' tiny cavalry. (Horses, which Jared Diamond terms "military assault vehicles," were also new to the Americas.)[7] Pestilence accompanying the avant-garde sometimes rendered the need for force unnecessary. In 1620, the Pilgrims founded Plymouth on the ruins of the Wampanoag settlement of Patuxet, a site abandoned in the aftermath of European raids and an epidemic

that had struck the Massachusetts coast a few years previously. But more often the greatest waves of mortality were registered long after first contact, and
their height depended on the severity of the ensuing disruptions imposed by
colonial regimes. Time and time again, the severest mortality struck years,
even decades, after European arrival, and almost always in the setting of sustained and conflictual contact.[8]

This was not, in other words, a history of inevitable mortality that resulted from ancient evolutionary forces, nor one of people born vulnerable
to European pathogens. It was the contingent history of a population made
vulnerable.[9]

In the face of indigenous collapse, Europeans in the Americas looked
to Africa for a supply of laborers to clear forests, work mines and plantations,
and transport and load the loot destined for Europe. By the 1520s, enslaved
Africans were being forced to help the Spanish and Portuguese grow sugar
in Haiti and Brazil, respectively. Many more Africans were dispatched to the
Caribbean coasts of South America, Mexico, and Peru. The Spanish had
even brought slaves to help them establish an outpost in what is today South
Carolina, although those Africans launched a rebellion that ended Spanish
plans for the neighborhood, ultimately opening it up to British traders and
settlers.[10]

The Iberian conquest of the Americas took decades, and the slave trade
grew as it advanced. But it was a complex, global web spun by British and
French concerns as well as Spanish and Portuguese ones. After 1570, to give
an example offered by the historian Patrick Manning, "Europeans used Mex-
ican silver to purchase textiles in India and cowries in the Maldives. These
commodities, after passing through Europe, went to West Africa in exchange
for slaves; some of the slaves became mine workers in the Americas."[11] When
the British began settling North America, in the first half of the seventeenth
century, they initially enslaved members of indigenous populations, but
those populations dwindled fast. At the end of the century, the Great Southeastern Smallpox Epidemic struck, hastening their decline. Subsequent wars
with the British all but finished them off.[12]

As slavery and serfdom began to loom large in the American colonies,

West Africa began to be brought slowly and reluctantly into what had been termed the "Atlantic world system." It was largely created for the benefit of Europeans, and by the middle of the seventeenth century, large numbers of their ships were prowling the estuaries, lagoons, and rivers of West Africa— waterways that the historian Walter Rodney has termed "the *autobahnen* of the Upper Guinea Coast." These waterways had sustained a complex rice economy and inland trade between coast and forest, and north toward the middle Niger and the western Sudan, but now increasingly were exploited by the Spanish and the Portuguese.

Part of the early Portuguese and Spanish dominance of the Atlantic world can be attributed to what would be today called their business plan, which was to focus their commercial ventures on acquiring free labor. But Iberian dominance can also be attributed to prudence. Wary of the flaming sword of deadly fevers, they mainly stuck to the coast, relying on local middle-men. "The ocean-going slavers remained in the coastal bays and estuaries," Rodney explains, "while the boats of the *lançados*"—the Portuguese who launched themselves into a social world made violent by slaving—"hovered like vultures in every river, waiting to take hold of the victims of the strug-gles."[13] If the Iberians were the first to look to Africa as a source of "resilient" and unpaid labor, the Dutch, Danes, British, and French weren't far behind. Europeans conducted the transatlantic slave trade from home and from out-posts from one end of the Atlantic to the other.

Most histories of the era have focused on the tropical and subtropical regions of the Americas to which most Africans were shipped. But the trade thoroughly shaped more temperate regions. New England, for example, sur-vived in part by trading in goods produced by far-off wretches and in part through treachery toward their weakened and thinned-out native neigh-bors.[14] Cautioning readers about the paucity of data, the historian Joseph Inikori notes,

> There was practically very little or no slave trading in Sierra Leone,
> the Windward Coast, the Gold Coast, and the Bight of Benin until the
> mid-seventeenth century . . . New England and the Middle Atlantic

colonies . . . were locked up in a subsistence production cul-de-
sac, because they lacked the natural resources needed to compete
effectively in the production of plantation commodities for Atlantic
commerce.[15]

So what pulled many European colonies out of that cul-de-sac? A triangular
trade that connected the Americas, Europe, and Africa from the middle of
the seventeenth century until well into the nineteenth century.

Enslaved Africans were brought to the Americas, where they were fed
with New England cod; sugar, indigo, tobacco, coffee, and cotton were
sent back to Europe; and textiles, rum, and manufactured goods, including
firearms, were sent to Africa, to be traded for more Africans.[16] Slaves were
purchased with iron bars, brass, salt, guns, and, infamously, cheap alcohol,
silk, hats, glass beads, and other trinkets. But the value of captives exported
from West Africa's estuaries and bays and peninsulas soon surpassed that
of gold, ivory, gum arabic (a treasured adhesive), kola nuts, peppers, camwood, and rice and other grains. As the price of slaves skyrocketed in the
late seventeenth century, an increasing number were captured inland, in
the middle Niger. But Europeans didn't have to go there to obtain them.
Instead, local African slavers either sold them for transport downriver or
made them walk, yoked or chained, all the way to the coast. Walter Rodney
describes this collaboration between the transatlantic slavers and European
and African on-shore agents as a "harmonization of the cupidity."[17]

The more prosperous trading states of West Africa, including those of
the Niger Bend, became exporters of young adults and children destined
for the increasingly depopulated Americas. In other African states and chiefdoms, slaves and serfs were used for agricultural work and domestic labor, or
to serve as soldiers without family ties to nearby rivalrous powers. These ruling families sold some slaves captured in raids beyond their borders but jeal-
ously guarded most of them for themselves. But regardless of export quotas,
the traffic sparked by European demand and African supply in turn sparked
raids and war.[18] And war, Rodney adds, was "the most prolific agency for the
recruiting of captives."

In the latter half of the seventeenth century, the British battled France, Spain, Holland, and Portugal for control of Atlantic commerce, and thus of the slave trade. Europeans during this period founded and fought over settlements and slave way stations all along West Africa's coast. These outposts became the foundation of their spheres of influence, which radiated inland from slave castles like Gorée, thrust into the Atlantic between the Senegal and Gambia Rivers, and Bunce (sometimes called Bance or Bence) Island, sheltered in the confluence of the Port Loko Creek and the Rokel River. Bunce had been under British control since the 1600s, when it boasted not only slave barracoons, prisons, and dungeons, but a shipyard and a small golf course.[19] Its lookouts were occasionally obliged to run up the Spanish flag in order to avoid attacks from partisans.

For many living in West Africa, the historian Emmanuel Akyeampong and colleagues have noted, "The answer to the question 'Why did Africa become poor?' is obvious: the slave trades."[20] Human trafficking ensured a great reversal of fortunes between Africa and the Americas. Perhaps the only more striking example of such a reversal was offered by the British pillage of India, which began at the same time and would endure even longer.

West Africa's reversal proceeded apace as Europeans came to dominate commerce across and along the Atlantic basin—then, as now, an epicenter of the world economy. Slave trading came to be the beating heart of that commerce, and to those involved in the trade, it seemed a good business to be in. One famous ship captain, whose cargo was mostly human when he traveled west across the ocean, observed that slave trading was "accounted a genteel employment."[21] Many of the crowded vessels that plied that trade, flying flags from what are today called "Western democracies," now lie with the enchained remains of their cargo below the surface of the ocean—and of memory, at least within Europe's still-rich former empires.

This traffic shaped the social worlds of West Africa in other enduring ways, ways not often studied by economists or historians. The slave trades shaped understandings of conflict and misfortune in general. If the Europeans had a well-founded fear of what lay inland of the Guinea Coast, West Africans (who also suffered the flaming sword of deadly fevers) learned to fear the white devilry reaching inland from the shoreline. The reputation of the coast and what lay beyond it—boats and ships that "ate" young men, women, and children, and captains rumored to cast captives to the train of sharks in their wakes if they were sick or troublesome—was quickly established among those at increasing risk of seizure and deportation to the Americas.

How did the West Africans involved in the slave trade justify the capture, sale, and export of their fellows? Some of those captured and sold were prisoners of war; others were seized for unpaid debts or claims of adultery. But all along the Upper Guinea Coast, accusations of sorcery and witchcraft—of indirect malevolent human agency as an explanation for misfortune and sudden death or disappearance—served as important justifications for the capture, sale, and export of people from across West Africa. These epidemics of accusation were part of everyday life and impossible to ignore. When leveled by those in league with the slavers, they led to dire punishments—or straight to the boats. One agent from an English slave-trading firm diagnosed a Sierra Leonean "addiction" to such accusations. "The best information I have been able to collect," he observed, is that "great numbers are prisoners taken in war, and are brought down, fifty or a hundred together, by the black slave merchants; that many are sold for witchcraft, and other real, or imputed, crimes; and are purchased in the country with European goods and salt."[22]

For certain West African publics, guilt or innocence was revealed by such methods as ordeal by sasswood, or "red water," which entailed ingesting poison concocted from the bark of a local tree and awaiting the uncertain outcome. For others, accusations of witchcraft often required confirmation by diviners, whom the anthropologist Michael Jackson has called "the most important intermediaries between social and extra-social domains."[23] The latter includes the unseen world, which always needs explaining. The transatlantic slave trade and its inland workings made the work of the diviners ever more important as arbiters of fate, because, as the anthropologist Rosalind Shaw has shown in her study of Freetown's early colonial archives, the diviners in confirming accusations were in effect dooming the accused to be "transformed into slaves."[24]

Today, in the regions most marked by slavery on both sides of the Atlantic, the enduring importance of witchcraft and sorcery in explaining sudden death and great misfortune is an enduring echo of the illegitimate trades. Shaw's work among the Temne at the close of the twentieth century, and her reading of fellow anthropologists' descriptions of similar understandings across West Africa, led her to interrogate claims about the origins of such beliefs in our times. "Given this imagery of the capture, transportation, and forced labor of the soul," she has wondered, is it possible that "the historical experience of the slave trade itself *produced* many of these understandings of witchcraft?"[25] Shaw goes on to answer that rhetorical question in no uncertain terms. "During the slave-trade centuries," she writes, "witchcraft and divination in much of the upper Guinea coast were part of an expanding Atlantic world in which inflows of European wealth and commodities were tied to the largest process of forced migration in world history."[26]

If they chose not to submit, those faced with forced migration had the usual options: to fight, flee, or die. Many millions did each. The slaves of Saint-Domingue fought, which is how Haiti became Latin America's first independent nation and the first to ban slavery. They did so at the height of the Enlightenment, the awakening of ideals regarding the rights of man. But the Haitians faced a hostile world in which wealthy white European men were able to propound in print their own unalienable right to freedom and franchise while overlooking not only women but also the global toll of slavery, which by then accounted for the majority of all transatlantic trade. "Slavery," the philosopher–historian Susan Buck-Morss has observed, "had become the root metaphor of Western political philosophy, connoting everything that was evil about power relations," but nonetheless the great Enlightenment thinkers and their forebears—Hegel, Hobbes, Locke, Voltaire, and even Rousseau— failed to see, or see clearly, the very nonmetaphorical slavery that had built their worlds.[27]

In his stirring account of the rise of British abolitionism at the close of the Enlightenment, the historian Adam Hochschild notes that "surprisingly few people saw a contradiction between freedom for whites and bondage for slaves." Instead, he writes, those who knew better indulged in a willful kind of white blindness:

> The philosopher John Locke, whose ideas about governments arising from the consent of the governed had done so much to lay the foundation for this century of revolutions, invested £600 in the Royal African Company, whose RAC brand was seared onto the breasts of thousands of slaves. In France, Voltaire mocked slaveholders in *Candide* and other works, yet when a leading French slave ship owner offered to name a vessel after him, he accepted with pleasure. Once the French Revolution erupted, merchants would promptly christen slave ships *Liberté*, *Égalité*, and *Fraternité*.[28]

The majority of those ships were then bound for Saint-Domingue, the world's most profitable slave colony, which by the time of the French Revolution was about to erupt.

According to Buck-Morss, the rebellion in Haiti was "the crucible, the trial by fire for the ideals of the French Enlightenment," but the rulers of the world's greatest empires were unable or unwilling to recognize that.[29] In the aftermath of the 1791 uprising, and as France was consumed by mayhem, Britain sent a massive armada to add Haiti as a jewel to its crown. The Haitians—and epidemic disease—humbled the expedition, killing off close to 12,500 or so redcoats, many of them impressed forcibly into the Royal Navy. As revolutionary France was reorganized under new management, Napoleon then made the same mistake on an even larger scale, sending a flotilla of hundreds of ships carrying 80,000 troops to the island under his brother-in-law's command. This 1801 expedition, the largest armada ever to set forth from Europe to the Americas, ended in disaster for the invaders. Napoleon's kinsman died in Haiti, along with more than half of those under his command. Haiti, declared independent on January 1, 1804, was Napoleon's Waterloo more than Waterloo itself.

Napoleon's defeat signaled the beginning of the end of the transatlantic trade. "More than anything," asserts Patrick Manning, "the uprising of slaves in Haiti and their assertion of freedom and, eventually, independence, created an anti-slavery movement that led ultimately to the emancipation of almost all those held in slavery."[30] Chastened British rulers, well aware of the magnitude of their rival's losses at the hands of the Haitians, and stinging from their own, would eventually heed increasingly vocal abolitionists from across Britain. By that time, its abolitionists were showering Parliament with petitions (one signed by up to a third of Manchester's residents), and hundreds of thousands of Britons had joined in a sugar boycott. A few years after the Haitian declaration of independence, both houses of Parliament banned the slave trade, and King George III made it official. "British self-congratulation," notes Hochschild, "knew no bounds."[31]

European and American abolitionists, to say nothing of myopic intellectuals and willfully blind politicians and merchants, would take decades to catch up with the Haitians. This was because, outside of Haiti, the abolition of the slave trade wasn't tied to the abolition of slavery. Slavery may have existed for millennia, but it had become, with the transatlantic trade, a hereditary status reserved for blacks. As their numbers grew within the United States, some of these states became slave exporters themselves. The British ban, and the American one that soon followed, didn't even slow the traffic between West Africa and Latin America. Nor did abolition by far-off decree improve (if that's the word) its wretched conditions. If there was, in the words of one historian, "an irony on which naval officers, antislavery activists, and slave traders could agree," it was that "the abolition of the slave trade and the subsequent policing of the seas by the British navy, in the face of surging demand for slaves from Brazil and Cuba, fomented social conditions at the factories and on the slave ships that were more violent, more degraded, and generally more horrifying than ever."[32]

These perverse effects arose in part because of the ambivalent and contradictory attitudes that the British and Americans held toward slavery, but also because Spanish, Portuguese, and French traffickers stepped up their game even after their governments agreed to ban the trade. This new cupidity—banning the slave trade but not slavery—would be tolerated or embraced by rulers on both sides of the Atlantic for the remainder of the nineteenth century. What would later become the nations of Sierra Leone and Liberia were founded in this period of official hypocrisy and an increasingly virulent strain of white supremacy.

The Atlantic slave trade required and buttressed a belief—taken for granted among traders and colonists and rulers, and most of the great intellectuals and religious leaders of the day—in the obvious superiority of white Europeans. There weren't many of those in West Africa, where they remained cloistered in coastal forts, which for the most part, like Bunce Island prior to Britain's ban, served as slave entrepôts. The flaming sword of fevers still kept most Europeans out of the interior. An 1805 British expedition to the supposed El Dorado of the Niger Bend counted forty-five Europeans at the start but only five by the time the expedition had traveled five hundred miles upriver from Timbuktu. Those five didn't make it much farther.

Subsequent expeditions would meet similar fates for years, until the latter half of the century, when Europeans started relying on quinine, an ancient prophylaxis that reliably prevented malaria when used religiously. The slave trades did not, however, require Europeans to chart the Niger, Congo, or other rivers, because by the early ninetenth century, many thousands of chained captives were being funneled each year from the interior through the Door of No Return in Bunce, Gorée, and other slave castles. As the historian Michael Crowder has explained,

> There had been no need for any other arrangement, since the only
> real interest of European traders at this time was the purchase of
> slaves, and sufficient supplies were available without the necessity
> of trading inland. The coastal Africans themselves would anyway
> have resisted any such move, being jealous of their monopoly of the
> middleman role in the trade; and Europeans had long since learnt
> that the briefer their stay on the "Fever Coast" the better for their
> health. Even if they could have overcome African opposition to
> penetration, they would have had difficulty in surviving the all-

pervading "fever" of which they did not know the cause but from which their compatriots in forts like that on James Island in the Gambia had died like proverbial flies.[33]

West Africa's economy had long been shaped by epidemics of all-pervading fever. These in turn were shaped by political economy, which in these parts is always both local and translocal. There can be little doubt that slavery and its disruptive machinery triggered raids and war while unleashing epidemics across the region and in the distant lands to which its sons and daughters were dispatched. Nor is there doubt that the racism underpinning and justifying slavery was rooted in an enduring belief that some lives matter less than others.

Why else would this part of West Africa be termed the White Man's Grave when whites were few in number and its graves so full of Africans?

The city now known as Freetown was originally established in 1787, at the behest of Britons who, in the words of one town historian, "condemned the activity of the slave trade which was very active towards the end of the 18th century."[34] Prior to Freetown's founding, the white men in question hadn't come to West Africa to be buried any more than they came to take in the sights and make new friends.

Famous names involved in Freetown's founding include the British abolitionists William Wilberforce, Granville Sharp, Thomas Clarkson, and Henry Thornton. Many of the chief allies of these men were Quakers, who played key roles in the movement to ban the slave trade across the empire and, after 1776, the United States. Although widely deemed eccentric—with their thees, thous, and refusals to doff hats for mere mortals—Quaker men and women were less wooly-minded than the great British philosophers who, in their long disquisitions on freedom, were able to overlook the traffic linking West Africa, Liverpool, Bristol, London, and Britain's American colonies. But it was formerly enslaved blacks who did the actual founding in West Africa.

The story begins after the U.S. war of independence, when "loyal blacks" who'd sided with the British upon promises of freedom were removed to Nova Scotia. These blacks had, in the words of one of them who twice escaped slavery, "taken refuge in the British lines" during the war.[35] The *Book of Negroes* lists the three thousand or so loyal blacks who left New York for Canada between April 23 and November 30, 1783. (George Washington and other American founding fathers were among those on the hunt for their personal Negroes.) The refugees didn't much care for frosty Nova Scotia—or the indentured servitude they faced there. "The wet, cold territory was crowded with white refugees from the war," writes Adam Hochschild. "Food, farm tools, and relief supplies were short, and the blacks were always last in line."[36]

After one of their number carried news of their grievances to Britain, many loyal blacks ended up in London, where they were re-dubbed "poor blacks." Conditions weren't much better for them in the empire's capital. In 1787, influential abolitionists (and variously motivated Britons looking to rid the city of a new nuisance) persuaded close to four hundred black subjects, most born in the Americas, to establish what they called "the Province of Freedom" at the mouth of the Sierra Leone River—a stone's throw from Bunce Island, then still open for business. They were joined by about seventy European women, disparaged as prostitutes rather than praised as intrepid colonists or loyal spouses.[37]

Britain's most famous ex-slave, the memoirist Olaudah Equiano, was to accompany the settlers as a superintendent. But while preparing for the journey, Equiano had a falling-out with a white colonist who had a similar job description. In a sign of things to come, Equiano was the one who lost his job, along with a couple dozen other "discontented persons." The party had plans to set out from Portsmouth in a four-ship convoy, but delays in provisioning meant that many of its pioneering members were cooped up aboard crowded vessels. Sixty died in the course of shipboard epidemics prior to departure; fourteen more perished between Portsmouth and Sierra Leone. When the "back to Africa" convoy finally reached the giant estuary where they planned to establish themselves, it was the height of the rainy season, which spelled not only waterlogged or washed-out gardens but also yellow fever, malaria, the bloody flux, and other ill-defined but often lethal afflictions.[38]

The settlers nonetheless established a small outpost they called Granville Town—named after the abolitionist Granville Sharp, who had helped inspire the expedition—only to have it torched in 1789 by a Temne chief angry that a British warship had shelled a village under his rule. Adam Hochschild describes what happened next:

> As supplies at Granville Town dwindled and crops failed, the increasingly frustrated settlers turned to the long-time mainstay of the local economy, the slave trade. Ever more of them, white and black, became clerks, carpenters, or shipyard workers at Bance Island, where there were always jobs for experienced and literate workers, whatever their color. Three white doctors from Granville Town ended up at the thriving slave depot also. When the frustrated white chaplain of the settlement could not persuade his parishioners to build him a church or house, he conducted worship under a tree; then, falling sick, he too sought shelter at Bance Island.[39]

Granville Sharp was horrified by such betrayal of the ideals upon which the settlement had been founded. British abolitionists (and other enthusiasts of colonization) were not, however, about to give up on the Province of Freedom.

In 1792, a naval officer named John Clarkson—the twenty-seven-year-old younger brother of the abolitionist hero Thomas Clarkson—led a fleet of fifteen ships to refound the settlement, this time with the name Freetown. Among the passengers was a contingent of 1,196 more blacks from Nova Scotia. (At least one of them had in fact escaped from George Washington.) Despite their greater numbers, Freetown's settlers didn't have it much easier than those who preceded them. Close to 200 of them died in their first year, most from unspecified fevers.

The fact that the colony was hard by Bunce Island also posed obvious dangers. In announcements of auctions in South Carolina and other southern states in the recently established United States, slavers advertised when their wares came from Africa's Rice Coast, as Sierra Leone and its neighbors were sometimes termed, and when they were immune to smallpox.[40] More poignant reminders of the worrisome proximity of the slavers occurred whenever settlers recognized settings in which they'd been seized, held captive, or from which they were deported—and, occasionally, when they were reunited with close relatives. Nor was the tiny British colony protected from their country's big feud with the French, who in 1794 burned much of the town to the ground.

Still, the ideal of a Province of Freedom refused to die. In 1800, about five hundred runaway Jamaican slaves—deported to Nova Scotia during the course of yet another costly British campaign to maintain control of its West Indian plantations—were resettled in rebuilt Freetown. After 1807, by which time free-floating British ambivalence about slavery had been linked to measures to enforce the ban on the trade, settlers from the diaspora (including Jamaican runaway slaves, or maroons) were further augmented by "recaptured" slaves bound west but intercepted by British antislavery patrols. Bolstered by maroons and recaptives, who hailed from across West Africa and often appeared by the hundreds, Freetown (and parts of it like Foulah Town) spread untidily from the left bank of the mighty estuary of the Sierra Leone River, and up into the neighboring hills.[41]

Freetown's first years were further marred by internal quarrels among and with the so-called Nova Scotians, and more feuds with the locals. The surviving colonists also found themselves afflicted with new private-sector patrons: in one of many instances of British trade leading the flag, Freetown was now under orders from the directors of a trading firm chartered by Parliament and known as the Sierra Leone Company. This formula had by then permitted the East India Company to bleed India, once the world's wealthiest region, for over a century. (The French, who were soon to relieve both Louis XVI and Marie Antoinette of their heads and declare war on Britain, often relied on similar arrangements; the Dutch were masters of the tradition, too.) The arrangements quashed promises of black self-rule, leading to recurring conflict over another common British practice, taxation without representation.

In what may be an apocryphal founding story, like those from Massachusetts and Nova Scotia some 150 years earlier, Freetown's settlers nonetheless celebrated Thanksgiving. As on the other side of the Atlantic, dates and intentions are unclear. Perhaps the only living witness to these events was a giant-trunked silk-cotton tree in the town's center, which has held fast over the ensuing centuries, untouched by fevers, feuds, or *forestiers*. In 1971, President Siaka Stevens named it the national symbol of independent Sierra Leone, stamping it on the national currency.

The Cotton Tree still towers over a small downtown street that Stevens named after himself.

Unlike Haiti, which openly supported antislavery struggles elsewhere in the Americas, Sierra Leone was not a nation but a crown colony. But like Haiti, Sierra Leone attracted widespread fascination on both sides of the Atlantic. That fascination was marked among abolitionists, many of whom favored removal of freedmen to some unspecified land of their own; whites who abhorred the idea of abolition; and free people of color in the United States, most of whom were intrigued by and dead-set against back-to-Africa schemes and some few of whom were for them.

Among the last group was Paul Cuffe, a successful ship captain and merchant from Westport, Massachusetts. Cuffe was born in 1759 to a freedman father and a Wampanoag mother. He, too, married a Wampanoag, but considered himself an African American. That was because he was fighting for his rights, a common enough New England hobby, and for the rights of others, which remained, as ever, a rare pastime. Cuffe and one of his brothers sought to use local legislatures and the courts to advance legal remedies for free blacks, who faced almost universal discrimination. These remedies often failed, even in the increasingly abolitionist (if persistently racist) northeast. After all, Article I, Section 2 of the newly inked U.S. Constitution had decreed slaves and others held in servitude equivalent to three-fifths of a person.

Unlike most black abolitionists, however, Paul Cuffe had anchors on both sides of the ocean, plying an increasingly lucrative trade throughout

New England, the Caribbean, and across the Atlantic. He had spiritual stanchions, too: at the age of forty-nine, Cuffe formally joined the Quakers, who, though not free of the racism plaguing all of white America, were in general deeply hostile to slavery. After single-handedly financing New Bedford's first school and chipping in for its Quaker meetinghouse, he turned toward the idea of the colonization of West Africa as a "humane substitute" for the slave trade, one that might "sustain black Africa's economy."[42]

The notion of colonization—of "sending them back where they came from"—may seem nonsensical. Most American blacks by then had been born in the Americas. Like Cuffe, many had been Americans for generations. But the same logic was applied to Native Americans in what would become the Indian removal acts. (In both instances, a separate-but-equal discourse often served as cover for the white supremacy of the day, which is why colonization was opposed by the majority of nonwhite people.) Captain Cuffe, who was later termed a father of black nationalism, set his sights and his sextant on Sierra Leone. He began planning an exploratory trip to Freetown on his favorite ship, the 109-ton *Traveller*. On January 2, 1811, it sailed from Philadelphia with nine crew—with the exception of a European apprentice, all men of color.

The *Traveller* reached Freetown after two months at sea, and Cuffe received a warm welcome from the governor, as well as from the settlers and local chiefs. But the British, who then numbered twenty of the colony's three thousand or so inhabitants, were lukewarm about the proposals of an American merchant, regardless of the color of his skin or his glowing letters of introduction from prominent New Englanders. So after a few days exploring the colony, Cuffe decided to head for the old England to take up his cause with Britain's abolitionists and its authorities. He set course for Liverpool, which until very recently had been the main port of British slavers. Between 1783 and 1804, an estimated 625,000 Africans had been shipped in chains from Liverpool's docks to plantations across the Americas, including Britain's colonies. Business was business.

Paul Cuffe, the consummate businessman, disagreed. He enjoyed little formal schooling but read widely, including Thomas Clarkson's newly famous history of the abolition of the slave trade.[43] Although the American assumed he could count on the support of the Clarksons, Wilberforce, and his fellow Quakers, he was likely unprepared for the mix of awe and adulation he received in England. (No one in Liverpool, certainly, had ever seen a well-kept ship like the *Traveller* captained and crewed entirely by black men.) Cuffe spent a few busy months in Liverpool, London, and the then-industrializing and staunchly abolitionist Manchester. He was received not only by fellow travelers in the abolitionist movement but also by the Duke of Gloucester—nephew to the king and president of an organization dedicated to "promoting the civilization" of Africans—and other nobles and notables.

The sea captain used his time in England not only to buy goods to trade but also to gather up antislavery tracts, Bibles, reams of advice about how his fellow merchant-missionaries should conduct themselves, and the fixings for smallpox vaccine (developed in 1796 by Edward Jenner and already well known among smart seafaring captains). Cuffe then set sail once again for Freetown, where he hoped to promote self-help projects and the legitimate trades in places such as Port Loko, rather than just doling out the standard emoluments used to placate or bribe local chiefs, which usually included firearms and firewater. Cuffe felt that such projects and trades, along with factories put in place to help improve local industry, would gradually wean Sierra Leoneans from being "so strongly influenced with the slave trade," which was then draining the region of its productive population.[44]

After returning to Sierra Leone, feeling sanguine about his odds of success, Cuffe set sail again for New England on February 11, 1812. He vowed to return with hundreds of free people of color from the United States. But world events eclipsed his plans. About the time Cuffe and the *Traveller* set sail from Freetown for Westport, the United States was gearing up for war with Britain and trade in British goods was declared illegal. On April 19, just a few days after the *Traveller* dropped anchor in its home berth and still laden with a cargo of camwood, ivory, and other bounty, a U.S. revenue cutter seized the ship. Cuffe's battle to recover his cargo took him all the way to the White House, where James Madison—who proposed the Three-Fifths Compromise, owned more than a hundred slaves, and also supported colonization—received him graciously. "This black man from Westport, Massachusetts," wrote one biographer, "became the first Negro known to have been both entertained as a guest by the President of the United States and received in his official residence."[45]

Captain Cuffe recovered his property in the end, but the War of 1812 kept him away from Sierra Leone for four long years, during which time he learned of widespread antipathy, among American blacks and white abolitionists alike, for the idea of colonization. A Quaker friend wrote to Cuffe at the time describing the prevailing sentiment in Philadelphia:

> The people of color here was very much frightened. At first they were afraid that all the free people would be compelled to go, particularly those in the southern states. We had a large meeting of males at the Rev. R. Allen's church the other evening. Three thousand at least attended, and there was not one soul that was in favor of going to Africa. They think that the slaveholders want to get rid of them so as to make their property more secure.[46]

The anxieties of free people of color were not misplaced. The pronouncements of plenty of American slaveholders and politicians, and also the courts, made that clear. When Cuffe finally did return to Freetown, in 1816, he'd recruited only thirty-eight settlers. His enthusiasm for back-to-Africa schemes faded as it became increasingly favored by antiabolitionists.

Cuffe spent the next few years, his last ones, railing against slavery and the transatlantic slave trade, which had grown after Britain's ban. "It is reported," he wrote to another Quaker friend, "that there are more than 200 sail of vessels cleared from Havana for the coast of Africa last year, 1815. Cannot anything be done to kill this clandestine traffic? The two months I was in Sierra Leone there was six vessels brought in who was taken in that abominable traffic. One of the six was under American colors, the others under Spanish colors, no doubt, under disguise."[47] Not all the vessels then flying American colors in the waters off the Upper Guinea Coast were traffickers, but the emerging naval power was internally torn regarding which trades could be considered legitimate.

As such constructions as North and South, free and slave, black and white came to be hardened—and as the agonies of Native Americans went down into the oubliette—the young republic's flagrant contradictions were on full display off West Africa. The USS *Alligator*, a sleek schooner outfitted with a dozen six-pound guns and launched on November 2, 1820, was sent to prowl that coast in order to block the traffic on which much of the U.S. economy depended. On one antislavery patrol, the *Alligator* carried a representative of the American Colonization Society, one of the best examples of these contradictions, to scout for land for a colony in what would soon be Liberia. The warship captured more than a half dozen slaving vessels—Spanish, French, and Portuguese—and rescued an American schooner from pirates off the coast of Cuba before running aground off the Florida Keys in 1822. Its remains are now part of a coral reef that bears its name.

It was a more wholesome reincarnation than others to follow. The U.S. Navy often recycled names, and, although the 1820 *Alligator* was not a submarine, these were already on naval drawing boards; a subsequent official launch was as one. Unofficial iterations as a submarine may have already been spawned, however, in the minds of those living along the Upper Guinea Coast and its rivers. Rumors of "human alligators" eager to snatch victims before diving below the surface of rivers and coasts spread inland across West Africa throughout the next century and into this one. Better to live on as a reef.

Whether or not malaria, sleeping sickness, smallpox, and other pestilence played an outsize role in West Africa's reversal of fortune is still debated.[48] Prior to the nineteenth century, the entire world was a medical desert, and great plagues shook the old world and the new. Secular trends revealing widening disparities in life expectancy between nations—much less continents—weren't well documented before they were linked through colonial rule. But it was the slave trade that first bound the Americas to West Africa.

Fever was never far from feud in Upper West Africa, and both were

linked to the slave trade. For many of Sierra Leone's settlers, the most common tribulations, once Bunce Island was shut down, were everyday feuds with
unseen microbes. For a century after Freetown's founding, little was known
about what made the place so unhealthy beyond clinically distinctive smallpox and a host of diseases termed, back then, the "bloody flux," yellow fever,
and—especially—malaria. Fevers continued to claim the majority of European
explorers of Africa's navigable rivers until 1854, when yet another attempt to
chart the course of the Niger included daily doses of quinine. No one died of
fevers on that expedition, although the reasons why were debated—and although, as the British writer and explorer Mary Kingsley later observed,
"there is no other region in the world that can match West Africa for the
steady kill, kill, kill that its malaria works on the white men who come under
its influence."[49] The problem in Sierra Leone wasn't simply malaria, which
couldn't be readily distinguished from a host of other sicknesses, including
typhoid and yellow fever (the bloody flux, similarly, was surely caused by
several species of bacteria and more than one parasite). Nor was the problem
of sudden febrile illness ever largely about whites and their immunity.

Virgin-soil theories continued to scant the impact of the violence and inequalities that determined the fates of many on the continent, whether or not
they were exposed to natural infection or lucky enough to receive the inocu-
lations of the day. But Freetown's settlers—black and white, men and women,
adults and children—did seem to lack resistance to these sicknesses, even
though they had long before reached the world deemed new. The story was
the same in similarly inspired settlements in Liberia. As one historian of the
period has written,

> The abolitionists proved that even African genes, sans an African
> childhood, provided only a flimsy shield against African pathogens.
> In the first year of the Province of Freedom, Sierra Leone, 46 percent
> of the whites died, but so did 39 percent of the black settlers. In
> Liberia between 1820 and 1843, 21 percent of all immigrants,
> presumably all or almost all of them black or mulatto, died during
> their first year of residence.[50]

In the first three decades after Freetown's founding, hapless early settlers "sans an African childhood" were increasingly replenished by returnees who'd had one. These were mostly recaptives taken by British interdiction patrols: well-armed and nimble ships flying the Union Jack outran overladen Spanish, Portuguese, and French slavers, liberating tens of thousands captured across West Africa and depositing them in settlements in and around Freetown.

The vast majority of Africans captured were never recaptured and returned to Africa, of course, but several who were wrote, or dictated, accounts of their travails. The Methodist minister Joseph Wright, for example, relates that he was born, in about 1815, "a heathen in a heathen Land." This was Yorubaland, in what is now Nigeria, as it was consumed by wars sparked by the slave trades. Writing from Freetown a dozen years after his capture, Wright described in gruesome detail the 1825 sack of his town, his capture by local raiders, and his forced march to Lagos, where he was sold to Portuguese slavers:

> We all were heavy and sorrowful in heart, because we were going
> to leave our land for another which we never knew; and not only
> so, but when we saw the waves of the salt water on which we were
> just to enter, it discouraged us the more, for we had heard that the
> Portuguese were going to eat us when we go to their country. This
> put us more to despair, and when they began to put us in canoes to
> bring us to the Brig, one of the canoes drowned and half of the slaves
> died. After they had done with loading the Brig, they stowed all the
> men under the deck; the boys and women were left on the deck. The
> Brig sailed in the evening. Next day we saw an English man-of-war
> coming. When the Portuguese saw this, it put them to disquietness
> and confusion. They then told us that these were the people which
> will eat us, if we suffered them to prize us.[51]

But the British were seeking to prize traffickers, not the trafficked. In 1827 alone, after the Crown beefed up its patrols, 5,393 recaptured slaves were landed—many in or around Freetown.[52]

The colony's population shortly thereafter was pegged at 30,000 souls, making it a large and unique outpost along a treacherous coast. Since the freed captives hailed from across a vast expanse of the continent, spoke scores of languages, and claimed several faith traditions—frequently, more than one at once—it's easy to imagine what a diverse (and Creole) place Freetown was in the decades when neighborhoods like Kissy and Foulah Town were established. The dangers of illness aside, the trauma of capture, recapture, and release, and the cultural upheaval of forced resettlement in a strange land, was associated with its own set of pathologies, which led the British to establish, in 1817, West Africa's first psychiatric facility, the Kissy Lunatic Asylum. Although many of the returnees retained strong ties to their linguistic and cultural traditions, and some sought to return home, most had little choice but to make a new one in Freetown: war wracked the inland reaches of the Upper Guinea Coast throughout the early nineteenth century.

It was the same story along the Gold Coast and the Bight of Benin, where kingdoms and chiefdoms engaged in the slave trades rose and fell. The violence of faction had by then overtaken most of West Africa. This was not tribal warfare, the doyen of Sierra Leonean historians, Arthur Abraham, has argued. Most feuds were between local chiefs struggling for commercial and political dominance, often with the assistance of powerful Europeans representing firms with ties to the slave trade:

> Captives of war became an accepted currency, a commodity of exchange, and continued to be such long after the British abolition and suppression of the slave trade during the first half of the nineteenth century. But it was the Europeans who introduced the demand for slaves on the coast, and their presence on the coasts of Africa from the 15th century onwards is to be seen as part of the direct cause of the capture of people . . . Having become a profitable occupation, warfare led directly to the emergence of a professional class of warriors. This increased the incidence of wars, because if the warriors were to be occupied, then they sought pretexts to cause or enter wars.[53]

During the first few decades after the founding of Freetown, Sierra Leone watchers—including residents of the colony and of other coastal settlements, and those engaged in the slave trade or opposed to it—heard stories of inland conflict and ongoing human trafficking.

These stories illustrated the relative impotence of British naval patrols as well as the cost of failure to abolish slavery itself. But inspiring stories of heroic resistance on the part of captives have survived. Among them is the now-famous tale of Sengbe Pieh, a young Mende man sold into slavery for failure to pay a debt. Engaged in local struggles over control of the slave trade, Sengbe was captured in January 1839. He and others seized with him were marched in fetters across difficult terrain to a slaving way station on the Galinhas coast, the no-man's-land between Freetown and Monrovia. Sengbe was imprisoned for months in Galinhas, thirty years after the British began policing the waters he could likely see from his cell. Slavers operating in the neighborhood—including a local warlord-king and an all-powerful Spanish agent representing a firm based in Havana—were far enough from Freetown's surveillance that their share of the traffic received a boost from the repurposing of Bunce Island after the 1807 ban.[54]

More or less twenty-six years old, Sengbe Pieh knew about British patrols. His "closest brother," he said, had been sold into slavery but was subsequently the beneficiary of the empire's new catch-and-release program. Since Sengbe was himself caught up in the region's trade wars, he also likely knew Britain hadn't been the only nation to abolish the slave trade, at least on paper. The 1814 Treaty of Ghent, which ended the Anglo-American feud delaying Paul Cuffe's return to Sierra Leone, had specified that both parties would enforce the ban. This was, in the eyes of some, a fool's errand in a time when the United States sent vessels like the *Alligator* on antislavery patrols to West Africa even as the country relied on slave labor. But the chief American negotiator in Belgium, a future U.S. president and the son of one, was no fool.

John Quincy Adams would draw on knowledge of Ghent and other treaties when his fate collided with Sengbe Pieh's, after both of theirs collided with Spain's. In spite of similar treaty obligations, Spain had reemerged as an engine of transatlantic trafficking after Britain gave it up. Sengbe was moved in chains, along with fellow prisoners hailing from across and beyond what would later become Sierra Leone, to the galley of the Spanish schooner *Teçora*. They joined more than five hundred other captives crammed into its holds and chained to its decks. The ship's first stop after the harrowing and cramped Middle Passage was Havana. (The kingdom of Spain had for years shipped the majority of its human cargo to work the sugar and tobacco plantations of Cuba.)[55] There, on June 16, 1839, Sengbe and forty-eight others were sold at auction to Jose Ruiz and another slave trader. Since the plantation to which they were to be sent was three hundred miles away, the still-bound West Africans were spirited under the cover of night aboard a smaller schooner anchored in Havana's harbor. They never reached their destination.

On July 1, after three days at sea, Sengbe managed to free himself and his fellow captives. Set loose, they killed the captain and the cook and seized control of the ship, taking Ruiz and the other slaver hostage. Adrift without guidance, several of the mutineers died of thirst or exposure. They drifted north, eventually making landfall on the tip of Long Island. There, while Sengbe and the others, who didn't speak English, were making plans to sell some of the ship's nonhuman cargo in order to hire a captain to pilot them home, the vessel was seized by the U.S. Navy. Arrested on charges of piracy and murder, the Africans were transported to a U.S. Navy brig, which towed the schooner to New London, Connecticut.

That schooner, as many now know, was the *Amistad*. But who were these prisoners and how were they seized? Who was Sengbe Pieh, who'd fought this new captivity tooth and nail and stood out as the ringleader? Although some contemporary accounts termed them "Mende men," many weren't Mende speakers, and several weren't men. Unlike most of the captors, the captives spoke more than one language, including Gbandi, Kono, Temne, Bullom, Gola, Loma, Kissi, and Kondo; Mende was the closest to a lingua franca they had. Linguistic diversity aside, most were poor farmers or the children of them. As one account puts it,

> Apart from three girls and two boys, all the "Amistads" were young
> or middle-aged men. They included two blacksmiths and one

hunter; but of the remaining 28, nearly all stated that growing rice
was their main occupation. One man claimed that his father had
been a chief and two said that their fathers were "gentlemen"; the
majority, however, were probably of lower social origins. Seven of the
Amistads were "seized in the road" while travelling from one town
to another: one of these was seized because a slave whom his uncle
had given to pay a debt had run away; the others could be said to
have been kidnapped. Four more were "seized in the bush" or on
their farms. Seven were captured in war by soldiers who attacked
their towns. Four were enslaved for adultery. Three were slaves
sold by their masters: these included one whose father had been a
"gentleman" but whose king had taken him as a slave after his father's
death. Two girls were pawned by their fathers; and one man was sold
by his mother's brother in exchange for a coat. Four did not explain
how they were enslaved.[56]

Such details usually went into the oubliette along with the names of the captives. But in Sengbe's case, this erasure wasn't simply about forgetting. According to those who had purchased him, Sengbe wasn't Sengbe. He was
Jose Cinque, a Spanish slave and not a freeborn man seized in West Africa.

The imposed pseudonym was an attempt by the Spanish Crown to show
that its planters in Cuba, and not the captives, were the victims in this affair.
If Cinque were a Spanish serf and not a free man, argued representatives of
Her Majesty the Queen—then exactly nine years old—the *Amistad* and its human cargo must be returned to Spain, meaning sent to the Cuban plantation
on which they'd never set fettered or unfettered foot. Thus began one of the
nineteenth century's epic legal battles.

United States v. Cinque began on November 19, 1839, in Connecticut's District Court, then and now based in Hartford. Sengbe and the others—whom
the press called "the Amistads"—had plenty to say on the matter of slavery,
but who could hear them? Few New Englanders (or free Americans of any

stripe) understood Mende or any West African languages. The first task facing defense lawyers was to find translators. They managed this by turning to Yale University, which boasted an ethnographically oriented linguist, and by turning back to the New London harbor, which boasted a handful of Mende-speaking stevedores.

Abolitionists from across New England raised funds to relieve the stevedores of their duties in order to help the Amistads. The Spanish put up a fight, aided by the U.S. federal government: in order to avoid a diplomatic fracas with Spain and its child sovereign, the Van Buren administration schemed quietly to return the *Amistad* and all of its cargo, including Cinque-Sengbe and the other captives, to Havana. Indeed, Washington had already dispatched to Connecticut a warship usually assigned to interdiction patrols in order to deport the mutineers—the sister ship of none other than the USS *Alligator.* These ironies and contradictions weren't lost on any American partisans. Fresh memories of Nat Turner's 1831 rebellion had upended illusions of peaceful compromises over American slavery.

Historians underlining the political economy of slavery and the diverse origins of the *Amistad* captives have argued that it's a mistake to read the struggle as a courtroom drama in which the American legal system was the protagonist. But it was a courtroom drama nonetheless: Sengbe Pieh and his shipmates, their fates having collided with those of John Quincy Adams and of Spain, had provoked what many termed the trial of one president by another. A broad American public was spellbound by Sengbe, who, in spite of his oft-reported inability to express himself properly in English—"Give us free! Give us free!" he shouted clearly enough in court—cut an imposing figure, even (or perhaps especially) in irons.

People traveled great distances to witness the proceedings, causing a good deal of ruckus in the courtroom. "Never before," observes one American historian of the period, "had a federal trial prompted the kind of popular fascination that surrounded the *Amistad* proceedings." Fascination cleaved along predictable lines—for or against slavery—as did reporting and commentary on the proceedings, and an explosion of art (and kitsch) inspired by them:

Newspapers detailed the seizure of the Africans and speculated
about the role of the charismatic Cinque. A theater on the Bowery in
New York City presented a melodrama about "The Black Schooner"
and the heroism of "the gallant tars" who rescued the Spanish
planters. Inexpensive mass-produced prints celebrated Cinque as
"the brave Congolese chief who prefers death to slavery" or as the
noble leader who inspired his compatriots.[57]

For those who couldn't travel to Hartford, one New Haven artist created a
replica of the decks of the *Amistad*, peopled with life-size wax sculptures of
the captives; abolitionists moved the display across New England. A massive panorama mural commemorating the revolt also made the rounds, and
museum-worthy portraits of Sengbe and the Amistads were painted or
sketched as they awaited trial.[58]

The most famous likeness of Sengbe was commissioned by a wealthy
Philadelphia freedman. Offered in 1840 for exhibition at the Pennsylvania
Academy of the Fine Arts, the portrait was declined for fear of violent reper-
cussions. Abolitionists, whose number included the artist, protested vigorously. "Why is that portrait denied a place in that gallery?" asked one of them.

> The plain English of it is, Cinque is a NEGRO. This is a Negro-
> hating and negro-stealing nation. A slaveholding people. The
> negro-haters of the north, and the negro-stealers of the south will not
> tolerate a portrait of a negro in a picture gallery. And such a negro!
> His dauntless look, as it appears on canvass, would make the souls of
> the slaveholders quake.[59]

The portrait was nothing if not stunning. Copies sold like hotcakes, as did
broadsides and biographies of several of the captives. The *Amistad* case (and
copies of the defendants' portraits) went all the way to the Supreme Court in
1841, pitting Adams, acting as counsel for the accused, against the administration of Martin Van Buren, up for reelection and anxious to win Southern
votes.

John Quincy Adams—the first U.S. president other than his father who owned no slaves—was an increasingly ardent foe of slavery. Rusty after thirty years outside a courtroom, he expressed doubts about serving as chief defense counsel, but insisted his reluctance "was founded entirely and exclusively upon the consciousness of my own incompetency to do justice to their cause. In every other point of view there is in my estimation no higher object upon earth of ambition than to occupy that position."[60] Adams proved more masterful than his modesty allowed. He drew on legal precedent, the treaty he'd signed in Ghent, and more than a bit of sarcasm:

> My clients are claimed under the treaty as merchandise, rescued
> from pirates and robbers. Who were the merchandise, and who
> were the robbers? According to the construction of the Spanish
> minister, the merchandise were the robbers, and the robbers were the
> merchandise. The merchandise was rescued out of its own hands,
> and the robbers were rescued out of the hands of the robbers. Is this
> the meaning of the treaty?

To the surprise of many, since most of its justices had upheld decisions favorable to slave owners and would do so in the future, the high court ruled in favor of the defendants. After eighteen months in U.S. custody, the Amistads were free. Jose Ruiz, the man who had purchased them and by then spent months in prison himself, returned to Cuba without his merchandise.

The *Amistad* trial was a landmark moment in the struggle against slavery. In neighboring Haiti, the verdict was cheered widely. But it struck fear among slaveholders in the Caribbean and the Americas.[61] The trial stoked antislavery sentiment in the North and led to the founding of hundreds of antislavery schools, but the Van Buren administration refused to provide the freed captives safe passage home. It took the better part of a year for them to reach Freetown, which they eventually managed to do in the company of American missionaries. Upon their return, according to the anthropologist Joseph Opala, Sengbe Pieh "found that his home town had been destroyed and most of his family wiped out." Soon afterward, Sengbe largely disappears from the historical record. For more than a century and a half, Sengbe was largely forgotten in Sierra Leone. "It is a pity," wrote Arthur Abraham in 1978, "that little recognition has hitherto been given to Sengbe in his own country, and continent, and whatever may have been his own shortcomings, he nevertheless remains a truly neglected hero in his own land."[62]

That's finally changed. Much of the world was reintroduced to Sengbe's story in 1997, when Steven Spielberg based his film *Amistad* on it. And Sierra Leoneans now know not only his story but his likeness well: Sengbe often appears on street murals and, like the great Cotton Tree, is featured on a Sierra Leonean banknote.

The *Amistad* case stirred long-term passions because the transatlantic slave trade, built over the course of centuries, took the better part of a full century to collapse. While this traffic persisted, few were truly free outside the boundaries of poverty-shackled Freetown. These chains were one reason an American journalist later termed the city's name "so ironic that no one even bothers to point it out." He did allow that its "founders, who had good intentions, however misplaced they may have been at the time, had certainly envisioned a different future."[63]

No doubt. But these intentions are worth remembering given the city's current, grim conditions. In spite of feuds and fevers, the Cotton Tree has been witness to greatness, at least as far as aspirations go, if tragedy in larger measure. Lofty ideals were an important part of the story of Freetown and other utopian settlements, but these settlements bore the seeds of dystopia within them. What dashed the era's hopes? The paradoxical attempt to abolish the slave trade without abolishing slavery. And nowhere was this paradox more powerfully at work than in Liberia. "Unlike the rest of the continent," writes the anthropologist Mary Moran, "Liberia was never formally colonized by a European power." But the country was born, she adds, "out of the contradictions inherent in the founding of the United States itself; a nation predicated on individual liberty which at the same time condoned and profited by chattel slavery."[64]

Those who founded Liberia's coastal settlements, including Harper and Monrovia, were black Americans sponsored by the American Colonization Society, an uneasy amalgam of white utopians who professed to black self-rule but preferred it occur elsewhere; missionaries out to convert heathens; abolitionists ambivalent about a multiracial America and for whom both Native Americans and freed slaves would be less "degraded" on their own turf; slave owners and Southern politicians who wished to send troublesome freedmen back to Africa and out of sight of those still in bondage (the very existence of Haiti was nightmare enough); and traders who wished to open up new regions of Africa to U.S. commerce.

By then, of course, the vast majority of those enslaved or recently freed in the Americas had been born there, as had their forebears. So, too, with the freeborn. The Maryland branch of the American Colonization Society, which sponsored the settlement of Harper, also counted free people of color who wanted to live in a country without slavery. But in the first half of the nineteenth century, the coast just south of Sierra Leone was anything but that. Like the rest of the neighborhood, what would become Liberia was a land long in the clutches of violent regionalism sparked by the slave trades. It was also in the clutches of microbes: close to half of the early settlers in Monrovia, founded in 1822, died in Liberia's early years. One recent assessment of mortality among these settlers concludes that they "experienced the highest mortality rates in accurately recorded human history."[65]

As in Freetown, the population of settlers in Monrovia was augmented by recaptives. But they were far fewer in number—about six thousand or so in the first several decades of colonization—than in Sierra Leone. Almost all settlers and recaptives lived in coastal settlements like Monrovia and Harper. When the boundaries of Liberia were traced more grandly, they joined a larger if uncounted number of natives said to belong to between sixteen and twenty tribes.[66] As elsewhere in West Africa, the term "tribe"—given broad currency by Europeans—usually referred to shape-shifting and sound-shifting ethnolinguistic groups whose members likely didn't know they were suddenly Liberian. In the words of Moran, "The Liberian national motto,

'The Love of Liberty Brought Us Here,' clearly did not recognize the presence of anyone of consequence 'here' before 1822."[67]

Many of the locals, happy to trade with the settlers on their own terms, were well aware of—and vocally irritated by—settlers' presumptions of superiority. Suspicious of the newcomers' intentions to acquire land as personal property, which clashed with longer-standing traditions governed by customary law, the natives threatened to attack settlers when they violated treaties or otherwise threatened local interests and institutions. In most outposts, given their numbers, colonists knew better than to flaunt these pretentions, or to grab land, unless backup from the U.S. or British navies was in clear view. Such was initially the case in the town of Harper, the capital of Maryland County, in the far southeastern corner of Liberia, where today Partners In Health has its home in the country.

Jungle and bush encircle Harper, which is surely one of the reasons it was spared the brunt of the Ebola crisis in 2014. Harper was founded in 1834 on Cape Palmas, the region's only high promontory, by a grand total of eighteen settlers sponsored by the Maryland State Colonization Society. Led by James Hall, a hardworking and hypochondriacal white doctor from Vermont, Harper's early colonists included free people of color and slaves freed on the condition they emigrate. (For the latter, it was a choice between unknown Africa or a return to the auction block.) Like other self-described American pioneers, the settlers showed up in already settled lands. Harper was singular, however, since it was planted on the edge of a bustling town inhabited by up to two thousand members of a tribe called the Glebo.[68]

The Gleboes—often spelled Greboes, a variant I will use—were one of dozens of communities that had long been settled along the coast, with boundaries that were mysterious to the newly arrived Americans. The coast itself proved far less fertile than its blindingly verdant and rain-drenched forests and mangrove swamps suggested, and Dr. Hall acquired land for his settlement from the Greboes in exchange for money and goods long familiar to the region's traders: bales of cloth, muskets and pistols and gunpowder, cutlasses, iron pots and assorted crockery, wash basins, looking glasses, decanters and stemware, razors, fishhooks, and, of course, hats, beads, and other trinkets.

In the course of long palavers, Hall threw in the promise of free schools for local children. To the disappointment of Grebo headmen, the Maryland Colonization Society initially refused to trade in spirits. Hall, an abstemious Yankee, warned that this might prove a deal breaker, but in the end, rum lubricated the sale.

According to many accounts, the local chiefs ceded Cape Palmas because they didn't believe the Americans would stick it out. But stick it out they did. In spite of unquestioned confidence in their own cultural superiority, the Marylanders knew—as correspondence and reports back to Baltimore revealed—that their survival depended not only on providence and hard work but also on avoiding all-out conflict with their new neighbors. The Greboes were subdivided by a dizzying array of distinctions made along lines of gender and age-grade structures, which conferred status as warriors in highly martial but gerontocratic communities. They and their native neighbors, who struggled over control of inland and coastal trade, were capable of forging alliances if their interests aligned.

Although the settlers saw themselves as bearing civilization and the Word to backward natives, trade and commerce had long shaped Grebo worldviews. For generations, a substantial fraction of the men had been, notes Mary Moran, "widely traveled and worldly, and up to half of them spoke some English or other European languages."[69] The Greboes were further subdivided according to membership in secret societies, which met mostly at night and in the bush. These societies were led not by hereditary chiefs, but by a sort of priesthood that appeared in public only behind masks and in full costume: these were the famous "bush devils." As in Sierra Leone, the more informed colonists and missionaries recognized the positive social functions of these esoteric societies, into which most were initiated during their early teens. Evidence from Cape Palmas suggests, however, that enlightened settlers and missionaries were in the minority. Most newcomers believed their new neighbors to display typically heathen and savage ways, which they were out to replace with Christian and civilized ones.

Around Harper, heathen ways were held to include ritual cannibalism and all manner of sorcery and witchcraft. According to the historian Richard

Hall, who read every letter and report sent from Harper back to the Maryland State Colonization Society, "Greboes firmly believed in the malignant agency of ghosts, and many lived in terror of necromancy. Furthermore, they held as an article of faith that witchcraft caused most deaths."[70] In some cases, guilt or innocence of those accused of witchcraft was established through ordeal by poison: the accused had to ingest the red water extracted from the bark of the sasswood tree. During the year after Harper's founding, colonists' testimonies suggest, four or five "sassy wood palavers" took place in the abutting Grebo settlement. "In notorious cases," recounts Hall, the historian, "whole populations would come out to watch and perhaps hasten the end. Scenes like this took on a special significance in relations between Greboes and Marylanders, for they often took place within the confines of the colony."[71]

These were tight confines, as now-Governor James Hall understood. Jostling for trade, land, and labor—and hemmed in along a narrow strip of coast—the settlers were suddenly part of a tenuous equation: "In signing the deed of cession, Hall and the Grebo kings committed their people to an arduous competition. Greboes must now share their territory with strangers who had radically different ideas of how to use it."[72] (Grebo farming methods relied on crop rotation, years-long fallow periods, and communal ownership of land.) Harper's early settlers were consigned to a penury far different from the agrarian idyll conjured by colonization enthusiasts. Competition over scarce land and its stewardship shaped the ensuing cultural struggles, as it did in other settler-native societies.

It's a marvel the Americans were able to survive there at all, since conflicts over land and trade were likely more significant than the cultural clashes dominating plaintive reports back to Maryland. Richard Hall summarizes the early years of the experiment:

> As in frontier America, settlers faced a challenge to their culture, not
> in the presence of Native Americans, but of Africans, who shared,
> more or less, skin color, but whose way of life scarcely corresponded,
> who spoke different languages, who had multiple wives instead of
> one, who farmed a different field every year or two instead of owning

and cultivating a single plot, who believed in sorcery and trial by ordeal, with persisting ritual killings, even on the public roads. Almost unbelievably, the two peoples coexisted without serious outbreak, despite mutual suspicion and animosity.[73]

The Americans might not have survived without regular resupply of trade goods from Baltimore. James Hall touted the agrarian idyll, but he hedged his bets by building ships for the legitimate trades, which he (like Paul Cuffe) believed would help sustain the colony in an often-hostile environment.

Then there were the fevers. As in other settlements along the Upper Guinea Coast, fevers felled colonists in Maryland, especially during the first year or so after arrival. But many survived thanks to Dr. Hall, who believed strongly in quinine. After two decades, close to 1,200 Americans lived in Harper.

In the twentieth century, the descendants of Harper's settlers, many of them members of Liberia's ruling clique, erected monuments to their own greatness and grit. One surges up from the beach just below Partners In Health's office. But Harper wasn't great when we first saw it. We found the statue, like many of the town's larger buildings, shrouded by weeds and vines. "Today," Richard Hall writes, "Maryland in Liberia scarcely exists: climate, economic change, and civil war have wiped away almost all trace of the bustling American expatriate community, which existed there in the mid-nineteenth century."[74]

Harper's decline didn't come at the hands of the Greboes. Their threats, it turned out, were largely bluster. Avoiding all-out conflict required mutual restraint, which prevailed for more than twenty years. Until independent Maryland was obliged to seek protection from Monrovia, the settlers had managed to forestall or quickly end armed conflict with the natives through tedious palavers. James Hall was a patient master of this West African tradition, although its true value (and his) may not have been appreciated until later. Conflict was nonetheless constant. A U.S. man-o'-war could and sometimes did flatten coastal villages in order to teach the locals a lesson or two.

The Cape Palmas Greboes were spared such instruction until 1856, when a headstrong governor, Boston J. Drayton, came to power in the colony's first coup and declared war on his neighbors. Why wage war in the face of precarity? Settler-native conflicts in 1856 weren't different from those in previous years. They stemmed, as ever, from competition for land and trade—and from cultural strife. Sasswood ordeals had been a bone of contention since Maryland's founding. ("The steady execution of innocents on superstitious pretexts," Richard Hall asserts, "confirmed Africans as 'savages' and did more than anything to harm relations between settlers and natives."[75]) But if the sources of conflict weren't new, a hothead at the helm of the colony was.

James Hall and the Grebo chiefs had often engaged in wars of words, but never had the Yankee doctor fired his cannons on his neighbors, and neither had the Bowdoin-educated black American who succeeded him. But shortly before noon on December 22, 1856, Governor Drayton ordered the old brass field pieces of the colony's eastern battery to open fire on the bustling Grebo town in the midst of which now-fortified Harper had been founded. The battery commander, Richard Hall writes, "could not believe his instructions and he asked to have them repeated." But he corrected his gunners' aim in order to flatten the settlement. Accustomed to being saved from war by last-minute palavers, residents were caught unawares. According to a report filed by the lieutenant-governor, "Less than 20 minutes after the first cannon was discharged, the town presented one sheet of flame." An hour later, it was "a heap of smoldering ashes."[76]

The Marylanders might win battles with superior weapons, a willingness to burn whole towns, and the help of antislavery patrols. But they knew they couldn't win an all-out war against a significantly larger population, especially if local enmities dividing neighboring groups were patched up to forge alliances—as was likely if the settlers sought to dominate inland or coastal trade by force or to seize more land. Nor could they win the war against hunger, which began to bite as homeless Greboes launched retaliatory raids on outlying homesteads. Beset on all sides and facing famine, the settlers called urgently for support from U.S. and British warships and interdiction vessels. As chance would have it, help was already on the way, in the form of the *Mary*

Caroline Stevens—a 142-foot clipper, 713 tons fully laden, built by James Hall and the American Colonization Society. It was the clipper's maiden voyage, and Dr. Hall was aboard.

When the *Stevens* hove to off the coast of Cape Mount, a newer American settlement up the coast, Dr. Hall got word of what had happened in Maryland. Devastated, he set sail toward Monrovia to plead for assistance to save the colony. There he convinced the Liberian president, Stephen Allen Benson, to lead an armed force, mustered and provisioned at the society's expense, in order to prevent Maryland's ruin and the destruction of more Grebo settlements; both were a serious possibility. Governor Drayton and a few others "were for exterminating the Africans," Richard Hall writes, but "the majority of Marylanders wanted to end the war. They knew the Greboes had suffered tremendously and were eager to have peace on any dignified terms." The chiefs refused to negotiate with the self-installed aggressor at the helm of the colony, demanding instead a parley with James Hall and the former president.

When the *Stevens* and reinforcements cast anchor off Cape Palmas, Dr. Hall risked a sentimental walk to the torched town. Where once he had engaged in palavers under a giant silk-cotton tree, sometimes partaking of "brimmers of the sweet palm wine" with the Grebo chiefs, he now saw "nothing but ashes and raised circles that had been house floors." The ruins were already disappearing under the shoots and tendrils that quickly follow fire. "His worst fears confirmed," Richard Hall writes, James Hall "wanted only to leave."[77] And that he did.

The parley began on February 23, 1857, the day after the colony's anniversary. A new treaty stipulated compensation for material losses on both sides, designated sites at which destroyed villages were to be rebuilt, forbade the plunder of wrecked ships, and reaffirmed the ban on the slave trade. "James Hall might have stayed to hear the palaver talked and to celebrate the colony's anniversary," Richard Hall continues, "but he could not bear to do so under such gloomy circumstances." The former governor was also distraught because he understood that the independent state of Maryland was about to dissolve, its citizens content to "throw ourselves into the arms of the

Republic." Liberia's sitting president, exhorting the legislature to endorse the annexation, predicted a time when "the vast multitudes of aborigines in this land shall have become as stone from the quarry, polished by art, and fully identified with us." Both houses of Liberia's legislature ratified the union without much debate but with much flowery speech, looking forward to the day "Christianity and civilization will soon be co-extensive on this continent with our geographical borders."[78]

Such outcomes were a long way off and still are. But it's clear from reading accounts of Liberia's early years that the roots of the conflicts of the late twentieth century and this one, including Ebola-related conflicts, were already growing a century and a half earlier. It's all there: the toll of feuds and fevers; palavers between feuding groups; ambition for power among settlers and natives alike; the former's belief in the inferiority of the heathens but the steady absorption of many of their ideas and practices (including the notion of power gained through juju ordeals and ritual cannibalism); struggles over land and land tenure; sedition and betrayal of both ideals and treaties; and the use of naval firepower to enforce colonists' wishes in a time when the bombardment of villages was "merely a tool of diplomacy in a violent environment."[79]

For a century, Harper, Buchanan, Monrovia, and the other Americo-Liberian colonies grew, creeping inland with the years. Liberia was diplomatically and socially isolated, despite the fact it produced coffee and other tropical produce for an international market. Even its ambivalent midwife, the United States, did not extend formal diplomatic recognition until 1862. The American Civil War slowed U.S. colonization, which saw a spike after a short-lived Reconstruction, the rise of the Ku Klux Klan, and the spread of lynching. But as the American Colonization Society and its branches folded, so did colonization, leaving the natives to swell these coastal settlements. It was an uneasy integration, since the Americo-Liberians remained paranoid of white encroachment from without and of native sedition from within.

Internally, the country had no unifying ideal, even if its occupants did share a skin color, more or less, and if its constitution, said to be drafted at Harvard, did forbid foreign ownership of land. The country's founding motto—"The Love of Liberty Brought Us Here"—certainly did nothing to protect or improve the lot of most of the natives on whom the Americo-Liberians depended. Like other colonial regimes in West Africa, Monrovia taxed the natives but built few schools, and almost no clinics or hospitals, in the hinterland. Liberia's consolidation and steady inland encroachment had little effect on the health of even the westward-facing Americo-Liberians along the coast.

Meanwhile, conflict simmered across colonial Sierra Leone, which was also self-aggrandizing. Both the crown colony of Freetown and the hinterland had expanding borders, as the British and their commercial agents were ever putting down a rebellion here, invoking an obscure treaty there. The colony was administered by British officers but dominated by Creole merchants, teachers, clergy, and bureaucrats. This was before blacks were excluded from leadership positions in the town's administration and clergy, as Joseph Wright's story suggests, and when the British founded Fourah Bay College—the first institution of higher learning built in West Africa since the decline of Islamic universities established in medieval times. It was established for the uplift of Africans, leading to proud comparisons with Athens.[80] Such comparisons were unintentionally apt, as far as social stratification went. The Creoles otherwise emulated British, not Athenian, cultural institutions, from bewigged judges to high tea, pink gin, and various dilute flavors of Christianity.

The hinterland population, hailing from a couple dozen tribes, didn't share Creole or white colonists' worldviews—which had designated them as fixed tribes in the first place—any more than they trusted or knew them. A century after Britain staked its first West African claims, many of those far from the coast had never met any of these overlords, in spite of stacks of treaties signed from the mid-nineteenth century on. Few were unaware, however, that the empire considered them subject to British law whenever indirect rule was applied with direct force. As the nineteenth century waned, and as disputes over borders and chiefly successions continued, social divisions beyond town and hinterland also caused trouble: British colonists began pursuing overtly discriminatory policies against the Creoles they'd once mentored.

This was a symptom of an increasingly codified white supremacy, linked to the rise of U.S. and European eugenics and related pseudoscientific regimes. In the face of competition from newly arrived traders from Syria, and mounting racism, Creole elites fought to maintain their privilege, which, by the last decades of the century, was tied to control of commerce and proximity to political rule. In West Africa, these were rarely local affairs. As telegraph cables encircled continents and spanned oceans, the boundaries of British rule across West Africa expanded. Since the empire's primary goal—commercial gain—was plenty clear, Britain delegated many aspects of its rule to private concerns. This neat mercantilist trick had deindustrialized and depleted India. Across the empire, it was widely adopted after the scandalous success of the British East India Company.

The Union Jack may have flapped or drooped over small embassies and consulates in the towns and cities on West Africa's navigable rivers, but it was often hoisted in the wake of trade deals inked by other imperial charter companies—the Royal African Company and the Sierra Leone Company were examples—serving as quasi-representatives of the Crown. A history of the formal European takeover of Africa explains why:

> The conventional wisdom at this period was that the British flag
> was a handicap to British trade. At any rate, it could only follow
> trade after several generations, when life was complicated enough
> to demand formal sovereignty and business was big enough to carry
> the costs. In the meantime, traders kept life simple and business
> blossomed in the political void. This was the secret and invisible
> empire, the network of trade supported by the network of informal
> power that British consuls and British gunboats extended around the
> coasts of Africa, invisible as an electrical field.[81]

The British network of power was not invisible, however, to Britain's neighbors across the English Channel, and the political void was soon filled by the formal and rivalrous European occupation of West Africa.

After the loss of Haiti and the close of the Napoleonic Wars, the French had been forced to surrender most of their American territories. Industrializing a few decades after perfidious Britain, France remained its chief rival for African markets and its raw materials throughout much of the nineteenth century. It had, however, proceeded somewhat differently from its rivals for hegemony in West Africa. Some French-sponsored, for-profit ventures weren't all that different from British ones. But when flag led trade under the tricolor, there was less dissembling about local autonomy and less feigned deference to indigenous institutions: Paris, which boasted a long-standing presence in Senegal, more honestly acknowledged that extending its influence and trade networks would require naked force. But there was little in the way of a standing French army elsewhere in West Africa in the mid-nineteenth century. (French forces were then busy suppressing Algerian revolts to the north.) The rainy season prevented inland travel, even as it reduced settlers and natives alike by unleashing deadly outbreaks of typhoid, malaria, dysentery, yellow fever, and pathogens as yet undescribed.

Often enough, in other words, French rule was also perforce indirect in much of West Africa. In the eyes of its elites, including those with military experience in its colonies, extending French cultural influence (an openly cherished goal of much foreign policy) and building back an empire (a more cloaked but likely more cherished goal) would not result from the efforts of the rivalrous explorers and amateur naturalists then hacking through forest, jungle, and savannah in search of navigable rivers and their disputed sources, or of new species of flora and fauna. Neither goal would result, in this view, from effete strains of Christian proselytizing such as those pursued by black Methodists in Freetown, by the likes of Joseph Wright, or by institutions like Fourah Bay College. Hardliners among the French who nursed Napoleonic dreams insisted that Africa required a more muscular formula of the three *c*'s: civilization, commerce, and Catholicism. Although telegraph cables bound imperial outposts into commercial networks, civilization and Catholicism required a more intimate connection.

If the British had invested scarcely any more effort in evangelizing Africa than had other European powers—they'd left that largely to the Muslims or, more recently, to American missionaries—its empire enthusiasts were not about to yield to French designs. Besides, the three *c*'s, with "Christianity" replacing Catholicism, was *their* idea, promoted by the missionary explorer Dr. David Livingstone, a Scotsman. Unlike post-Haiti France, however, Britain still had a real jewel in its crown.[82] An immense flow of loot—a Hindi word—hadn't slowed after Queen Victoria, promising Britons and Indians alike to address the abuses of the East India Company, established the Raj in 1858. But trade still led flag, and abuse continued as formal colonial rule hardened. As protests mounted in India, there was no assurance that the colony would keep generating cash. The empire looked to expand its sway elsewhere, turning once again toward Africa. Some politicians in London may have been, by the late nineteenth century, more cautious about further imperial expansion, but many British elites in the worldwide colonial service seemed to feel "a proprietary right to most of the continent."[83]

Prince Otto von Bismarck, the German chancellor, had similar pretensions. His boss, Wilhelm II, was Victoria's eldest grandchild, but both chancellor and emperor chafed with *ressentiment* over British and French colonial holdings. In the final quarter of the nineteenth century, a unified Germany had the economic might to realize long-nursed dreams of distant colonies. Even without West African footholds like Dakar and Freetown, German merchants were giving French and British competitors a run for their money. As for military might, Germany could call up large armies if it turned away from war with its neighbors.

Nor was it just the big three who wanted in on the spoils. King Leopold of Belgium, Queen Victoria's cousin, had dark designs on the vast Congo River basin. The leaders of a recently unified Italy also wanted a piece of African pie, and were already ogling Ethiopia. (This proved a bad idea for the Italians.) Even the sovereigns of run-down Portugal and Spain considered themselves due for another go at empire. Many European subjects objected to their takeover of another continent, and for varied reasons. Costly pacification campaigns, replete with ample evidence of war crimes and other outrages, were held up by European fiscal skeptics and by pacifists as fodder for their arguments. But nothing, it seems, could stop the train of empire once it left the station for Africa. The three *c*'s thus required a fourth: conquest.

This would in turn require—to the dismay of cautious bureaucrats and of Europe's historically minded and more progressive subjects—boots on the ground. Echoes of the occupation's footfalls were soon heard across the last uncolonized continent excepting Antarctica.

The Great Scramble for Africa had begun.

6.

The Great Scramble and the Rise of the Pasteurians

In the whole of Africa's nearly twelve million odd square miles there are probably not more than 1,200,000 whites to 150,000,000 natives. Of the former 750,000 are in Africa, south of the Zambezi, and over 300,000 in Algeria and Tunis, leaving 150,000 for all the rest of the continent. Of the continent between the tropics, all experience up to present goes to show that it can never be colonized by white races, but must be developed by the natives under white supervision.

—Sir John Scott Keltie, "The Partition of Africa," *The Independent*, 1898

Suddenly, in half a generation, the Scramble gave Europe virtually the whole continent: including thirty new colonies and protectorates, 10 million square miles of new territory and 110 million dazed new subjects, acquired by one method or another. Africa was sliced up like a cake, the pieces swallowed by five rival nations—Germany, Italy, Portugal, France and Britain (with Spain taking some scraps)—and Britain and France were at each other's throats.

—Thomas Pakenham, *The Scramble for Africa*, 1991

UNDER THE BANNER OF THE "INTERNATIONAL AFRICAN ASSOCIATION," THE Berlin Conference opened in 1884 in Radziwill Palace, now better remembered as headquarters of the Third Reich. In commissioned portraits, Otto von Bismarck looks the rearguard-ready Prussian general—stout and bald; festooned with a droopy white mustache, bristling eyebrows, and a chestful of medals; and girt with a sword. Like his guests and his Kaiser, the chancellor was ready to fight for his bit of Africa, which conferees regarded as the globe's last unclaimed turf. Needless to say, no Africans were invited.

The conference was Europe's attempt to avoid warring over Africa while ramping up exploitation of its resources. Since war had long been the favored sport of Europe's sovereigns, even when related by blood and marriage, it's notable that fourteen countries signed the accords. U.S. envoys, setting aside tepid American disparagement of European imperialism, went to Berlin to take notes. (These soon proved useful in the Philippines, Cuba, and Hawaii. Their own natives mostly down the oubliette, the Americans knew that taking over an entire continent wasn't straightforward.) French, British, and German empire enthusiasts faced objection from their more principled subjects, of course, but most official reticence about seizing another continent came from the exchequers. The masters of coin worried about the costs of occupying and administering vast and unruly regions of varied promise, as far as return on investments went. And there were other reasons Europe's top bureaucrats feared being dispatched to West Africa.

The flaming sword of deadly fevers loomed large. "Up to the year 1885," according to a British factotum writing of Sierra Leone, "no less than ten Governors (in addition to eight Acting Governors) died while on the coast, or on their way to England."[1] Occupying savage lands further required boots on the ground, and cautious generals feared they might not have enough of them. Midcentury expansion in Algeria had required France to muster a force of two hundred thousand to suppress "Islamic revolts," and Britain's extractive occupation of India, which was where the great majority of the world's colonized people then lived, demanded a massive standing army. The jewel in Britain's crown footed the bill for its own occupation while financing many imperial misadventures far from the subcontinent, and early British efforts to drain loot from Africa had sought to follow a similar model. But British forces had been routed by the Ashanti nation in 1824; they fought to a draw between 1863 and 1864. Although the empire finally prevailed in its third war against the Ashanti, 1873 to 1874, it cost many lives—and close to a million pounds sterling. The British also lost the First Boer War in 1881, two years after their defeat at the hands of the Zulu in nearby Isandlwana.

Europe's rulers knew, from these and scores of similar conflicts, that the likelihood of pacific acceptance of white rule was scant across Africa.

A unified Germany, having become Britain's largest trading partner, might compete militarily, but there was little hope of Portugal, Italy, Spain, or Belgium assembling tens of thousands of troops in order to subdue and administer the territories claimed from Berlin. There were, however, new (or newish) technologies that favored a new imperialism based on old ideas. Enhanced by telegraph—which one historian termed the "invisible weapon" of empire—and rail networks, policies of divide-conquer-keep had permitted the pillage and deindustrialization of India.[2] As French, British, and German cable ships laid the trunk lines that would connect the African coast to the era's worldwide web, gung-ho conferees in Berlin came up with talking points, which they titled "Principle of Effective Occupation," to dampen objections from the bean (and boot) counters. These talking points promised to make African colonies self-financing while shipping surplus and taxes north. This was new language for old tricks: with the help of slave labor and conscripts, Europeans had used this formula in the Americas to enrich themselves and whiten North America. This formula worked in Africa, too—just not for the Africans.

The partition hatched in Berlin had swift and profound effects across the continent. Colonial powers chiseled new polities out of slender or specious claims made during decades when explorers, envoys, and traders—along with the occasional missionary doctor—were dispatched inland with trade goods, weapons, liquor, and fill-in-the-blank treaties to be signed by chiefs, kings, sultans, and other African rulers. Across West Africa, Britain divided its claims into colonies (lands claimed before the Scramble) and protectorates (the vast hinterlands divvied up during it). The enormous parcel of earth suddenly termed French West Africa had a similar pedigree. A decade before Berlin, less than 10 percent of the continent was colonized by foreign powers, and the number was lower than that across West and North Africa. By 1902, 90 percent of Africa—ten million square miles—was under nominal European control.

The always-humming imperial propaganda machine kicked into high gear after European rulers proclaimed their rule a civilizing mission, with disease control and "hygiene" offered as important justifications. Precisely in the years colonial powers gathered in Berlin to plan Africa's partition after

1884, European scientists were developing revolutionary new tools to control the pestilence that had for centuries threatened towns, cities, and global commerce. At the time, much of the world was a medical desert, and the Pasteurian revolution under way in Europe and North America was decades off for colonial subjects in Africa. That didn't mean that people living on the continent were unenthusiastic about preventing the epidemics that periodically devastated its cities, towns, and villages. Many African communities had long practiced forms of variolation and self-imposed quarantine in the face of smallpox.[3]

As the century drew to a close, many Africans sought access to new vaccines. But the manner in which these and other preventives were shared mattered, a great deal; much of that sharing was martial or imposed. The establishment of formal European rule across Africa saw the imposition of quarantine, isolation, and varied schemes of social segregation, as well as attempts to vaccinate by force. In West Africa, as elsewhere on the continent, the control-over-care paradigm became entrenched in the early twentieth century. Adverse events and unexplained deaths during the course of imposed public-health campaigns sparked fear and resistance.[4] This was especially true when and where European notions of hygiene were less effective than advertised, which was often.

The empire builders who gathered in Bismarck's palace also promised economic development and the uplift of Africa's benighted natives—until they could manage their own affairs, if they wished to do so. Europe's grandees threw in a pledge to ban slavery by "African and Islamic powers," by which they meant the Swahili-speaking Arab traders who'd supplanted them as that black market moved east. With millions shipped west to the Americas during the same century, and almost none of them on the ships of the Islamic powers in question, the historically minded found this hard to swallow. In *The Heart of Darkness*, Joseph Conrad mocked the Berlin Conference as a gathering of the "International Society for the Suppression of Savage Customs."[5]

"Suppression" was the right word, and it was plenty savage. The idea that the takeover of West Africa was achieved by fulfilling treaties signed while toasting the mutual benefits to ensue sends history down into the oubliette. Treaties (to paraphrase a Haitian expression) are made of paper; bayonets are made of steel. Across the region, rulers who resisted European rule were tamed, toppled, exiled, or killed.

The accumulation of capital and other wealth in Europe—much of it, India aside, extracted from the Americas with the help of twelve million Africans and their tens of millions of unfree descendants—occurred in tandem with ongoing state militarization and the uptake of new weapons of war. By the time of the Berlin Conference, both Europe and West Africa were armed to the teeth, if with different weapons. Although rifles and other guns had long since infested both continents, they were of European provenance and had (most historians of the place and time argue) uneven effects on the martial cultures of West Africa.[6] But some of its rulers had developed a great fondness for firearms, and they began to resist the three *c*'s—commerce, civilization, Christianity—well before the violent clash of partition.

Throughout the nineteenth century, British and French military forces had been held at bay by a series of sultans, emirs, almamies and imams, viziers, qadis, damels, caliphs, kabakas, pashas, suzerains, and other Defenders of the Faith. "For Muslim societies of West Africa," explains the historian Michael Crowder, "the imposition of white rule meant submission to the infidel, which was intolerable to any good Muslim."[7] Although some of these societies had been fairly recent converts to Islam, its roots in the region were deep. The Tukolor, who resisted French military incursions from the 1850s to the 1880s, had been Muslim since the eleventh century; Timbuktu boasted mosques dating from before medieval times, as did other cities along the Niger Bend.

Nor was resistance to white rule an exclusively Muslim affair. The great Mossi empire, for example, extended its sway from the ancient city of Ouagadougou, on the upper Volta River; its rulers had "resisted Islamicization and indeed any foreign penetration for more than two centuries."[8] From holy north to pagan south, and from fortified cities and towns, those who'd traded spears and arrows for rifles and horses resisted European rule. Looking at developments in West Africa during the decade just before and after Berlin, it's possible to count hundreds of feuding factions and signed treaties, and many more battles, skirmishes, ambushes, raids, rebellions, and sieges.

There were, of course, differences in the manner in which the colonizers of West Africa proceeded. When historians assert that France's occupation was more of a military exercise than British rule, inquiring minds want to know: Just how military an exercise was it? Since the architects of European rule were fond of unburdening themselves in print, forests were felled to publish their accounts of this chapter of imperial history and to constitute the awesome, numbing detail of colonial archives. Although much of this trove was self-serving, there wasn't often a problem of too little candor. The views of the suppressed savages, on the other hand, are harder to uncover. In the eyes of the occupied, there was likely more similarity between the methods of the occupiers than its chroniclers allow. There may have been different flavors of conquest and rule, but all tasted violent, and European.

By all accounts, meek was not on the menu.

How did these developments square with French tales of *missions civilisatrices* or British sighs about colonialism as the "white man's burden"? The noisome flower of racism, planted long ago, had grown into maturity by the late nineteenth century. That's when many of today's notions of race, which have no basis in human genetics but found one in eugenics, were hardened.

Colonial whitewash, some of it slopped on by the academics of the day, helped keep the myth of civilizing missions alive. Michael Crowder has summarized European justifications for colonial rule: "Some believed that the children they watched over could grow up into good Europeans; others believed they were permanently children, or, rather, immutably separate and inferior to the Europeans."[9] The details of the period he calls "Conquest and Occupation" leave readers wishing for some form of paternalism (or maternalism) rather than the savage repression then in evidence. It wasn't disdain or condescension, much less time-outs or spankings, awaiting those who resisted. It was the lash, the gaol, the gallows, the firing squad, the torch, the artillery, and the protracted siege. When fortifications crumbled or burned, it was fight or flight. Many fought.

London and Paris may have wanted the pacification of West Africa to end quickly, but French commanders didn't seem to have received that memo. (Several of them blamed cable communications inferior to those of the British and Germans.) Headquartered in Dakar—thrust into the ocean across which captive-laden vessels had sailed toward Haiti, Martinique, Guyana, and New Orleans—the commanders looked inland for other targets, setting their sights on the middle Niger and western Sudan. The region's reputation as an African El Dorado had faded: the French historian Jean Suret-Canale, later chastised for discrediting his country's colonial narrative, described the region as an "ungrateful, punishing setting, even if the wounds of sleeping sickness and, more recently, of onchocerciasis were likely opened by the violent disruption of colonization."[10]

The part about violence was certainly indisputable. West African leaders were used to it, but they hadn't counted on Maxim and Gatling guns able to turn whole platoons into mincemeat, or on artillery that could breach their walls within hours. Nor had they counted on European commanders finally catching on to quinine. Powerful West African polities, shaped by the slave trades and their attendant miseries, began to collapse. In 1891, French forces seized Kankan—the major trade hub on the Milo River—from their nemesis, Samory Touré. They stormed the city of Djenné, leveling its thirteenth-century great mosque. When the rulers of the Mossi empire declined the "protection" of France, French troops took Ouagadougou by force in 1896. They then invaded the Imamate of Futa Jallon, in the highlands of Guinea, where Samory was born.

Although he took the flourish Emperor of the Believers, Samory— sometimes spelled Samori—was more warlord than religious leader. He may have lacked artillery and repeating rifles, but he had mastered the art of guerrilla warfare. The French warlords knew they'd have trouble with him, as suggested by the grudging admiration of commanders in Dakar:

Who were these half-armed black soldiers who could withstand the fire of machine gun and artillery without flinching? Who, indeed, was Samori, the great warlord from the Milo, who had trained these pagans to fight with even more desperate courage than the soldiers of a Muslim jihad, only a swordthrust away from paradise?[11]

Samory hailed from a Mandinka family farming the wooded highlands and savannah on either side of the Milo, which—like the Little Scarcies, the Mano, the Saint Paul, and other major rivers running south to the Upper Guinea Coast—springs from the highlands of the Futa Jallon. Prior to the transatlantic slave trade, the Futa had seen the continent's "longest development of agriculture, of markets and long-distance trade, and of complex political systems."[12] Such development required, as did mere survival, powerful patrons. Samory became one as a young man, after uniting Milo villages and towns to repulse Islamic invaders from Kankan.

Spurred by youthful success, Samory trained and equipped a growing army between the 1860s and 1880s. At the height of his power, he could muster an army of more than thirty thousand, many of them mounted. (Taking Kankan, he transformed it and other towns into the capitals of a far-flung caliphate after he turned, or turned back, to Islam. French forces were initially stretched too thin to force themselves on his realm.) By 1890, Samory's rule stretched across what are today northwest Guinea, Mali, and parts of Sierra Leone and the Ivory Coast. At the insistence of Paris, whose envoys had signed numerous accords with Samory during the era of promiscuous treaties, French commanders first tried diplomacy. When this failed, in 1891, they embarked on a campaign to bring him down. "From then until 1898," reports Michael Crowder, "it was war to the bitter end."[13]

The French campaign against Samory Touré and his allies was just one among many. But its details and dénouement say a lot about the intended and unintended consequences of the European project in West Africa. Armed resistance to that project, even when translated into wars between African rulers, disrupted or ended the lives of many farming and trading across the region.

Epidemics stirred up by the conflict shortened even more of them. French efforts to bring down Samory were associated with the usual camp epidemics and with the introduction of pathogens from one part of a vast theater of conquest to others. Men and horses drew tsetse flies from Kankan into what are now the Ivory Coast and southern Burkina Faso, where African sleeping sickness—said in one recent review to be previously unknown—wiped out entire villages.[14] (Onchocerciasis, a fly-transmitted disease widely termed river blindness, followed similar trajectories.) When the dry season permitted French incursions inland, Samory deployed part of his army to stop them, turning the rest of it east to conquer new territories. Upon faring the worst in a skirmish, he withdrew his army and his subjects—along with portable treasures and belongings, including horses and beasts of burden—after razing ceded territory. These retreats required "a fantastic administrative ability," in the opinion of Crowder, "for not only was an army on the move, but a whole empire."[15]

There was less evidence of fantastic abilities in administering relief to the hungry, sick, or injured in Samory's train, or to those displaced from scorched lands or gang-pressed into feeding either his mobile empire or French-controlled forces, who were of course also mostly African. As the French pursued Samory, a swath of illness, injury, despoliation, and displacement was driven steadily south across the forest-savannah mosaic toward the tropical forest (an immense green wall between the belligerents and the coast) and east toward the Volta River and Ashanti (which, having twice dealt defeat to the British, was finally falling). Beyond the eastern shores of the river, north of Nigeria's lowland rain forest, sprawled Dahomey, Yoruba, and Benin—rich states long hubs of the slave trades, and soon to succumb. To the north rose the walled cities of the western Sudan, which were also implicated in these trades.

European rulers gathered in Berlin had held up "domestic" or "internal" slavery as evidence that they weren't the instigators of the peculiar institution.[16] Although Guinean and Malian nationalists would later burnish Samory's

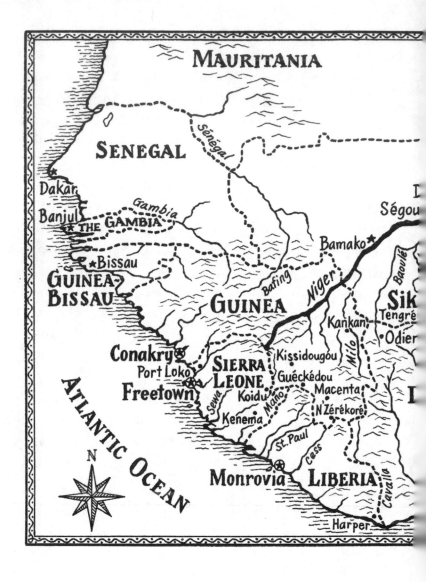

memory as a leader of the resistance to French occupation, there's little doubt that his subjects included serfs and slaves. A history of partition lays out his strategy to acquire rifles and other weapons:

> To pay for them, he sent pack mules loaded with gold and ivory back over the mountains. He also paid, indirectly, in slaves: rebels or men captured in war, whom he sold to the wild tribes of the eastern plains

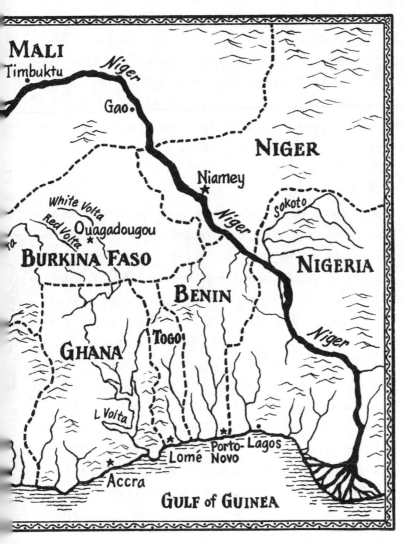

West Africa in a time of changing borders and threatened cities

in exchange for horses. He could never get enough modern rifles, even though his village blacksmiths had been trained to produce their own efficient copies of the Gras repeater. Nor did he ever succeed in training his men to use their rifles as the Europeans did. Disciplined though they were, his warriors were too excited to co-ordinate their fire—or even to fire straight—unlike the Africans trained by the French.[17]

As Samory was driven eastward—his forces thinned by raids, wounds of war, defections, hunger, and illness—he sought British protection, informing Freetown that he could no longer abide by the terms of his treaties with France. The governor wished to shield him, but was overruled by London.[18] Desperate, Samory sued for peace, asking to remain the titular head of his empire. The French responded by pushing their weakened foe farther east and south, trespassing Sierra Leone's new borders and provoking a European diplomatic row.

Samory next retreated north and east toward the drier Sahel, forging a last-ditch alliance with Babemba Traoré, the king of Kenedougou. Established in the late eighteenth century, this prosperous trading state encompassed a significant region within the boundaries of modern-day Mali. The great fortified city of Sikasso, Kenedougou's capital, lay athwart the crossroads leading south (to Kong), north (to Ségou, Djenné, Mopti, and Bamako), east (to Ouagadougou), and west (to Tengréla and Kankan). These were the major trading towns of the era, and most of them were ancient. Sikasso, in contrast, hadn't been chosen as a capital until 1877. During the subsequent two decades, Babemba's elder brother—who, while king, had adopted an appeasement strategy with the French—invested capital and labor to erect the city's massive walls. Initially built of mud, but later reinforced or rebuilt with clay and stone, Sikasso's fortifications offered refuge for the nobles and their households of kin, servants, and courtiers. Horses, mules, livestock, and the granaries, storehouses, and souks of traders and artisans—all were sheltered within.

Samory knew this, having himself laid siege to Sikasso at a time French reports described it as "a powerful and sprawling fortress."[19] In 1888, at the height of his sway, his forces had surrounded the city for over a year but were defeated by outer ramparts that topped, in most stretches, twenty feet. The war cost Samory dearly, and not just in terms of prestige: his army was reduced by as many as ten thousand; his entire cavalry, destroyed. Although Kenedougou's losses were also steep—the kingdom was estimated to count five thousand deaths—impregnable Sikasso still stood. The success of its walls in protecting the many thousands living within them from the era's most powerful warlord led Kenedougou's rulers to expand the city's rings of protection. By the time of Babemba's rule, which began in 1893, its outer walls—an unbroken chain of crenellated towers pierced by countless embrasures for snipers—were more than ten kilometers long.

Sikasso under Babemba was the strongest fortress in the western Sudan. Rising above the plain in all its pride and might, the city was, notes the Malian historian Alpha Konaré, ever "on war-footing." Within its walls lived some thirty-five thousand souls, and thousands more were in and out of the city to conduct seasonal trade or to pay tribute as vassals of the king. As the French took over other once-powerful states, and hounded his rival from Milo, Babemba grew more suspicious of their intentions. Their plan, he concluded after receiving French envoys, was "to soften me up in order to take away my birthright." That would happen, he famously told another of his brothers, over his dead body: "I will never give up, to anyone, even a morsel of my ancestors' land."[20] Now, in 1898, Babemba's kingdom and its walled redoubt lay squarely within territory declared French as French forces were moving to attack Sikasso. Although Samory had forged an anti-French alliance with Babemba, the king sealed Sikasso's gates, denying Samory refuge within its walls. He retreated south to his own keep in the town of Boribana.

By April 15, 1898, French-led troops had surrounded Sikasso. According to French military reports, spies within it provided crucial information about the fortress. The besieging commanders knew it was well provisioned and defended by a militia of ten thousand to twelve thousand men, some two thousand of them cavalry. After a two-week siege, punctuated by sorties, Babemba could likely see from the top of his many-storied keep that his forces outnumbered French ones. What he couldn't see was where "the white man's thunder" came from.[21] Atop the siege wagons was the artillery, which counted brand-new 95 mm Lahitolle cannons, made of tempered steel and able to launch two mortars per minute from a distance of more than four miles. This was the weapon, reports Konaré, that got the best of Sikasso.

The city's defenders scrambled each night to repair the wall, but could not keep pace with the Lahitolles. At dawn on May 1, French commanders launched the final assault. It was over by nightfall. By their accounts, they breached the walls and executed Babemba. Survivors of the siege of Sikasso, including members of the royal family, told a different story. They said the king took his own life upon seeing his walls crumble and was laid to rest in a secret place. As refugees fled the sacked city, Samory knew Boribana was next and sought to negotiate an honorable surrender. Retreating west and south, he was seized by French forces in a town closer to Monrovia than to Sikasso. Under the headline "African Chieftain Captured," *The New York Times* reported that "the most dangerous antagonist the Europeans have had to deal with" had at last been subdued.[22] Touré was exiled to a prison in newly French Gabon, where he soon died of pneumonia.

A century later, Malian officials and scholars sought to "erase the myth that Africans offered no resistance to colonization" by marking the centennial of Sikasso's fall. "African heroes like Babemba and Samory did fight," explained Mali's event planners to a BBC reporter in 1998, "and it is this that we want the world to know."[23] They discovered that some of Sikasso's residents knew their history all too well, even if a heedless world did not. The city boasted modern monuments to both rulers, but marking Babemba's final resting place proved impossible: his descendants still protected knowledge of its whereabouts. For them, according to the reporter, "the anniversary marked only defeat and death." The ceremony, in any case, didn't go as planned. Live from Sikasso, the reporter described what happened next.

The rebuilt city's municipal stadium was packed shortly after "the historic day dawned to the thudding boom of cannon fire." The commemoration came to a "quick and shaky end" when the throng realized the program was to include revelation of the hidden tomb's location. "Instantly," she reported, "all the solemn old men in the stands—Babemba's own grandchildren and great-grandchildren—were on their feet, waving their fists and shouting that the whereabouts of the king's real grave would never, ever be divulged to anyone."[24]

If resistance to European occupation was fierce, how did such small armies—a fraction of British forces in India, or of French expeditions to retake Haiti or subdue Algeria—come to conquer West Africa?

Medical advances helped European commanders prevail, as did steam-ships and new communication technologies. But, as Michael Crowder writes, new weaponry and old regional feuds were bigger parts of the equation:

> Superior weapons, a skillful manipulation of hostilities between
> African states or the internal divisions within them, enabled the
> Europeans to conquer West Africa with small forces and with
> comparative ease. For the most part Africans were cut off from
> sources of supply of modern European weapons and even had they
> been available lacked instructors to teach them how to use them. Too
> often they met the invaders with the same military tactics they used
> against each other. Cavalry charges, hails of arrows or spears, and
> hand-to-hand fighting were no use against repeater rifles and Maxim
> guns. The great mud walls that would withstand a six-month siege by
> an African army crumbled before the European artillery.

European victors now set out to disarm their new subjects, a project not lim-ited to seizing weapons and leaders of the resistance. They also seized or dis-mantled West Africa's fortresses. Sikasso's walls may have been exceptional in height and girth, but circular stockaded towns and palisaded villages had long been the rule in raid-prone West Africa. In some regions, walls that didn't crumble upon bombardment were victim to bureaucratic assault—a highly honed European skill.

In the early years of their occupation of Sierra Leone, the British disman-tled, then banned, fortified ring towns from coast to forest. "As towns moved and stretched in lines along the colonial roads and railway," Rosalind Shaw writes in *Memories of the Slave Trade*, stockaded settlements soon gave way "to ribbon development."[25] The word "development" suggests significant investments in infrastructure but also in the freedoms and services—freedom from want and services like education and health care—that anticolonial forces later claimed to be fighting for, along with the dignity of self-rule. But were colonial health and educational systems a successful part of the civi-lizing mission, as has so often been claimed? Were they more reliable than the disintegrating mess that followed independence in the latter half of the twentieth century?

It's doubtful. Fourah Bay College and Kissy Lunatic Asylum aside, there was little in the way of postprimary education or medical care in occupied West Africa. Such services were often relegated to missionaries—some of them Americans with slightly more meritocratic notions than their European cousins—or to no one at all. Colonial efforts to provide health services, even those designed to protect public health rather than respond to individual ailments, were equally paltry. (The Kissy asylum was, in the words of one historian, "established as a depository for the mentally disordered," including those deemed by the British to be "socially disordered" or violent, two diagnoses that proliferated under formal colonial rule.)[26] When they were for West Africans, the first objection from the occupiers tended to be about who was going to pay for them. Britain's treasury was more tightfisted than that of France, but both empires had long embraced policies to ensure that local surpluses and levies were used to finance colonial administration (including policing, justice, and public health) and infrastructure projects (including railways, ports, and telegraph cables as well as roads and sanitation in coastal capitals).

Some of these projects were financed initially by loans from the metropole. They were paid back in spades. In order to enjoy the privilege of belonging to a glorious empire, in other words, colonial subjects were expected to defray their own expenses, including the cost of promised health and educational services that mostly failed to arrive, while defraying the expenses of unknown others in increasingly opulent European cities. In practice, this was easier said than done without forced labor and fabulous booty—the spoils of conquest in previous centuries. Whether flag-led or trade-led, both colonial administrations relied on forced labor. The hated *corvée*, forced labor in lieu or on top of taxes, continued in French West Africa until the end of World War II, and "existing slavery" wasn't formally abolished in Sierra Leone until 1928.[27] So in practice, and in spite of sanctimonious denials, slaves and serfs and plunder continued to figure among the rewards of loyal service to the occupiers.

To supplement its resources, since regimes of forced labor often failed, colonial authorities turned to taxation. Efforts to collect taxes also often failed, especially on British turf. But amnestic colonials had forgotten, it seems, the turmoil sparked by taxation without representation in both the Province of Freedom and in their North American colonies. Shortly after retracing the boundaries of its empire to include the hinterlands of Sierra Leone, Ghana (née the Gold Coast), the Gambia, and Nigeria, Britain sought to impose household levies on its new subjects. In Sierra Leone, authorities attempted to collect this house tax—more widely and honestly termed the "hut tax"—within three of five districts at the beginning of 1898. Resistance was fierce and immediate.

Thus began the Hut Tax War. Insurrection in the south included, in the words of one British historian, "a series of savage attacks" on Britons and Americans living in the Mende hinterlands.[28] British officers and their foot soldiers responded savagely and with far superior firepower: Maxim guns and artillery, of course, but also the old-school firepower of arson. Manned by the Third Battalion of the West Indian regiment, gunboats traveled up navigable rivers in the south to level "enemy positions"—meaning riverine settlements said to house recalcitrant chiefs and other troublemakers. Across the south, punitive raids forced thousands to flee their farms and rice paddies; food was soon scarce across the ill-named protectorate. It was worse in the north, where Temne-speaking chiefs, including Port Loko's Bai Bureh, were said by the stiff-necked new governor—a military officer knighted after subduing unruly natives in India and South Africa—to have declared war on the British.[29] Sierra Leonean historians would later denounce this as self-serving colonial calumny. One of twenty-four chiefs to sign one of a "plethora of petitions" protesting the tax as beyond the means of the rural poor, Bureh was, in the words of Arthur Abraham, "an innocent victim of the prejudices and designs of the frontiersmen of Pax Britannica."[30]

There were many more victims in 1899, when the governor sought to make an example of Bai Bureh by leveling scores of settlements around Port Loko. Progressives back in Britain took the trouble to dismantle colonial claims, and to deplore Freetown's methods, in no uncertain terms. One prominent English pacifist wrote of the "monstrous unfairness" of the tax, naming it the cause of the violence spreading across Sierra Leone:

> Upon ethnological grounds the Hut-Tax was a risky measure at
> best, and should only have been applied by gradual stages: suddenly
> thrust, as it was, upon the natives distributed over a wide area, it
> became a preeminently unwise and foolish measure. Viewed from
> an historical standpoint its morality was doubtful. Upon financial
> grounds it was manifestly unjust.[31]

Even a Royal Commission sent to investigate the conflict termed the tax "sudden, uncompromising, and harsh."[32] American Quakers following developments in Sierra Leone were indignant at the governor's feckless and brutal reprisals. "The best natives in the whole of the protectorate," one of them wrote at the time, "the most law-abiding, the most energetic, the best, if not the only, agriculturists, are being shot and hunted down like rabbits. Why? Because an official made an administrative blunder, and followed up that blunder by a display of force."[33]

And what a display it was. T. J. Alldridge, who spent decades as a British officer in Sierra Leone, did not express (at least in his memoirs) ambivalence about razing rebellious towns and villages to the ground. He felt he gave fair warning to the enemies of progress, including chiefs who continued their slaving ways or refused to collect taxes. "I sent messages by the people," wrote Alldridge of one insubordinate headman,

> and had it loudly called out that if he would return to the town by four
> o'clock that I would not destroy that place, but that if he did not appear
> before me by that time it would be burnt. As he did not do so and I
> could get no information whatever, the straggling and outlying parts of
> the town were fired, and in the morning the town itself was destroyed.

The point of these dramatic expressions of imperial firepower was unabashedly laid out by Alldridge for the British public and any literate victims of his arson and ammo. But the natives didn't need to read his book to read his message. A series of punitive expeditions into another rebellious area, he wrote, "effectually reduced that country and left there a practical example of British power that will not soon be effaced from the memories of the West Coast people."[34] And it wasn't.

Many have parsed this chapter of conquest, which offers, as does the siege of Sikasso, an early snapshot of formal European rule and responses to it. The Berlin Conference had called for signatories to extend their civilizing reach by establishing protectorates, their borders cooked up by conflict and with the acquiescence of rivers. For the British, this meant making the neighborhood safe for trade deemed legitimate and profitable—and collecting funds to pay for law enforcement. Hence the hut tax. To enforce borders and tax collection, and to complement West Indian troops, the British created the Frontier Police in 1890. It consisted of about five hundred African rank-and-file soldiers led by a dozen British officers. Less than a decade later, most rural people, regardless of tribe or creed, had endured much policing but enjoyed little in the way of tangible benefits of belonging to the world's most powerful empire. Hence the Hut Tax War.[35]

The pattern of white officers leading African infantry against domestic foes would leave a poisonous legacy upon independence, by which time the armed forces would be widely feared as a coup-sponsoring, tribute-collecting threat to civilian rule. But within turn-of-the-century Sierra Leone, it spelled danger when the Frontier Police, even with the backup of troops from elsewhere in the empire, overreached in a setting of resentful diversity. "In a region the size of Ireland," observed one British historian,

> there were well over a hundred independent chiefdoms, inhabited by peoples of some fourteen tribal groups. No single African ruler approached the status of a Sultan of Sokoto or a Kabaka of Buganda, or even of the Mandinka warrior chief Samori on the northern border. The establishment of the Protectorate implied an arbitrary work of political unification.[36]

If political unification of the protectorate remained a consummation devoutly to be wished, social unification was even less likely. (The British made even less effort in this regard than they did in Ireland.) In British West Africa, the sun set on generations of subjects who lived and died in the manner of their ancestors.

Which is to say, often at the hands of others and without the benefit of any mission that might be termed civilized, much less civilizing. The colonial record is replete with instances in which the occupiers, unable to understand their rural subjects, used native underlings to impose British law and order with little to show for it beyond mutual incomprehension and dead bodies. African dead bodies.

Throughout the first years of formal colonial administration, West Africa's main occupying powers whittled away at the prestige and honor of local chiefs, if in different ways. As in India, the British openly embraced indirect rule, carving the Sierra Leone protectorate into 149 chiefdoms and naming a paramount chief to lead each of them. The selection of chiefs was loosely based on hereditary succession within noble houses. This may have squared with practice in the House of Lords, but it clashed with much local tradition.

When succession was contested, which it often was, the British stepped in to reward loyal leaders. That's how Madam Yoko—widely known as Mammy, although she never bore children of her own—came to have a hotel named after her. In the course of three astute marriages to Mende chiefs, and by establishing a celebrated bush school for girls hoping to marry into prominent families, Yoko consolidated power and influence during the last three decades of the nineteenth century.[37] She first attracted British attention in 1875, when she took up the cause of her third husband, a chief clapped in irons after making war on a prominent family of Creole merchants. Authorities in Freetown were taken by her elegance and savvy, and her husband (who'd previously sent Mende mercenaries to fight Ashanti alongside the British) was let off with a flogging. Three of his peers, jailed for the same transgression, were hanged by the neck—after seeing their towns put to the torch.

Mammy Yoko's husband requested that she rule Senehun after his death, which came to pass in 1878. The British hadn't yet claimed their full protectorate but had the influence to favor someone else; Yoko wasn't named a chief until 1884. A Methodist missionary visiting Senehun the next year made the following observations, which speak volumes about Freetown's accommodation of domestic slavery:

> In the evening we paid a visit to the most wealthy and influential
> native in town, named Yoko, the widow of the late chief of Sennehoo.
> She is about thirty-five years of age, has a good appearance, is very
> reserved in manners, shrewd, thoughtful, and dignified, and has
> all the semblance of superiority to her surroundings, befitting her
> for her elevated position. As is customary in these places, she is the
> possessor of many slaves, who live in small towns owned by her,
> near and around Sennehoo. These work on her farms, and she is
> supported solely by their labour and industry. About her person is a
> train of female attendants—about twenty in number, all slaves—who
> are her ladies-in-waiting, and ministers of her wants and wishes.[38]

The Hut Tax War strengthened the queen of Senehun. Having made shrewd analysis of the likely outcome of continued conflict with the British, Yoko sided with them during the war, receiving a silver medal of honor from Queen Victoria. With British backing and through patronage—she often supplied the Frontier Police with wives—Mammy Yoko came to rule over a veritable Mende confederation.[39]

The French claimed to reject expedients like indirect rule with a heavy hand—not infrequently, a balled fist. In their own fashion, however, they, too, pursued a divide-and-rule strategy, which included the dismemberment of several previously independent, if warring, states and empires. There's little doubt that Samory, Babemba, and other pre-partition rulers imposed heavy burdens on their subjects; they were, after all, warrior chieftains. But traditional rulers propped up by France found themselves increasingly despised as the "white's man's children," and soon bore "little resemblance to those who had been conquered at the end of the 19th century."[40] By the end of the period of conquest and pacification, the things-fall-apart anomie seen in the Americas in previous centuries was endemic in the inner reaches of newly French West Africa. *Et voilà*. The Pax Gallica had begun.

What to make of the deadly hypocrisies of France, which had famously rejected both monarchy and slavery, the hated *ancien régime*, a century before the Berlin Conference? Slaves and free people of color on French plantations in Haiti heard clearly the 1790 declaration of the new National Assembly— "The French nation renounces to undertake any war of conquest and will never use its force against the liberty of any people." But they also recognized Napoleon's intention to undertake many new wars of conquest, and to restore slavery (in Haiti, at least). Still, that was Napoleon, not the modern and democratic Third Republic, which in 1870 claimed to be inspired by "an emancipatory and universalistic impulse that resists tyranny." Yet it took republican forces about as much time to invade the western Sudan as it had taken Napoleon to attempt the reconquest of Haiti.

Many French republicans, including those declaiming the rights of the citizen, readily embraced the retrograde ideals underpinning their occupation of West Africa. That much comes across clearly in some of the high-handed directives issued by an expanding bureaucracy in Dakar. Some of these edicts were reminders of why colonial rule was for the good of native subjects, but most concerned taxes, labor, public health, agriculture, and trade; the rest addressed what were thought of as cultural matters. As one historian put it, "Four African institutions were singled out for eradication: indigenous languages, slavery, barbaric customary law, and 'feudal' chieftaincies. The republican virtues of a common language, freedom, social equality, and liberal justice were to take their place."[41]

How much chastened chiefs bought into French fatwas was and is subject to debate. But the echoes of these instructions, and reactions to them, resounded in Senegal, Guinea, Mali, and elsewhere after independence, when republican virtues remained elusive, but deep ambivalence about African social institutions did not. The high modernism of the French colonial project in West Africa wouldn't have surprised many Haitians, certainly, and shouldn't have surprised any historians. "Colonization under the Third Republic was in large part an act of state-sanctioned violence," allows one of the latter. French republicans never identified "any contradiction," she adds, "between their democratic institutions and the acquisition and administration of their empire." That's because they saw their African subjects as "barbarians, and were continually undertaking—or claiming to undertake, as the case may be—civilizing measures on behalf of their subjects that appeared to make democracy and colonialism compatible."[42]

It was a distressingly similar story in contemplating the views, if not the resources, of the Americo-Liberians. Monrovia also relied on force to impose a hut tax, soon the republic's largest source of revenue, and launched campaigns to eradicate native institutions deemed barbaric—pretty much the same ones that bothered the French. Colonial barbarism in West Africa was surpassed only by German campaigns farther south, where Kaiser Wilhelm's lieutenants offered a foretaste of the Third Reich's methods by launching a genocidal spree against the Herero and Nama tribes in what is now Namibia. Into the oubliette went the missing millions, torched villages, deported or executed resistance leaders, and famine resulting from farmers' inability to plant, harvest, and trade in the midst of turmoil. Into the oubliette went the epidemics sparked or fanned by this mayhem, even as the Europeans claimed to introduce hygiene to their savage subjects.

Much of this chapter of African history reads as a case study in unvarnished racism of the white-supremacy hue. Its role in the intertwined institutions of slavery and colonialism (and the hygiene regimes associated with both) has been studied and parsed and studied again as new archives became available, or as fresh eyes reconsidered old ones. Although most Americo-Liberians rejected the formal racism of the color bar, they were slow to assimilate the natives, in some instances slower than the Europeans. In Freetown, assimilation wasn't regarded with hostility for most of the nineteenth century, as evidenced by scores of African mayors, doctors, lawyers, bishops, and even colonial officials; in urban Senegal, some subjects became voting citizens. By the close of the century, however, there were many objections to social integration. Two came to the fore, and both turned about Europeans' changing conceptions of demography, biology, and culture—meaning their changing conceptions of race.

First, and even after varied and violent African-reduction campaigns, the population of colonizing nations was often smaller than that of the colonies. This implied, as Michael Crowder notes, that a "full-scale policy of assimilation would mean that both France and Portugal would be politically dominated by the peoples they were assimilating." A second strain of objection to assimilation, he continues, was the notion that Africans and Europeans were fundamentally distinct:

> Some argued this in terms of biology, asserting that the African was irremediably inferior and therefore could not be assimilated. Most of those who talked in terms of culture insisted that even though the African *qua* human being was equal to the European he was culturally separate and could not be assimilated to an alien culture.[43]

A common understanding of the relationship between subjugation and immutable essentialisms—common, at least, among those ruling the colonies and apparently disinclined to bother with dog whistling—was laid out in a 1901 report from authorities in Dakar to the French minister of commerce:

> The black does not like work and the notion of thrift is completely foreign to him; he does not realise that idleness keeps him in a state of absolute economic inferiority. We must therefore use the institutions (if that's the word) by which he is ruled, in this case slavery, to improve his circumstances and afterwards gently lead him into an apprenticeship of freedom.[44]

Thus did the new century dawn. With most natives gently led to still their opposition to European rule, civilian administrators announced the real work of high modernism could begin. In the view of French administrators based in Dakar—and in new capitals like Abidjan and Conakry, conjured from scratch by work-averse blacks—their civilizing mission would be advanced through public works and public health.

Railroads, the ranking emblem of social progress in Europe as in the United States, received the lion's share of investment, much of it floated as large loans from Paris. In today's policyspeak, these were public-private partnerships in which the public took significant risks (whether financial or, for those obliged to lay down track, physical) while huge profits were privatized.[45] France's sleek black trains must have been awe-inspiring in regions in which footpaths and camel trails had until recently been the primary overland means of travel. But many public-health interventions inspired more fear than awe. The sanitarians' grand plans, then as now termed "health reforms," were often as ill-conceived as they were ham-fisted. They focused from the very start on disease containment.

Throughout decades of French rule, health authorities responded to varied epidemics with less varied measures, including the destruction of housing, highly restrictive and segregationist building codes, quarantine, isolation, fines, and other penalties for infractions. Disease-control algorithms were applied in discriminatory fashion, sparing Europeans—and their businesses—in a manner that rankled Creole elites. As for the majority, medical care for sick natives was always the neglected stepchild of these zealous Pasteurians. Yet in spite of the arrival of a wave of eager sanitarians with an ability to enforce health regulations unmatched in Europe, the control-over-care paradigm never amounted to much. Outbreaks of yellow fever, smallpox, typhoid, sleeping sickness, and epidemic meningitis ripped through French West Africa.

The new capital of the Ivory Coast, Abidjan, was established after a 1903 epidemic of yellow fever killed thousands of Europeans in the old capital, and an unknown fraction of Africans resident there; Conakry had also been planned with these scourges in mind.[46] As these outbreaks joined the chronic insults of malaria, onchocerciasis, schistosomiasis, tuberculosis, and a host of venereal diseases, three pathogens alleged to be new to the region—cholera, plague caused by *Yersinia pestis*, and (later but not least) influenza—heightened fears of the White Man's Grave and contradicted imperial boasts of public-health prowess in Africa. This bragging nonetheless gained traction in Europe, where it was fashioned into narratives for broad dissemination and reexported to literate African audiences reluctant to denounce them as propaganda while living under colonial rule.[47]

The views of the chief victims of these plagues were seldom solicited and rarely reported, but some of the locals clearly feared the Pasteurians more than the pathogens. When the first—meaning first identified—outbreak of bubonic plague hit Dakar in 1914, locals were offered rewards of cash or kola nuts for dead rats and mice. According to a French naval physician sympathetic to the natives, the bounty "produced poor results because the Africans feared that discovery of an infected rat would bring down on their property and their homes the fire and brimstone of the sanitary brigades."[48] French Pasteurians surely knew the vastly differing life cycles of many of these pathogens, some vector-borne and some not, some zoonoses and some not. But they (the Pasteurians, not the pathogens) were working from a purposely rudimentary playbook. Its control-over-care chapters would remain influential for over a century—as those unlucky enough to contract Ebola would later learn.

The impact of similarly punitive policies was registered in Britain's territories, if perhaps at a more irregular pace and with greater geographic variation. "In attempting to explain the uneven success of health reform measures in British West Africa in this period," asserted one British historian, "it is worth recalling that the Colonial Empire did not function as a centralized system: the keynote of British rule, in contrast to that of other European overseas empires, was decentralized improvisation."[49] It's possible, however, to exaggerate local variation in Britain's sanitary policies. As regards "urban segregation, discrimination and the metaphoric equation of disease with so-called inferior races," a Sierra Leonean historian later countered, colonial "policy and practice bore the peculiar badge of consistency."[50] These policies and practices consistently favored control over care as much as French ones did. As far as the natives went, medical care from doctors and nurses remained mere footnotes in the British sanitarians' playbook.

Not that there were many clinicians there to provide care. Beginning in 1902, African physicians were excluded from the West African medical service. A ban on black doctors, including those trained in Europe's best medical schools, was a self-inflicted wound. The colonial medical service lacked staff as much as stuff and space, and some of the excluded or demoted sound like titans. The degrees trailing the name of one Sierra Leonean physician qualified in England in 1880 signaled additional diplomas earned in Ireland and Belgium. When the medical service was established, he was "excluded on account of his colour and placed in a new category, that of Native Medical Officers, and automatically became junior to the latest joined member."[51] Since this eminent physician had already served as the colony's assistant colonial surgeon for twenty years when demoted, one imagines his white peers would be mortified. To judge by their published complaints, not so much.

In print, at least, British doctors in West Africa griped mostly about low salaries and insufficient time for private practice, which was almost always for white patients.[52] While medical officers whinged about not having enough time to care for fee-paying employees of commercial firms or the colonial administration, they managed to neglect duties protecting the broader public from even vaccine-preventable disease. Pathogens against which there were no effective vaccines, but which called for vector control by the colonial medical service, caused even more mayhem. After surveying epidemics attributed to pathogens new to the region, the historian Emmanuel Akyeampong concludes that two old foes, malaria and trypanosomiasis, "posed the greatest challenge to the European colonization of Africa."[53]

Trypanosomiasis sickens cattle and other beasts of cloven hoof, but is, in West Africa, primarily a disease of humans. In 1803, a century before its etiologic agent and life cycle were identified, it had been described as "African sleeping sickness" by Thomas Winterbottom, Freetown's first medical officer:

> The Africans are very subject to a species of lethargy, which they are
> much afraid of, as it proves fatal in every instance . . . This disease
> is very frequent in the Foola country, and it is said to be much more

common in the interior parts of the country than upon the sea coast. Children are very rarely, or never, affected with this complaint, nor is it more common among slaves than among free people, though it is asserted that the slaves from Benin are very subject to it . . . Small glandular tumors are sometimes observed in the neck a little before the commencement of this complaint, though probably depending rather upon accidental circumstances than upon the disease itself. Slave traders, however, appear to consider these tumors as a symptom indicating a disposition to lethargy, and they either never buy such slaves, or get quit of them as soon as they observe any such appearances. The disposition to sleep is so strong, as scarcely to leave a sufficient respite for the taking of food; even the repeated application of a whip, a remedy which has been frequently used, is hardly sufficient to keep the poor wretch awake.[54]

One hundred years later, the world's most powerful empire hadn't whipped African sleeping sickness or its vector into submission. The first decade of the twentieth century was marked by cataclysmic trypanosomiasis outbreaks, including one that brought British East Africa to its knees. Between 1901 and 1905, colonial authorities estimated that two hundred thousand Ugandans perished along with their all-important cattle.[55]

Epidemics of what had been previously considered an indolent infection also exploded across northern Rhodesia (present-day Zambia) and Nyasaland (now Malawi). One prominent British authority insisted that trypanosomiasis was new to Nyasaland, noting in 1910 that the first medical officer to investigate rumors of mounting cases was himself bitten by tsetse flies during the investigation. He was soon dead of the disease.[56] Across the colonies, afflicted subjects were removed to "treatment units" after much assurance that new medications derived from arsenic were miracle drugs—even after their failure and toxicity became evident. The director of one lazaret in the Belgian Congo put it this way as the plague moved north: "Strictly speaking, it was a permanent prison and should bear the inscription, 'Abandon all hope, ye who enter here.'"[57]

Sleeping sickness surged across areas of the Sudan not known to be infested with tsetse flies until linked by French rail—and by campaigns to bring down Samory, Babemba, and others resisting European rule. Neither were German nor Belgian colonies spared. Across the continent, vector control had failed. This was common knowledge among the few European physicians actually providing clinical care for the natives. Along with his wife and unnamed nurses and local laborers, Albert Schweitzer had established a mission hospital in the interior of French Gabon. A few patients with signs and symptoms of trypanosomiasis could, the Alsatian doctor complained in 1914, "tie me for a whole morning to the microscope, while outside there are sitting a score of sick people who want to be seen before dinnertime!"

Dr. Schweitzer had many flaws, which his critics weren't shy to underline. Yet even if he famously wouldn't hurt a fly—and was thus unable to do much in the way of preventing trypanosomiasis—the future Nobel laureate had more sophisticated notions of integrating prevention and care than many of his contemporaries in the colonial health services. Schweitzer's inclination to scale up treatment of afflicted natives, and deny thirsty tsetse flies infested blood meals from the humans, was more sophisticated than some of the schemes of hard-line disease controllers a century later. As regards sleeping sickness, he waxed philosophic in this peroration, as was his wont:

> Shall we now conquer it? A systematic campaign against it over
> this wide district would need many doctors and the cost would be
> enormous . . . Yet, where death already stalks about as conqueror,
> the European States provide in most niggardly fashion the means of
> stopping it, and merely undertake stupid defensive measures which
> only give it a chance of reaping a fresh harvest in Europe itself.[58]

Of stupid defensive measures there were many. One of the stupidest and most costly of them, the nighttime segregation of Europeans from the native population to protect the former from malaria and funded in nonniggardly fashion, was hatched in Freetown. Beyond the obvious insult to the city's abolitionist roots, the scheme revealed a sharp divorce between policy and evidence—another badge of consistency in Britain's colonial medical service.

Fruitless efforts to stop malaria through segregation came to pass even as discoveries about malaria should have compelled the integration of disease control and medical care. As the name suggests, malaria was long held to be caused by bad air—"marsh miasma"—and environmental filth. Although mortality among European explorers, administrators, and soldiers dropped sharply when they took quinine, they weren't sure why. But at the close of the nineteenth century, the British physician Ronald Ross laid out the parasite's life cycle; he, too, was awarded a Nobel for this work.[59] Ross began his research while a colonial health officer in India, where he was born to privilege and where malaria joined cholera and plague as leading causes of death among Indians and resident Britons. By late nineteenth-century estimates, an entire company from each British regiment stationed there was lost to malaria every twenty months.[60]

A few years before his Nobel, Ross left the service for a post at the newly created Liverpool School of Tropical Medicine. In 1899, he headed to the most malarious outpost of the empire with the charge of recommending policies to make it less so. He reached Freetown as the spasms of the Hut Tax War continued. Weeks earlier, martial law had been declared in the area around Port Loko, and Bai Bureh was exiled to a Gold Coast prison. The protectorate faced food shortages as conflict rendered farming impossible in many areas, while colonists across West Africa—and on Spanish and Portuguese islands in the Bight of Benin—fought over scarce labor.

This turmoil, covered in the international press and the subject of a royal inquiry, was of scant concern, it would seem, to the Ross posse: it was all about the fevers, and mostly about the British. According to an unnamed correspondent from *The British Medical Journal* reporting back from the colony:

> Freetown is a charming town built on and between small richly-wooded hills, sloping somewhat abruptly to the sea. The houses are

mostly made of wood, and are generally of two storeys. They are however small, and in the town overcrowded. There is an excellent water supply, and dysentery and typhoid are comparatively scarce—the latter, indeed, being said to be absent. Nevertheless, the place is certainly very unhealthy to Europeans.[61]

Ross didn't really find Freetown charming—he termed it pestilential in private correspondence—and didn't dispute its danger to expatriates of African descent. Death rates among soldiers posted to Sierra Leone, who included close to a thousand West Indians at the turn of the century, were alleged to be higher than in the empire's malarious outposts in the Caribbean, tropical Asia, and India. Explaining this variation required just the sort of expertise Ross possessed, as long as it could be linked to broader analysis of the social pathologies of colonial rule, which had enveloped him since birth.

Understanding the interplay between colonial pathologies and the epidemics they fostered would have required firm grounding in social medicine. As with other epidemics, much more than immunity was at play. There was growing awareness of the fact that, although adults in malaria-endemic areas enjoyed at least partial immunity to the parasite, children—then as now, malaria's chief victims—were often infected and infectious. Once Ross implicated the female *Anopheles* mosquito, a nighttime feeder, policies needed to focus on the integration of prevention and care for all, especially children.[62] Such integration would require changes in policies and culture—not the culture of the natives, whether little people or not, but of the colonial medical service.

Ronald Ross knew that a significant medical discovery is not automatically translated into practice. After all, quinine had been around for centuries but wasn't faithfully used by the British, except during expeditions and military campaigns, and in their homeopathically dosed gin-and-tonics. Given his experience in India, Ross also knew that he faced medical officers deeply attached to the notion that the torrid climate made the region unhealthy for the fairer races. West Africa's reputation as the White Man's

Grave, which qualified physicians for hardship pay and long leaves, had been bolstered by sensationalist European dispatches and by medical officers' self-interested depictions of their own heroism. But in spite of control-over-care leanings, on-the-spot medical officers in West Africa weren't quick to embrace mosquito control, either—even after it and quinine had been shown to result in a decline in malaria deaths across the region, including Sierra Leone.[63] Nor did they issue mea culpas about their failures to recommend quinine as prophylaxis.

Colonial medical officers also complained when contradicted on technical matters by experts in the "new tropical medicine"—sometimes and more honestly termed imperial medicine—sallying forth from Liverpool and London. Aware of disgruntlement and mistrust within the West African medical service, Ross focused on the mosquitoes. On leaving Freetown in December, 1899, he recommended four nonpharmaceutical interventions: "obliteration of the breeding pools of *Anopheles* by drainage," the use of "kerosene or of an agent (i.e., a person) to destroy" larvae, and the installation of screens and bed nets. Finally, Ross suggested—in the words of one historian, "only briefly and well down on the list of several recommendations"—that "houses of Europeans should be built on elevated sites."[64] The first three suggestions would protect all British subjects, including its African majority. The fourth, if effective, would protect only the colony's white minority. In the view of Sierra Leone's governor, that was precisely the point, and one that he could make.

Freetown had something most other coastal towns in West Africa did not: high hills. Taking a leaf from the book of the British Raj, which hadn't bothered with medical justifications for segregation, the governor proposed to move the white population and part of the West Indian regiment up to two "hill stations" hundreds of feet above the mosquito-infested coastline. Somehow, such a feat seemed less daunting than spiking gin cocktails with higher doses of quinine—or rapid diagnosis and treatment of children with malaria and the drainage of standing water. The next imperial feat rubbed salt in the wound. In 1902, after a second Ross expedition reported that "not a puddle, not a ditch had been drained" in mosquito-ridden Freetown, the British built a small train line to carry them (the white people, not the mosquitoes) back and forth from the hill station to the commercial districts clustered around the port.[65]

Even among British officials, Freetown's segregated hill station and barracks were soon acknowledged as malaria-ridden by all but ardent propagandists. In 1904, referring to the barracks, the Royal Army Medical Corps insisted "Mount Aureol is not healthy." The cause remained "fevers," which each year led to an admission rate of 1,955 per 1,000 Europeans and 1,329 per 1,000 West Indian troops—meaning most nonnatives were hospitalized more than once a year for febrile illness.[66] Laboratory studies conducted in the hill stations, and in military sickbays, suggested these fevers were due largely to falciparum malaria. (Viral etiologies could not, at the time, be excluded.) The inquiries further suggested that wingèd *Anopheles* had little trouble crossing an open space between bungalows, barracks, and the shores of nearby streams. The mosquitoes could also ride the train, fare-free, up the hill.

Perhaps Ronald Ross shouldn't be blamed for the empire's stupid malaria policies, even if they were rolled out at the height of his influence.[67] But a number of British governors refused to implement them, arguing that segregation would waste resources and harden native resentment. The governor of Lagos, a Scottish physician, asserted that "the primary aim of tropical medicine should be to treat people who lived in the tropics—that is, Africans—and that the employment of African taxes to develop luxurious segregated areas for Europeans was indefensible."[68] A number of expert panels and at least one commission of the Royal Society disagreed with such heresy, as did Sierra Leone's flinty chief executive.[69]

The course of events was different in Dakar. During the first decades of formal colonial rule, some French authorities also called for the city's segregation in order to control malaria, plague, and yellow fever. But they'd built their administrative offices in public squares in the middle of towns new and old, not in hill stations. The French also made the mistake, during an earlier and more assimilationist period, of granting civil and political rights to a select group of Africans in the city. Once empowered, however partially, French-speaking and prosperous Senegalese used every means available to protect their property:

> The urge to segregate residential neighborhoods in the towns of Senegal resonated throughout the thirty years of endo-endemic plague. What made Dakar and the other communes of Senegal different from virtually every other urban setting in Africa, however, was the ability of African citizens to use the law and, if necessary, the streets, to resist forced relocation.[70]

If granting of rights to some citizens tempered the fire and brimstone of French sanitary brigades, timid steps toward the franchise didn't lead to the integration of prevention and care for Africans under colonial rule.

This blind spot endured for decades. When, during World War II, American soldiers arrived bearing DDT, they also brought newly discovered antibiotics effective against plague. There's not much evidence, however, that authorities in Dakar asked that their sickened subjects benefit from these wonder drugs. It was much the same story in other parts of the continent under British rule, and in India.[71]

Colonial medical services had pasteurized caregiving right out of their practice and policies.

The outcomes of control-over-care policies—like the attitudes of individual Pasteurians, governors, and other colonial administrators—were varied, if sometimes less varied than advertised. But it's not difficult to discern their conflicted echoes in the region's subsequent epidemics, including recent ones of Ebola.

That's in part because disease control in West Africa had been linked under colonial rule to vigorous efforts to extract profits from these lands and their people. That quest, which continues, always sparks conflict. Every chapter of the history of West Africa under European rule seems to include yet another cataclysmic outbreak of disease or conflict (or both) followed by ineffective or repressive measures (or both) and linked in an unbroken chain of profiteering. Punishment plus profiteering in turn triggered social epidemics among African subjects. During the transatlantic slave trade, wild rumors proliferated on both sides of the ocean—the side on which young Africans were seized and the side on which they'd been forced to work and die. Both shores spawned cannibals, witches, zombies, were-animals, and even that quintessential European specter, the vampire. These spectral spawn flourished in the colonies after the decline of the transatlantic slave trade made the inner workings of forced labor regimes a more locally visible affair.

To take one example, the growth of legitimate commerce through illegitimate means—requisitioned or underpaid labor to complete public works or private ventures right there in Sierra Leone—often sparked accusations of ritual cannibalism. Across Upper West Africa, colonial authorities trafficked in rumors of a ritual cannibalism that emanated (in the recent assessment of one anthropologist) from "those parts of the forest zone most thoroughly transformed by commercial contacts."[72] A murderous secret society existed deep in the untamed bush (so some authorities claimed), the members of which would don the guise of leopards in order to acquire victims' blood and body parts and gain earthly power. British officials, keen to extract profits from the forest, gave shape and substance (and capital letters) to this network by calling it the Human Leopard Society—and, having done so, engaged in efforts to stamp it out.

The society's members (so some authorities claimed) not only practiced cannibalism but also carried out ritual murders in the guise of baboons, gorillas, chimpanzees, crocodiles, and alligators.[73] There was considerable disagreement among the British regarding these secret societies and about cannibalism, ritual or otherwise.[74] In 1803, Thomas Winterbottom—whose interests were broader than describing sleeping sickness and other plagues—offered one of the first detailed descriptions of the ubiquitous societies, underlining their role in local governance and the enforcement of social norms. As regards cannibalism, Winterbottom protested with some heat that there was no evidence for it: "That this horrid practice does not exist in the neighbourhood of Sierra Leone, nor for many hundred leagues along the coast to the northward and southward of that place, may be asserted with the utmost confidence; nor is there any tradition among the natives which can prove that it was ever the custom."[75]

A century later, T. J. Alldridge advanced a similar view as regards the Mende, noting that allegations of cannibalism were received as hurtful calumny. The question of shapeshifting with malevolent intent—including *ritual* cannibalism—was, however, a different one. These accusations surfaced in several mid-nineteenth-century British accounts. "The Temnes believe that, by witchcraft a man may turn himself into an animal, and, in that form, may injure an enemy," wrote an Anglican bishop posted to Freetown. "A man was burnt at Port Lokkoh in 1854 for having turned himself into a leopard."[76] During that era, Freetown's authorities had tried, mostly successfully, to leave such matters to customary law. But with the launch of formal colonial rule, accusations of ritual cannibalism and membership in the Human Leopard Society proliferated. They could be construed as part of the cultural arsenal of populations newly subjected to colonial rule, but they were the weapons of the weak. As during the Hut Tax War—believed by many colonials to have been coordinated by the Poro and other secret societies—the victims were almost never British.

In the last years of the century, Captain Kenneth James Beatty, an Australian resident in Freetown when Australia was a commonwealth of the empire, was charged with stemming "the expansion and increased activity of the Society during the past twenty years."[77] Beatty thought that earlier examples, such as the Port Loko case, may or may not have been an instance of mere shapeshifting, which was not, in his eyes, a capital offense. In the case of human-leopard murders, however, there was often an actual body involved. Sometimes more than one: deaths attributed to human leopards by the natives led to revenge killings and even the occasional mass immolation. In 1891, officials were shocked, reported Beatty in a 1915 book called *Human Leopards*, that "a number of cannibals had been burnt to death" in Mende country after a group of divinatory specialists called Tongo players declared them guilty.[78]

Captain Kenneth Beatty took pains to note that "one of the first to be cast into the flames was the principal chief who had been instrumental in calling in the Tongo players." Among the appalled was the Australian's fire-loving mentor, T. J. Alldridge, who traveled to Mende country to investigate. "The pyramid of calcined bones which he saw at the junction of two roads just outside Bogo," Beatty wrote, "was about four feet high."[79] The Crown, he insisted, "could not view with indifference such a crude and barbarous administration of justice."[80] Its representatives preferred to administer their own, with death by hanging the favored method. This deterrent failed; human-leopard accusations continued to mount, and the administration escalated its campaign. To deal with this threat to law and order during the first years in which they sought to show themselves able to rule their hinterland, soon to be crossed by the railroad reaching from Freetown to the eaves of the eastern forest, the authorities began to issue new and curiously specific regulations.

They started by going after the Tongo players. In a proclamation issued on May 5, 1892, one of the first in a series of decrees seeking to control (*à la française*) customary law and ritual in the hinterlands, authorities banished "every Tongo person" from the colony, giving them twenty-one days to leave.[81] With the players reportedly expelled, British authorities became the diviners, forming a Special Court to adjudicate hundreds of allegations against what they called "unlawful societies." That "unlawful" was a nod to sodalities not prohibited: Poro, Sande, Bundu, and other secret societies were still viewed by many officials as performing useful regulatory functions in everyday life. Even Poro-hating Captain Beatty knew that attempts to ban the region's most prevalent social institutions would trigger explosive revolt.

If the Hut Tax War was a result of British overreach in the realm of taxation, and the failure of malaria control through segregation was a result of poorly conceived and overtly racist public-health policies, the obsession with ritual murders, and with secret societies, was their equivalent in the realm of jurisprudence. Beatty set his prosecutorial sights not on diviners but on those accused of abusing delegated authority, political or otherworldly: refractory chiefs and headmen who resisted British notions of law and order regarding capital crimes.

The Special Court came into full flower after the Human Leopard Society Ordinance, Number 15 of 1895, banned "a leopard skin shaped so as to make a man wearing it resemble a leopard," the oft-described (but never seen) three-clawed knives held to be used by human leopards, and "a native medicine known as 'Borfima.'" While Alldridge observed that "medicine" was "a word of terror all over the country," Beatty explained that *borfima* is the Mende term for medicine bag:

> This package contains, amongst other things, the white of an egg, the blood, fat, and other parts of a human being, the blood of a cock, and a few grains of rice; but to make it efficacious it must occasionally be anointed with human fat and smeared with human blood. So anointed and smeared, it is an all-powerful instrument in the hands of its owner, it will make him rich and powerful, it will make people hold him in honour, it will help him in cases in the White Man's Court, and it certainly has the effect of instilling in the native mind great respect for its owner and a terrible fear lest he should use it hostilely.

In other words, the *borfima*—a supernatural aid to the quest for self-promotion—demanded human sacrifice as recompense for the elevation of chiefs and for ostentatious personal gain. Beatty, Alldridge, and others were unfazed when their ordinances failed to curb their subjects' unruly desires to leave poverty and powerlessness behind.

The authorities soon turned their attention to other demonic animal guises. In 1901, the purported rise of Human Alligator Societies led to a ban on "alligator skin shaped or made so as to make a man wearing the same resemble an alligator." An amendment to the Human Leopard and Alligator Societies Ordinance, Number 17 of 1912, extended the ban to include "a dress made of baboon skins," a special whistle "commonly used for calling together the members of an unlawful society," and "an iron needle commonly used for branding" its members.[82] And so forth. But who was wearing the pelts, blowing the whistles, and wielding the needles? Beatty had his ideas. There were the insubordinate chiefs, of course, and the Tongo players, and a group of Muslim ritual specialists he termed Mohammedan Mori. The latter may have denied involvement in such "a heathen custom as the Poro," but were, he alleged, "associated with every form of secret society, magic, witch-craft, 'medicine,' and every sort of trickery."

Captain Beatty also knew that colonial officers weren't above trickery themselves. The tribunal they administered demanded that "pagan Mende witnesses" swear an oath prior to testifying. Every Monday morning, a "medicine"—that terror-inspiring term—consisting of a watery sludge of salt, pepper, and ashes was compounded by the Special Court's interpreter:

> The oath administered in the presence of the Court and repeated by each witness was, in its English translation, as follows: "I (*name of witness*) swear by this medicine to speak the truth, the whole truth, and nothing but the truth. Should I tell a lie, if I go to the farm may a snake bite me, if I travel by canoe may the canoe sink, and may my belly be swollen. I swear by my liver, my lungs, my kidneys, and my heart that, should I tell a lie, may I never be saved, but may I die suddenly."[83]

How on earth did folks like Kenneth Beatty come to be engaged in explain-ing, much less adjudicating, the lethal effects of human-fat-soaked medicine bundles brandished by bush devils in drag? To divine whether, yea or nay, ritual cannibalism was being practiced?

The rise of the Human Leopard Society occurred during the years the British sought to replace internal slavery with legitimate trade (in palm oil, camwood, coffee, cacao, groundnuts, and the like) that might be taxed, and from which a long chain of merchants and middlemen might extract surplus. Colonial officials continued to rely on trade leading flag, which meant they dragged their political and commercial proxies into conflicts of interest lead-ing commoners to despise many headmen. (Some of them women: Mammy Yoko, said to have a lion-tongue talisman with cosmic powers, had many detractors because of such conflicts.) The epidemic of human-leopard accusations was also linked to forced labor: the chiefs, not the diviners, were called to force their subjects to provide free or near-free labor for public works and to pay the obnoxious hut tax.

Like Bai Bureh, some chiefs spent months trying to convince their new overlords that such projects and policies were not only unfair but impossible to implement, in part because they feared popular retribution in the form of precisely such allegations. On the other side of the ledger, the Crown's attempts to ban domestic slavery had been vigorously opposed by Creole elites in Freetown and by many chiefs. Imperial authorities lived in unequal symbiosis with both groups, but increasingly depended on the chiefs when requisitioning labor to work the mines, to clear bush, and to build barracks, bridges, roads, and railroads. All this talk of punishment for donning pelts in order to feed the *borfima* might have been seen as a jape by some, or seem like one now. But that such cross-species cross-dressing was no joke to the authorities is suggested by the gravity of their penalties. Between 1903 and 1912, 17 human-leopard cases—involving 186 persons charged with ritual murder—were prosecuted under these ordinances. Eighty-seven of them were convicted and sentenced to death by hanging. In time-honored English tradition, "the sentence was duly carried out publicly in the vicinity of the place where the murder was committed."[84]

Then as now—since accusations of ritual murder are still a thing in this part of West Africa—readers want to know how solid these capital cases were. Kenneth Beatty insisted the guilty parties were readily identified; the cases against them, airtight. Then again, he was both judge and jury in the White Man's Court: Captain Beatty's account of the proceedings of the Kale case does little to dispel British fog. In the Mende village of that name, a fourteen-year-old named Kalfalla was going through initiation into the Poro society when he was killed—"in or about the month of March, 1911"—in a mysterious attack that left him mutilated about the throat and chest.[85] The boy was buried surreptitiously and not exhumed for autopsy. Little would have come of it, according to Beatty, if sharp-eared locals in the pay of the district commissioner hadn't attributed Kalfalla's death to ritual murder.

The boy's father, a minor subchief, was among those fingered by informants. He and two other Mende headmen were arrested and taken to a town in

Sherbro District, one setting of Alldridge's incendiary hobbies. Charged with murder, they were held in a stockade enclosed by a thicket of lashed stakes and guarded by the Frontier Force. The three-man Special Court commenced its sittings on December 16, 1912. It was presided over by one Sir William Brandford Griffith, recently arrived from Britain's Gold Coast, where he'd served as that colony's chief justice. For two weeks, Beatty and his colleagues sought to decipher evidence previously spurned by courts priding themselves on robust empiricism, a tradition newer to colonial jurisprudence than the judges let on.

Among witnesses called to testify were the boys secluded with Kalfalla in the Poro bush. According to Beatty, the boys readily "described how they had been captured by the Poro Devils and taken to a Poro bush at the town of Senehun," not far from several riverfront villages leveled by British gunboats before Mammy Yoko rose to power. The defendants protested that they'd gone after the boys not to rescue them from what was then sometimes a years-long process but rather to bring them home in order to help with agricultural work, disastrously disrupted by renewed conflict. Upon the premature end to the boys' seclusion, they lodged in a sleeping hut behind Kalfalla's father's house. Roused before daybreak by a commotion, the boys espied (reported Beatty) one of the accused "holding the deceased boy by the legs, whilst another of them, who had a leopard skin over the top of his head and hanging down his back, was bending over the body."[86]

The defendants, including Kalfalla's father, insisted the boy had been killed by a leopard, even though they'd initially implicated a snake:

> Their reason for doing so was in order to save the father of the deceased, the first accused in the case, from certain penalties which he would have incurred had it come to the ears of the Poro Headman that he had allowed a "bush-boy" who was still in the Poro to sleep in an open place outside of the Poro bush.

Kalfalla *had* to have been killed by a leopard, argued Creole defense lawyers from Freetown—unlike their medical peers still permitted to practice alongside white folks—because "it was contrary to nature that the first accused would have murdered his own son in such a cold-blooded manner." Although Beatty allowed that the accused were ably defended, their counsel "did not create doubt as to the main facts deposed to by the witnesses for the Crown."[87] The Special Court found the boy's father and a second defendant guilty of murder. They were hanged by the neck in the town of Mattru, heart of the Jong chiefdom, on January 25, 1913. The third was given life in prison.

Sir William Brandford Griffith, veteran of many colonial courts, was spooked by the human-leopard cases. "I have been in many forests," he wrote in an introduction to Beatty's book, "but in none which seemed to me to be so uncanny as the Sierra Leone bush." There was something about its villages "which makes one's flesh creep," he continued. "It may be the low hills with enclosed swampy valleys, or the associations of the slave trade."[88] Mayhaps. Others may feel that the court's methods (circumstantial proofs, an absence of forensic evidence, elevation of rumor and hearsay, testimony from paid informants and children, torture-forced confessions) were enough to make one's flesh creep, given the penalties exacted. But by then, colonial officials—stung by mass immolations, the Hut Tax War, and other apocalyptic manifestations of upheaval in an agrarian society shaped by the slave trades—had declared war on ritual murder. In for a penny, in for a pound.

In the years following Captain Beatty's reign, the authorities became skeptical about such accusations, which surged during political and economic turmoil. But no one put Beatty in a corner. "Every member of the Human Leopard Society is a member of the Poro," he declaimed. "The main supporters of both societies are the chiefs, the place of meeting for both societies is the Poro bush—this suffices to show how easily the Poro organization can be used, and no doubt has been used, for many of the purposes of the human leopards."[89] Sierra Leone's suffering subjects, especially women and young men, had ample reason to resent headmen. But most of them accepted the societies—to which they all belonged—as one forum for resolving disputes, airing grievances, and addressing new misfortunes. The latter included such bush exotica as unfair taxation, forced labor for public works, personal enrichment at the expense of others, and massive land grabs.

The idea that the societies and their bush business were unrelated to colonial practices—or to the great reversal of the Atlantic World—is given the lie by the black-and-white plates illustrating Beatty's book. Facing the page on which the underaged Kale witnesses detailed their capture by Poro devils is a photograph labeled "Poro Devil." This sad sack is festooned in what looks like a feather-tufted, cowrie-encrusted Halloween costume. Another plate features five devils in full regalia. Although Beatty reported that the bespoke loin cloth was standard menswear across the region, the first of them sports a T-shirt, shorts, and porkpie hat; slung over his shoulder is a model of an accordion fashioned from cloth and feathers. The second is wrapped in a hunting net, accessorized with a raffia skirt and whisk. The face and arms of the third devil are painted white; he is costumed in a florid re-creation of the uniform of an early nineteenth-century European military officer. A fourth is similarly bedecked. The last devil sports prisoner's muslin, another tribute to cloth and custom of European origin.

A less frightening set of diviner-devils might possibly be found in a carnival parade in Brazil, Haiti, or New Orleans—a fitting comparison, since the human-leopard trials, like the divinatory practices of the natives, rang more like morality plays or carnival displays than judicial proceedings. In replacing the Tongo players as diviners-in-chief, British authorities sought to put a lid on the simmering resentment that Beatty hints at by citing dramatis personae such as "the Temne boys"—presumably men—massed around the stockade in which the Kale defendants were held. "It was absurd to waste so much time over the prisoners," sang the chorus. They recommended instead burning alive "all the persons charged with human leopard offences together with their villages and families" in order to "stamp out the practice as it had been stamped out in the Temne country."[90]

Even if well versed in such methods, British officers couldn't continue torching villages after claiming to have pacified them. If the point was to tamp down the upheaval that had led to massive loss of life and property in the early years of colonial rule, the judges of the Special Court felt compelled to decipher the social subtext of an epidemic of accusation. They were amateur anthropologists armed with nooses.

7.

A World at War

THE MAKING OF A CLINICAL DESERT

With medicine we come to one of the most tragic features of the colonial situation.

—Frantz Fanon, *A Dying Colonialism*, 1959

The influenza pandemic of 1918–1919 was almost certainly the single greatest short-term demographic catastrophe in the continent's history. Nothing else, not slaving, colonial conquest, smallpox, cerebrospinal meningitis, the rinderpest panzootics of the 1880s and 1890s, nor the great trypanosomiasis outbreaks in East and Equatorial Africa after 1900 killed so many Africans in so short a time.

—K. David Patterson, "The Demographic Impact of the 1918–19 Influenza Pandemic in Sub-Saharan Africa: A Preliminary Assessment," in *African Historical Demography*, 1981

ALTHOUGH THE FORMAL EUROPEAN TAKEOVER OF AFRICA WAS LAUNCHED in order to avert warring over its spoils, that didn't mean the Europeans couldn't find other reasons to fight. They always had. In 1914, they found another, and soon dragged their African subjects into the dispute. Boasts about civilizing missions to the Dark Continent had already caused eyes to roll among the alleged beneficiaries of colonial rule, who were now called to gear up for history's most savage war.

The Great War shook colonial West Africa to its core. Many of those pushed and pulled into it knew that colonial rule had not led to improved health for its subjects, who remained prey to epidemics periodically thinning the ranks of natives and Europeans, if not alike. The war brought excess native mortality into relief when the assets of Europe's colonial possessions— much of the world and almost all of Africa—were surveyed and counted in order to fuel the empire-sponsored war machine. The redirection of labor toward the war economy after years of local and lethal conflict spelled food insecurity and deep trade deficits. Across West Africa, these stretched from the decade following the Berlin Conference to that following World War I.

Throughout its vast dependencies, France made the draft obligatory for all able-bodied male subjects nineteen years and older. But able bodies were in shorter supply than officials in Paris and Dakar believed, even though they'd had a direct hand in reducing that supply. What's more, many French subjects in West Africa remained unfree, this in spite of a 1905 decree abolishing slavery, which those paragons of *liberté*, *égalité*, and *fraternité* had abolished repeatedly and would abolish some more. That decree, echoing proclamations regarding Freetown's ambivalence about such matters, banned future enslavement but didn't free the already indentured. Authorities estimated that two million or more inhabitants of French West Africa were *non-libre*, the euphemism deployed to avoid—in the words of historian Jean Suret-Canale—"protestations triggered by using the actual term." In some regions, he added, almost half the population could be classed as enslaved, pawned, indentured, or otherwise unfree.[1]

Thousands of unfree West Africans, skeptical of French proclamations, fled their territories for Sierra Leone, which hung on to its abolitionist reputation longer than was warranted—or wished, since these fugitives were turned away as Freetown's overlords continued to manage their own ambivalence about freedom for the natives. In 1906, the governor announced that, while his administration frowned on slavery, its formal policy was to dither:

> You are aware that although the Government has not abolished
> existing slavery in the Protectorate, the policy has been to stand from
> the system: in other words, the power of the Government is never

used to back up the system of slavery. The system of existing slavery is left to work itself out, and, in a decade or two, will probably cease to exist.[2]

During the course of those decades, the administration—responding to pressure from the Creole business elite and from many chiefs in the protectorate—continued to pass legislation designed to keep peasants and serfs, including fugitive ones, out of Freetown.[3] As with responses to human leopards, colonialism's stew of contradictions was apparent to all parties with any proximity to its practice. Revolt, evasions, and work stoppages continued, as did grudging and reactive attempts to limit human trafficking. "By the outbreak of World War I," in the assessment of one of the best chroniclers of its impact in West Africa, "the slave trade had gone under cover."[4]

Meanwhile, in the American South, the authorities didn't even bother to hide their system of serfdom. In the aftermath of the Civil War, Reconstruction had promised civil and political rights, and physical protection, to African Americans. Upholding this bargain—which, along with women's suffrage, might have led to the founding of a real American democracy—would have required ceaseless monitoring by Freedmen's Bureaus established with these rights and protection in mind.[5] But their watch was neither ceaseless nor long enforced, dashing promises made during Lincoln's costly war and affirmed in a thrice-revised Constitution. The rollback of black enfranchisement went hand in hand with the project of restoring to whites their previous advantages, and of celebrating the Confederacy that fought to preserve slavery in the United States by sundering the nation. The monuments that proliferated across the South weren't erected by grieving widows at war's end but by the architects and enforcers of Jim Crow, bent on restoring antebellum labor arrangements and on stripping blacks of the franchise.

Both projects were a success. After 1901, it became impossible for African Americans to vote across the South, where more than 90 percent of them then lived and where neoslavery occurred on farms and plantations, in mines deep underground, and in lumber camps hidden deep in southern forests.

Forced labor also mined quarries and fired foundries, kilns, and brickworks in full view of local authorities. Across Alabama, Georgia, Mississippi, Louisiana, the Carolinas, northern Florida, Arkansas, and parts of Texas, these industries relied on the uncompensated work of teenage and young-adult descendants of those shipped over from Africa. So did the revenues of state and local governments. In the last decade of the nineteenth century, more than 10 percent of Alabama's state budget was financed by convict or slave labor; a decade later, such labor generated the equivalent of 25 percent of all taxes collected in the state. As in West Africa, black men were often detained for imaginary or exaggerated offenses; inability to pay penalties led to debt peonage under armed guard. During these years, notes one account of American neoslavery, "the seizure of black men on the back roads of the South was no longer even a brazen act."[6]

Neoslavery was further enforced by tortures running the gamut from the lash to waterboarding (already a thing) and by the ever-present threat of attack by "night riders." White vigilantes could burn down black homesteads, businesses, and churches without fear of legal retribution, since their numbers often included those charged with law enforcement. T. J. Alldridge and other British colonial officers might have been appalled by comparisons to night riders but would have been familiar with their tactics. The era's klansmen discovered that, "of all their methods, torches and kerosene worked best, since a fire created a blazing sign for all to see and left the victims no place to ever come back to."[7] For daytime murder, there was the festival-like atmosphere of public lynching, replete with grisly relics, some of which circulated as widely as those of martyred saints. White residents of some areas didn't even bother to resubjugate black labor. In what was soon to be all-white Forsyth County, Georgia, night riders used arson, lynching, and other methods to spearhead a successful effort at racial cleansing.

After completing an 1895 dissertation on the history of the North American slave trade, and doubtful of finding a university post in his native New England, the sociologist William Edward Burghardt Du Bois—the first African American to receive a doctoral degree from Harvard—moved to all-black

Atlanta University, about forty miles south of Forsyth County. W.E.B. Du Bois's goal was to teach and to investigate the social conditions of black Americans. This research was not, to use his expression, car-window sociology. It was empirical inquiry in the spirit of the emerging discipline and deeply informed by history and political economy.

With meager federal funding, Dr. Du Bois and his team conducted a complex survey of labor conditions across part of the "Black Belt." This research confirmed impressions that, while some captives were held on family-owned farms, many toiled in the industrial economy that made Alabama a force in the global steel industry even as the region continued to grow cotton, sugar cane, and timber, and to expand rail networks with the help of chain gangs and the like. Du Bois wrote up a report based on these findings—hundreds of handwritten pages that he then sent off for publication and dissemination. (It was, he recalled after decades of prodigious scholarly production, the best work he'd ever done.)[8] But the report was suppressed by the federal agency that had funded his research. He shouldn't have been surprised. It was the Gilded Age in America.

Federal authorities may have been willing to bury such findings, but they were beacons of enlightenment compared to elected officials in the South. "Not a single Southern legislature stood ready to admit a Negro, under any conditions, to the polls," wrote Du Bois. "Not a single Southern legislature believed free Negro labor was possible without a system of restrictions that took all its freedom away; there was scarcely a white man in the South who did not honestly regard Emancipation as a crime, and its practical nullification as a duty."[9] Doubts about Du Bois's conclusions, and his integrity, were raised by civic leaders and officials—all white, of course—as they raised Confederate flags and statuary in and around Southern capitols, courthouses, legislatures, and parks.

After a dozen years in Atlanta, Du Bois left for New York City, where he became a driving force behind the National Association for the Advancement of Colored People and a number of small but influential publications. But change would come slowly to the region he left behind, even after America's tardy civil rights movement. In 1999, *The New York Times* described Forsyth

as "the whitest of the country's 600 most populous counties."[10] Across the
South, Confederate statuary remains firmly affixed to its plinths.

W.E.B. Du Bois's frustration as a second-class American, and his close study
of a strain of capitalism relying on apartheid and even ethnic cleansing, led
him eventually to socialism and to such destinations as China and the Soviet Union. Having renounced his citizenship after the U.S. government renounced him, Du Bois followed his passions to Liberia.

The political class in Monrovia—largely comprised of Americo-Liberians,
no matter what part of the first three-quarters of the twentieth century one
considers—still sought to impose civilizing rule on an uncivilized majority.
The first decades of that century were punctuated by Monrovia's repeated attacks on those who resisted. The politically excluded natives stood accused,
as were rural inhabitants of neighboring colonies, of cannibalism, slaving, and
the sundry other hobbies of unreconstructed savages. These included holding
land communally (and socialistically), speaking their own languages, and (as
in Georgia) participating in their own fraternities and sororities.

W.E.B. Du Bois must have been unsettled by the Liberian variant of Jim
Crow. But he turned a blind or clouded eye to it, and instead focused on the
economic and political attacks launched against the country by those with imperial designs on its territory. In 1909, Monrovia faced a serious challenge to
its sovereignty from European creditors, while the great powers (soon to be a
lot less great, thanks to an ill-named war) further tinkered with the map: Britain affixed the Galinhas area, where Sengbe Pieh had once been imprisoned,
to Sierra Leone; France folded part of Liberia into Guinea and annexed a parcel of Maryland County to the Ivory Coast. Both empires sought to conscript
Liberian labor, as did European and African cacao planters on the Spanish
territory of Fernando Po, the largest of a handful of islands in the Bight of
Biafra. Perhaps because it was busy massing military might back in the fa-
therland, Germany projected soft power in Liberia—trade and aid, including
supplying a few doctors and laying down cable lines from Brazil to Monrovia
and on to telegraph stations in Togoland and other German territories.

There was also the pressing matter of the actions of Du Bois's own government, which took new interest in Liberia. Debt to private banks was considered a matter of state by the American rulers, who often used their military and diplomatic corps as muscle for Wall Street and the colossal firms of its Gilded Age. As in Haiti and at the same time, U.S. forces seized control of Liberia's customs houses and treasury, proposed a $1.7 million loan to pay its arrears, and settled in for the long haul. That the notion of black self-rule remained as troubling to American elites as German saber-rattling, and far more worrisome than colonial rule, is suggested by U.S. diplomats' calls for the Liberian government to cede control of its finances to the curious cartel of the United States, Britain, France, and Germany. The Great War would annul this proposal of convenience, if not the logic of white supremacy underpinning it.

World War I afforded, in Michael Crowder's view, "an opportunity for revolt to many peoples only recently subjugated."[11] But its impact in West Africa was mostly dire. Liberia, never recognized diplomatically by the United States during slavery, was suddenly if informally an American protectorate, which allowed the Americans to set up a West African naval outpost. Like many Liberian estuaries, that of the St. Paul River—home to the port of Monrovia—was surrounded by sandbars and reefs. It was nonetheless transformed by the U.S. Navy and its contractors into an important coaling station for oceangoing vessels. After Washington pushed for the expulsion of German merchants from Liberia, the country's trade shrank considerably.[12] As global conflict slowed legitimate commerce, smuggling and other illicit trade received a commensurate boost.

Then there were the fevers, which continued to afflict Liberians in Monrovia, as in towns and villages across the hinterland. It was a similar story in the neighboring colonies, where the long-standing mobility of the population heightened risks of epidemic spread from crowded towns to previously isolated regions now linked by rail; zoonoses became epizootics (the animal equivalent of epidemics) as livestock was transported along similar routes. In addition to the draft that eventually engaged close to half a million African men in military service to France, many as porters, the war economy crowded tens of thousands of poor farmers into insalubrious barracks in coastal cities and towns. These developments unleashed new waves of smallpox, yellow fever, plague, sleeping sickness, and malaria.

It was a similar story in the colonies of other warring powers. Sierra Leone may not have instituted mandatory conscription, and sent far fewer African troops abroad than did France, but it engaged thousands of workers, most from rural regions, in Freetown's port. Barracks were erected and filled, while informal settlements sprouted in the margins of the city.[13] The colony's arsenal of public-health measures was also plenty martial. These included penalties (a two-pound fine was levied on households "hiding" a smallpox victim); the threat of quarantine within contagious-disease "hospitals" that offered little in the way of medical or nursing care; legal actions against the locals (in Freetown, where ditches and puddles remained ubiquitous, there were 1,333 "mosquito larvae court cases" in 1914–1915 alone); more futile and corrosive attempts to segregate the city; and ongoing efforts to restrict free movement of the populace, which came to include many fleeing French impressment. The colonial medical service continued to exclude black physicians, even when, in 1914, overstretched health officers were dispatched to Cameroon to tend to those wounded or sickened in an early campaign against German forces.

Wait, what? Germans in Cameroon? Yes. The Scramble had made it Kamerun, a German colony lying between British Nigeria, French Equatorial Africa, and the Belgian Congo. British forces, mustered largely from southern Nigeria, joined Belgian and French ones—of course also mostly African subjects—in an assault on the German territory in August 1914. With amphibious support from the Royal Navy, the Allies soon prevailed in Cameroon's capital, its chief port city, and elsewhere along the coast. German forces retreated north to fortified posts such as Mora, which their foes besieged in the months that followed.

Like Sikasso prior to its fall, Mora was a walled town transformed into a fort, its outer defenses measuring some thirty miles in circumference. Unlike Sikasso, Mora was perched 1,700 feet above the plain; enemies could be descried from miles away. Also unlike Babemba's keep, this one was defended by

European artillery, booby-trapped trenches, and "five self-contained circular works, positioned to give each other supporting fire."[14] But Mora's human defenders were, once again, mostly African. Photos show them barefoot in khaki uniforms, waists cinched by ammo belts. After a year-long siege, their supplies of food and ammunition had dwindled, and British and Nigerian artillery had reduced the siege towers to rubble. It was the threat of famine that led to Mora's fall, on February 18, 1916. Although German forces held on to a couple of Cameroonian outposts, the French and British eventually divided the colony between themselves.

While Allied forces were laying siege to pieces of rock, reducing them to rock rubble, the work of providing health care to Sierra Leoneans in need of it went undone. "Between August 1914 and December 1915," relates the historian Festus Cole, "seven European medical personnel left for the Cameroons, one each from Freetown, Batkanu, Daru, Kaballa, Kailahun, Pujehun and Waterloo. Kissy, Makeni, Moyamba, Bonthe and Bo were without medical officers."[15] In other words, most of the white doctors outside of the capital left the colony. But if the great majority of Sierra Leoneans lived outside of towns and cities, why mourn the absence of distracted, demoralized, and under-supplied health officers if their performance to date had been poor? Well, the doctors did have a couple of items in their bags that really did work, including the fixings for smallpox vaccination.

The production of heat-stable smallpox vaccine was just beginning when the Great War began, and health officers in West Africa reported that some of their "lymph" failed to generate the visible scars signaling a protective immune response. But poor coverage during that war was sometimes due to failure to vaccinate rather than vaccine failure. In 1916, smallpox spread across the doctor-free (and largely nurse-free) districts of Sierra Leone and adjacent colonies. In terms strikingly similar to those heard during the Ebola epidemic a century later, many officials blamed smallpox outbreaks on superstitious, backward, and rebellious natives. When blaming local anti-vaxxers didn't work, other health authorities disparaged their African subordinates, mostly nurses. Native-blaming officials were contradicted by peers, missionaries, and employers, who reported that Africans—long familiar with the disfiguring, deadly disease—were lining up to supplant their own practice of variolation with safer and more effective vaccination.

Some British officials were more self-critical. A new reform-minded (and remarkably frank) governor in Freetown acknowledged in 1916 that the results of public-health efforts, even in the city, were "meagre" at best. In the protectorate, he wrote, where 95 percent of the population resided, it was "an exaggeration to say that one percent" of them had benefited from the administration's medical efforts.[16] In French West Africa, similarly, public-health resources and medical care were concentrated in coastal cities, where press-ganged conscripts continued to be crowded into barracks of their own hasty confection. Building them was quite a feat, given that many had been forced to walk, sometimes hundreds of miles, in order to report for duty. It wasn't until many hundreds died en route that the conscripted men were transported by truck or train.

As French subjects from across West Africa were called up for military service or steered to the construction of barracks, ports, armories, and warehouses—or herded into iron, gold, and coal mines—too little attention was paid to the subsistence agriculture that allowed folks to subsist. The draft also meant that land newly dedicated to cash crops lay fallow. By 1917, "a chorus of protest against the effects of conscription was raised by colonial administrators," including the governor-general himself. He complained to Paris that

> extensive and brutal recruiting of men was ruining the economy of
> the colony, both on its traditional subsistence base and in its fledging
> modern sector. Labour was in short supply and the people hopelessly
> demoralized by forced recruitment, shortages of food and related
> difficulties. Not only were thousands of men being drained off by the
> war, but thousands more were fleeing, sometimes with their families
> and even entire communities, across the frontiers to British West
> Africa to escape the recruiters.

The governor-general predicted that continued conscription would lead to widespread revolt and the loss of the colonies. When the French president, having already made cannon fodder of French Frenchmen, chose to ignore this warning—and instead ordered the immediate levy of fifty thousand more Africans, arguing that "France needed soldiers more than groundnuts"—his chief representative in Africa "resigned in disgust and marched off to the trenches, perhaps in search of martyrdom."[17]

That quest, at least, was successful in short order.

As the war drew to a close, West Africa's frail health systems were almost delivered the coup de grâce by a virulent new strain of influenza. With limited understanding of viruses, health authorities across the world initially misdiagnosed this pandemic flu as a host of pathologies with varied signs and symptoms: bacterial pneumonia and purulent bronchitis, which influenza often triggered, but also pneumonic plague, measles, dengue, "galloping consumption" due to tuberculosis, and even gastrointestinal afflictions like cholera and typhoid.

Although they didn't know its viral etiology, international health authorities recognized influenza's explosive spread as novel and apocalyptic. In three waves between 1918 and 1919, it killed more than fifty million people, many of them adults in their prime.[18] In the worldwide fog of world war, however, the origins of the pandemic were disputed. Origin stories implicated China, India, Britain, an Allied army post in France, and even Sierra Leone. Deaths in Spain were reported more openly than in countries at war, a candor rewarded with the nickname Spanish flu. Influenza had, in retrospect, shared genetic material with other strains and species. It's what these viruses do, and why flu shots are reformulated each year. By 1918, when pandemic flu seemed to be striking simultaneously in New England, France, and West Africa, Emmanuel Akyeampong observes, "the disease was unrecognizable in its new form."[19]

The dissemination of the mutant strains was rapid; its nature, disputed. In a widely read account of the American pandemic, one eminent medical historian asked how Spanish flu appeared in separate "explosions" in "three port cities thousands of miles apart." Were these due to a single point mutation and rapid spread in a time of war, a conflict that had drawn the ports of Boston, Brest, and Freetown into a single social web? Or to three different and almost simultaneous mutations? "All we can say," he concluded, "is that the first hypothesis is improbable and the second extremely improbable."[20] But historians knew, or should have known, that it was the triangular trade, not the Great War, that long linked these ports, making the first hypothesis the plausible one.

Review of the evidence suggests that hitherto (and once again) unknown Haskell County, Kansas—with a population, just prior to the war, of about 1,800 souls—offered "the first recorded instance suggesting that a new virus was adapting, violently, to man." The bucolic county was transformed by Camp Funston, a military base home to, on average, 56,222 troops. The first case later deemed consistent with the new strain (the alleged Patient Zero in the dominant origin story) fell ill at Funston on March 4, 1918. Within a month, many thousands more were sickened on the base. Previously healthy young recruits were, in the words of yet another historian of the pandemic, "struck down as suddenly as if they had been shot." Immune therapy for pneumococcal pneumonia, deemed the magic bullet of the day, had little or no effect. Meanwhile, Funston "fed a constant stream of men to other American locations and to Europe, men whose business was killing. They would be more proficient at it than they knew."[21]

From the fruited plains of the heavily armed American heartlands, the virus moved with stunning speed across a world upended by the business of killing. By 1918, more than 450,000 soldiers from "French Africa" had served during the war, some in rock-pounding campaigns like the siege of Mora, others on North African and Mediterranean fronts, and most in formal service to local militias or as porters. Perhaps three-quarters of them had been, prior to the draft, domestic slaves, serfs, or otherwise unfree. Although other colonial powers may not have reached French levels of impressment in Africa, their troops had similar backgrounds. These were the millions who'd benefited not at all from colonial rule, and influenza was widely seen as another noxious export, one largely impervious to what was then deemed modern medicine. The flu was, in the view of the historian Sandra Tomkins, "unquestionably the greatest challenge to Western imperialism from this quarter."

That challenge was especially forceful in Sierra Leone. The pandemic, Tomkins explains, "appeared to originate in British West Africa. As a result, questions of both its origins and imperial administrators' responsibilities were particularly acute and controversial."[22] It's not likely, however, that Freetown was much more than a flu destination and way station. Nor did West African soldiers returning from European fronts bring the new strain home with them. Spanish flu probably appeared to originate in British West Africa because it had traveled there aboard HMS *Mantua*, a 540-foot-long commercial liner that had been converted into an armed merchant cruiser. It was assigned to protect a convoy of merchant vessels headed through the U-boat-infested waters between England and West Africa and to return with gold to help finance a final push against Germany and its allies.

With the Suez Canal threatened by Germany and its Ottoman partners, the old route between England, Australia, and British colonies in Asia—via South Africa's Cape of Good Hope—had taken on renewed significance. This shipping lane led right past Sierra Leone.[23] Well before the discovery of diamonds, its mineral wealth still included gold, but also iron ore and coal, the primary fuels of the British Empire. During a war fought on land, at sea, and from the sky, Freetown's vast estuary—now protected by extensive boom defenses—became the empire's deepest mid-Atlantic port and an important coaling station for oceangoing steamers. Influenza's spread from Funston to Freetown was, in other words, another episode in the saga of an unequal global economy and the feuds and fevers it fostered.

On August 1, six months after the mysterious affliction erupted in Kansas and at the outset of the second European wave of mortality, the *Mantua* left Plymouth, Tomkins reports, with "many mild cases of influenza aboard."[24] The ship entered Freetown's harbor, another historian writes, "with 200 of her sailors sick or just recovering from influenza . . . apparently a mild variety of the disease, because there was no other variety to contract in England and there is no mention of deaths among the 200."[25] But declassified records—the *Mantua*'s log is now available online—do mention on-board deaths, as well as explosive shipboard spread in the days prior to reaching Freetown. The sailors were sickened by anything but a mild strain, as Sierra Leone and the entire continent were about to discover.

On the day of its departure from Plymouth, the *Mantua*'s log reads as follows: "Commenced coaling" at 3:00 a.m.; "Stopped coaling" at 5:20 a.m.; at 5:50 a.m., "Up anchor." On the alert for U-boats, the cruiser "commenced No. 51 zigzag" at 11:00 a.m. The only clue that something was amiss on board was the report of 4 sailors on the sick list. With 44 officers and a crew of 320, just 4 couldn't have seemed like a lot. But by August 10, the sick list ran to 25; the next day, to 38; and the next, 72. On August 14, at 5:50 p.m., the giant cruiser and its convoy churned into a harbor sheltering converted ocean liners, battleships, destroyers, dreadnoughts, corvettes, and hundreds of smaller craft. With 124 sick on board, according to the log, "Vessel ordered in strict quarantine."[26]

The quarantine was neither strict nor effective, as events were to prove. It was, however, typically British. Festus Cole reminds us that, at the close of the war, Freetown's responses to epidemics "remained largely authoritarian, revolving around quarantine measures, enacting ordinances and punishment for Africans who breached sanitary regulations." Before the war, such measures were often honored in the breach when it came to maritime trade, since hoisting the yellow jack meant short-term losses for the customs houses flying it and for shipping lines unable to discharge or take on passengers and cargo. Smallpox, rat-borne disease, and epidemics of yellow fever were attributed to lax enforcement just before the war led to a sharp rise in the number of vessels docking there. "It was clearly necessary," asserts Cole, "to examine all ships calling at Freetown (as most were rarely disinfected before coaling), to protect labourers employed on or in their vicinity." The "most effective way of disinfecting a ship," he adds, "was by using Clayton gas, which Freetown's harbor lacked."[27]

It's unlikely that all the king's Clayton (whatever that was) or the enforcement of quarantine in the absence of palliative measures would have made much of a difference in the days following the *Mantua*'s arrival. At 9:40 on the morning of its docking, "coal-lighters came alongside" the *Mantua*. Twenty minutes later, "native labour" from the Sierra Leone Coaling Company commenced coaling. On board, the sick list reached 132, and a young merchant marine, Patrick McFarlane, died from "pneumonia"—listed as the cause of death for most flu victims.[28] The number on the sick list continued to mount: 159 on the second day in harbor, 164 on the third, 176 on the fourth, 170 on the fifth. On August 20, Able Seaman William Sutton died, and then William Glazzard of the Royal Marine Light Infantry and Ordinary Seaman H. Tilling, followed a couple of days later by Petty Officer Gilbert Brown.

The bodies of three more sailors were landed on August 24 while the *Mantua* took on forty-eight crates of gold bullion. By the time the ship left for Plymouth on August 26, her crew had buried ten of their mates in Freetown's King Tom Cemetery. The sick list dwindled as the convoy zigzagged back to Plymouth, but not before losing more men, their bodies committed to the deep. On September 2, gunners fired the howitzers for practice and sent medical staff and stuff to a cargo ship transporting troops from New Zealand; they, too, had been laid low by influenza. But by September 5, the sick list had dropped to five, and no more deaths were reported. That the *Mantua* "lost one paint brush by accident" while docked in Freetown did, however, make the daily report.[29]

His Majesty's ship had let loose more than a stray paint brush before bringing home the bullion. Wartime Freetown's port counted thousands more dockworkers than were employed when Ibrahim Kamara's father spent his days counting those who showed up to work. Within a week of the *Mantua*'s arrival, more than five hundred employees of the Sierra Leone Coaling Company, their names undocumented, reported in sick. Leaping from person to person, influenza spread from the packed harbor to the rest of the city. Within three weeks, 4 percent of Freetown's residents were dead.

Influenza leapt quickly from Freetown to other major West African ports. If maritime spread of communicable disease was nothing new, wartime spread of influenza to the hinterlands via rail was.[30]

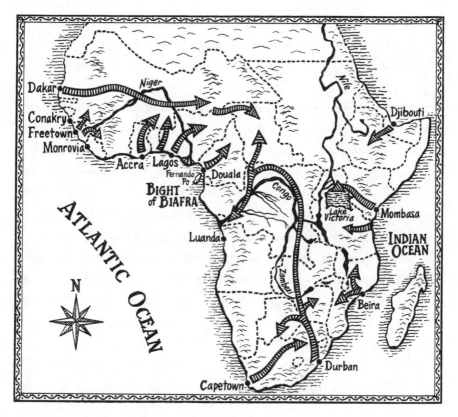

Old overland and newer rail networks sped the spread of influenza
across Africa. (Map after Patterson and Pyle, *Social Science and
Medicine*, 1983)

The virus was coughed overland from Freetown to military bases like the
one in Daru, in Kailahun District. Soon, old trade routes afforded the disease
other means of moving across the Kissi Triangle, and then east, north, and
south. Although Freetown was among the most catastrophically flu-stricken
cities, the entire region was devastated, as described by Sandra Tomkins:

> Not less than 1.5 percent of the population of Lagos died, and the
> toll in the provinces of Nigeria was thought to be even greater, with
> about 200,000 deaths in the northern provinces and 260,000 in
> the south (about three percent of the population). Deaths in the
> Gold Coast totalled at least four percent of the population, and the

Gambia, by far the smallest colony, sustained about 10,000 deaths. The West African colonies were a scene of abject misery and social dislocation.[31]

The death tolls were guestimates, of course. As war's end approached, the public-health service was much thinned out and, sanitarian inclinations aside, unable to count the dead. According to Sierra Leone's governor, its doctors spent a good deal of time bickering and blaming others—including each other—for the parlous state of the colony's health. There was plenty of blame to go around, and the Creole press, initially unaware influenza was racing across the world's transportation hubs, heaped it on slow-to-act authorities.

In the absence of a vaccine, which wouldn't come along until the 1940s, the sanitary measures of the day, even if uncontested, wouldn't have stopped pandemic influenza—not during war, not in Africa, not anywhere.[32] Spanish flu, Tomkins claims, was "completely impervious to the methods and practices of European—or any other—medicine."[33] If British authorities couldn't have stopped influenza, however, they could have done a better job organizing relief efforts. These might have rendered conventional public-health measures—including social distancing and voluntary isolation, decreased work hours, school closings, and even formal quarantine—more effective. But as another wave of therapeutic nihilism crashed on the colonies, the control-over-care mania of imperial health authorities swept over Britain itself.

It's sure that these tactics were resented, and also pretty clear that many of the therapies of the day were harmful. But therapeutic nihilism was dying a slow death in industrialized nations, and its resurgence in Britain was remarkable. By the start of the war, from Germany to England and across the pond, immune therapy for pneumococcal pneumonia had inspired the growth of a public-health apparatus concerned with the treatment of this common killer, and of commercial networks of labs able to produce anti-serum.[34] By war's end, several other interventions were believed to lower death rates among those stricken with infectious pathogens. Most were nonspecific (replacement of lost fluids and electrolytes, reduction of fever and inflammation, nutritional support, supplemental oxygen, and above all good nursing care) and a few were specific (in addition to transfusion of convalescent sera from those who had survived plague or pneumococcal pneumonia, reactive vaccination with "lymph" for smallpox, and immune therapy for toxin-mediated diseases like diphtheria and tetanus). In the absence of specific antiviral therapies for influenza, supportive and nonspecific care saved many lives. They might have saved many more.

Several of these interventions, along with social support and relief of hunger and crowding, constituted the mainstay of well-organized responses to the pandemic in most affluent nations. Not so in the United Kingdom. Obsessed with containment, and aware of the failure of antipneumococcal therapy on U.S. Army bases like Camp Funston, British sanitarians, Tomkins writes, paid scant heed to caregiving. Theirs was a control-over-care strategy familiar to their African subjects:

> With remarkable uniformity, other policy makers in the United
> States, Canada, Australia, New Zealand, and South Africa
> recognized the futility of influenza prevention and overwhelmingly
> directed their efforts to the relief of epidemic-related distress through
> the provision of nursing assistance, home helps, soup kitchens, and
> dispensaries . . . Britain, which had by far the most sophisticated
> public health machinery among those societies where the epidemic
> has been chronicled, mounted the least effective response.[35]

Across their African colonies, British authorities initially adhered to failed control-over-care policies, with the expected results. In what will remind many of the recent Ebola response—or of sleeping sickness isolation centers—attempts to corral suspected influenza cases within understaffed and under-supplied isolation units were met with stiff resistance and attempts to flee.

These responses were not to be attributed to native ignorance or superstition, argued the editors of the *Lagos Standard* on October 2, 1918, but to widespread awareness of "the reckless disregard for human Native life displayed by the Authorities." Residents of Lagos were especially mistrustful of an "infectious disease hospital" offering little in the way of care, and a quarantine station in the neighborhood of Abekun offering even less. Isolation centers had become a feature of colonial medicine, and would persist in the postcolony. Indeed, the *Standard*'s editors might have been writing in response to the West Africa Ebola outbreak:

> People are hustled out to practically certain death in a building
> where . . . those sent are obliged to lie on bare cement floor with
> no bed nor anything, and one is not allowed to carry his own bed
> with him . . . It is not a wise thing to depend on Force as the most
> essential weapon for stamping out an epidemic. The co-operation
> of the people with the work of the Sanitary Authorities is very
> essential, and that co-operation cannot be secured by the present
> methods of the Sanitary Authorities which make people run away
> not from dread of the disease, but from fear of sanitary officials and
> their ways.[36]

In the face of widespread resistance to sanitarians and their ways—and after the obvious failure of containment—health officers and other authorities in British colonies caught on. Available resources were finally turned to "relieving distress through the provision of medicines, hospital accommodations, foodstuffs, and health visits."[37] This relief didn't reach the rural majority. But had dispirited and contentious officials followed London's policy directives to the letter, the toll in colonial capitals might have been even steeper.

What accounts for Britain's embrace of policies that clearly conveyed indifference to the suffering of those already sick? Influenza in Britain aside, these polices were crafted for colonial subjects, not the fair folk of the Emerald Isle. Although clinical infectious disease did not yet exist as a field, and although critical care, as practiced in field hospitals on the fringes of Europe's battlefields, was in its infancy, there was still a lot one might do to save lives imperiled by hypovolemic shock caused by infectious pathogens. The most reliably life-saving intervention is often the simple intravenous replacement of lost fluids and electrolytes. Even in the preantibiotic era, and even in the White Man's Grave, one finds little evidence that the non-poor ever faced the same risks as the poor—whether we're speaking of risk of infection or of poor outcomes once infected.

Control-over-care policies still bear the obvious stamp of the fire-and-brimstone colonial sanitarians of the early twentieth century. For them, influenza, smallpox, plague, yellow fever, epidemic meningitis, and even pneumococcal pneumonia were the Ebolas of the day. Once subjects were sickened, there was little to be done about them beyond promoting "better hygiene," which usually spelled more containment efforts. In Europe's African colonies, disease control was too rarely leavened by professional caregiving. In Sierra Leone, greater attention to caregiving and other supportive measures might have lessened the impact of smallpox in 1916 and of influenza two years later. In the absence of such measures, however, these epidemics compounded other afflictions common there prior to the war but worsened by it.

Consider the years-long synergy of plagues that afflicted the town of Port Loko and its surroundings in the months after war's end. Influenza in West Africa was catastrophic for many reasons: the nature of the pathogen, the failure of preventive efforts, ineffective therapies, and a dearth of supportive and critical care. But the catastrophe was compounded by wartime follies, among them the campaign that pulled Sierra Leone's medical officers to Cameroon. The people of Port Loko would come to see their farmers and petty traders lose their livelihood and livestock (and thus know hunger and despair), then an explosive smallpox epidemic (and more hunger and despair) and, finally, the mother of all pandemics.

Port Loko had known little but hard times in the years since its first Spanish (and Portuguese) affliction. Although *lançados* no longer prowled the area's rivers and estuaries, legitimate trade there remained under threat long after the Loko-speakers themselves had faded into memory through displacement and assimilation or into the hulls of hungry ships—or, in the case of Bai Bureh and other chiefs resisting the hut tax, into British jails or nooses. Legitimate commerce had been further complicated in Port Loko and other towns by the late nineteenth-century arrival of traders from the Levant, as the region between the Mediterranean and the Arabian Desert was known at the time, before the victors of the Great War traced the still-disputed borders of Syria, Lebanon, and Turkey.

Levantine influence in West Africa was established through control of long-haul commerce, some of it reaching (as in previous centuries) into the Middle East, Europe, and Asia. Along the Upper Guinea Coast, Syrians came to control the commodity trade, including that in rice—the staff of life in what later became the three most Ebola-affected countries. Once established, many Syrians resisted social integration through marriage, the adoption of local customs, and cultivation of Africans for leadership positions in their businesses. Syrian assimilation was further thwarted by traditions and laws restricting their integration as subjects or citizens. These would come to favor behind-the-scenes political patronage, the offshoring of profits, and deft avoidance of taxes.

The Spanish flu's toll around Port Loko and its war-depleted hinterland was worsened by a years-long string of misfortunes and by sharp tensions between Syrian traders, local farmers, Creole merchants, and colonial authorities. Many Sierra Leoneans—including some enrolled in the military—considered the Great War a "white man's palaver." But the Syrians' chief business rivals, Freetown Creoles, often expressed empire loyalism to Britain; some were quick to observe that Syrians were subjects of the Ottoman Empire. Trade feuds and related conflicts deepened as the war drew to a close, spilling over among farmers already facing devastating dislocations. These were worsened by regional epidemics, not all of them afflicting humans directly.

In 1913, an outbreak lethal to cattle began in then-French Chad. Although the culprit wasn't identified initially, whatever was killing the cows (and their antelope cousins) was stalled by the mighty Niger and by quarantine measures on its western shore. When the latter faltered, the cattle killer raced toward French Guinea and its neighbors. The cause of the calamity was revealed in 1915, when a German veterinarian diagnosed the disease as rinderpest. (He was a prisoner of war in that high-stakes battle zone of Niger, where veterinarians were evidently deemed to pose security threats.) A viral disease of cattle and other ungulates believed by evolutionary biologists to be related to measles, rinderpest was also prevented by a vaccine. Doughty French veterinarians introduced it across their empire. They'd claimed rinderpest was of little concern in their territories, alleging the disease had been eradicated from French West Africa since 1893.[38] But by war's end, four-fifths of Senegal's cattle were dead, and French Guinea's were dying.

It was inevitable that cattle-loving pathogens would leap the Anglo-French frontier, since Karene District had a busy marketplace dedicated largely to cross-border trade with Guinea, including trade in livestock and game from the grasslands and forest-savannah mosaic to the north of its border. Authorities in Port Loko and Freetown made the usual noises about closing borders, seizing and destroying livestock and bushmeat, and fining or jailing violators—always, of course, of the African persuasion. Local traders and chiefs were loath to shut down the bazaar on the orders of health officials who weren't around to care for the sick or to inoculate man or beast. This was true whether or not British sanitarians had been dispatched to the rock-pounding campaign in Cameroon; by the time Allied forces claimed the great prize of Mora, rinderpest and other pestilence had claimed Karene's cattle.

In the dry season of 1915, smallpox hit Karene's human population, a disease for which sanitarians actually had something to offer in the midst of an epidemic. Karene's authorities did not, however, enjoy enthusiastic cooperation from chiefs (minor or paramount) even when people, not cattle, were viral targets. Although the noises from Freetown were more insistent this time, the health service was too weak to enforce its genuinely protective regulations as opposed to its stupidly punitive ones. Within a year, all of Karene's fifty chiefdoms were reporting cases of smallpox. Quarantine and travel restrictions, along with the toll taken by recruitment of farmers into the war economy and by the disease itself, made it harder to plant and tend fields and paddies, harvest and thresh the rice crop, and bring it to market. In the past, according to Walter Rodney, only giant locust swarms could destroy carefully tended rice paddies. Desert-loving locusts, unlike other plagues, were rare in Sierra Leone. But when Levantine traders began to hoard stockpiles of rice, and to raise prices as hunger deepened first in the countryside and then in the towns, comparisons between Syrians and a plague of locusts were bound to ensue. Creoles still controlled much of the Freetown press and had, explains historian Ismail Rashid, "sufficiently focused on the 'Syrian Peril' to strengthen popular belief that Syrian merchants were acting outside legitimate limits."[39]

Into this years-long synergy of plagues came the Spanish flu. Having hitched a ride south on the *Mantua*, influenza was offloaded by colliers formerly engaged in the primary activity of the hinterlands. In September, days after the infected ship headed back to Plymouth, influenza struck Port Loko, Karene, and Kambia, a region afflicted by catastrophic food shortages and still reeling from livestock losses and smallpox. Although the Pasteurian hobby of disease surveillance had been weakened before influenza laid waste to Freetown, it was estimated that three-quarters of those without prior exposure to the mutant strain—meaning most everyone—was sickened by it. Thousands died in Port Loko, Kambia, and the other towns of Karene. Overwhelmed families were further traumatized by an inability to afford their felled kin dignified interment. "Many areas had mass burials with twenty to thirty corpses sharing the same grave," writes Rashid. "In Kambia, the graves of the dead stretched for a quarter mile."

Although Ebola responders and public-health authorities are short-memoried—in 2014, none of us knew mass graves had been dug before in Kambia and Port Loko, except during the civil war that ended a dozen years earlier—the noxious synergy between feuds and fevers has long been well known to the area's farmers. During the Great War, British authorities may not have forcibly conscripted unwilling African men and youth into the army, but siphoning them off to the urban war economy, or to mines, meant that more land than usual lay fallow. (Although women did and do most of the work in farming communities, men were responsible for clearing exuberant bush and mangrove thickets in order to prepare paddies. They also did some of the threshing.) If empire loyalism was difficult to discern anywhere in rural Sierra Leone as memories of the Hut Tax War faded, it was decidedly absent among small-scale farmers by the close of World War I.

The disruption of subsistence agriculture didn't end with the armistice of November 11, 1918, or in the months that followed. Around Port Loko, this was due in part to influenza's toll. As far back as the region's collective memories reached, the start of the rains marked the beginning of the hungry season. In the aftermath of war, that season was upon them throughout the dry harmattan months beginning in November, when in good years granaries and larders were filled and shops and warehouses replenished. But 1918 was not a good year. After a meager harvest, 1919 looked ominous from the point of view of Karene's surviving farmers. "Early rains interfered with clearing and burning of farms," explains Rashid. "Peasants sowed rice on only sixty to seventy percent of land cleared. Influenza made it impossible for them to keep pace with weeds, which in some cases choked the crop. Without labour to drive them away, birds devoured a great deal more than in a normal year."[40]

Karene's paramount chief, aware of the threat of famine, reported dire food shortages as people were forced to uproot cassava three months before it was ready to harvest. But the rice crop, their potential salvation, was already in the warehouses of Levantine traders. British authorities attempted to halt hoarding and speculation by fixing the price of rice, a measure sublimely ignored by the Syrians. In Port Loko and its Maforki chiefdom, as the rains continued, "the river trade stood still and there were 'a lot of idle people' around." With catastrophe looming, there were "signs of restlessness and readiness to raid Syrian stores." A century before Ebola burial teams were to face a hail of stones during the unceremonious collection of the dead in the village of Matweng, the hungry people of the same neighborhood launched a brief intifada against those stockpiling rice and other edibles.

Maforki, the setting of the mortal dramas related in previous chapters, made it into the sorry annals of history from below long before the Ebola crisis. "The gathering of three chiefs and their supporters in Port Loko to sign the decree book on the ascension of a new Bai Forki of Maforki Chiefdom on August 1, 1919," Rashid reports, "provided opportunity for the 'rioters.'"[41] The new chief was likely sympathetic to the hungry farmers, as were native troops tasked with protecting the foodstuffs piled in warehouses scattered throughout the town. On August 3, the district commissioner—cloistered in his hill station—declared a curfew, recommending that Syrian traders bulk their rice in the home and courtyard of a town official. The farmers shifted their attention to the house, and the next night, about a hundred of them began to loot it. The African soldiers sought to stand down, but their British commander fired on the crowd, killing four. Shops were also raided in Kambia.

No Syrians were harmed, however, in the making of these riots. Throughout these postepidemic uprisings, the intention of those rioting was to eat, not harm. But when the government was faulted by farmers for "its failure to restrain private enterprise during the epidemic, especially widespread profiteering in medicine and food," they were referring to Syrian-owned businesses.[42] Although Levantine traders discerned the dark designs of their Creole competitors in this critique, the plight of the famished looters, and of the population from which they hailed, wasn't lost on colonial authorities. No less a man than the governor, pointing to food scarcity and to Syrian hoarding, "discounted the notion of a Creole or Freetown-based conspiracy," even though members of his administration "retained the view that the Creoles had directed the animosity of a 'half-starved people' to injure Syrians because of 'trade jealousy.'"[43]

Colonial rule in West Africa would endure for decades after the Great War. But in the view of historians writing in recent years, overlapping outbreaks of rinderpest, trypanosomiasis, malaria, smallpox, plague, yellow fever, and influenza sounded the death knell of accommodation to colonial rule among people already sapped by endemic disease, taxation, coerced labor, the draft, and wartime food shortages. "Regional and global disease epidemics, which followed in the wake of World War I," concludes Ismail Rashid, "became the crucial tipping point in the balance between resistance and accommodation that had been established between British and colonized people of the Sierra Leone Protectorate."[44] Nor were the Sierra Leoneans the only victims of misguided and punitive policies, or of hunger and epidemics worsened by wartime ones. These were the lot of many millions of Africans far from Europe's epic slaughter.

Some demographers peg the population of Africa south of the Sahara at about 200 million souls just prior to the Scramble unleashed in the 1880s. The violent and disease-inciting shocks of occupation, and the engagement of African subjects in the Great War and its long tail in the colonies, may have reduced the region's population to 150 million before Europe descended once again into chaos in the 1930s.[45] That might make the first few decades of the colonial enterprise in Africa as deadly as the 1919 influenza pandemic, the world's first mechanized war, or the Atlantic slave trade. In fact, these noxious events are readily bound up into a single storyline, which continued to unfold as a world of colonies and colonizers became ever more unequal.

In recounting the Great War's untold African chapters, historians of epidemic disease—and of famine, flight, riot, and revolt—resist the allure of agency by pointing out where it really lay: among those who conceived colonial extractive empires and then prosecuted "total war" to preserve them.

If Europe was wrecked, it was also a wrecking ball. Yet the war's carnage brought down only the flimsiest wings of the colonial edifice. Radziwill Palace was still standing, awaiting its Third Reich tenants and another cycle of wreck and ruin. Germany's noxious experiment in Africa may have seemed over—it wasn't—but France and Britain clung tightly to their empires and, like Germany, to the conviction that some lives mattered less than others.

Surveying the devastation en route to sign the Treaty of Versailles, the continent's sovereigns—leaders of the nations represented at the Berlin Conference—had more weighty concerns than the prospects of peasants, porters, miners, dockworkers, and petty traders in the colonies. Surviving African soldiers, even those who'd fought in the heart of Europe, were also mostly forgotten. Although the postwar French government understood it could not continue the draft within France proper, it long retained the unpopular policy in West Africa in an attempt to address the loss of a generation of young Frenchmen. Across its battered empire, the United Kingdom wearily raised its trade-led flag even before its dead were buried. But the real trade-led flag was now the Stars and Stripes.

Spared the material destruction and much of the carnage of the war, the United States was increasingly dominant in global affairs and global trade. American investments overseas grew twentyfold between 1900 and 1926. Washington, claiming an aversion to European brands of colonialism, may have participated as a mere observer in the Berlin Conference. But the American plutocracy—which included some politicians and bankrolled many others—had already been keen to switch from gunboat diplomacy to dollar diplomacy. The latter relied less on occupation of distant lands and more on dominating global commerce through technological and scientific advances, vaunted business know-how, and an ever-increasing demand for American products. Products like automobiles. There was, in the postwar period, one big problem for a booming U.S. auto industry: rubber.

By the 1920s, Americans owned 85 percent of the world's cars and consumed 75 percent of its rubber. But latex remained a British monopoly. When the war-savaged empire sought to drive up rubber prices by restricting flow to the States, the titans of its auto and tire industry—notably, Henry Ford and Harvey Firestone—cried foul. Predicting an annual surcharge to American consumers of $300 million, they were especially irked with Britain's newly appointed chancellor of the exchequer, the India-looting Winston Churchill. ("It was only natural to expect Lord Churchill to use his power looking to the rigid enforcement of the Restriction act," fumed Firestone in *The New York Times*, "as he was Colonial Secretary at the time the legislation was enacted.")[46] Taking a cue from their former sovereigns, the American industrialists sought to break the monopoly the British way—by establishing tropical colonies while using government muscle to jack up private profits.[47]

Henry Ford had attempted to start rubber plantations in Brazil, the largest of them named Fordlandia. But these and other Latin American essays failed in the face of political upheaval, labor strife, and agricultural blights. That left Harvey Firestone to note that a British firm had abandoned a small Liberian plantation after the war. In 1925, the Ohio-based Firestone Tire and Rubber Company began negotiating its famous million-acre, century-long concession:

Ultimately, only Firestone would succeed in creating a viable rubber supply for the United States that was largely free from foreign production and control. He did so by bringing the forces of industrial capital, foreign diplomacy, and science and medicine to bear on the transformation of the West African republic of Liberia into the United States' rubber empire.[48]

"Science and medicine" did not include, just then, much in the way of either social science or social medicine. Unlike the Liberian imaginary and its cannibalistic denizens, transnational rubber empires—and the offshore shoots of multinational corporations in general—enjoyed little in the way of critical oversight from the professoriate.

One exception was W.E.B. Du Bois's exposé of Firestone's early years in Liberia. The sociologist may have abandoned his post in Atlanta, but he was as prolific as ever, and increasingly influential in intellectual and political circles. By the late twenties, Du Bois was also an avowed socialist and surprised, understandably, when Calvin Coolidge named him Special Minister Plenipotentiary and Envoy Extraordinary to Liberia. "The appointment was purely ornamental," he explained in *Foreign Affairs*, "but I did all I could to coöperate with Hood"—the U.S. envoy to Liberia, an African American—"and Africa and Liberia and tell them of the tremendous interest which American colored people had in them." The sociologist soon discovered that the mandarins of dollar diplomacy also had a growing interest in Liberia: compound interest.

The rubber magnate, it transpires, had insisted on financing a $2.5 million loan to service the country's debt. "When I heard of the terms which Firestone demanded in Liberia," Du Bois wrote, "my heart began to fall."[49] One needn't be a cardiologist to understand the Envoy Extraordinary's palpitations. Indeed, medical training seemed to confer no special sympathy for the plight of Liberian negotiators. One of my predecessors at Harvard Medical School, Richard Pearson Strong—who founded Harvard's Department of Tropical Medicine, the country's oldest—led a scientific and medical mission to Liberia as Firestone negotiated his deal. Dr. Strong disagreed with Du Bois regarding both the deal and the intentions of the Americo-Liberians. Then again, Professor Strong's expedition was funded in large part by Firestone, and not merely because he'd previously served as the head of the Philippines Bureau of Science's Biological Laboratory and had worked extensively, even from his Harvard perch, with United Fruit, another giant U.S. multinational.

Experience in the Philippines and Latin America taught Richard Strong that barriers to commercial investment in the tropics were as political and economic as they were medical and ecological. His conclusions were entirely compatible with the lessons of social medicine, although the uses to which his insights were put may have troubled colleagues in that discipline. In 1925, he reached out to Harvey Firestone to propose "an extensive medical and biological survey" of inland Liberia:

> Firestone was highly receptive to the idea, having grown ever more interested in a small, two thousand–acre rubber plantation in Liberia when, in the 1920s, his prospects of securing land in the Philippines for rubber production were dashed by anti-American sentiments and an experimental plantation in the state of Chiapas, Mexico, became engulfed in revolution and flames . . . But while the political and economic climate seemed relatively congenial to U.S. investment in 1925, natural obstacles nevertheless had the potential to stand in the way of Firestone's success in Liberia. Most significantly, endemic human and plant diseases threatened both the healthy survival and growth of rubber plants imported from Southeast Asia and the health and well-being of the native Liberian population that Firestone was counting on to harvest and process the raw latex these plants produced.[50]

Strong and his colleagues, once Firestone funding was secured, went on to describe some of the worst health conditions on the planet, gathering evidence of endemic sleeping sickness, schistosomiasis, onchocerciasis, malaria, leprosy, yaws, diverse venereal afflictions, and lymphatic filariasis.

Surveys of Liberian children suggested that 90 percent of them suffered from blood-sapping hookworms and the like. The list went on.

Even prior to the antibiotic era, all of these pathologies could be prevented, palliated, or cured. But Liberians weren't often on the receiving end of control over care. Usually they received neither. Outbreaks of smallpox and yellow fever were common in Liberia; preventive and containment measures were not. "The history of Liberia has been simple in respect to hygiene and sanitation," Strong summarized. "Preventative measures have been few, and the survival of many of the Americo-Liberian people in Monrovia and the vicinity has often apparently depended, in the main, on the tolerance or immunity which they have acquired in respect to infectious disease." A visit to the city's, and the country's, sole public hospital revealed a handful of beds attended by a single "poorly qualified Liberian physician" with almost nothing in the way of supplies.[51] Liberia's rural and indigenous population, with whom Strong's sympathies lay, had even less access to health professionals of any sort. His team reported "no doctor of medicine in the interior of Liberia and no pharmacy of any description."

These details and thousands more were collected in a handsome, two-volume report that was dedicated to—wait for it—Harvey Firestone. Team Harvard catalogued important discoveries made in Liberia and in the course of overland travels across the Belgian Congo. The expedition had done its best (one would like to think) to help the afflicted from its base camps, even though only two of its members were experienced clinicians. And even though they were in Liberia for only four months. And even though medical historians later questioned the ethics of some of Strong's medical experiments.[52] And even though he, at least, was an ardent cheerleader for the proposed Firestone deal.

In Monrovia, Strong met with his patron's son. Harvey Jr. was there to push forward the loan, which Americo-Liberian politicians—keen as they were to rent out others' land and labor—recognized as poisonous usury. In a letter of thanks to Harvey Sr. "for all the courtesy and assistance" extended to him by his son and their company, the professor added that "what you are doing and trying to do will undoubtedly bring great benefit to the country and redound to the welfare of its people."[53] Richard Strong laid out even stronger opinions about the loan in his diary: "If the Liberian people have any sense they will certainly accept the terms, which are however far too favorable to the Liberian people."[54]

Whether or not Firestone's investment in that country would redound to its benefit, it's hard to imagine the Liberians had ever been offered overly generous terms for anything. But Strong was referring to the Americo-Liberians, not the natives:

> No one has stressed the responsibility of the Americo-Liberians
> toward the indigenous people. Clearly, the most important source of
> internal revenue for the Government lies, as we have seen, in the labor
> that the natives of the interior can furnish and the taxes that they can
> pay, but they receive from the state practically nothing in return.[55]

Sometimes less than nothing: Strong tipped off contacts in the U.S. State Department about evidence of an international slavery racket run on Fernando Po—the largest of a series of islands not far off the Upper Guinea Coast—by influential Americo-Liberians. Native labor had long been in short supply for all the reasons already mentioned and because of competition for it on cacao plantations cultivated by Fernando Po's shrinking indigenous population and by migrants from Sierra Leone and elsewhere on the mainland, including Liberia. This labor famine hadn't subsided after the Great War. The Liberian Labor Bureau, which rounded up contract labor, was rumored to receive kickbacks from middlemen in the pay of plantation owners and of in-house concessions within Liberia.

British and other colonial governments had complained about such schemes for years, since they were competing for the same workers. Now, in 1928—141 years after the founding of the Province of Freedom—Sierra Leone's government took the monumental step of abolishing slavery across the protectorate, sharpening the competition. The allegations against Liberia, fanned by short-handed colonial neighbors and by Firestone, led the League of Nations to launch an official inquiry into these charges. The republic's shaky sovereignty was again on the line. The "black slavery scandal," as it was termed, forced Liberia's president from office and further tarnished the country's sketchy reputation as a beacon of decency in a racist world.[56] Its legislature, seeking relief from bad press and the threat of hostile takeover by the League as much as Mr. Firestone's proposed terms, made the export of contract labor illegal. This did not suffice for the tire titan, who insisted the loan be signed before any bailout or further investments in Liberia were to proceed.

This time around, the colonial cartel deferred to Firestone and his countrymen. In lockstep with the Ohio company, the Hoover administration refused to recognize the new government. Over the objections of Liberian negotiators—who included the rainmaker and future president William Tubman—the local Firestone bank became the financial agent for both sides of the deal. According to Liberian officials, their government caved because "the State Department of the United States told us to accept this loan."[57] In tedious detail, W.E.B. Du Bois explained what came to pass: "The first instalment was marketed at 90, giving $2,027,700 in actual receipts. This sum was expended to repay $1,146,715 in outstanding 5 percent bonds, $175,000 in internal bonds, mostly at 3 percent, and to meet various other debts. Of the balance, $11,730 was spent for health and sanitation and $156,439 for public works."[58] Even a Harvard medical professor can see this was bad math.

It gets worse. As in previous years, Liberia's foreign creditors joined forces to demand that a group of "financial experts" report to a "financial adviser" of their choosing. Salaries for said experts, who happened to be white Americans, added $44,500—four times the amount pledged to health and sanitation—to Liberia's tab. On paper, Firestone Rubber Company was soon the largest taxpayer in Liberia. But the company extracted its pound of flesh along with tons of latex:

> The loan charges, including interest on the bonds, amortization expenses, and salaries of fiscal officers, in 1928 absorbed 20 percent of the total revenue of Liberia; in 1929, 26 percent; in 1930, 32 percent; in 1931, 54.9 percent; and for 1932, according to an official statement, "nearly the whole revenue of the government."

The financial advisor, in the opinion of a 1932 report from the League of Nations, offered "deplorable advice." He was, added Du Bois bitterly, "subsequently transferred to Haiti by the United States Government to take care of that country's American debt."[59] The world's oldest black republic, then in the seventeenth year of its own U.S. military occupation, was about to get another lesson in voodoo economics, American-style.

Liberia, the world's second-oldest black republic, was soon so mired in debt that Washington again pressed for receivership. Britain and Germany (its merchants now back in Liberia) joined in this request. Making Liberia a U.S. protectorate would have suited Harvey Sr. just fine. The hard-nosed tycoon continued to support research in tropical medicine. In 1933, he built a hospital in Harbel, the new company town, staffing it (as his employees requested) with white doctors. One of Firestone's first hires was a German medic who doubled as head of the local branch of the Nazi party.

So there was that.

The non-Nazi German contingent in Liberia included a handful of medical missionaries. One of them was the surgeon Werner Junge, who in 1931 reached the northern town of Bolahun—not far from the Kissi Triangle—where he worked as a medical jack-of-all-trades in a fifty-bed mission hospital.[60] For the better part of his time there, Junge was the sole physician at the hospital, which each day faced a wave of the sick, the injured, and the curious.

Like Team Harvard, Dr. Junge found the Liberian residents of the trizone region—tribes, he wrote, from "the great family of the Mandingos"—to be swimming in a sea of endemic and epidemic disease. Unlike the folks from Boston, the German surgeon and a crackerjack team of nurses and orderlies from Bolahun kept an operating room busy with elective surgeries while receiving up to a thousand outpatients a day. This allowed them to see not only infections unique to the tropics but "all the long list of ailments familiar in Europe, with the difference that owing to neglect they appeared often in chronic forms."[61] Also unlike Strong, Junge had the gift for the vivid anecdote and illustrative tale. That didn't mean the surgeon's tales weren't misinterpreted. A *New York*

Times review of his memoir alleged that "patients were afraid to come to him lest they antagonize their witch doctors."[62] But unless something besides the title was lost in translation—it originally appeared as *Bolahun: An African Adventure*, but my treasured copy is called *African Jungle Doctor*—local reticence and fear of the unfamiliar were far from the main story.

Though unimpressed with germ theory, those who showed up in droves at the Bolahun hospital were stunned by the success of yaws treatment and by the magic of anesthesia. This willingness to be prodded, poked, put under, and sliced open spoke to a hard-nosed empiricism regarding what sort of magic works. (Plenty of Junge's patients might have been classed as witch doctors.) "Again and again," he wrote of those crowding his waiting rooms, "their desire to have injections and operations instead of merely taking pills and tablets proved almost invincible."[63] In contrast to the colonial sanitarians who complained of the natives' adamant rejection of what was good for them, the German complained of his patients' long-winded narratives and simulations of false symptoms in order to partake in the modern medical care of the day. That's why they lined up for it, trading tips on what stories might impress the doctor and his translators. Worn-out Junge had good reason to thank the Lord when finally joined by a young German medic he described as "shamelessly healthy."[64]

Perhaps because vaccines were given as injections, or perhaps because they recognized Dr. Junge as a caregiver also interested in preventing affliction, the folks living not far from Macenta and Kailahun didn't come off as *réticent* about vaccination campaigns, either. His experience of struggling as the sole credentialed physician on the Liberian side of the trizone region during a devastating 1932 outbreak of smallpox—the disease had, the German was informed, "obviously come from over the nearby French border"— laid out the cost and consequences of therapeutic nihilism in a time when a heat-stable vaccine might be complemented by nursing care, smallpox antiserum or lymph, and passion for the easement of suffering. It was smallpox, and Junge's reputation as a death-defying medicine man, that allowed him to enter bush schools previously closed to outsiders—whether from Monrovia, Europe, rival societies or tribes, or the rival sex.

Back then, cohorts of boys were sometimes sequestered for years, emerging as young men. Smallpox had no trouble infiltrating these sacred groves. Werner Junge and his team went to the assistance of one bush school, and not merely to administer vaccines to those not yet afflicted:

> When, with the chief and the utterly desperate and bewildered medicine-man, I penetrated to the Bush, I found eighteen of the twenty-two boys seriously ill. Those who were still unaffected had in their terror withdrawn to a distance and left their unfortunate companions to their fate. So there they lay in the blazing sun, covered with pustules, in some cases confluent, forming large septic ulcers, upon which flies had settled in hundreds. Some of the boys could scarcely move for the agony they were in. Others had crept under a wretched palm-leaf shelter to find shade, whimpering for water they were unable to swallow. They lay uncared for in all their dirt and filth. No one had dared to touch them, and so it was a true deliverance for them when all day long we bandaged, washed, and tended them, made them beds with mosquito curtains, and soothed their pain. I have rarely been rewarded with such thankful looks as I was that day.[65]

It's too easy to dismiss Junge's depiction of this suffering, and its alleviation with supportive care, as a self-serving tale of heroism. He and his mobile team spent untold hours in tedious palavers with local chiefs in order to muster support for vaccination. In two weeks and in difficult conditions, they'd inoculated more people than had Edward Jenner—father of the smallpox vaccine and beneficiary of official patronage and wide renown—in the course of several years.

The folks in and around Bolahun certainly sound more receptive to disease-control efforts than the merchant class Junge later got to know when assigned to rebuild another mission hospital in Cape Mount, a settlement in which the natives mixed uneasily with Americo-Liberians, missionaries, and traders willing to brave the reef off the coast. Those living and trading there were more rankled by the notion of quarantine than were the forest folk.

Clearly unfamiliar with the history of Dutch commerce, Junge was surprised when a trading company based in the Netherlands sued him for £1,000 for hoisting the yellow jack over the dock of a nearby trading post. The litigious merchants only stopped hassling him when the Liberian health ministry retroactively named him district health commissioner.

Dr. Junge was appalled and fascinated by the human-leopard furor that struck his new catchment area. Unlike the British in Freetown, he saw ritual cannibalism as a colonial pathology. After a decade in Liberia, the German surgeon worked his way up to a strong condemnation of colonialism by asserting his belief that racism was a sickness—ironically enough by deploring Americo-Liberian disdain for the natives. He pegged grasping aspirations, and the envy they stirred, as the reasons accusations of ritual cannibalism were mostly leveled at Americo-Liberians. His book resounds with the exoticism of his memoir-writing contemporaries, but his reflections on ritual cannibalism are intended to explain, in functionalist fashion, its origins (colonial clash) and purpose (power play by those seeking material advancement).

Junge was an amateur anthropologist with a scalpel, not a noose.

As the Harvard expedition suggested, academics could have conflicts. So could missionary doctors. If the latter had conflicts of interest, however, they were more likely to be in service to the sick than to for-profit concerns or empires.

W.E.B. Du Bois may have been overly sympathetic to Americo-Liberian politicians, averting his usually keen gaze from their long-standing abuse of the natives. A "race man," he'd offered Haitian elites a similar pass. But Du Bois generally sided with the underdogs, including those in the two black republics. In his own country, he attacked neoslavery in the American South, nationwide and institutionalized racism, gunboat and dollar diplomacy, and Red Scares. For the stance he took on these various American excesses and outrages, he was rewarded with calumny and severe official penalties.[66] Perhaps as tragically, his eloquent if dour harangues about dollar diplomacy were drowned out by more entertaining propaganda from transnational corporations. The largest ones received PR assistance from journalists-turned-flacks, filmmakers, philanthropists, more than a few academics, and—most significantly—politicians and government officials.

Firestone Tire and Rubber Company enjoyed ample help from all these sources. Not long after his inauguration, when Franklin Roosevelt was preparing to end the U.S. occupation of Haiti, he could have withdrawn Washington's support for the demands of Firestone and of Liberia's other creditors—there was no way for Liberia to meet these demands, because its debt service was by then larger than its receipts, which were largely from its hut tax. Tied up with addressing the Great Depression, however, Roosevelt chose a different course of action. As Du Bois put it, he assented to "a dying gesture of the Hoover Administration," which included replacement of the African American ambassador with a major general who underlined fealty to U.S. commercial interests. "Liberia is not faultless," Du Bois concluded:

> She lacks training, experience and thrift. But her chief crime is to be black and poor in a rich, white world; and in precisely that portion of the world where color is ruthlessly exploited as a foundation for American and European wealth. The success of Liberia as a Negro republic would be a blow to the whole colonial slave labor system. Are we starting the United States Army toward Liberia to guarantee the Firestone Company's profits in a falling rubber market or smash another Haiti in the attempt?[67]

Historical oblivion—and reading W.E.B. Du Bois on Firestone was, I'm ashamed to say, a personal revelation—is one way that structural violence is cloaked, and why it's worth looking for accounts from those unlikely to have the chance to air their views or relate their experience.

That's why the first third of this book relies so heavily on the testimony of Ebola survivors, and why its historical chapters draw on the memoirs and correspondence of former slaves, recaptives, and black abolitionist ship captains, and on the works of dissident African American writers, radically revisionist historians from the colonizing nations, West African scholars, and the odd novelist or poet. Those best poised to teach us about fevers, feuds, and (soon) diamonds—those who endured, fought, or panned for them—left few memoirs or other testimony. Between world wars, however, a rich trove of detailed information about the social lives of those living in rural West Africa began to come from anthropologists. This wasn't the paltry detail offered in ships' logs, in detailed but dull reports from colonial administrators, or in the self-serving memoirs of European officials. Nor was this the experience-distant farrago of a previous generation of historians: ethnographers set out to detail the minutiae of everyday life.

Newly professionalized Africanist anthropology rapidly developed its own jargon, obsessions, and omissions. Its focus on specific "tribes"—a term variably describing groups of people speaking the same language and communities forged in the wake of displacement, assimilation, and Creolization—scanted class and gender differences. Anthropologists were often mute or muted on the savagery of colonialism and its role in shaping (and even creating) tribes, tribalism, and the discipline itself. The extractive trades, too, received scant attention from colonial-era ethnography. These were blind spots, since formal colonial rule had enabled European researchers' access to the rural reaches of Africa. Similarly, the growth of concessions like Firestone facilitated American ethnographers and other social scientists seeking to penetrate the Liberian interior. That didn't mean there wasn't much to learn from scholars with debts to powerful interests. Most had them.

For example, George Schwab's 1928 expedition was funded in part by Firestone. His *Tribes of the Liberian Hinterland* was published by Harvard's Peabody Museum (a good place to study, I later learned, if you could concentrate in close proximity to displays of masks, drums, and other diverse artifacts from West Africa). The distracting menagerie of human leopards, alligators, baboons, gorillas, and chimpanzees was discussed by Schwab, an American missionary and anthropologist. So was funerary ritual, rendered even more exotic and tribe-specific by the passive voice and matter-of-fact tone typical of the genre:

Formerly, only chiefs and big men were washed after they died. In Half-Grebo the corpse of a warrior who died from the effects of a

gunshot wound was taken to a stream and washed. In both Half-
Grebo and Sapā, the shot was extracted in order to prevent his being
reincarnated with a wound. Now, all the dead are washed. The corpse
is then laid on a mat and rolled up in it. With the corpse are put some
cloths, the number varying with the rank of the person. (Mano.)[68]

That gunshot wounds were still common enough to lead to special rituals,
which didn't include the attentions of a Werner Junge, suggests that rural Liberia remained a violent clinical desert in the years before much of Europe
was again reduced to one. But the question of how and why twentieth-century
"warriors," whether Mano or Grebo or whatever, died from gunshot wounds
received too little attention from the era's anthropologists.

If some early ethnographies were the work of amateurs distracted by day
jobs, not all of them were the fruit of passing expeditions led by armchair
anthropologists. Beginning in early 1934, a German anthropologist named Etta
Donner spent eighteen months in eastern Liberia, through which she hacked,
hiked, and trotted on horseback; she returned undaunted for a second stint a
couple of years later. An initiate of the Snake Society, naturally, Donner whacked
through dense bush, dressed wounds, and dosed her "boys" for dysentery and
other ailments. She breezily described the region's secret societies, but had a bit
less to say about the roots of Liberian conflict over land and labor, which
throughout her account threatens to explode in lethal raids. The patient reader
interested in the social lives of the Mano, Dan, Krahn, and Mandingo "peoples"
can, however, learn a great deal from Donner's *Hinterland Liberia*, a small-font,
three-hundred-page report illustrated by her own black-and-white plates.

Like most ethnographies of the era, Donner's book is replete with the usual
harvest of healing ceremonies, funerary ritual, and dietary preferences. En-
chanting pages are devoted to blood rituals, trance ceremonies, magic powders
and elixirs, fire medicines, trial by ordeal—beware the sasswood, as ever—and
to descriptions of masks, headdresses, amulets, fetishes, feather-magic, tattoos,
and scarification. Donner wasn't above prideful displays of arcane knowledge
as she explored witchcraft. ("I took a wicked delight," she wrote of one young
informant, "in being able to instruct Seweh in native magic.")[69] There's also

report (and photos) of distractions afforded by wrestlers, acrobats, and stilt walkers, and by dancing, drumming, gossiping, weaving cloth, plaiting hair, and, one is tempted to exclaim, much, much more.

Those disinclined to sift through voluminous ethnographic or historical studies, or to wander through tottering stacks of paperwork submitted to colonial bureaucracies, can turn to the works of Graham Greene.

Several of Greene's essays and novels, and at least one travelogue, reveal a familiarity with West Africa rare among colonial-era European writers. Some of it was acquired by trekking across the Kissi Triangle in the mid-thirties. *Journey Without Maps* never made bestseller lists, in part because the Liberian government threatened him with a libel action: prey to a childhood fascination with Africa, aware of secret societies, and uncharacteristically credulous in the presence of credible authorities, Greene alleged that cannibalism had not disappeared from the region.[70] The book was pulped after eighteen months on the shelves; the edition now in circulation was revised with lawsuits in mind. The Englishman nonetheless managed to serve up a damning assessment of Britain's civilizing mission.

Although Greene grew fond of Freetown, and would choose to return, he was struck mostly by the inadequacy and absurdity of empire. Sierra Leoneans were *British* subjects, so why hadn't its civilizing mission and the colony's mineral wealth led to anything remotely resembling British standards of living there? "This was an English capital city," Greene wrote of Freetown:

England had planted the town, the tin shacks and the Remembrance
Day posters, and had then withdrawn up the hillside to smart
bungalows, with wide windows and electric fans and perfect service.
Every call one paid on a white man cost ten shillings in taxi fares, for
the railway to Hill Station no longer ran.

In spite of a failure to maintain the train up to the hill station, investment in railways remained unquestioned in West Africa. The writer and his entourage reached the eaves of the forest on the same train as a district commissioner called to Pendembu "to investigate a Gorilla Society murder. A child had been carried off and killed, and a woman had sworn she had seen the gorilla and that he wore trousers."[71]

Britain's civilizing mission, Greene concluded crisply, "remained exploitation." Its Sierra Leonean discontents were subject to attacks from gorillas in trousers, leopards armed with Freddy Krueger knives, and a basket of deplorables including coerced labor, regular irruptions of famine and feud, and microbial plagues largely vanquished or unknown in Europe. Would the young writer find the citizens of independent Liberia any better off, or were they as sunk in superstition, poverty, and disease as British subjects next door? At the time of Greene's visit, Liberia was condemned in the court of world opinion for human trafficking and described as lacking little in terms of disease but almost everything in terms of health care and sanitation. Visitors from the powers that had taken over Liberia's finances and forests, draining them both of vital sap, offered a steady stream of commentary about its misfortunes— fever, feuds, misrule—and attributed them mostly to the people they visited.[72]

The received wisdom then had it that little was known of Liberia's interior.[73] Werner Junge claimed to be the first European to have traversed one stretch of forest between the trizone region and the coast near Cape Mount. But he reached northeast Liberia the same way Greene did—by train, via Pendembu—and had reason during the previously mentioned smallpox outbreak to pop over to French Guinea. There, we learn, Junge could pop the cork on a well-deserved bottle of champagne. The British may have preferred gin to champagne, but they also seemed to know a lot about the region, especially after discovering diamonds nearby. They were unearthed thanks to a geological survey costing only a few thousand pounds sterling. In 1932, a paltry 749 carats of diamond were found in Kono's riverbeds. By 1949, the yield reached 10,153,154 carats, including a stone decreed to be "the largest diamond ever to be recovered from any alluvial deposit."[74]

The source of all this portable wealth was a couple of glittering kimberlite pipes linking the bowels of the protectorate to the still lush world above. "Gaseous explosions probably blew through the jungle canopy as the pipes surfaced, showering diamonds and everything else for miles around like so much birdshot," explains the journalist Greg Campbell in *Blood Diamonds*:

> The kimberlites that blasted into what would eventually become Sierra Leone—two small chimneys that are about a billion years old and likely stood more than 1,500 feet above the plains—bore beautiful, innumerable diamonds. Millennia of erosion and lavish summer rains on the tropical forests that grip Africa from The Gambia to Somalia have hidden the diamonds under the region's red and yellow dirt like so many undiscovered Easter eggs.

The British find helped seal the fates of millions. "For most of its postslavery history, there was nothing remarkable about Sierra Leone, and Freetown likely lived up to its name," Campbell continues. "Those living there got along well with their neighbors and their British overseers. It wasn't until diamonds were discovered in the 1930s that Sierra Leone's course toward self-destruction was set."[75]

A history of Sierra Leone from below—the slave trade going on under the noses, or prows, of interdiction patrols; the raids and regional wars sparked by the project of moving young captives to Bunce Island and through the Door of No Return along the coast; the Scramble and the death of thousands who resisted British rule; the incineration of villages by gunboats and arson during the Hut Tax War; the punitive control-over-care policies of the sanitarians, including the attempted segregation of Freetown in order to protect Europeans from malaria and the failure of smallpox and rinderpest inoculation; forced labor regimes and widespread hunger, death, and epidemic disease when the empire was on war footing; wartime hoarding of rice and medicines by Syrian merchants; and the British export of influenza—suggests that Freetown never lived up to its name or to the majestic Cotton Tree surging skyward from its heart, a silent witness to long years during which Freetown failed to be truly free. But the hastening of the country's decline by the discovery of diamonds is heart-wrenching enough without quibbling over hyperbole.

Graham Greene may not have known all this, of course, but he knew a lot. He was, from the outset, doubtful about the imperial project, suspicious of British sanctimony about conditions in (and migrant labor from) Liberia, and curious about black self-rule in a world so hostile to it. Some of his insights were distilled from his skeptical reading of the U.K. Foreign Office's regularly published bulletins about the wide world, including Liberia. One of these Government Blue Books, issued just before Greene's trip, complained of the "absence of any attempt by the Government, not only to take effective steps to control yellow fever or plague, but even to arrange for the notification of yellow fever."[76] This was deliberate, according to one Liberian historian, who alleged that Monrovia "intentionally feigned attempts of cooperation with the West to develop sanitation measures in order to maintain an image of the nation as undesirable to white settlement."[77]

If true, it worked. But the pathogens did their bit, too. One major outbreak of yellow fever in 1929 killed an American diplomat from Minnesota and sickened many of Firestone's expatriate employees. Undiplomatic diplomatic demands for improved sanitary conditions in Monrovia and other towns with foreign residents only seemed to harden the views of Americo-Liberian officials, who kept up their stonewalling. They were doing a lot more than stonewalling unruly natives. The same Blue Book went on to describe the burning of forty-one villages—a feat that did not surpass British reprisals during the Hut Tax War, although this obvious resonance went unmentioned by the Foreign Office—and the murder of scores of civilians by the Liberian armed forces, whose methods differed little from those used by flame-throwing T. J. Alldridge.[78]

Such dire detail only deepened Greene's fascination and heightened his suspicions of imperial and racist propaganda. "The agony was piled on in the British Government Blue Book with a real effect of grandeur," he wrote. "The little injustices of Kenya became shoddy and suburban beside it."[79]

After disembarking from the train at its terminus in eastern Sierra Leone and avoiding human gorillas, Graham Greene and his cousin Barbara were off in search of the shabby, the shoddy, and the vivid. On this score, Liberia did not disappoint. They found the country to be dirt-poor, abundantly troubled by colonial cleavages (white-black, settler-native, civilized-savage, Christian-pagan, coast-forest), and beset with internecine conflict between tribes. Its authorities remained hostile to censorious white opinion and faced sharp tensions over their own land grabs, forced labor schemes, and taxes.

What struck Greene most immediately, however, was rural Liberian hospitality. "One was aware the whole time," he wrote, "of a standard of courtesy to which it was one's responsibility to conform." It's not as if Greene romanticized either the Liberians or their penury. He didn't care for some of the Americo-Liberians he met any more than Richard Strong did, and was dismayed by rampant poverty and disease. But he enjoyed his time in the remote hamlets strung between the trizone forest and the coast:

> However tired I became of the seven-hour trek through the untidy and unbeautiful forest, I never wearied of the villages in which I spent the night: the sense of a small courageous community barely existing above the desert of trees, hemmed in by a sun too fierce to work under and a darkness filled with evil spirits—love was an arm round the neck, a cramped embrace in the smoke, wealth a little pile of palm-nuts, old age sores and leprosy, religion a few stones in the centre of the village where the dead chiefs lay, a grove of trees where the rice-birds, like yellow and green canaries, built their nests, a man in a mask with the raffia skirts dancing at burials. This never varied, only their kindness to strangers, the extent of their poverty and the immediacy of their terrors.[80]

The immediacy of Greene's own terrors was attenuated by (more or less) twenty-six porters and hammock bearers, two personal attendants, and a full-time cook.[81] He and his cousin had ample reason to be grateful for the kindness of those who helped them cross 350 miles of rough terrain in the course of a month.

The posse of porters was recruited largely by the missionaries in Bolahun. There the cousins met a couple of Germans—including Werner Junge's successor, already looking a good deal less shamelessly healthy than on arrival. But Graham Greene was more interested in the health of the natives. As one American writer later observed, "There is no big game in Greene's Africa but there are predatory people—whites usually—and there is illness."[82] Lots and lots of illness. *Journey Without Maps* mentions the following diseases in the course of 242 terse pages: malaria, yellow fever, leprosy, and yaws, of course, but also plague, typhus, trichinosis, infectious jaundice (this was decades before the identification of its viral etiology), trench fever, foot-and-mouth disease, equine influenza, "rat-bite fever," bacillary dysentery, Guinea worm, tungiasis ("jiggers"), ringworm, river blindness due to onchocerciasis ("craw-craw"), and all manner of venereal diseases.

Great though Greene's medical lore may have been, it must have had a source. He can't have read Werner Junge's memoir or the report of the Harvard expedition, because they had yet to appear in print, but he did read *Rats, Lice and History*, by the bacteriologist and social-medicine guru Hans Zinsser, and he plowed through medical and public-health reports. Greene's sources about matters medical and otherworldly also included key informants—the term used by both anthropologists and spies, about whom he would later learn a great deal—who had long experience in Liberia. George Way Harley, an American missionary doctor who toiled not far from Liberia's border with French Guinea and the Ivory Coast, was one of these.

Dr. Harley sounds little like his energetic and wry German contemporaries, Junge and Donner, who wrote of similar experiences and understandings in a strikingly different tone. He was, Greene wrote, "a man with a body and nerves worn thread-bare by ten years' unselfish work, cutting away the pus from the huge swollen genitals, injecting for yaws, anointing from craw-craw, injecting two hundred natives a week for venereal disease."[83] After years in Ganta among Mano and Dan speakers, Harley more than dabbled in anthropology, collecting the sort of local lore about illness and injury for which ethnographers were already known. His writings about the snake cult—the one Donner joined—advanced the hypothesis that it served to diminish anxiety about snake bites and, through regular ingestion of tiny doses of venom, their lethality.

Enthralled with (and perhaps in thrall to) bush societies, George Harley acquired hundreds of ceremonial masks, selling many to Harvard's Peabody Museum to form a collection well known today among scholars and curators.[84] So, too, are his essays about the roles of these masks in initiation ceremonies, and the social functions of these sodalities across West Africa. Greene knew of the doctor's obsession before he met him:

> All the way along the Liberian border I had heard of him; he was
> the man in Liberia who knew most about the bush societies—the
> little time that the long hopeless fight against disease allowed him
> was devoted to these investigations. But he did not care to talk about
> them before his servants for fear of poison.

Each time Greene brought up bush societies, Harley "sheered away from them." The doctor had his reasons for sheering away from discussions of either Poro or poison. (His first years in Ganta had been marked by the death of one of his children, a four-year-old boy who downed a bottleful of quinine tablets by his febrile brother's bedside.) But on the Greenes' last night in Ganta, he relented, showing them his "grotesquely horrible collection of devils' masks."[85] Once unburdened of his reticence, Harley gave the Greene cousins an impromptu lecture.

Dr. Harley didn't share Richard Strong's view that the bush devils' tricks were for kids any more than he shared Donner's or Junge's dry wit. The masks were serious business, as were the bush schools. The stakes were high in the hinterlands. Legislation banning societies held by Liberian officials to practice cannibalism—they could say so, even if famous white visitors could not— had been passed just prior to the First World War. Up until the second one, bush societies were fiercely repressed.[86] Aware of such campaigns, Greene took pains to make comparisons that might make sense to a reading public in whose name the empire limped on: Etta Donner likened bush schools to freemasonry; Greene compared the rigors of initiation to hazing in elite English schools.[87]

Greene's cousin also wrote about secret societies in a memoir, but confessed to having dozed off as nerve-wracked George Harley unloaded his lore.

"The doctor told us many tales of the Leopard Societies, and the Alligator Societies, strange, dark, and horrible," Barbara Greene recalled. "With all honesty I confess I was incapable of understanding nearly everything that Dr. Harley said to us. Sleepiness, so overpowering that it became an agony, crowded into my brain."[88] Her 1938 *Land Benighted* is described (in the introduction to a recent edition) as "modest and a bit self-mocking."[89] Greene's modesty served her well, as did her curiosity. When after one disorienting hike she stumbled into a recently abandoned settlement, she asked the right questions: "Most of the houses had fallen almost into ruins, but a few were standing more or less complete. I wondered why it had been deserted. Had there been a fight, or had some horrid disease emptied this village of human life?"[90]

Who knows what might have emptied out the settlement? Conflict was everywhere, but so was epidemic disease. Even a great man like Harley lacked the staff, stuff, space, and systems to confront it: he had no laboratory; penicillin and other nontoxic antibiotics recently developed in Europe were largely unavailable in West Africa. His long tenure in Liberia had been further marked by the loss of countless fearful patients whose families and neighbors accounted for most deaths by invoking poison, violations of taboos, witchcraft, sorcery, or other incursions from the shadow world.[91] With the exception of a few medical missionaries like Harley and Junge—and a handful of German physicians, including Junge's successor in Bolahun and Firestone's Nazi enthusiast—the rural sick of Liberia were on their own unless their afflictions could be countered by spells, divination and propitiation, or herbal concoctions. The Greene cousins shared Epsom's salts with the natives but kept their quinine for themselves.

Across Liberia, serious illness, injury, snakebites, and obstructed labor ran their course. But just as Graham Greene's time in Sierra Leone didn't improve his initial impressions of British colonialism, neither did the republic's sorry state of health leaven his assessment of colonial medicine's control-without-care formula. "Even the poorer tribes beyond the Buzie country, the Gios and the Manos, with their loin-cloths and sores," he wrote, "were not more neglected than were the natives of a Protectorate under the care of a single sanitary inspector."[92]

If colonial rule in West Africa, including its Liberian variant, was a demographic and political failure, it was, for some few, a profitable and protracted one. As its neighbors disgorged minerals, diamonds, and ores, Liberia became America's largest supplier of latex.

The plantation expanding around Harbel allowed American automobile manufacturers to break Britain's rubber monopoly. But there were no cars or paved roads to speak of outside Monrovia, and Firestone's good fortune hadn't broken microbial monopolies over Liberian bodies. As another world war approached, so, too, did the antibiotic era. But not in Liberia.[93] Just as illness among its poor and vulnerable was often attributed to their own misdeeds or missteps, so, too, was sickness in the body politic attributed to local misrule. When the League of Nations report on its slavery scandal referred to cannibalism, however, it was to Firestone's insatiable appetite for able black labor and to creditors' unquenchable thirst for blood drained from a stone.[94] The report soon went down the oubliette, as did, with a helping hand from the Nazis, the League itself.[95]

Across the region, the intensification of extraction—of latex, timber, iron ore, bauxite, gold, diamonds, and labor—was once again stepped up to meet the demands of the war economy. In West Africa, only Liberia sought to remain officially neutral during the war, even after Pearl Harbor, since Germany was again its largest trading partner. But the United States kept a small standing force in Monrovia, sometimes (in Du Bois's phrase) starting the army toward the protection of expanding American interests. Now, with the Mediterranean closed to Allied ships by Axis forces, Franklin Roosevelt wanted Liberia to give the Germans the boot. Having been named Cape Mount's district health commissioner, poor Werner Junge was pushed out after being told he couldn't hire more than one German doctor at a time. They might be spies.

Dr. Junge would survive the war to write his book.[96] But his shamelessly healthy assistant in Bolahun, having returned abruptly to Germany in 1935, was to meet the fate of several naval medics: he went down with the *Bismarck*. Launched by Hitler himself, Europe's largest battleship was of course named after the man who hosted the meetings that created the borders of Liberia and much of the rest of the continent; only 110 of the 2,200 or so on board were rescued from the icy Atlantic. Far worse was yet to come during an Armageddon even more fully mechanized and industrialized than the previous one. As during the First World War, the colonies—and the waters off them and the skies above—were theaters of conflict throughout the Second.

In 1943, FDR became the first U.S. president to set foot in "Black Africa," when he traveled to Monrovia to secure Allied landing and docking rights in Liberia. The Americans had of course more or less enjoyed such rights for decades. By the time Roosevelt arrived, they were dredging the artificial harbor that would become Monrovia's freeport and had built—at the cost of $20 million in today's currency—the longest runway of any African airport so that B-47 bombers could land there. (It was sited close to Firestone's Harbel headquarters and, like Sierra Leone's international airfield, far from the capital city.) But with rain-drenched Liberia holding several world records as a clinical and public-health desert, the Americo-Liberians needed more than military assistance to bolster their shaky supremacy. If part of their plan to keep out foreigners was to leave public-health crises unaddressed, it had largely worked. But Liberia's new president-elect—the Convivial Cannibal from Harper himself—was a forward-looking fellow.

On January 31, 1943, William Tubman wrote to FDR to request support for a five-year plan to launch what would amount to Liberia's first healthcare system. Roosevelt gave the nod, instructing the State Department, Lend-Lease, and the War Department to "confer jointly on the ways and means of implementing the plan."[97] Some American generals expressed concern about establishing bases so far behind the front lines of the microbes' war on humans. When the U.S. health mission reached Monrovia in October, they "found no supplies or equipment available for starting our work." On the bright side, optimists from the Army Medical Corps underlined how much bang for the buck Liberia offered those willing to invest in basic public-health measures:

A rapid survey and casual observation by Colonel Fox in 1942 revealed that malaria was rampant, venereal disease played an important part in both morbidity and mortality, enteric diseases and helminthiasis were rife, and there was no general vaccination program, thus rendering the public susceptible to a smallpox outbreak. In addition, water supply and sewage disposal were individual and primitive. Flies, mosquitoes, and other vectors were abundant. All these findings could but lead to the conclusion that a public health program here would yield at least as much per dollar spent as could be expected in any part of the world.[98]

Sierra Leone could have used assistance launching a real health system, too. But even during the blitz and after humbling military setbacks across the empire—and after Lend-Lease—a haughty imperialist like Winston Churchill was unlikely to ask FDR for medical missions like the one dispatched to Liberia.

The two parted ways over old-school colonialism, as their shipboard tussle over the Atlantic Charter—a rough road map for decolonization drafted by FDR and signed reluctantly by Churchill—suggested. Besides, it wasn't the health of Sierra Leone's natives that most interested the U.K. War Office. It was mines and minerals, and, especially, diamonds. Nowadays, locals readily make the connection between diamonds and conflict, as does pretty much everyone who's studied Sierra Leone's recent civil war and its antecedents. But Graham Greene made the fever-feud-diamond connection in real time. During World War II he returned to Sierra Leone, Britain's most malarious possession, which was becoming one of its most diamondiferous, as a government employee, quite possibly a spy. Greene drafted *The Heart of the Matter* in Freetown's City Hotel, a fixture in the jumbled port city and just the sort of place he loved. Set in an unnamed West African British colony, the novel is about one man's losing struggle to keep to the code—Catholic, law-and-order, marital fidelity, generosity to the weak.

The Heart of the Matter stands as a primer of colonial life during war, introducing a cast of unmistakably Greene characters: Scobie, the tortured and devout police chief (doomed, of course); his hard-hearted nemesis (who also proves to be tortured); a young and shipwrecked waif, wounded enough to be a temptress in a Greene novel; a shrewish and chronically disappointed wife; shady but lovable Syrian merchants; soldiers and spies of war; the gossipy priest who delivers when it counts.[99] Some would later opine that the natives served largely as backdrop in this novel and others Greene set in Africa. But there's a lot to be learned from what they saw when they looked at the strange folk who lived among or in the hill stations above them. These folk included many drawn to diamonds, the fictional colony's chief obsession. Much police effort is wasted on pursuing rumors of their diversion to the Germans, since the Syrians had a new commodity to trade, smuggle, and hoard.

Decades later, we found a related cast of characters, and similar intrigue, in Kono District. We also found its Ebola survivors quick to make connections between their own low-yield mining and their losses to the disease.[100] But if during the Ebola epidemic many condemned the failure to invest mineral wealth in health and education, it's unlikely that Greene-era officials of the nonfictional variety voiced similar opinions: diamonds helped to fund the British war effort, especially after Lend-Lease made it unnecessary to spend time looking for gold, or to transport it on floating bull's-eyes like HMS *Mantua*. Local chiefs in Kono were unlikely to agree that diamonds were all bad, since that traffic restored some of their chiefly power—they were assigned the task of regulating concessions, distributing small-time licenses, and collecting fees and other tribute—if not their moral authority.

Neither did poor Sierra Leoneans complain. British efforts to regulate the trade there proved more difficult than in South Africa, since alluvial diamonds could be recovered by those equipped with little more than shovels and flat woven baskets called shake-shakes. The banks and beds of rivers that had yielded largely the sting of mosquitoes and tsetse flies, and once facilitated the removal of children and young adults to the Americas, now yielded a potential path out of poverty; the tiny village of Koidu became a rush town. If, on his first visit to Sierra Leone, Graham Greene had gotten off the train to Pendembu at the right longitude, he might have found a hamlet consisting of precisely six thatched dwellings a few days' hike to the north. During the war, and the years shortly after it, more than twenty thousand settled there.[101]

As the population of Kono and its capital exploded, explosive outbreaks of several afflictions mentioned to date—including smallpox, yellow fever, and sleeping sickness—were registered across the region. Malaria, typhoid, tuberculosis, and the same zoo of greedy parasites described by Werner Junge, the Greene cousins, and Team Harvard levied heavy taxes on the humans who converged first on Kono and then on Kenema, after another stream of diamonds was found to have trickled across that district. With new mineral wealth and assistance from their overlords, paramount chiefs might have organized vaccination campaigns against some of these pathogens and medical care for those afflicted by any of them. Like their overlords, however, the chiefs spent little time or treasure on public health or medical care.

Some native aristocrats picked up the nasty British habit of blaming epidemics on local superstition, a feat of analytic legerdemain in the diamond-rich east, since the locals had been submerged under a decidedly nonlocal influx. Koidu's residents now counted Mandingo and Fula traders from Guinea, *forestiers* galore, Syrian-to-Lebanese diamond dealers, and the odd British geologist pottering about with pickax and duster in hand (or, more likely, in his boy's hand). The Kono people for whom the district was named were few and far between, and rarely able to display intransigence, superstitions, or other local cultural wares.

Many previously mentioned fevers (and some local feuds) persisted or flared in West Africa during World War II. These epidemics have since gone down the memory hole, to the dismay, surely, of those who offered firsthand accounts of them—and to the grim satisfaction, perhaps, of those who later rescued such accounts from the dungeon of oblivion.

In the fall of 2014, at the height of Ebola's western surge and when experimental therapies like ZMapp were front-page news, the historian Guillaume Lachenal wrote about a zoonosis fatal to both man and beast:

It was the first time the disease appeared in Sierra Leone. It began to make the news in June. Dozens of British newspapers covered the story over the summer. The *Liverpool Post* started on June 7, announcing an "investigation" from a "Medical Research Council research worker who has gone to Sierra Leone to investigate an abnormal prevalence" of the disease. A month later, the first reports were received. "Research workers on their way to scene" read the *Liverpool Post* on July 7; the "outbreak" was located in the Sierra Leone hinterland and neighboring Guinea. In August, alarming news came from the eastern region of Sierra Leone: "Reports appear to indicate that the outbreak is assuming the proportion of an epidemic"; 500 cases, all of them potentially fatal, had been discovered during an extensive survey of only 9,500 persons. There were the usual journalists' approximations about African geography . . . There were the usual heroes, like the MRC researcher Dr. Lourie, who went onsite alone and set up the first "treatment centers" with very limited means. And there were the first signs of mobilization and hope. "It is anticipated," read the *Liverpool Daily Post*, "that the Sierra Leone government will organize measures to deal with the epidemic and that more doctors and trained staff will be available. Dispensaries are being set up in the districts worst affected, and it is hoped that the use of new drugs will conquer the epidemic."[102]

Lachenal wants the reader to believe, at least for a long paragraph, that he's writing about Ebola. But the June in question was June 1939. The epidemic was African sleeping sickness, which had already afflicted hundreds of thousands, if not millions, of French, Belgian, and British subjects by the outbreak of war.[103]

The new drugs in question in 1939 included pentamidine, one of the world's first effective antiparasitics since the "magic bullets" derived a couple of decades earlier from arsenic. Though effective against trypanosomiasis, these bullets had the unfortunate side effect of ricocheting into the eyes: many Africans treated with arsenicals went blind. The development of pentamidine by researchers in a London company with roots in France's first modern pharmaceutical concern—Rhône-Poulenc, which later begat Sanofi—offered new hope in the fight against the lethal affliction. It also led to some of the world's first major clinical trials, one of which took place in that small bit of real estate spanning eastern Liberia, Sierra Leone, and Guinea.[104] Because mass treatment of trypanosomiasis with arsenicals had failed prior to World War II, trizone health officials subjected mass prophylaxis with pentamidine to a trial without what they termed "subsidiary means"—meaning control of population movements, still a colonial favorite in spite of limited effectiveness against diseases transmitted by vectors with wings.

One account of this effort, and of the outbreak that prompted it, was published in the *Transactions of the Royal Society of Tropical Medicine and Hygiene* by R. D. Harding and M. P. Hutchinson, both of Sierra Leone's Yaws and Sleeping Sickness Service. Like Lachenal, they unfurl their outbreak narrative as a medical mystery. In 1942, in the region of Fuero—not far from Meliandou, where Ebola's spillover event was later held to occur, or the Liberian towns and villages in which Werner Junge battled smallpox, and about thirty miles north of the town in which Humarr Khan would meet his end—a British sanitarian reported an "atypical strain" of trypanosomiasis, alleged to cause a more fulminant and lethal course of the typically chronic disease. Blood smears revealed, he reported, a higher-grade parasitemia than previously noted in the region.

The reader of their article knows Harding and Hutchinson will turn, in seeking to explain this atypical disease course, to strain variation caused by genetic mutation—a default logic later to shape discussions of Ebola's wildly varying case-fatality rates and one closely related to that underpinning virgin-soil hypotheses. But any good outbreak narrative requires taking down alternative explanations, and the British doctors felt obliged to dismiss potential changes in the habits or habitats of the vector, as well as cross-border introduction from French Guinea. In seeking to make their case, a team from the Yaws and Sleeping Sickness Service went from village to village, drawing blood, aspirating lymph nodes, performing lumbar punctures, and collecting tsetse flies.

Regarding the vector, Harding and Hutchinson found "no striking seasonal changes in its overall density."[105] As proof of this claim there was the obvious metric of "flies per boy-hour," which today's incredulous reader should assume to mean precisely what it sounds like: How many bites would a boy endure along this or that river in the course of an hour? Along the Meli

River, we learn, "a figure of about six flies per boy-hour (FBH) has been obtained except in the heavy rains when the figure was lower."[106] It's not clear from British accounts if the boys were boys, since the term was still used to describe grown men, or if the poor wretches were forced to stand out in the rain, awaiting their insect tormentors at the behest of their white ones.

After the fly-boys exculpated the tsetse fly, the sanitarians dispensed with the notion of a novel strain of trypanosomiasis introduced from Guinea or Liberia. It's a curious dismissal, given human and fly disregard for these borders. Graham Greene had marveled at the former a few years earlier, when he saw the post delivered by mail-boys holding aloft cleft sticks into which even diplomatic correspondence was inserted.[107] Just over the watery border he and his cousin crossed by raft a few years earlier, sleeping sickness was alleged to affect a majority of those living in the Liberian patch of the trizone region. Neither did Harding and Hutchinson pay much attention to the other extenuating factors laid out concisely by the novelist. (The natives, Greene wrote, were "as worn out with fever as before the white man . . . introduced new diseases and weakened their resistance to the old.") Thus were the sanitarians able to conclude that "it seemed more probable that a spontaneous mutation had arisen in the strain itself."[108]

In the case of trypanosomiasis, invoking mutation as the cause of new disease patterns was entirely reasonable, given the parasite's famous ability to mutate in order to camouflage itself from host immune responses. But exclusive focus on the pathogen leads us astray. Social and economic factors, and the health of human hosts, also determine, then as now, the dimensions of an epidemic and clinical course among the afflicted. This is, of course, the crux of the virgin-soil debate, which called for the sort of analysis native to social medicine. The attribution of devastating New World epidemics solely to immunological naïveté was simplistic when this debate began centuries ago; attributing increased microbial virulence to novel mutations is contested even with full knowledge of a pathogen's genome. None had yet been sequenced at the time of World War II.

It wasn't even clear whether or not a novel strain of sleeping sickness had invaded the Fuero region. Reports of a higher-grade parasitemia and a more fulminant course suggests greater capacity to measure change than then existed. Enterprising field teams aside, there was little in the way of either surveillance or lab capacity in the trizone area in the years preceding the war or during it. The rural poor of the region had endured plenty of deadly epidemics without triggering much sympathetic attention from the authorities—concerned though they then were to protect livestock, the labor force required by the extractive trades, and city folk, especially white ones. The fly-boys, not so much: at least one of them was featured in a subsequent issue of *Transactions of the Royal Society of Tropical Medicine and Hygiene* after he was sickened during his tour of duty as a mineshaft canary.

The story of epidemic trypanosomiasis at the dawn of the antibiotic era points, Guillaume Lachenal concludes, "to the simple fact that the global health infrastructure now at work in the region has a long history: a history of treatment centers, of catastrophic mortality and saved lives, of people seeking or fleeing medical teams, and of medical heroes and foreign journalists, which started long before the summer of 2014."[109] His exercise suggests we're doomed to repeat at least some errors responding to epidemics because we can't seem to remember what happened before. The "we" here aren't the afflicted; those of us spared such horrors don't have to recall much about them. But a look at bubonic plague in Senegal suggests (to invoke another Haitian proverb) that while he who strikes the blow forgets, he who bears the scar remembers.

Plague caused by *Yersinia pestis* showed up in Senegal's towns and cities at about the same time the Pasteurians did, and likely via the same lousy and rat-infested means of transportation. A few decades later, the advent of new classes of antibiotics spelled another chance to break the bonds of the control-over-care paradigm: just before pentamidine came penicillin and the miraculous sulfa drugs, and shortly thereafter, streptomycin. Although plague could be cured by more than one of the new miracle drugs, French sanitarians continued to rely on a playbook that still featured—at least for the natives—quarantine, isolation, and other intrusive or draconian measures, including the destruction of infested houses and the banning of funerals and wakes. The historian Myron Echenberg reminds us why such measures were unlikely to prove a panacea for plague:

> Isolation of index cases, suspects, and so-called "healthy carriers" remained an important control measure in smallpox and typhoid epidemics, when disease could spread directly from person to person. Quarantine was ineffective, however, for diseases like bubonic plague. While it isolated some humans thought to be infective from others, it had little or no effect on the main vehicle of infection, the biting insect.

If martial measures were unbuttressed by evidence of effectiveness in slowing the diverse epidemics to which they were indiscriminately applied, they reliably deepened mistrust of the colonial medical service.

The control-over-care tactics of the Pasteurians left indelible social residue. Interviews with elderly men some forty years after Senegal's last outbreaks revealed many to have vivid memories of plague-control efforts of French authorities. What these men didn't recall were efforts to provide care for the afflicted, even after American military medics showed up with both pesticides and antibiotics. "Armed with DDT and sulfa drugs," writes Echenberg, "American medics were prepared to entirely transform plague control and therapy, providing they could overcome the bureaucratic and political obstacles placed in their way."[110] They could not. Prevention had finally worked, thanks to DDT, but the case-fatality rate of plague was as high in Senegal's last outbreaks as it was in its first documented ones.

Neither were American medics able (or their superiors willing) to help Liberian authorities link disease control to care. U.S. support for President Tubman's health plan came to an end just as it was beginning to yield results—at least as measured by disease-control enthusiasts anxious to protect American troops stationed there. The State Department canceled the medical mission to Liberia not long after the war, citing a lack of funds. (This must have sounded like satire in Monrovia and theater of the absurd in the hinterlands.) The mission's leaders hadn't much concerned themselves with training health professionals, even though the army medic leading it reported only six doctors practicing in a country the size of Virginia. A Liberian returning from medical training in the States counted, just after war's end, a dozen physicians practicing there. Not one of them was Liberian.[111]

One assumes that Firestone's Nazi doctor had been let go during these interesting years. But it's too bad Werner Junge was.

By most lights, the end of World War II marked the end of African accommodation of formal colonial rule. The rulers of war-depleted empires continued to resist calls for independence. They weren't often moved by their West African subjects' demands for health care and education, but rising political activists in Africa promised bright futures for their countries as independent nations.

Aspirations ran high in Guinea, which in 1958 irritated prickly France by declaring independence before being invited to do so. Its first president, Ahmed Sékou Touré, claimed to be a direct descendant of Samory himself. He settled in for the long haul in spite (and because) of withdrawal of French support for an orderly transfer of power. Touré turned to other potential allies by looking to France's foes. Although the United Nations cheerfully declared 1960 to be "The Year of Africa," the rollout of independence in West Africa occurred in the context of deeply conflicted global trade and a new kind of global conflict. The Cold War delayed the dismantling of colonial institutions—and the decolonization of at least some hearts and minds—as weak states were called to align themselves with one superpower or the other. If President Touré couldn't point to a single university after a century and a half of French control, small wonder he looked for help from the Soviet Union.

For African leaders on the development bandwagon, alignment with a superpower patron held the promise of access to resources and know-how that might replace those stripped or undeveloped during colonial rule. Unsurprisingly, the weaker and more plundered the new nation, the less independent its independence. The vast Congo, suddenly Zaire, was bereft of higher education, so who could blame its bumbling new elites, Patrice Lumumba aside, for seeking ties with American cold warriors? (The Congo played a part in launching the Cold War, having supplied the fissile materials that ripped apart Hiroshima and Nagasaki.) As for taking sides, the Americo-Liberians had made their choice in a previous century. Sierra Leone may have had an easier transition than Guinea or the Congo, but the notion that its independence was a tidy and peaceful affair doesn't stand close scrutiny much more than does the claim that Freetown lived up to its name prior to the discovery of the diamonds that later fueled its civil war.

As the British in Sierra Leone planned a gradual hand-off in the decade prior to the actual event, they continued to exclude—with the collusion of many chiefs and Creole elites—the poor majority. Long-simmering resentments eventually boiled over in a Freetown workers' strike, the formation of a pro-poor political movement in Kono District, and what Ismail Rashid terms the "peasant war of 1955–56," which had as its theater the northwest chiefdoms around the Scarcies River. Port Loko, Maforki, and Bantoro were, once again, in the middle of the action:

> While the workers' strike had erupted over pay and conditions of
> service in Freetown, the peasant insurrection was directed against
> the excessive colonial taxation and the pecuniary demands of
> paramount chiefs in Port Loko, Kambia, Tonko Limba and Bombali
> districts. By the time the dust settled in early 1956, the insurrection
> had led to the death of over a hundred people and the deposition of a
> dozen chieftains.[112]

A decade after independence, and Fourah Bay College aside, Sierra Leone had not channeled taxes or mineral wealth toward meeting demands for social services long deemed basic within industrialized democracies—as the former colonial powers were suddenly and unironically termed. Increasingly, similar demands were made (and sometimes met) across broad swaths of Latin America and Asia, providing the counterpoint for those advocating narrowly measured economic growth as the one true measure of development and modernity. GDP growth became the lodestar of pretty much every newly independent West African nation, and of Liberia, whose Open Door Policy made it tantamount to a state religion.

I've claimed in this book that epidemic disease rarely collided with modern medicine within Upper West Africa, in spite of superpower promises of development assistance to attain whatever happened to be defined at any given moment as modernity. This general rule held true during the Cold War, a feud during which the body count was high only in former colonies. Until the advent of cell phones, collisions with material modernity in Upper West Africa were more likely to consist of encounters with the machinery of mechanized extraction of mineral wealth—or with automatic weapons and rocket-propelled grenades—than with X-ray or surgical suites, or modern laboratories.

The identity crises of postcolonial West African elites after a century of retrograde and racist notions of modernity—laid out in French fatwas flowing from Conakry, Abidjan, and Dakar, as well as British diktats issued from Freetown, Lagos, and Accra—had their tightest hold on those who sought to supplant European rulers. Imperious instruction didn't stop after independence, but the high formalism of the postcolony took on Cold War coloring. Guinea's politicians and bureaucrats, explains an anthropologist with long experience in the forest districts, "mobilized a third cosmopolitan form that partially resolved the contradictions within and between traditional Marxism and Pan-Africanism," further irritating their former masters.[113] If imitation is a form of flattery, however, President Touré's adoption of socialism as the path to modernity didn't preclude pursuit of certain French ambitions. Embarrassed by the same cultural practices and social institutions that had vexed colonial authorities, he launched a series of "iconoclastic sweeps aimed at eradicating religious 'fetishism' and social 'mystification.'"[114]

Touré's anti-mystification campaign recalled not only the goals of heavy-handed colonial campaigns but also their methods. The sweeps destroyed masks and other ritual objects while calling for social and religious conversion—meaning choosing a monotheistic religion and sticking with it. Needless to say, the effort had unintended consequences, many of them registered in Macenta, Guéckédou, and other so-called forest regions already known for *réticence* about policies imposed from Conakry. Guinea's commercial concessions also had unintended consequences. Given its insertion into a socialist network, it might seem plausible to assume its mineral wealth would be traded largely with the Second World. But Guinea's tiny political and merchant class sold its wares not only to China and the Soviet Union but also to customers from officially vindictive France and to high bidders from all over.

Sékou Touré's pragmatism, rather than his Africanized Marxism, was one reason Guinea's neighbors sped up their own races to the bottom. Lowball bidders got bargains after Liberia's leader, a veteran of the League of Nations scandal, adopted less obviously exploitative labor practices to staff its concessions. Firestone remained the largest of these, but President Tubman had other partners besides the tire and rubber company. His Open Door Policy encouraged direct foreign investment by companies trading in iron ore, timber, and other treasures under the earth or on top of it. The intended consequences of this way of doing business included great private profit. Between 1952 and 1957, according to some estimates, the Liberian economy—as myopically measured by growth in GDP per capita—grew faster than the economy of any country other than Japan. The unintended consequences of many Americo-Liberian business deals included a rising tide of complaint from citizens largely deprived, after 120 years of alleged independence, of health care and higher education.

One of Liberia's few postsecondary schools, Cuttington University, was founded by American missionaries in the nineteenth century. In 1952, it boasted a graduating class of five; few other institutions of higher learning were much bigger. The restless young men of the Liberian hinterlands, excluded from even secondary education and from political participation, hadn't forgotten the martial past. Nor did they fail to chafe over long-standing local resentments. As more of them were willing to work as day laborers, the "resulting transfer of labor from the subsistence sector to the concessions tended to undermine the traditional social mechanisms of rural areas, where male elders exercised authority through their monopoly control of land, trade, and women."[115] A turn from rigid, age-based, and gendered hierarchies toward an uncertain future of migrant or poorly salaried manual labor set the stage for violence once Liberia was awash in modern weapons and aspiring warlords.

Independent Sierra Leone followed a different path to the same violent end. Its new prime minister, Milton Margai, was the first medical graduate from "upline," the new word for the hinterland after the railroads opened for business. (He attended medical school in Britain, since there wasn't one in its colony.) Like many other young professionals in short supply, Margai was drawn into politics. In the eyes of the British, whose queen knighted him before her own state visit, Sir Milton led a proper transition from colony to statehood. But he had many rivals, including a former police officer named Siaka Stevens.[116] Elected in 1967, and overthrown and reinstalled by the army in the course of a single tumultuous year, Stevens was the fellow who named Freetown's Cotton Tree a national icon. He was considerably less sentimental when it came to political opposition: Pademba Road Prison was filled in no time and kept full to bursting after Stevens formally declared Sierra Leone a one-party state—his—in 1978.

By that time, the majority of the country's diamond and mineral revenues—meaning the majority of all public revenues—were enriching those who dodged taxes or lived elsewhere. Opposition to kleptocracy in the diamond districts included a new political movement among what was left of the Kono people, who fought to invest diamond wealth in health care, education, sanitation, and roads within the rich-poor district. The Kono Progressive Movement, one of the first of its sort anywhere in rural Africa, was derided by politicians in Freetown. Its Robin Hoods, accused of banditry, were persecuted. Then they, too, disbanded.[117]

The collection of more standardized data about health and well-being within the boundaries of newly sovereign nations brought into relief the generally miserable conditions—and short lives—endured by citizens of Sierra Leone and Guinea during the second half of the twentieth century. As far as health indicators went, these countries were, along with Liberia, down near the bottom of the world's barrel.

This was true even when brisk sales of diamonds, minerals, rubber, timber, and other commodities meant that all three countries regularly posted high rates of economic growth as conventionally measured. Returns on this traffic were seldom invested in promised upgrades to colonial health systems, and rarely met local aspirations when they were. Health ministries in Upper West Africa continued to receive slim pickings after independence, with most of their tiny budgets going to pay personnel in urban areas. Not that there were many to pay: colonial authorities, their general views on black doctors plenty clear, hadn't bothered much with medical or nursing education in West Africa. Some few of the region's best and brightest were offered scholarships to study in Europe, North America, and the Soviet Union. They weren't always keen to return to the clinical desert, even if the cities of northern Russian held little appeal when buried under six feet of snow.

Those whose itineraries were limited to West Africa remained bent under the weight of infectious pathogens. "Older diseases such as malaria, trypanosomiasis, schistosomiasis (bilharzia), and onchocerciasis (river blindness) remained potent challenges at the time of independence," explains the historian Emmanuel Akyeampong. "Diseases such as tuberculosis, described by health officials as a relatively minor threat in the earlier colonial years and often restricted to coastal towns, had begun to grow in prominence in the colonial era, with the rise of underground mining and increased overcrowding in towns."[118] There were also newly identified pathogens to worry about: Lassa fever was first described in 1969 after it took the life of a missionary nurse in Nigeria. Spread by a species of rat common across West Africa, the causative virus leaps, like Ebola, from human to human within medical facilities (and households) with weak infection control. Humarr Khan's predecessor—who died of Lassa after a needle stick sustained while caring for a pregnant patient—revealed the region around Kenema to be an epicenter of both rat-to-human transmission and human-to-human spread.[119]

In addition to newly recognized causes for anxiety, old ones beyond tuberculosis resurged. The great seventh pandemic of cholera, which began its world tour in Indonesia in 1961, reached Conakry in August 1970. Guineans studying in Soviet cities had taken a brief Black Sea break as cholera was passing through once-Russian and again-Russian Crimea. As soon as they returned, by one account, this horseman of the apocalypse galloped off:

> On August 18, Guinea reported a significant number of suspected cholera cases to the WHO. When the WHO confirmed these as cholera, Guinea refused to make the announcement official, and when the WHO unilaterally announced cholera's presence in the country on September 4, 1970, Guinea resigned from the WHO in a huff. That first epidemic resulted in at least 2,000 cases and 60 deaths.

The author of this account calls Conakry "the capital of the remote and re-clusive West African Republic of Guinea."[120] But Guinea was more politically iconoclastic than remote, as its trade receipts and cholera's spread revealed. Within six months, all of West Africa knew cholera's sting. During the next two decades—phase one of the seventh pandemic's African tour—close to half a million cases were reported in regions connected to the Upper Guinea Coast in long-standing ways.

Trypanosomiasis followed similarly well-worn routes, reemerging during these years as a major threat across West Africa and buttressing false narratives about the collapse of once-sturdy health systems established under colonial rule. There was, however, some good news from the region: small-pox was in sharp decline. Even at the height of the Cold War, the leaders of a fractured world could agree that the disease—with no nonhuman reservoir and prevented by an effective, safe vaccine—had to go. As eradication became a likely outcome of a massive and targeted campaign, significant outbreaks of the once global scourge were seen mostly in rural African villages. In both 1967 and 1968, Sierra Leone had the world's highest incidence of smallpox among countries reporting cases to the World Health Organization.[121]

As with social responses to the Ebola control-over-care paradigm, so, too, with smallpox. The biggest difference in officialdom's replies to the two plagues was of course the existence of a highly effective smallpox vaccine. It was deployed rapidly during the course of sporadic outbreaks by offering vaccine to all known contacts and, for good measure, within the households ringing afflicted ones. This was called "ring vaccination." Although the case-fatality rate of smallpox varied, and—as Werner Junge had noted from rural Liberia—much could be done to ease the suffering and save the lives of the afflicted, the approach to smallpox within laggard countries remained classic control-over-care: quarantine, isolation, ring vaccination, and the walling off of affected villages, which were sometimes razed along with the inhabitants' meager possessions. Since person-to-person spread is the rule with both smallpox and Ebola, many such measures made sense in responding to them. But that doesn't mean sanitarian SWAT teams were welcomed warmly in the absence of medical care, social assistance for the afflicted and quarantined, and personal protective gear for those bound to care for them.

Across Upper West Africa, both nursing of the sick and last rites remained largely in the hands of families and traditional healers. Unsurprisingly, most of them resisted authoritarian moves to ban caregiving, and quarantines and travel bans weren't welcomed by anyone obliged to scout for food and water without ring-fenced hamlets. Smallpox brigades were greeted with deep distrust by the children and grandchildren of those who had openly resisted colonial-era sanitarians, some of them surely future grandparents of those who would later flee, or attack, twenty-first-century sanitarians seeking to contain Ebola. But old is the new new whenever history goes down the drain. Writing of Ebola, journalists reported in 2014 that quarantine and *cordons sanitaires* were "a disease-fighting tactic not used in nearly a century." Anthropologists familiar with the region countered that "governments that have long been experienced as deeply detached from their publics, and perceived not to act in their interests, are now the enforcers of biomedicine at its most authoritarian."[122]

The control-over-care paradigm—its lineage readily traced to colonial Pasteurians—was really *public health*, not biomedicine, at its most authoritarian. By the 1960s, sanitarians responsible for smallpox eradication were mostly epidemiologists and other species or strains of public-health specialists, some the bearers of underutilized medical degrees. Few of them were

African. But regardless of pedigree, the global-health experts of the Cold War era complained about the West African villagers offering stiff resistance to their tender ministrations. Smallpox sanitarians paid less attention to structural barriers to the villagers' embrace of modernity. Among these barriers was an embryonic health-care system (reviews of Sierra Leone's national budgets at the time revealed health-related expenditures to be among its lowest priorities, with rural regions last in line), and a lack of professional and financial assistance with burying the dead—to say nothing of insurance or amenities like electricity, roads, and running water.[123] In the absence of a safety net, villagers were of course forced to rely on their own social institutions.

That's one reason the causes of resistance to disease-control efforts were again deemed by these international experts to be less material and structural than local and cultural and cognitive, with superstition and membership in secret societies at the top of the list. Since control-over-care tactics ultimately proved successful in the fight against smallpox, only medical historians and West Africans of a certain age dwell on these details. But they reveal striking similarities between the epidemiology of—and social responses to—Sierra Leone's last smallpox outbreaks and its first documented ones of Ebola. In 1968, two smallpox outbreaks occurred in Kailahun District. Patient Zero in one smallpox flare-up was a forty-year-old trader from a village there. She was, we read in the *American Journal of Epidemiology*, "the local head of a secret society, and she received several visitors during her illness." The term "superspreader" hadn't yet come into vogue, but that was the idea: according to the article, "Villagers reported that 243 persons attended her funeral."

The man cited as the index case in the second smallpox outbreak was tarred by the *American Journal of Epidemiology* authors in a similar fashion. He was a farmer, like most men in the village of Naiaguehun, population 114. He was cared for by his two wives, as might be hoped in the case of sick men fortunate enough to have two wives. When he died, "almost the entire adult population" of the village attended his funeral, as might be hoped in a small, close-knit community. "Apparently," the authors add without revealing the source of their insight, the stricken man "was an important secret society official, although villagers denied it."[124] Why villagers in the trizone area would deny such affiliations upon being interrogated by rapid-response teams— who swooped in to conquer, confirm, count, isolate, and vaccinate, and soon departed to report and publish—was unexplored.

Expatriate smallpox controllers were likely as knowledgeable about officialdom's various campaigns against secret societies as I was in 2014. But since both smallpox and Ebola may be thought of as diseases of caregivers, with smallpox transmitted predominantly via respiratory secretions to those within a few feet of the afflicted, associations with nursing and last rites are unsurprising. In Europe, several of the previous decade's handful of smallpox cases had been registered within hospitals with inadequate infection control; in decades before that, funeral-associated transmission was known to occur there, too. In eastern Sierra Leone (in 1968 as in 2014) there were no modern hospitals or funeral homes to speak of. Family and friends who provided care or paid last respects, whether in secret or not, were of course those most likely to fall ill. Sentiments such as grief, sorrow, and neighborly sympathy also receive short shrift in epidemiology journals. But as regards "cultural factors," everyone was an expert, it would seem.

After noting the deceased farmer from Naiaguehun likely belonged to the Poro society, the smallpox-experts-cum-anthropologists added that its sway reached "over large contiguous areas of Guinea, Liberia, and Ivory Coast, as well as Sierra Leone." They then arrived at a memorable conclusion:

> The involvement of secret societies in funeral ceremonies is
> significant insofar as societies increase the likelihood of a prolonged,
> widely attended funeral, or otherwise increase the opportunities for
> smallpox transmission by rites peculiar to the societies. The role
> of secret societies in such funerals is also important because secret
> societies are ubiquitous in West Africa.[125]

Thus did the peculiarities of bush societies, and the diviners and healers tasked with explaining and addressing misfortune, come to be thought of as superspreaders—a pattern established during the colonial era and to recur during the Ebola years.

Old is the new new.

In the latter third of the twentieth century, close observers, some of them real anthropologists, remained convinced that many in West Africa feared assault from malefactors who drew power from the unseen world with the help of ritual cannibalism. Yes, it was still a thing.

If such accusations had been given a boost by civilizing missions claiming to uproot slavery, serfdom, cannibalism, and other pagan practices—like speaking one's mother tongue, clinging to caregiving and its final act, propitiating ancestors, and sharing land communally—the slow dissolution of colonial institutions didn't lead to a decline in magical thinking among national elites. As colonial voodoo was replaced by its neoliberal variant, an uptick in accusations of ritual murder was registered among and against those most tightly enmeshed in cosmopolitan trade networks, and in the political networks enmeshed in those. What fraction of an emerging postcolonial elite believed in power conferred by the consumption of another's vital parts is unclear. What is clear is that rumors of ritual murder proliferated as the intensity of the struggle to simply get by once again deepened.

Global markets for African exports, the same commodities extracted during the colonial era, collapsed in the sixties, followed by an oil crisis and a worldwide recession beginning in the next decade. This occurred as West Africa, having survived three waves of depopulation—the first swelled by the slave trades, the second by violence sparked by European occupation, and the third by coerced participation in World War I—began to register record rates of population growth. The success of the extractive trades, as gauged by loudly trumpeted growth in GDP per capita and conspicuous enrichment of authorities with a hand in the public cookie jar, had already been harnessed to widespread impressions of more being spread among fewer and less being spread among more. Now, as banks crashed and debt rose, rich-world leaders and postwar international financial institutions—like the World Bank and the International Monetary Fund—began banging the drum of austerity. To mix metaphors, a heaping helping of the neoliberal juju of millennial capitalism was followed by a dessert course of accusations against those seen to benefit from it.[126]

Many descendants of Liberia's American settlers fell squarely in this class of beneficiaries. A century and a half after the founding of Maryland County, in the decade before things fell apart, allegations of assaults along darkened roads resounded as the struggle for earthly power intensified in and around its capital. Now hemmed in by the invading green of weeds and vines, trees erupting within burned-out and abandoned buildings, Harper looked much different before 1989, when insurgents led by Charles Taylor invaded from across the nearby border with the Ivory Coast. A *New York Times* article about a spate of ritual killings describes the county as it appeared just before the war: "Today, with its red dirt roads, old country churches, Masonic lodges, antebellum-style plantation houses and familiar place names—Rock Town, Fish Town, Barclayville—Maryland County seems like part of the rural American South lost in Africa."[127]

Shortly after Ebola's western surge, colleagues of mine from Partners In Health reopened Harper's decrepit public hospital and completed construction of a nearby health center. We also worked with nursing students at Tubman University, just outside of town, and renovated its small clinic. The bucolic campus is smothered in hues of bright green by the light of day. But one (at least this one) can imagine it smothered in fear at night, the dark deepened by the encircling forest. Parts of it are dominated by crowded stands of rubber trees strangely angled skyward, and blacker than the night above when the moon is more than a quarter full. They're hung with buckets, into which drips sticky white latex, luminescent above an even blacker forest floor: for a New Englander, a tropical-nightmare negative of spile-studded maples leaking fragrant sap into pails offset by a carpet of fresh-fallen snow.

Tubman University was of course named after Harper's leading son. The forebears of William Vacanarat Shadrach Tubman were themselves named after a Georgia plantation owner, who, on his deathbed, called for the release of his slaves on the condition they emigrate to Liberia. Several took his widow up on the offer, and boarded an American Colonization Society ship that reached Cape Palmas in 1837. Many of their descendants flourished there. Having cut his teeth as a lawyer for Firestone, Tubman rose rapidly to prominence in the True Whig Party, becoming Liberia's youngest-ever senator. (He resigned in order to represent its government during the black slavery scandal.) Like FDR, Tubman would win four consecutive presidential elections. He accomplished this mostly through clientelism and by dabbling in the occult.

William Tubman hadn't called himself the Convivial Cannibal from the Downcast Hinterlands as a campaign stunt. Cultivating a reputation as a living link between affluent Americo-Liberians and the excluded majority within Liberia's modern borders, the urbane and grandiloquent lawyer assumed the ceremonial title of Supreme Zo of the Poro society. (When visiting the hinterlands, observed an unnamed writer in a 1947 edition of *The New Yorker*, Tubman "takes a witch doctor with him, just in case.")[128] Covering his bases, the president was also Grand Master of Liberia's Masonic Order, erecting a massive lodge just across the street from his Harper mansion. The formula worked for him: Tubman died in 1971, shortly after a surgical procedure in London, rather than, as was soon to be common among Liberian statesmen, at the hand of his rivals.

President Tubman's sudden disappearance led to years of intense competition for control of the True Whig Party and thus the ship of state—if that's the right metaphor for a country becoming famous for promiscuous bestowal of flags of convenience on variably seaworthy vessels from all over. William Tolbert, who'd served as vice president for twenty years, assumed the presidency. A Baptist minister with a hand in the till, he sought to remain in the post by being elected outright. He needed such legitimation in a time when African leaders' every move was viewed through a Cold War prism. Tolbert was already suspect in the eyes of his country's primary patron. He'd renegotiated the Firestone contract along lines not to the company's liking, insisted Liberia chart a neutral course in the Cold War, and railed against the neocolonialism from which he and his had profited handsomely.

There was really only one neocolonial power in Liberia, and none of

Tolbert's posturing pleased Washington. But its druthers and displeasure were fickle things that changed, or didn't, with each new administration. The issues of the seventies weren't those of FDR's day. Sure, Liberia's port and ship registry were still managed by Americans who expected fealty from their wards, and the same was true of Firestone. But it's not as if one source of rubber among many, or the cargo of the world's rustbuckets, remained ranking concerns in the State Department. It was Tolbert's establishment of stronger ties with the Soviet Union and China, and his sermons against neocolonialism, that were viewed as high treason by America's cold warriors. These had been sprinkled in both major political parties since the beginning of the Cold War, and their ideas remained influential as it neared its finale. (During the late seventies, the civics course required in my small-town Florida high school was called AVC, short for "Americanism Versus Communism.")

The cold warriors and their proxies were often in and out of the U.S. embassy in Monrovia, just then the largest one, surprisingly, in all of Africa. That's why many politically savvy Liberians thought Tolbert, long overshadowed by Tubman, likely to lose the 1975 election. When he didn't, some within the ruling clique predicted a rapid end to Tolbert's administration, and to Tolbert. But Jimmy Carter's election the next year upset Americo-Liberian political calculations. If the White House was going to tolerate Tolbert, they'd better get and stay on his good side. The biggest obstacle was that there weren't enough seats at the True Whig high table, even though the resentful majority had never been seated.

What happened next was drawn from an old and well-thumbed playbook, but it shook up the Maryland aristocracy and reminded Liberia-watchers what all Liberians knew: the country sat on a major social fault line, and even recent arrivals could see it yawning. Fred van der Kraaij, a Dutch diplomat and aid official, was living in Harper while conducting research on Tubman's economic policies. During the summer of 1977, he felt "as if an earthquake struck the country."[129] The temblor was triggered by the June 26 kidnapping of Moses Tweh, a fisherman and singer from Grand Cess, up the coast toward Monrovia. As van der Kraaij tells it:

His mutilated body was found a week later, on July 3, near the "Devil Rock" in Harper. Missing from Tweh's body were his eyes, ears, nose, armpits, testicles and tongue, among other parts. Police investigation revealed that the arrested persons admitted of being involved in the murder of Moses Tweh and that they divided certain parts of the body among themselves for "juju" purposes in order to obtain higher positions in the government.[130]

As in previous decades, such murders were said to be the work of a group of "heartmen" after body parts. But what the Harper heartmen were really after was personal and political gain. Those with privilege had sought more of it by opening a supernatural front in the war for secular power.

The quake's aftershocks spread along the fault line, away from the epicenter. This was to be found not in the bush or its sacred groves, but in the county's and the nation's administrative and commercial districts. In gatekeeper states like Liberia, control of scarce or unjustly hoarded resources was conferred through public office, and Moses Tweh had been abducted in a vehicle with government plates. Subsequent legal proceedings unfurled like a suspense novel set in the hometown of the Convivial Cannibal, with the suspense more about what would happen to the accused than about whodunnit. It didn't take long for someone to sing the names of the alleged human leopards.

The list of those arrested read like a Who's Who of Maryland County, the home or vacation resort of many Liberian grandees during Tubman's long reign. Among those charged with murder were the recently sacked county superintendent (the most important post at the county level); the son of a former vice president then serving in the House of Representatives (and a Tubman cousin); the Kru governor; the chief representing residents of Grand Cess living in Maryland; the assistant supervisor of schools (bearer of a master's degree in education from Howard University); the senior inspector of the Ministry of Commerce; and the chief security officer of the Liberia Sugar Company. Tweh's dismemberment required the skills of a seasoned butcher, which is why a cook rounded out the list of the twelve accused. The crime's mastermind was alleged to be the fired superintendent, none other than the son of the chairman of the True Whig Party.

In the struggle between the Tubman and Tolbert camps, the accused—who included a few who'd predicted the U.S. government would block Tolbert's ascent—were alleged to be trying to work their way from the former to the latter, by any means necessary. Several confessed, under the enhanced interrogation techniques of the Harper police, to quite specific political ambitions. In an effort to save their skins, other detainees enumerated these strivings in detail. A sampling: Maryland County's assistant supervisor of schools was required to pass a "traditional juju ordeal" in order to be promoted to supervisor; the superintendent recently fired by Tolbert wanted to be named an ambassador; the congressman wished to trade a seat in the House of Representatives for one in the Senate. And so on.

The Harper trial made international headlines, if usually filed under miscellany or African exotica. Free to print what they wished as long as they didn't question the Americo-Liberian supremacy, the Liberian tabloids had a heyday, although even their editorial standards were taxed by the lurid details uncovered during legal proceedings. Font sizes only got larger with developments. On October 28, 1977, the single-word headline "Guilty!" ran over a photo of the defendants in a lineup. (One of them was stripped down to his briefs.) All but one appealed to the Supreme Court, whose justices ruled that a mistrial had indeed occurred in Maryland County, many of the confessions having been obtained by torture and whatnot.

The high court elected to retry the case. The initial gang of twelve was further reduced by the deaths of two of the accused. The jury again ordered the seven remaining defendants who had appealed to the gallows. Only Liberia's president had the authority to stay the executions, the end result of most death sentences under Tubman's long rule. In January 1979, however, Tolbert signed all seven death warrants, which meant Harper's authorities had to build gibbets. These were erected over a platform high enough above one of the town's public squares to be visible to the expected throng. The Dutch diplomat was there at dawn—along with his camera and in the company of more than fifteen thousand other spectators—when the sheriff sounded a whistle. Strangled bodies jerked and then dangled as a cheer rose from the crowd.[131]

Like his hosts, Fred van der Kraaij wondered if Tolbert had pursued the Harper case in order to "reduce the power of some influential Maryland families, in particular those who had been close to former President Tubman."[132] Questions of motive were never answered: Tolbert himself was shortly thereafter murdered in the executive mansion he often avoided on grounds of bad juju, which he'd attributed to the Convivial Cannibal. His killer was Sergeant Samuel Kanyon Doe, a twenty-eight-year-old who ended 133 years of Americo-Liberian rule by toppling Tolbert. (The president was disemboweled and stabbed repeatedly in the face with a bayonet, a decidedly un-Tubmanesque flourish.) A Krahn-speaker from Zwedru, Doe hadn't benefited from higher education. But he had been the beneficiary of training by American army officers and deemed "exceedingly pro-American" by the chargé d'affaires representing the new administration of Ronald Reagan in Monrovia.[133]

Naturally, Doe, too, was later accused of participating in ritual murders. But there was nothing ritualistic about what came next: a summary and public execution of almost the entire Tolbert cabinet.[134] (One of those spared was the finance minister, the future president Ellen Johnson Sirleaf, the first woman to win that rank in Africa; she was technically on loan from the World Bank.) It's true that many in the U.S. embassy thought Doe's cabinet reshuffle overkill. But if American officials were cross, or appalled, they seemed to get over it quickly. The day after Tolbert's assassination, Americans had assigned—yes, again—advisors to key government agencies, promising increased financial assistance and substantial military aid. This began to flow shortly after the blood did.[135]

The assassination of President Tolbert may have "started the decline of Americo-Liberian supremacy," observed Fred van der Kraaij, "but it did not stop ritualistic killings in the country."[136] In 1980, the year Tolbert was killed, the mayor of Harper was among those arrested on such charges. More tremors—ritual killings attributed once again to "pillars of the local establishment," as *The New York Times* had it, but also to aspiring warlords—arose from the same social fault lines, and would do so even after the big quake of civil war broke apart the country.[137] In the decade before it started, bad juju abounded from coast to forest, and (as ever with juju) proved difficult to control. The yellow neo-Georgian Tubman mansion, allegedly connected by a tunnel to the monumental Masonic temple across the street, was looted thoroughly during the war. But passersby have long skirted the lodge at night.

To this day, wooden gavels gather dust on desks and daises.

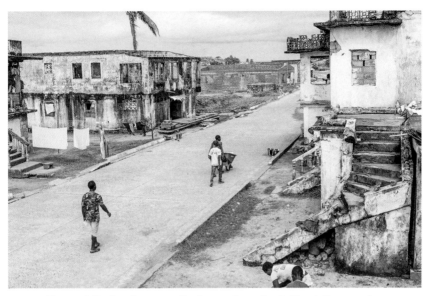

Harper, Liberia, nine years after it was almost leveled by civil war, and as Ebola swept through the countryside (MACKENZIE KNOWLES-COURSIN)

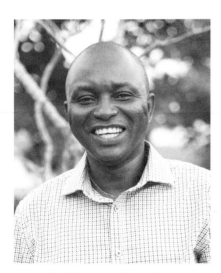

Dr. Sheik Humarr Khan in Kenema, Sierra Leone, shortly before his demise (PARDIS SABETI)

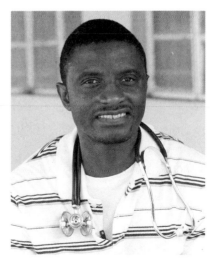

The surgeon Dr. Martin Salia shortly before his death from Ebola in November 2014 (MIKE DuBOSE, UNITED METHODIST NEWS SERVICE)

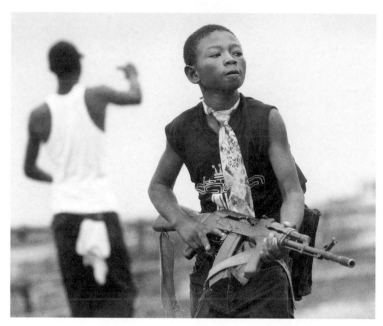

Child soldiers became a feature of the West African "blood diamond" wars that lasted into the twenty-first century. (CHRIS HONDROS / GETTY IMAGES)

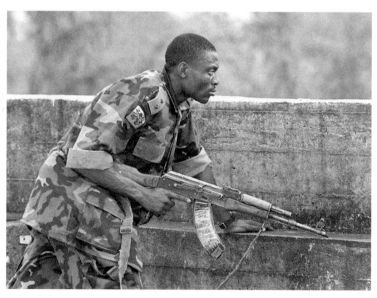

A Nigerian peacekeeper prepares to take aim from the rooftop of Freetown's Mammy Yoko Hotel as it is besieged by rebels in 1997.

(ISSOUF SANOGO / AFP VIA GETTY IMAGES)

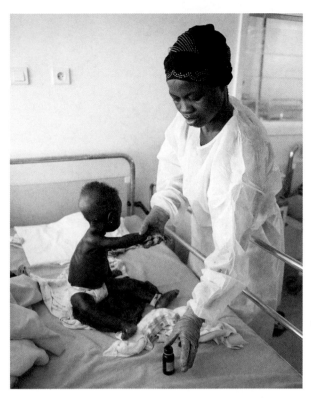

A nursing aide tends to "Miracle Baby" Jariatu, at Port Loko's hospital in January 2015. (PARTNERS IN HEALTH)

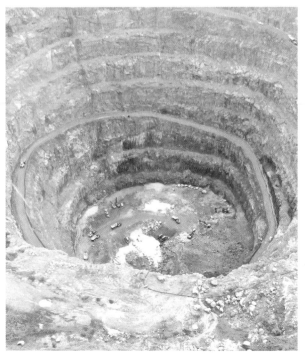

The Mordor pits of Kono District's diamond mines continued to operate during the height of the West African Ebola epidemic. (PARTNERS IN HEALTH)

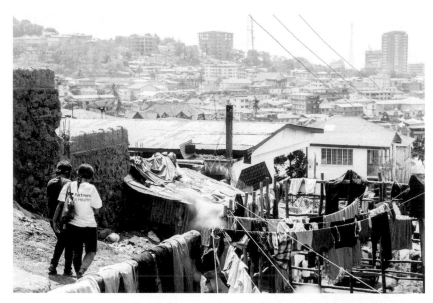

Contact tracers from Partners In Health do home visits in a Freetown neighborhood during the fall of 2015. (PARTNERS IN HEALTH)

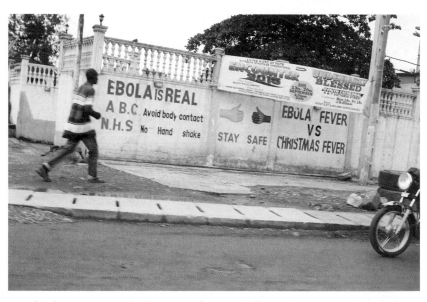

Cautionary messages in Freetown, where social-distancing measures—branded with the slogan "Avoid Body Contact"—were complemented by exhortations that "Ebola Is Real" (PARTNERS IN HEALTH)

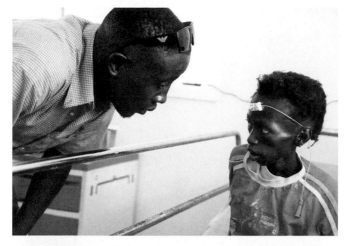

Ibrahim Kamara, shortly after his recovery from Ebola, visits still-sick Mariatu in the pediatric ward of Port Loko's hospital. (PARTNERS IN HEALTH)

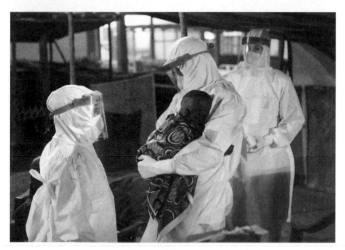

Volunteer clinicians provide care for a child with Ebola during the night shift at Maforki's Ebola treatment unit. (PARTNERS IN HEALTH)

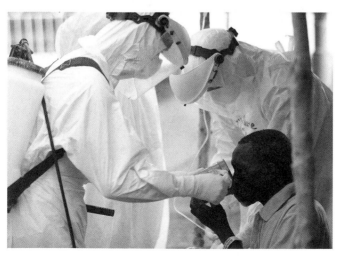

A young man with Ebola receives oral rehydration salts and encouragement in Maforki in November 2014. (PARTNERS IN HEALTH)

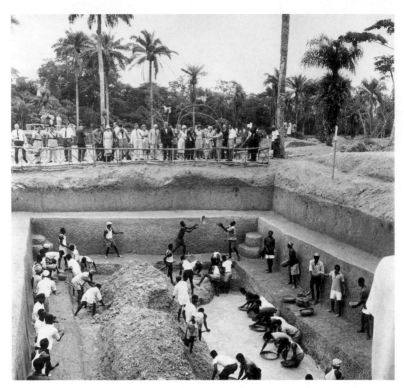

Queen Elizabeth II visits Kenema to admire her former subjects' diamonds.
(BETTMANN / GETTY IMAGES)

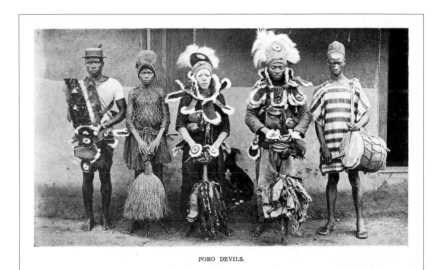

PORO DEVILS.

Five Poro devils in "traditional African garb," echoing the cloth and
customs of Europeans. The photo appeared in Captain Kenneth Beatty's
1915 book, *Human Leopards*. (KENNETH BEATTY, *HUMAN LEOPARDS*)

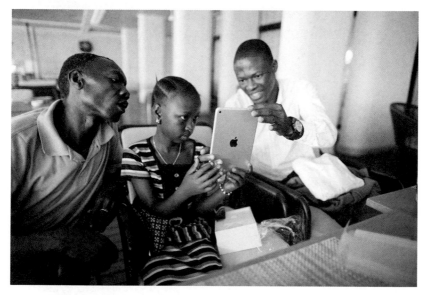

After a near-death experience, Mariatu announced that what she wanted most was an iPad, a wish granted in the summer of 2015, shortly before she began school. She is seen with her father and Partners In Health's Gibrilla Sheriff. (PARTNERS IN HEALTH)

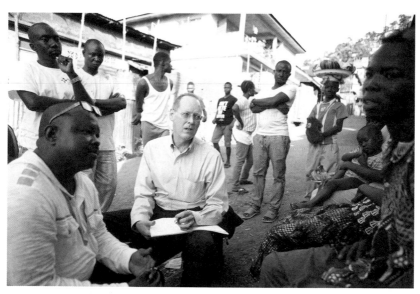

Bailor Barrie and Paul Farmer visit just-discharged Ebola patients in Freetown in October 2014. (PARTNERS IN HEALTH)

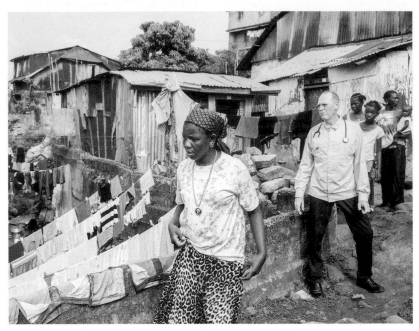

Yabom Koroma and Paul Farmer in the courtyard of Yabom's house
in the Mountain Cut neighborhood of Freetown, spring 2015
(PARTNERS IN HEALTH)

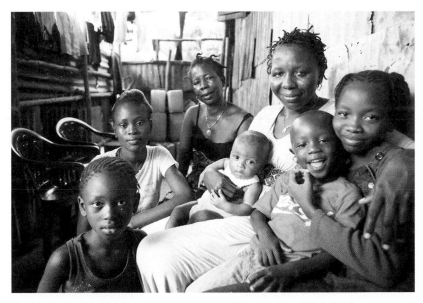

Yabom Koroma and her sister with what remains of their family
after Ebola mowed through its ranks (PARTNERS IN HEALTH)

8.

Things Fall Apart

CIVIL WAR AND ITS AFTERMATH

Large hemorrhagic fever virus outbreaks almost invariably occur in areas in which the economy and public health system have been decimated from years of civil conflict or failed development.

—Daniel G. Bausch and Lara Schwarz, "Outbreak of Ebola Virus Disease in Guinea: Where Ecology Meets Economy," in *Ebola's Message*, 2016

The epicenter of the outbreak was also ground zero for a decade of civil wars spanning the 1990s and early 2000s. In Liberia and Sierra Leone, tens of thousands were killed, and millions were displaced internally and to other countries in the region. Health facilities in Liberia and Sierra Leone were among the institutions destroyed or left to deteriorate during the war. Training for health workers, along with much tertiary-level education, was suspended or severely limited in the most affected areas, and the most well-trained health workers fled as the war intensified.

—Adia Benton and Kim Yi Dionne, "International Political Economy and the 2014 West Africa Ebola Outbreak," *African Studies Review*, 2015

THE TUMULT OF THE SEVENTIES AND EIGHTIES—AUSTERITY POLICIES THAT fed long-standing grievances while starving education and health care; British-style hangings of human leopards in Harper and struggles over diamonds in Koidu; strikes, riots, political thuggery, and coups d'état in Liberia, Sierra Leone, and Guinea—was a mere shade of the violence to follow. And it was the civil strife that after 1989 consumed two of these countries, and swamped the third with a flood of refugees, that set the stage for the world's first major urban epidemic of Ebola, or at least its first documented one.

There are many preconditions to any metaphorically perfect epidemic storm. But for big outbreaks of Ebola, Marburg, and many other pathogens, conflict sits at the top of the list. In Ebola's case, war traced the same hectic paths followed by the virus two decades later—from the trizone area to the coast, and on both sides of the Mano River. And the conflict, like the epidemic, started small. Launched by groups of insurgents numbering a hundred or so rebels and mercenaries each, armed strife quickly engulfed Liberia and Sierra Leone, throwing lethal tendrils into a dozen other nations. The epidemic of violence, however, reached a different order of magnitude than the plague: before it was over, more than 150,000 combatants—not counting 20,000 Nigerian soldiers and a similarly numerous contingent of UN peacekeepers called up late in the game—left up to 450,000 dead or maimed, pushed six million refugees into camps or slums, and destroyed already weak health systems.

These rough numbers aside, it's hard to answer the inevitable question, *But why?* It's also hard to know where and when these wars started, what fueled them, or whether they were in fact two wars or one. Just as West Africa's coups and trade wars weren't local affairs, the strife that laid waste to Liberia and Sierra Leone were interlocking feuds, sustained by receipts from global commerce and prosecuted by armies, allegiance-shifting factions, international peacekeepers, and guns-for-hire from across the continent and later the world.[1] But because, as with epidemics and responses to them, analyses commonly frame war in the bounds of nation-states—the Liberian civil war, the Sierra Leonean Ebola epidemic, the Guinean Ebola response—it becomes difficult to recall that war and pestilence are reliably transnational when and where commerce is.

Recognition of this fact doesn't really answer the why question, of course. Was Liberia's conflagration triggered by the fecklessness, corruption, and violence of Samuel Doe's regime? Was it a dying spasm of the Cold War? Or was it caused by over a century of political exclusion of the majority, including young and unemployed men? Could this last response explain the roots of Sierra Leone's conflict, as insurrectionary propaganda alleged—even as rebel forces twice swept west to loot and burn Freetown after consuming villages and towns to the east? Or did its civil war have more to do with control of the diamond fields, where kimberlite pipes had done their spewing two billion years previously, and with lucrative concessions to international mining and other interests?

Were these conflicts, in other words, about greed or grievance?

The anthropologist Paul Richards's *Fighting for the Rain Forest*— published shortly before the 1997 assault on Freetown—seemed to favor the grievance perspective. "The war in Sierra Leone drags on essentially because there are social factors feeding the conflict," he wrote. "The main rebel group feels it has not yet had a chance to get its political point of view across, and that it needs to do so to honour activists who died in its cause."[2] Many Sierra Leonean scholars and journalists begged to differ. They underlined greed, as do most invoking such frameworks. Although the rebels (as they were and still are termed) reliably underlined grievance, the true interests of Revolutionary United Front (RUF) commanders—increasingly the soldiers-turned-rebels known as sobels, an epithet applicable to the faction's founder—were revealed by their repeated seizure of the diamond fields.

As so often in war, greed and grievance came to be inseparable in Upper West Africa.[3] In the first years of these conflicts, however, greed-versus-grievance debates received little play in the international press. By the latter quarter of the twentieth century, the default logic in attempts to make sense of most African conflicts turned about ethnicity and tribal affiliations. This interpretive logic was honed under colonial rule and increasingly shaped local understandings of conflict. Looters-in-chief on both sides of the Mano River reliably raised tribal fig leaves to advance their aims. Liberia was held to be in the grips of ethnic conflict, and soon was, even when and where that conflict was manifestly about pillage.[4] Politics in Sierra Leone had been similarly rooted in an "ethnoregionalism" fanned and exploited by self-serving politicians and future warlords alike.[5]

There are many reasons to resist rigidly identitarian readings of war in West Africa, but that doesn't mean identity politics of one sort or another weren't salient (if malleable) during fifteen years of war. Excluded young foot soldiers from both sides of the Mano switched allegiances and even ethnic and national identities as they pursued the perilous work of war—and the precarious project of living off its spoils.[6] Greed-versus-grievance debates, and claims of tribal conflict as the root cause of war, were eventually informed by deeper understanding of cash flows from the global retail trade—worth $80 billion annually—in glittering diamonds. That trade, like others in the region, is fundamentally transnational. It was one means by which the district of Kono, scarred with a thousand pits and massive heaps of tailings, reached into the homes of Americans who believed, and still do, that diamonds are forever. There were plenty of other valuables under the earth, and plenty of timber and rubber on top of it.

Scrutiny of the extractive trades lends credence to arguments that this was a single war while implicating the titans of industries orchestrating operations from locations far from the Mano or any other West African river. As Sierra Leone's legal diamond exports plummeted after blood diamonds, amputations, and child soldiers gave the country new and grisly renown, Liberia suddenly became a major exporter of these gems.[7] Without international supply lines, kept open with receipts from once-again illegitimate trades, rebellious factions would not have long survived determined counterattacks from national security forces. Still less would these factions have become major players in a global conflict involving a couple hundred thousand combatants. These included, by the end, a quarter of the Nigerian army, the world's largest deployment of UN peacekeepers, and shadowy terrorist groups operating not only across West Africa, but in Kenya, Lebanon, Afghanistan, Libya, and—as revealed after September 11, 2001—the United States.

What does all this have to do with Ebola? A long and sorry chain of events ending in war constituted the storied perfect storm that led to its runaway epidemic—and to others, in spite of claims of singularity made with each major outbreak, including the one now unfurling in the Congo.

The best way to understand armed conflict in West Africa is to link firsthand accounts to analyses alive to the region's history and political economy—the causes of the causes laid out in previous chapters. Easier said than done: in spite of journalists' front-line dispatches, comprehensive first-hand accounts of the region's recent wars remain few and far between. There are, of course, thousands of personal testimonies gathered during postwar legal proceedings, or by Sierra Leone's Truth and Reconciliation Commission. But Liberia had a more partial reckoning, and partisan accounts from both sides of the Mano await careful vetting, interpretation, and a stitching together. Another problem with eyewitness accounts of war is that much of it is ethnographically invisible. Those seeking to learn *who* was prosecuting the war could see that, as elsewhere, a majority of combatants were young men. Numerically, they were likely to belong to militias or factions rather than to the armed forces. But why were they at war? Where were they from? How did they come to be armed, and with what weapons?

If none of those questions could be addressed thoroughly from the midst of the mayhem, the outlines of compelling answers could be discerned there during it. One reason to rely on anthropologists is that the best of them rely on their own firsthand observations *and* on knowledge of history and political economy. They insist, as did Mary Moran after war pushed her out of Harper, "on returning local histories of conflict, and their relationship with global political and economic forces, back to the center of the analysis."[8] The rise and fall of factions and warlords were tied to control of the labor required to fell timber or to extract diamonds, latex, bauxite, iron, titanium dioxide, and rutile ores. (Titanium dioxide is a pigment known for its bright white color; rutile is its precursor. They're used in manufacturing everything from paint to electronic components.) As these were commodities for an international market, the warlords, rebels, and sobels also required airports, seaports, and overland routes, as well as middlemen and foreign contractors.

Arms dealers and private security contractors also played outsize roles in West Africa. War (and peace after it) required weapons—the kind that can lay waste to staff, stuff, space, and systems. Machetes, cutlasses, and muskets had been around forever, but during and after the Cold War, military-grade munitions reached the region from the era's rival superpowers—one less powerful than alleged but bristling with fearsome weaponry nonetheless. Weapons of war also flowed in from Europe. In the global arms trade, the chief competitors of the United States and Soviet-bloc nations were not Libya or Nigeria but the martial artists formerly known as the colonial powers. These were the same Western democracies, their colonial histories sanitized, that later imposed arms and petroleum embargoes on Liberia and Sierra Leone, boycotted trade with them, and froze warlords' bank accounts while seeking to ban their international travel.

It's hard not to wonder what Liberia and Sierra Leone might look like today had the region not been flooded with weapons of war from these nations—a thought exercise fitting for this book, since my own country was one of the biggest offenders. "During the height of Cold War tensions in the first Reagan administration," marvels Moran, "tiny Liberia, with a population of two and a half million people and an area the size of the state of Ohio, was the 'beneficiary' of the second largest package of United States military aid in the world (after Israel)."[9] Since such largesse seems, at least in retrospect, to have no other likely outcome, and since these armaments have few other uses, the novice again asks, But why? Surely Liberia was more than a pawn on the Cold War chessboard?

Yes, but it was also that. In addition to a supersize U.S. embassy, Liberia was home to the Africa-based relay station for the Central Intelligence Agency and other spy networks, U.S. satellite tracking and navigation systems, a Voice of America transmitter, and a number of U.S.-built military bases and airfields. When, at the onset of the conflict, George H.W. Bush asked his new assistant secretary of state for African affairs why it was necessary to tolerate such a violent and erratic buffoon as Samuel Doe, the diplomat reminded Bush that Liberia was America's gateway to Africa. An estimated twelve U.S. government planes on sundry unnamed errands, many of them elsewhere on the continent, landed each month at the big airfield near the Firestone plantation. Extravagant "aid" was not aimed at benefiting Liberia's population, he explained, but at protecting American interests after "the Cold War tilted us in favour of supporting Doe because we got reciprocal treatment."[10]

That war's victors had significant economic interests on the continent that furnished much of the labor that built the Americas; reciprocal treatment might come in handy. There was West African oil, or the promise of it, and American businesses and banks headquartered far from West Africa still held sway in Monrovia and in the State Department. By the time Harper and much of the rest of Liberia went up in flames, the majority of the country's businesses—five out of every seven firms—was foreign-owned.[11] As Liberia's civil war broke out, Firestone remained headquartered in Ohio but had just been sold to a Tokyo-based conglomerate. (The sale marked the largest Japanese acquisition in the history of American commerce.) The venerable if troubled company would play a significant role in the early years of the war, even though rubber wasn't the chief accelerant for the fire and even though Liberia no longer counted as a top supplier of latex to U.S. manufacturers.

Nor did swollen military aid toward the close of the Cold War sustain these particular conflicts well into the twenty-first century. What, then, was their chief accelerant? When weapons come as commodities rather than part of aid packages, they have to be paid for; they're often paid for even when billed as aid. Portable diamonds were a warlord's best friend. That trade, which catered to an American clientele (in Ohio, say) convinced that diamonds were the way to seal a marriage pact, generated the cash used to buy munitions. The arms trade, which catered to a warlord clientele (in West Africa, say) convinced that it needed no social pact with civilians outside their patronage networks, was linked less to ideological struggles than to the fight to seize diamonds, mineral wealth, and other natural resources.

As various parties were alleged to traffic in blood diamonds, protestations of innocence from Monrovia, Freetown, Pretoria, Antwerp, New York, and London strained credulity. But few of the consumers back in Ohio showed much interest in allegedly tribal conflicts or in the provenance of their baubles. What did pique passing outrage among those in the market for diamonds—and a touch of fear among those cutting, polishing, or hawking them—were the tactics used by irregular forces on both sides of the border. These included (most infamously) mass amputations, rape as a weapon of war, and the conscription of child soldiers. When ideas *were* accelerants, the Liberian warlords' grisly playbooks were copied not only from various guerrilla and terrorist groups but also from the governments of independent

Sierra Leone and Guinea and from the administration that employed Charles Taylor almost a decade before he launched his years-long takeover of Liberia. Many chapters of these playbooks clearly echoed colonial practices, including those of Americo-Liberian settlers.

Divide and conquer remained a recurrent theme. In this war's origin stories, political rifts and economically motivated patronage were often passed off as tribalism—a conflation that would have been difficult to mask in the course of trade-related conflicts on other continents.

The chessboard of West Africa had long been set with pawns but has counted its heavy pieces, too. Charles Taylor, now a guest in a British maximum-security prison, is a central character of a war that ranks among Africa's most destructive. It's not the first prison he's known, nor was The Hague his first dock.

Educated, if not very well, at Boston's Bentley College—he majored in economics, naturally—Taylor returned to Monrovia to work in the Doe administration, and was soon running its procurement activities. Sacked in 1983 after wiring close to $1 million to a U.S. bank account, Taylor fled back to Massachusetts. New England's abolitionists, had there been any supporting Liberia's colonization, must have been turning in their graves. The storied Pilgrims, too: arrested on an extradition warrant in the town of Somerville, a student-heavy suburb hard by Harvard Yard, Taylor was sent to Plymouth County Correctional Facility, which proved to be anything but maximum-security. Astoundingly—in some eyes, downright supernaturally—the future warlord escaped from an open window on September 15, 1985. (In other accounts, Taylor and other inmates sawed through iron bars and lowered themselves down knotted sheets to the ground twenty feet below.)

The fugitive made for the parking lot of a local hospital to be picked up, Taylor testified during his Hague sabbatical, by two men he believed to be "agents of the U.S. government."[12] The American chauffeurs, whoever they were, drove Taylor to Staten Island, where he disappeared (in the words of press accounts) into thin air. He would later boast in some detail of assistance from the CIA, which would only admit that he'd indeed been working with the agency in Monrovia. If true, the blowback was severe, since these events would result in the destruction of two nations, badly cripple a third, and draw a significant portion of West Africa's largest standing army, and several others, into a decade of costly and warlike peacekeeping. War left control of Sierra Leone's diamond fields in the hands of Taylor allies for the better part of the decade. And conflict diamonds, *The Washington Post* later revealed, were one of the means by which al-Qaeda financed its attacks on American targets from Nairobi to New York.

Leaving aside the why, *how* on earth did all this lethal nuttiness come to pass? By the close of the Cold War, Samuel Doe had fallen from favor among the architects of U.S. policy in West Africa. He was supposed to *plan* civilian elections, not run in and win them. What's more, and in spite of lavish aid, the Doe junta had been as bad as any True Whig administration in managing its finances. In 1987, as in the days bemoaned by W.E.B. Du Bois, no less than the U.S. secretary of state himself persuaded Doe to accept a team of U.S. "financial experts" (they were still a thing, too) with the power to sign off on all major government transactions. The assassin-turned-president declared them personae non gratae within a year. Not a smart move for Doe, whose patrons began looking for a more presentable alternative.

Surprisingly, given his post-Plymouth travel itinerary and outstanding warrants, Charles Taylor's name cropped up in these discussions. The embezzler and future warlord had disappeared not into thin air but into the smog of Mexico City, and thence to Ghana, where he was arrested as a suspected CIA mole. Again Taylor's prison stay was brief. A couple of years later, he could be found in the Ivory Coast with the nascent National Patriotic Front of Liberia (NPFL), a splinter group pledged to dislodge Doe. Somewhere in the course of Taylor's grand tour was a stop in Libya, which helped train and equip the NPFL. The faction also received a helping hand from grateful friends in Burkina Faso, where in 1987 Liberian exiles had been involved in a military coup and the murder of the sitting president. Covering all its bases, the NPFL was also in touch, according to later testimony from its officials, with the U.S. government. This after it was known that its cadres had been trained in Libya.

It didn't take Taylor long to purge the faction's leadership of rivals. But in order to depose his former boss, he, too, required staff, stuff, space, and systems. Staff like young and unemployed men and boys (real boys), mercenaries, and soldiers. Stuff like weapons, ammo, vehicles, gas, and radios, but also stuff to sell. Space like houses, barracks, and warehouses—preferably with electricity and plumbing, surrounded by forests in which to hide, and close to an airport able to receive weapons shipments and to export commodities across a far-flung international market. Systems, including at least rudimentary knowledge of shipping and receiving and the care and feeding of thousands of combatant-workers. Taylor headed, naturally, for the town of Harbel—named in a contraction of Harvey and Idabelle. As in Firestone.

The plantation's big house had a less creative name, but House 53 boasted a nine-hole golf course and a full bar, and was close to the airport built thanks to FDR. Taylor reckoned Harbel would make excellent headquarters from which to launch repeated attacks on the capital, where his ultimate objective—the real Liberian Big House—lay. As a growing, ragtag militia invested the neighborhood in June 1990, Firestone's expatriate executives (according to one recent investigation) retreated to House 53, "playing cards and listening to BBC reports about the war" while the managing director "smoked his pipe and practiced his golf game, using a pitching wedge to place short chip shots into nearby buckets."[13] Such distractions aside, the folks sheltered in House 53 were in a pickle.

Samuel Doe had previously ingratiated himself to Firestone by scrapping his predecessor's proposed terms for the concession. When unable to pay his clients, including the armed forces, the dictator convinced company executives to advance him funds from future taxes. Now, glued to the radio station Taylor periodically updated by satellite phone—one of his chief weapons of war—the expatriates stranded in Harbel knew the NPFL was each day augmented by unemployed youth, members of ethnic groups mistreated by Doe, returned exiles, mercenaries, and the steady defection of opportunistic military officers.[14] After acceding to rebel demands to borrow or buy trucks and warehouse space (and more satellite phones) did not confer protection, Firestone's managers pulled out under escort by U.S. special forces. The Pentagon, skeptical of the State Department's varied schemes—which still included scenarios in which American operatives would put Taylor in power—had by then dispatched the Marine Amphibious Group to Liberian waters.

There are, of course, many versions of this story. Taylor still claims he received not only Firestone's support but also assistance from the U.S. government. But so had an all-African military force mustered to oppose him. In August, the region-wide alliance called the Economic Community of West African States, or ECOWAS, dispatched its first-ever peacekeeping force to protect civilians, evacuate refugees, and keep Taylor out of the palace. The assignment would lead this largely Nigerian force—the one known by the unholy acronym ECOMOG—to a decade-long deployment there and in Sierra Leone. The U.S. State Department announced a "symbolic" $3.3 million donation to ECOMOG in order to display "solidarity with an important African initiative." The force had, added a high-ranking diplomat, "the extra merit of involving Africans working to solve an African problem."[15]

It's hard to think of war in Liberia as a strictly African problem. It was a country bristling with American matériel, some of it bound to end up in warlord hands. Within weeks of overrunning Harbel—an American company town more than a Liberian or Japanese one—Taylor's army was closing in on the giant palace erected by Americo-Liberians and paid for in American dollars, a legal tender of Liberia. He was beaten to the task of toppling the American-trained Samuel Doe by a former Taylor ally named Prince Johnson, who had a background in military intelligence and had also benefited from U.S. tutelage. Doe's unannounced September 9 visit to Monrovia's Freeport, an American-built and American-run shipping complex of cranes and containers, proved his undoing. Johnson's irregulars killed Doe's bodyguards while (U.S.-supported) ECOMOG troops stood by. They took the president to their base, where they tortured him while videotaping the proceedings. In the video, Johnson, who currently serves in the Liberian

Senate, is seen sipping a Budweiser, an American beer, as Doe's ears are severed. In the next act, Doe's mutilated corpse is paraded through the streets of a city founded by American settlers and named after the fifth president of the United States.

By then, all of Liberia had been engulfed in war, and as many as seven hundred thousand of its citizens had fled to Guinea, Sierra Leone, Nigeria, and the Ivory Coast. Now *that* was an African problem.

The generals at the helm of Africa's most populous nation understood this, which is one of the reasons Nigerian forces opposed the man who'd launched the war in Liberia and was soon to foment one on the far side of the Mano River. Another reason the oil-rich junta footed the bill for ECOMOG, and for the evacuation of tens of thousands of refugees, was to burnish Nigeria's reputation as the ranking and stable regional power in the face of local and international calls for civilian rule there. The generals in Abuja sought to broker a cease-fire and supported (as did Western powers) an interim government formed to plan the elections required to establish in Liberia the civilian rule repeatedly deferred in Nigeria.

In 1992, Charles Taylor—denied the palace by ECOMOG—launched another wave of war to oust the provisional government. By then, receipts from diamonds and other treasures from under or just on top of the earth were known to be fueling conflict in both Sierra Leone and Liberia. One of these treasures was latex. Although Firestone's Liberia operations were no longer critical to the automotive industry, sales of condoms surged early in the AIDS era, leading to something of a rubber renaissance in Harbel. Now the NPFL controlled much of the countryside, including parts of it covered by rubber trees. Taylor, the erstwhile economics major, declared himself ready to halt the pillage of Firestone assets—for a price.

Several of the Liberia hands now stuck in Ohio warned against dealing with the warlord. They knew that what was happening in and around Harbel was a lot uglier than the rebels' garish red paint job on the white Corinthian columns of House 53, or the neglect of the vast and orderly groves surrounding it. But executives advocating an accommodation with the warlord could also claim to be worried less about infrastructure and trees than about thousands of Liberian employees, some of whom had worked for the operation for decades. If Taylor were to prevail, they claimed, these employees would face peril if the company was seen to be against him. Arguments for a shift in support from a shambolic interim government to Taylor were given heft by attention to the bottom line: the Firestone acquisition was proving a bad deal for its new owners. As the Japanese conglomerate hemorrhaged money, Tokyo pressed Akron to cut a new deal with Taylor. Executives in both cities feared that, without an agreement, Firestone was likely to lose forests, processing plants, warehouses, housing, and other infrastructure that had taken decades to build. Looting aside, all of it would molder or die without maintenance.

In the end, orders from the C-suites were followed; critics of any sort of truck with Taylor were pushed out or silenced in golden retirement. A recently published investigative report—based on declassified diplomatic cables, internal corporate documents, and interviews—reveals what happened next:

> The company signed a deal in 1992 to pay taxes to Taylor's rebel government. Over the next year, the company doled out more than $2.3 million in cash, checks and food to Taylor, according to an accounting in court files. Between 1990 and 1993, the company invested $35.3 million in the plantation. In return, Taylor's forces provided security to the plantation that allowed Firestone to produce rubber and safeguard its assets. Taylor's rebel government offered lower export taxes that gave the company a financial break on rubber shipments. For Taylor, the relationship with Firestone was about more than money. It helped provide him with the political capital and recognition he needed as he sought to establish his credentials as Liberia's future leader.[16]

Just as the Firestone acquisition was costly to its Japanese parent company, so, too, was the Taylor arrangement costly to its Liberian assets, including many employees. Nigerian alpha jets bombed the Harbel plantation once they knew Taylor's forces were based there.

The crack-up of Sierra Leone was right behind Liberia's. On March 23, 1991, a small band of malcontents calling themselves the Revolutionary United Front crossed their shared border into Sierra Leone near Kailahun. The RUF was led by a Charles Taylor protégé named Foday Sankoh, formerly of the Sierra Leonean armed forces and long a guest in Pademba Road Prison for his role in a coup attempt or two. Sankoh, the original sobel, was also rumored to have been a guest of Muammar Gaddafi. But even with Liberian and Libyan material support, the RUF consisted of only a hundred or so Sierra Leoneans, and a score of sellswords from Liberia and Burkina Faso.[17]

This small group did plenty of damage around Kailahun, Koidu, Bo, and Kenema, eastern towns familiar to anyone who's read about Ebola or blood diamonds. When invaded, Kailahun was a small town with fewer than ten thousand inhabitants, most of them farmers or petty traders serving the diamond trade. They didn't know what was about to hit them. Then again, neither did the central government, then helmed by one Joseph Momoh, head of the Sierra Leonean army and a protégé of Siaka Stevens. General Momoh's ascension had required Stevens to tinker with the country's constitution, which stipulated civilian rule. This led to loud opposition from certain civilians, including politicians and political aspirants wishing to expand their own patronage networks. There were also objections from rowdy students at Fourah Bay College, some with ties to their age-mates dispatched to quell the insurrection and others whose sympathies lay with the RUF.

It's hard to imagine such a small faction, or a bunch of fractious politicos and students, would have posed a serious threat during Stevens's salad days. As my friends Ibrahim Kamara and Yabom Koroma both observed, however, the RUF invasion occurred in the heyday of austerity measures peddled by powerful development banks—powerful because of cash and credit, but also because their policies shaped those of government bureaucracies, public and private banks, and development organizations. These policies, loosely termed structural adjustment, meant structurally adjusting many of Momoh's clients right out of a job, and dashing the dreams of those who'd hoped for one. In the formulation of one political scientist, "State payouts to clients were already declining with implementation of a harsh structural adjustment program after 1991, which laid off 15,000 workers, 40 percent of the country's civil service. Much of the savings went to debt service."[18]

The general and his cabinet, and coup-savvy military officers, were surely well aware of the threat posed by measures that almost halved a modest civil service. They knew for sure that austerity policies would mean already malnourished health-care and educational systems would be left to starve. So why had Momoh acceded to such demands? Faced with an already growing insurgency in the east, which threatened income from mining, he needed cash flow to regain control of the diamond fields, the key to his government's survival. The armed forces then counted perhaps three thousand troops, and they weren't much use in putting down armed rebellions: Stevens had dealt with the constant threat of coups by depriving the army of heavy weapons. Given the rumored growth of the RUF through the recruitment or capture of young people with little hope of higher education or formal employment but drawn to the siren call of the diamond fields, the general-president needed financial assistance to enlarge and arm the army, even if aid came with strings capable of garroting him.

So Momoh signed up for austerity.

The results were certainly austere across the public sector. By 1992, in the words of the previously cited political scientist, "creditor-sponsored efforts to reduce corrupt state intervention in the economy" were associated with a sharp drop in revenue collection—from 30 percent of Sierra Leone's GNP in 1982 to 20.6 percent of a much lower GNP as war began to bite a decade later.[19] Among the corrupt clients to suffer most were schoolchildren and sick people. Spending on basic services such as education and health care quickly plummeted to less than a fifth of the already meager levels of the early eighties. Many of the neglected patients (and would-be patients) became the deceased. But some of the children no longer in school were soon enrolled in less academic pursuits, as first the rebels and then the army targeted them as recruits. Through terror and forced conscription, but also because they were swimming in an ocean of young prospects with few prospects, the rebels controlled a fifth of the country within a year of their unpromising incursion.

Foiled coup attempts had been common in the years around the 1968 election of Siaka Stevens—Sankoh's Pademba sabbatical was the result of his involvement in at least one such attempt—and became so again after the RUF invasion, which led to the rearming and growth of the institution responsible for previous attempts to overthrow civilian governments, in Freetown as across West Africa. It's hard (at least for me) to keep the details, names, and acronyms straight, much less to count the power grabs and plots hatched in Monrovia, Freetown, Conakry, Abuja, Tripoli, and other capitals. But if the goal is to understand how war rolled out the red carpet for Ebola, it's worth dissecting Sierra Leone's coups d'état, which, along with a decade of pillage, finished off a health system reeling from austerity measures.

The first coup occurred in 1992. A group of junior officers, hammered in the east by the superior weaponry and woodcraft of the insurgents, marched on the palace to demand back pay and better provisions. The young soldiers scared off Momoh without much effort and established, as if by accident, the National Provisional Ruling Council. The NPRC was led by Captain Valentine Strasser, at age twenty-five suddenly the world's youngest head of state, having won the title from the late (if largely unregretted) Samuel Doe. Though warmly welcomed in Freetown after promising the restoration of civilian rule, these are the fellows who gave birth to the neologism "sobel."[20] The junta of the young took an ostentatious shine to the high life. "Suddenly, they had unimpeded access to the diamond fields, to BMWs and Mercedes, and to Siaka Stevens's old presidential palace," reported one astute observer. The sobels transformed the latter into "a private disco where they danced, smoked pot, and snorted cocaine through the night. They also seemed to have forgotten that they were at war."[21]

Maybe they hadn't forgotten. Collusion between the NPRC and the RUF had been reported by many residing in towns and villages to the east, and the epithet "sobel" was current in Freetown in the early years of the war, well before sobels joined the big leagues. It seemed to some observers there, including several Sierra Leonean journalists and scholars, that the army had abandoned its stated goal of defeating the RUF. "Government soldiers could use rebel tactics pure and simple," explained the historian Arthur Abraham, "or reach an accommodation with the RUF, exchanging arms and uniforms for cash or diamonds."[22] Suspicions of a Faustian pact between the RUF and the NPRC deepened as both groups accessed the diamond fields, supplying their own and Taylor's war machines with fungible wealth. How else could both rebels and the junta enjoy access, unimpeded or otherwise, to Sierra Leone's diamonds?

There were other hints, drug-fueled raves and newly acquired bling aside, that defeating the RUF was not a ranking NPRC priority. Pademba Road Prison was soon full, as well it might be if there was any interest in punishing violent crime. But marauding gangs remained mostly at large, while the junta's detractors seemed to end up behind bars, self-deported, or disappeared altogether. Some were hanged, and a couple dozen alleged coup plotters were publicly executed on a city beach, in full view of an approving mob and (likely) of diplomats and aid workers staying in the Mammy Yoko—or of anyone with a good set of binoculars on the diamond freighters offshore.

Notably absent from Pademba were members of the RUF or their sympathizers in Freetown. According to NPRC propagandists, this was because so many rebels had been killed in pitched battles and ambushes on the eastern front. But as evidence of staged conflict between the junta and the RUF mounted, so did civilian, not military, casualties. By 1995, there was little doubt in Freetown or Monrovia—and surely none in strafed and burned eastern towns—what much of the misery was about. Diamonds in the rough were being smuggled to parts of Liberia controlled by Taylor, and thence to cities across the region and the world, by a diverse cast of rebels, army officers, Lebanese merchants, and sundry middlemen hailing from Israel, South Africa, Poland, and the Ukraine. The occasional diamond finisher from Antwerp, London, or New York also had a hand in this traffic, if press accounts of Valentine Strasser's mysterious trips to Antwerp are to be credited. He, too, was rumored to have profited from the sale of blood diamonds, including a few giant gems—one pale blue and worth a fortune.

Beyond the diamond fields, other instances of sobel collusion included ambushes along major roads linking Freetown to the provinces. Some were spectacular. In August 1995, a seventy-vehicle World Food Programme convoy escorted by a helicopter gunship and armored personnel carriers was stopped by soldiers ostensibly hunting for rebels. The sobels revealed their true colors when they opened fire on the convoy, leaving at least thirty dead, twenty vehicles in flames, and most of the rest of them in RUF hands.

As the junta of the young radically expanded the Sierra Leonean armed forces, it paid scant attention to training and even less to discipline. The numbers are telling. Prior to the war, as noted, the army numbered no more than two thousand. By early 1996, in the last days of the NPRC, it included fourteen thousand troops and an unknown number of irregulars, some of them children. Most new recruits had little secondary schooling and many had troubled histories, leading several Sierra Leonean scholars, echoing Marx, to term the new recruits "lumpen youth."[23]

Having more than sextupled the size of the army as his bling diplomacy faltered, Captain Strasser faced an increasingly serious domestic and international PR problem in a time when many of the war's spectacles were fashioned for an unseen and global audience. It was clear to even casual observers that undisciplined new recruits weren't keen on fighting *any* group bearing arms. In spite of the army's rapid growth—and its initial grievance that its infantry was underpaid and undersupplied—NPRC initiatives to restore order came to rely heavily on outsourcing security to private firms. These included Frontline Security Services (under contract with Sierra Rutile, a U.S.-owned mining concern) and Gurkha Security Guards, Ltd. (under contract with the Sierra Leonean government). But Sierra Rutile was soon overrun by the RUF, and Gurkha's commander, an American Vietnam veteran rather than a Gurkha, was killed in an ambush not far from Port Loko.[24] The Gurkha wannabes packed up their kit and turned tail in February 1995.

It was a good time to quit Sierra Leone. By then, as the American journalist Elizabeth Rubin observed, "there were no coherent front lines, no political causes, and for the terrorized public no place was safe. What began as a civil war had become civil chaos." By year's end, Rubin continued,

> rebels and renegade soldiers had overrun Sierra Leone's diamond, bauxite, and titanium dioxide mines—the three main sources of foreign revenue; locals and expatriates had been taken hostage; foreign investors had pulled out; tens of thousands of people had been maimed or killed; and one quarter of the prewar population of 4.5 million were living in overcrowded refugee camps.

Determining what led to what is a fraught exercise in the midst of civil chaos. But the sobel masquerade was up well before January 1996, when Captain Strasser left the country for golden (or diamondiferous) exile, and, just as likely, for the oubliette. One of his last actions in office—a gambit, said some, to stay on by actually doing his job—has nonetheless been hotly debated since.

Perhaps because he'd so publicly pledged to bring the country back under government control, Valentine Strasser cut a deal with one last mercenary group. He had read about Executive Outcomes in *Soldier of Fortune* magazine and cold-called its CEO, formerly of the South African armed forces, to offer him $15 million and a big cut in diamond operations in return for ridding Kono and environs of the RUF—at least for a while. Executive Outcomes' troops included black Namibians and Angolans who'd served in an apartheid-era battalion, as well as the white South African and Rhodesian officers who'd led it. The force dispatched in response to Strasser's invitation was, in Rubin's words, "a collection of former spies, assassins, and crack bush guerillas, most of whom had served for 15 to 20 years in South Africa's most notorious counterinsurgency units." This rent-an-army was worth its weight in rough, and likely more than accustomed to being paid that way: many of its fighters, who netted between $2,000 and $7,000 a month, were flown in from diamond-rich Angola, where Executive Outcomes had performed similar chores. (War there had rolled out the red carpet for a couple of large outbreaks of Marburg.)

The mercenaries from the south received uniforms from the Sierra Leonean army upon arrival. "No passports were stamped," Rubin adds, and "no customs procedures needed." Discretion was hardly possible, however, since the white mercenaries cut quite the figure in Kono's towns and villages, where they set up camp Afrikaaner-style, replete with a bar and barbeque. More to the point, their kit included a big, loud arsenal:

> The force came equipped with two MI17s and an MI24 Hind—
> Russian helicopter gunships similar to American Apaches—a radio
> intercept system, two Boeing 727s to transport troops and supplies,
> an Andover casualty-evacuation aircraft, and fuel-air explosives,
> bombs that suck out oxygen upon detonation, killing all life within a
> square-mile radius.

Of all the death-dealing predators in a forest long depleted of wild beasts, the Russian-made Hinds were soon the most feared by those flitting through the trees or cowering on the ground. They could swoop within a few feet of the forest canopy, shredding bodies, trees, and huts indiscriminately. To call in air strikes, adds Rubin, Executive Outcomes relied upon "traditional Sierra Leonean hunters, known as Kammah Joes—a witchcraft battalion armed with old single-barrel muskets, special herbal potions, and supernatural war garments believed to repel bullets."[25]

Members of this largely Mende militia, colloquially termed Kamajors, were young—too young, some observed, to have mastered woodcraft and hunting techniques, much less the alleged mystical powers of hunting societies' elders. Nor did they traditionally hunt in groups.[26] Then again, these untraditional Kamajors were armed with a lot more than hunting nets, arrows, cutlasses, antique rifles, and amulets. The white pilots could claim at least a personal and professional tradition of using military-grade armaments against black Africans scurrying below. Some airborne hunters' rituals included (Rubin reports) flipping a coin before each sortie to see who would man the helicopters' four-barreled Gatling guns, which fired up to four thousand rounds per minute. These apartheid warriors were goaded on by their new paymasters: "When the pilots told the Sierra Leone military commander that they were having difficulty distinguishing between the rebels and civilians camped under the impenetrable canopy of vines and trees, the reply was, 'Kill everybody.' So they did."[27]

Proving the jungle canopy plenty penetrable, Executive Outcomes and the Kamajors routed RUF forces, who likely then numbered no more than a couple of thousand conscripts, some of them children loyal to—or detained and drugged by—Foday Sankoh and his commanders. The crazy scheme to restore the diamond fields to the government and its fair-weather friends actually seemed to work. Output again flowed to private mining concerns from all over, often through the hands of locally based diamond dealers, many of them Lebanese. For the first time in years, it seemed in February 1996 that peace or something closer to it might be given a chance. Although insecurity and structural violence reigned from Freetown to dwindling forest, the citizenry clamored for democratic elections. So did that diverse constellation termed "the international community."

The remnants of the NPRC, on the other hand, insisted conditions were unpropitious for voting, despite Strasser's docile exit. Ominously enough, his successor's sister was a high-ranking RUF official, and their elder brother was rumored to procure weapons for the NPRC *and* the rebels: a Gold Star sobel family. Even more ominously, the RUF had been driven east, not defeated. Nursing wounds in their forest redoubts, its commanders wanted elections even less than did the army. They stepped up a hand-amputation campaign in order to send a clear message about voting, which was done by pressing one's ink-drenched thumb on a ballot.

Foday Sankoh would later describe this spree of mutilation in an unapologetic apology: "Fighters in the bush went on the rampage and as their own way of stating their objection to the planned elections, they proceeded on a campaign to cut off the hands of innocent villagers as a message that no voting should occur." Arthur Abraham (who described Sankoh's pronouncements as "a smattering of disarticulated and undigested ideological droppings drawn mainly from Gaddafi's populist formulations") couldn't resist sarcasm: "The indiscriminate amputations, which extended to babies and children of non-voting age, raise serious doubts about whether the RUF was 'making a political statement,' or whether this was just another exhibition of its character as a terrorist organisation pure and simple."[28]

The number of civilians maimed this way was disputed, but they loomed large as the conflict menaced Freetown. The anthropologist Michael Jackson later spoke with some thus mutilated, as have many who work in places like Kono or stop to converse with an all-amputee soccer team that enlivens a pitch not far from the Mammy Yoko. His interview with one young woman from a village not far from the town of Kabala, where he'd conducted fieldwork over the course of decades, goes on for pages. In contrast to the inhabitants of Bantoro, the villagers around Kabala had been in and out of hiding for months when rebels attacked. "They shot many people," she told Jackson. "They stacked the bodies under the cotton tree. Then they grabbed us. Their leader said they were going to kill us, too. But then they sent their boys to bring a knife. My daughter Damba was six. They took her from me and cut off her hand. After that they cut off all our hands."

Like Yabom, the woman and other survivors from the Kabala region fled into the bush as their village went up in flames. And like the people of Bantoro, this woman was soon forced to think about food, shelter, and returning to the scorched and desecrated land. On the day she was fleeing it, it took a while to find her husband and uncle. "Everyone was crying," she said. "I told them to stop crying."[29]

The hacking campaign did not meet its goal, if preventing elections was indeed its goal. Although the army provided little in the way of security, a nominally democratic vote was held for the first time in almost three decades on February 26, 1996. This ended the reign of the NPRC, an event that civilians not beholden to its patronage—that is, most Sierra Leoneans—welcomed warmly.

Ahmad Tejan Kabbah, who had studied law in the U.K. before going to work for the United Nations Development Programme, was inaugurated president a month later. The anthropologist Joe Opala, who'd come to Sierra Leone from Oklahoma as a Peace Corps volunteer and returned after graduate studies to teach at Fourah Bay College, was deeply moved by these developments. "On a bright day in March 1996, I stood outside the American Embassy in Freetown," he wrote in *The Washington Post*, "with tears of pride streaming down my face. In defiance of the guns and grenades of an angry junta, the people of this beleaguered West African nation had just held democratic elections." Since the angry junta and its sobel foot soldiers were still on hand, as were guns and grenades and machetes, those celebrating the rebirth of democracy in Sierra Leone might have mixed some water with the wine.

Plenty of sobels were bound to be unhappy with this turn of events. A peace agreement Kabbah signed in Abidjan a few months later treated the RUF as an equal partner to the elected government. Sankoh and the bush sobels demanded the expulsion of Executive Outcomes, and suggested the same treatment for much of ECOMOG. Many Sierra Leoneans regarded rejection of these concessions as sure to shorten Kabbah's life span. But he and his party hoped to counter a bush-Freetown alliance by outsourcing security to ECOMOG and to progovernment militias. The latter included the shape-shifting groups loosely termed Kamajors, which had morphed into a large "civilian defense force," further irritating the swollen army.

Kabbah's bet didn't pay off. The Abidjan accords served largely to strengthen the bonds of the sobel alliance. But his hand was forced when it came to the mercenaries of choice. Influential representatives of multilateral development banks were more squeamish about Executive Outcomes than about the adverse effects, mostly ignored or denied, of the policies that had led to the outsourcing craze in the first place. Complaints from the high priests of privatization about the security force's cut in diamond profits and loans might have sounded rich to unarmed civilians—one sobel spree was called "Operation Pay Yourself"—but some first-world and UN diplomats sided with the world's bankers. Fragile shoots of democratic rule would be better protected, insisted influential voices in the international community, by a reformed national army and police force, with backup from a more neutral

peacekeeping force from across West Africa. Much of the army agreed, naturally, as long as the Nigerians could be neutered.

Since civilians from Freetown to forest had a long and unpleasant experience with their own army, and a bitter taste of Nigerian methods, there was
little popular support for this move. Expatriate squeamishness about Executive Outcomes wasn't widely registered in the diamond districts. After
flying gunships and cowrie-talismaned militias drove off the rebels, Kono
and Kenema were flooded by panhandlers from across the hungry, wrecked
country. Locals, newcomers, and returning refugees clearly preferred the
shake-shake invaders to the machete-bearing ones immediately preceding
them. The global bankers' ambivalence about the public bankrolling of Executive Outcomes wasn't shared by the region's paramount chiefs, either.
They, too, depended on the diamond trade.

Failure to restore basic services and to halt violence and pillage as the
country's only growth industries had led to widespread popular resolve that
sobel coups had to stop. But who would stop the next one without an army
willing to protect civilian rule? ECOMOG forces had already been unable
to do so on either side of the Mano River. (Although the Nigerians had kept
Taylor out of the palace, rumor then had it that he was planning a run for
it through the ballot box.) The banker-sovereigns were again, however, in a
position to insist. In spite of mounting infusions of foreign aid, the treasury
had again been emptied, and Kabbah needed access to credit to restore even
the most rudimentary services. In January 1997, Executive Outcomes—
predicting another coup within months—faded into the harmattan haze
above the Lungi airfield like a secret society into the forest.

The South African–led force, which left several team members behind to
look after its investments in Kono and other eastern districts, had, in effect,
made an easy prophecy. The means to unseat an elected government were
available to quisling soldiers and aspiring warlords in Freetown—including
officers with sobel leanings then stowed in packed but porous Pademba.
Rumors that the Kabbah administration intended to shrink the army, or to
abolish it, emboldened disgruntled officers and foot soldiers with little to
lose. The whole lot of them were against even a modest force reduction; some

openly warned that attempts to upset their gravy train would be met with extreme prejudice. Nor was the RUF so weakened that it couldn't violate a treaty signed in Abidjan or anywhere else. If allowed to regroup, the rebels could again divert proceeds from diamonds, minerals, and rubber to acquire weapons and the fighters to wield them—if barely in the case of the pint-size soldiers increasingly visible on all sides of the conflict and on either side of the Mano.

The RUF was allowed to regroup. Their resolve stiffened by weapons from Taylor—purchased with proceeds from the sale of the gems its two-handed serfs had won from Sierra Leonean soil—rebel units crept back toward towns like Kailahun and Koidu and took back the diamond fields. They then headed west. Joe Opala, like many others on the Fourah Bay faculty, would soon be crying again, "but this time, tears of rage and sorrow."[30]

It wasn't long after Executive Outcomes withdrew that the pits and washing stations of the diamond district were again manned in part by RUF captives. But the verb "manned" isn't quite right, since so many of the miners were minors: another page from the Taylor doomsday manual stipulated the use of forced labor (for porterage, mining, and logging) and the recruitment of boys and girls as spies and combatants. "Small-boy units" were also formed by officers in the regular armies of Liberia and Sierra Leone, and their fates weren't always different from those gang-pressed into rebel factions.

The very existence of child soldiers triggered the question, How are children turned into ruthless killers? A better question was, How were *these* boys and girls turned into killers, with or without scruples? The roots of the West African child-soldier phenomenon ran deep. War-boys had been armed for centuries, and youth thuggery had long been a staple of electoral politics in both Sierra Leone and Liberia. Freetown and Monrovia, like other West African cities and like Fourah Bay College, were incubators of rebellious youth culture, which informed or shaped insurgent groups. Culture aside, war pushed people out of villages and into larger towns and cities, where there was little for the young to do. Not all underage combatants were abducted, for they needed jobs or something that might lead to them. But it was a shortage of able-bodied men willing to kill (or be killed) that spurred the RUF and the armed forces to recruit minors.[31]

The recruitment of children as combatants, or the conclusion that joining the RUF (or any another faction) was the only way out of mortal peril, eroded social norms demanding respect for elders and for rules limiting young men's access to land, prestige, and women. Why go through a years-long initiation in some godforsaken backwater populated by bush devils when power and booty were available instantly to those with automatic weapons? Many tried to get at the heart of these matters after complaining that most reporting on child soldiers was as unhelpful as decontextualized descriptions of the voodoo antics of exotically festooned Kamajors.[32] The usual case in point was the Rambo iconography that crops up in any extended discussion of child soldiers in West Africa. One anthropologist, who'd worked extensively in both Sierra Leone and Liberia prior to war, warned against focusing overmuch on "the dramaturgy of youthful violence." Like other correctives from the discipline, his review attempts to avoid "exoticizing, decontextualizing, or essentializing child soldier behavior."[33]

I found the review helpful—I think. It's possible to be at once stupefied, appalled, mystified, and pained when contemplating "child soldier behavior." Or the experience, atrocities, and fates of child soldiers. Or the means by which they were recruited and trained in clandestine bush schools with overlapping curricula from what might be termed peacetime initiation—had there been much peace in recent memory. And even with sociological and historical understandings, making meaning out of these developments was a tall order for even seasoned students of the execrable.

Like Yabom Koroma, journalists and anthropologists alike were often moved by mercurial transformations from kid into killer and, sometimes, back again. Reporting from what was left of Kailahun, Greg Campbell, the American journalist, was sickened by blood-smeared and gangrenous scenes under the eaves of the forest. But he saw pathos, too:

> There are few things more terrifying than having a blank-eyed
> 12-year-old girl stick the barrel of a loaded AK-58 in your stomach,
> but there are also few things more satisfying than seeing her drop
> the weapon and squeal with long-lost childhood joy at the news that
> she'll soon be flying away from the frontline.[34]

When psychological speculation about the motivations of others fails, and since philosophical musings almost always do, it's important to get back to weapons. Guns make killing easier; for children, guns make killing possible.[35]

The experience of a child soldier named Ishmael Beah is detailed in *A Long Way Gone*, a widely read memoir of the years following his 1993 conscription into the Sierra Leonean Army, back when at least part of it was locked in a genuine struggle with the RUF. As with accounts of teenagers faced with the tasks of caregiving and heeding the illegal, dying wishes of their Ebola-stricken kin, Beah's story is one of impossible choices. When he was twelve or so, he and a group of schoolmates suddenly found themselves fleeing rebel forces advancing to "liberate" them. Escapees from that advance left little doubt about what the rebels had in mind. As Beah put it,

> Young boys were immediately recruited, and the initials RUF were
> carved wherever it pleased the rebels, with a hot bayonet. This not
> only meant that you were scarred for life but that you could never
> escape from them, because escaping with the carving of the rebels'
> initials was asking for death, as soldiers would kill you without any
> questions and militant civilians would do the same.[36]

Beah's account reveals that the Sierra Leonean army took on boys as young as seven, plying them with drugs—amphetamines, prodigious amounts of marijuana, and an admixture of cocaine or heroin and gunpowder they called *brown-brown*—in order to goad them into killing. Before the army was in open collusion with the RUF, the units with which Beah served razed villages, shot civilians, and tortured and executed bound prisoners, some of them his age or younger.

Army officers spared the boys none of these tasks. (And the RUF, especially, spared few of the girls, who were often used as sex slaves, or "bush wives.")[37] Beah recounts that the army's underage irregulars, terrified, tried to fit into their units. But many were simply too small. His first gun battle was in the company of two boys, one eleven and the other seven. "Josiah and Sheku dragged the tip of their guns," he recalled, "as they still weren't strong enough to carry them and the guns were taller than they were." The boys were instructed to carry extra ammunition on quoits atop their heads. "As we tied our head cloths, Sheku, standing next to me, fell backward," details Beah. "He had taken too much ammunition." Josiah, the eleven-year-old, was dead of a broken back during the first hour of his combat career: "An RPG had tossed his tiny body off the ground and he had landed on a tree stump."[38]

This is only the beginning of Beah's nightmarish descent, and far from the most disturbing event he chooses to share. By his account, he was a hardened killer by the time his commanding officer, following orders received just after Tejan Kabbah's election, sent him and several other boys to a rehabilitation center in Freetown. The center had been established by the United Nations and a couple of nongovernmental organizations to "de-program" child soldiers from the army and the RUF. Beah's first weeks in the center were marred by knife fights and brawls as kids from both sides of the conflict fought withdrawal from a steady diet of drugs, the awakening of remorse, and diverse new symptoms associated with both.

Ishmael Beah recovered, thanks to the hard work of several persistent Sierra Leoneans, including a remarkable young nurse who tended visible wounds from on-campus fights and front lines—and the less visible wounds sustained by all the children. After every enraged outburst or brawl, and after ducking hurled objects and epithets, the nurse insisted, *It's not your fault*. At first, this mantra angered the boys. But some of them began to believe it. In his first months of rehabilitation, one of the few pleasures Beah knew was listening to music, mostly rap and reggae, after the nurse bought him a Sony Walkman. She and others working in the center reintroduced him and the other feral boys to civilian life. Fewer girls benefited from these efforts, a shortcoming to be repeated at scale during nationwide demobilization efforts.

By the time Beah reached Freetown, the city was swollen with refugees, its tenuous peace about to be shattered by another coup. It seemed a tranquil haven to the war-battered boys. Most had never been to Freetown, nor did they claim to know much about why they were fighting—except to find work or avenge their families—or for whom. During one of Beah's first outings, a motorcade chock-full of Mercedes-Benzes whizzed by him and a couple of friends as they walked the city streets. When he learned that President Kabbah was in it, he notes only this: "I had never heard of this man."

Other city sights, especially ones they'd heard of, impressed Ishmael Beah and his companions. On one field trip, they walked to the Cotton Tree. "We stared openmouthed at the huge tree that we had seen only on the back of currency," he wrote. "We now stood under it at the intersection of Siaka Stevens Street and Pademba Road, the center of the city." One of his companions, who'd seen pretty much everything war had on offer, thought of their friends still caught up in combat as he took in the towering green cathedral: "No one will believe us when we tell them this."[39]

Even were God dead—and what child soldier doesn't have the right to conclude as much?—the fact these boys raised their faces in wonder at the living monument reminds us that faith is hope in things unseen. Not faith in the permanence of a national symbol, but in a nurse's faith that the redemption of these children was worth fighting for.

As Ishmael Beah and his friends marveled at the Cotton Tree rising from the center of Freetown, hope was withering on the vine across the country and among refugees hoping to return to it. By early 1997, according to the United Nations—which had launched an effort to bring home those displaced beyond national borders—there were 340,000 Sierra Leonean refugees in Guinea, 120,000 in Liberia (where Charles Taylor had just announced himself a candidate in presidential elections), and tens of thousands more scattered across Mali, Nigeria, the Ivory Coast, and Guinea-Bissau.

These were the numbers of officially registered displaced persons; the number fleeing to the Guinean side of the Kissi Triangle was significantly larger. (At one point, the majority of those living in Macenta District were refugees.) Repatriation efforts were abandoned during the first weeks of May, when humanitarian agencies and UN staff began to retreat as they, too, were targeted by rebels, sobels, and other armed groups. A murderous merry-go-round continued to spin in the east, throwing off gems and conflict like a nightmare pipe of kimberlite. Pitched battles between the army and the Kamajors—erstwhile allies—left close to a hundred dead in Kenema alone. Bo, the largest city to the east, was also fiercely contested. As for peace in Freetown, the auguries were poor. Executive Outcomes' prediction of another coup was about to come true, and right on schedule.

On May 25, 1997, elements of the armed forces joined the RUF to topple President Kabbah in the course of an explosive attack on refugee-packed Freetown. It was this long-prophesied sobel coup that led, in Lansana Gberie's words, "to a complete normative collapse."[40] The attack began when sobels used antitank rockets to blast open the gates of Pademba Road Prison, springing hundreds of soldiers detained on charges of sedition. Hearing fell voices in the air, the clatter of automatic weapons, and the thud of mortars, Kabbah—his Nigerian guard quickly overwhelmed—fled to Conakry in a helicopter. Members of his cabinet were arrested by sobels now more or less under the command of Major Johnny Paul Koroma, one of those army officers stashed in Pademba.

Major Koroma was described by one British journalist as "largely unknown even inside the country."[41] Some within Her Majesty's army must have known him, however, since he'd been the beneficiary of training at their famous military academy in Sandhurst. And even if most Sierra Leoneans couldn't pick him out of a lineup, Koroma boasted a strong sobel pedigree, having been implicated in previous insurrectionary plots and the looting of the headquarters of the Sierra Rutile mines. His first executive order, issued on national radio, was to ban Kamajor and other civilian militias; his second demanded the liberation and repatriation of Foday Sankoh, recently detained in Nigeria on charges of gunrunning. The worst part of it, for many who had braved mutilation and death to vote, with whatever limbs remained to them, was that military officers and the RUF had clearly planned and carried out the coup together.

That's the thing about coups, as a friend observed about one in Haiti: they don't just happen. Many of the sobels responsible for its opening salvos, Arthur Abraham has written, were from the army's Kailahun barracks, which the RUF had infiltrated and coached using (it would seem) the Taylor playbook:

> The nature of the take-over conformed exactly to the standard
> RUF carbon-copy from Charles Taylor's National Patriotic Front of
> Liberia doomsday manual: indiscriminate looting and destruction of
> that which could not be looted; disregard for all diplomatic immunity
> in the looting process; raping of women (a sore point in Freetown)
> and harassing of civilians; recruitment through jail breaks; use of
> civilian clothing as camouflage; communication through gun shots;
> battle cries mostly in Liberian dialects; graffiti-like death squad
> inscriptions and death angels painted on vehicles and walls.[42]

As regards previous attacks to the east, it had been possible for some in Freetown to argue (at least with a good poker face) that these were rebel, not army, tactics. Now the capital's more insular citizens—including prosperous Creoles, Lebanese, and expatriates—could see for themselves that those who used these tactics had just seized the ship of state. This meant the sobel alliance had access to a new cache of weapons. The unmasked army invited the RUF in to use them, and to loot the city.

As the end of civilian rule in Sierra Leone was condemned across West Africa, and by governments around the world, the bush-Freetown alliance now taking power faced stiff resistance only from ECOMOG and the rebranded Kamajors, who were increasingly revealed to have little in common with Mende hunting societies. Although the Nigerian guard responsible for Kabbah's security had been swiftly overrun on May 25, Nigerian commanders were determined to beat back the marauders. On day four of the coup, the peacekeepers fought off yet another attempt to seize the Lungi airfield. Although the affray was sharp, they held on to the runway, enabling Britain to evacuate 392 of its citizens, and sundry others, on a Boeing 747. The jumbo jet required every inch of tarmac for lift-off.

Outnumbered ECOMOG forces were soon pushed back to a smaller patch of Lungi. In Freetown, the peacekeepers retreated to their headquarters in a hotel and conference center built for diplomats before the war. The generals huddled in Abuja, dispatching more troops from their Liberian bases, decided to send in the big guns. Two amphibious assault ships, close to three hundred feet long and bristling with antiaircraft batteries and heavy machine guns, steamed toward Sierra Leone, where the seven-story Mammy Yoko towered over the neighborhood. (The warships had been involved in previous ECOMOG operations, including the epic evacuation of seventy-two thousand Liberian refugees to Nigeria.) As the vessels throttled west, rebels and their sleeper cells had moved in from the east and north to loot the city. Once the commercial districts had been picked clean, some of the rebels made for the hotel.

The Mammy Yoko was a rich target, and appeared to be a soft one. A few days after the coup, the hotel was packed. Although lightly defended, it had been designated as the staging point for the rescue of AMCITs, and others deemed worthy, in the obscurely titled Operation Noble Obelisk. To this end, President Clinton sent in the really big guns: the USS *Kearsarge*, a floating airfield and military base almost a thousand feet long, was redirected north from the shores of the Congo, where a coup against Mobutu had just taken place. (Zaire had just become, in name at least, the Democratic Republic of the Congo.) Though far more modest than Nigerian rescue efforts in Liberia, Noble Obelisk would prove to be one of the largest noncombatant evacuations in U.S. military history.

The operation didn't sound like much at first. Noble Obelisk's commanders had been instructed to rescue about four hundred civilians from the Mammy Yoko and ferry them to Guinea. But by May 30, as the *Kearsarge* drew close enough to Lumley to launch helicopters and marines, the U.S. embassy had fielded requests from more than forty governments for safe passage of their citizens to Conakry, and an advance team sent to the hotel found "over 2,000 people present and more arriving."[43]

The Mammy Yoko was where I'd first met Ibrahim Kamara, and heard him toast Yabom Koroma and their fellow Ebola survivors within earshot of scores of public-health professionals dispatched to join the fight against the virus then surging through the city. A very different crowd, and a different fear, inhabited the hotel on May 30, 1997. When the sun rose that morning, the Mammy Yoko sheltered not public-health specialists, but a small contingent of Nigerian peace-keepers, hundreds of terrified expatriates, perhaps as many Sierra Leoneans with dual nationalities or homes abroad, a handful of diplomats and reporters, scores of well-to-do Lebanese businessmen and their families, and an anxious staff.

Also tucked away in the hotel, and elsewhere in the city, were a handful of "security experts." Some had been engaged until recently with Executive Outcomes, others were vying for its contract to train and equip the civilian militias coalescing under the Kamajor brand, and still others were guarding their clients' investments in gold and diamond mines. One of these experts, formerly of the British Special Forces, had the misfortune to show up in Sierra Leone nine days before the coup. His passport was seized during a sobel raid on the headquarters of a planned operation to strengthen the shapeshifting Kamajors, whom he was to help train and arm with the contents of the ar-mories suddenly in the hands of the bush-Freetown alliance. Now he had turned his attention to extracting his team and himself from Sierra Leone.

Fleeing Sierra Leone wasn't a straightforward matter. It would take cash to escape, the Briton believed, whether by boat or by chopper. To acquire some, he'd reached out to a friend of a friend for a loan. This proved to be the manager and part-owner of the Mammy Yoko, so he went there in hopes of collecting some, and bolting. He described the scene that awaited him:

> There were hundreds of people milling around in the lobby and in
> the drive outside the hotel . . . They were all getting ready for the
> American evacuation . . . In fine contrast, more hundreds of locals

were hanging around outside the hotel on the road and among the trees in the hollow ground on the opposite side of the road. They sensed something was going to happen at the hotel and there was a buzz of excited chatter.[44]

Separating those inside the gates from those hanging around the perimeter with unknown (but troubling) intent was a group of Nigerian soldiers. Watching them triage passports and fight back the crowd, the former British special forces soldier termed them "arrogant," but he must have known they, too, were terrified: with large parts of the city looted and burned, and many of their fellows killed or taken hostage, the Mammy Yoko was a dangerous place for anyone in a Nigerian uniform.

Many of the hotel's unexpected guests had arrived with not only their valuables and cash but also with their children. Edgar Thomas, the future chief financial officer of Partners In Health in Sierra Leone, was among those trying to get into the hotel to get out. Born to an American mother and a Sierra Leonean father, Thomas and his younger brother—then fourteen and twelve, respectively—were hustled to the Mammy Yoko in order to be there well before 8:00 a.m., when processing for the first airlift to the *Kearsarge* was to begin. "We received the announcement that all Americans were to go down to the beach," recalled Thomas in 2015.

> I was with my mom and brother as we argued who was going to go, who was going to stay. It was still dark. We were scared when we left the house, but we wanted to stay with our dad to protect it. Our mom said "No way, boys." The rebels had declared they were going to fight the Americans. We were all scared that more civilians were going to be caught in the cross fire.

With more than a thousand refugees, guests, and staff cowering in and around the hotel, fear of civilians caught in cross fire was entirely reasonable. It had been the war's signature from the outset.

As the Thomas family reached the Mammy Yoko, a nervous line of Nigerian soldiers was still trying to hold back a surging crowd. Edgar recalled the scene awaiting them as the sun climbed in a blackened sky:

> The city had already been assaulted for days, and there was smoke coming from around the beach next to the Mammy Yoko. We saw uniformed soldiers on the beach, but it wasn't until we saw white faces that we knew they were Americans and not sobels. The sobels had ceased their attacks, but we could see them with their shoulder-mounted RPGs. The Americans had snipers on the roof. They processed us at the hotel and airlifted us to the aircraft carrier. They just checked our passports and to see if we had any weapons, but it took hours to process everyone, and all night to reach Conakry.

Thomas and his brother worried about their father, who remained behind, but were no longer frightened once aboard the carrier. "You saw the full force of the Americans and felt safe," he recalled years later. (Our exchange occurred in the dining room of the rehabbed Mammy Yoko.) "All their military might was on display in huge hangars, and they invited the kids to come see it. One young soldier from North Carolina, who was showing us tanks and weapons, asked us, 'What the hell's going on over there?' He had no idea why they'd been sent to Sierra Leone."

The colossal carrier, which thanks to its choppers and landing craft could remain just over the horizon, couldn't take all the AMCITs and other expatriate civilians to Conakry in a single run. On May 31, the *Kearsarge* reversed course to make a second rescue the following morning. The French navy had by then evacuated hundreds of Europeans in a corvette stationed off the coast, and similar operations brought the total of rescued expatriates to three thousand. But the 162-bed Mammy Yoko still had more than a thousand refugees crammed in the basement and lower floors. The hotel was now surrounded by insurgents; they eyed it hungrily (as did the vultures congregated in the stand of trees just across from the compound gates). The former

British special forces soldier, having obtained the cash to escape in a boat to Conakry, was suddenly face-to-face with three rebels who burst into the lobby:

> Maybe 200 people stood frozen where they were, lying on the floor among their luggage, sitting on the few chairs or boxes they had brought, or standing in groups talking, and they were all staring at the front entrance. There, by the glass doors, were three rebels, glaring round at everyone, in filthy mixed combats and civvy shirts, one in a skirt. Two carried AKs and the third carried an RPG.[45]

The insurgents, having scoped out the scene, slipped back out the door as fear mounted inside, and chaos without. The real assault would begin later.

On June 2, the Nigerians attacked the sobels by sea. "Nigerian warships off Sierra Leone bombarded the capital today," reported the *Washington Post* correspondent. The rebels, in turn, "attacked Nigerian troops defending a luxury hotel full of foreigners seeking to flee the city." The Mammy Yoko was growing less luxurious by the minute. Guests, staff, and refugees "scurried to the hotel's basement and hid as attacking Sierra Leoneans fired rifles into the building, shattering windows in the lower floors."[46] The British military contractor, pinned down on the hotel's roof with what was left of the Nigerian contingent, heard the familiar and reassuring sound of a gunship. It proved to be one of the Russian Hinds favored by Executive Outcomes. But its pilots were now sobels; he and other rooftop defenders were its targets.

It wasn't rifles or gunships that threatened to roast those sheltered below them. The Freetown-bush alliance now had military-grade machine guns and plenty of RPGs, and grenades launched through shattered windows gave the hotel's bucket brigade plenty of fires to extinguish. As those awaiting rescue headed toward the basement, the Mammy Yoko's owner-manager called contacts in Washington to announce parts of the hotel were in flames, with hundreds still sheltered in the basement. By then, he reported, two Nigerian soldiers had "been killed, a British military liaison officer had been shot, the temperature in the basement was over 100 degrees, and people were suffering from dehydration."[47] Aware that their fellows inside were under attack, Nigerian commanders directed a sustained barrage on other parts of the city, including the headquarters of the pariah junta. The shelling missed the military barracks in western Freetown, but, according to certain journalists and staff at Connaught, killed close to a hundred civilians.

The bombardment had begun, recalled Bailor Barrie, then in his first year of medical school, just after dawn. "There were hundreds of sobels around the Mammy Yoko," he told me, "but they were all over the rest of the city, too. Many of the bombs were aimed at the area not far from Lumley Beach." One needn't be a medical student to offer a grim prognosis for Freetown, which is why all those who could were trying to flee. Barrie, who was plenty hostile to the RUF, had nonetheless joined hundreds protesting the Nigerian assault perilously close to the hotel. When asked why he chose to join them, he credited an opposition leader who'd polled behind Kabbah in the recent elections:

> He was very well educated, a doctor, had lectured at Harvard,
> and was a professor at Fourah Bay College. He said that the exiled
> government had invited the Nigerian government to come and bomb
> the city, and that people should not sit and see Freetown destroyed
> because of politics. They should find ways to negotiate with the
> rebels. It may not have been possible to negotiate with them, but I
> subscribed to the idea that talks were better than bombs.

Barrie wasn't alone in this view, but the city was thick with heavily armed belligerents who couldn't come to terms.

The commander of Operation Noble Obelisk deemed the once-luxurious Mammy Yoko too dangerous a rendezvous, but hinted he'd be back for a third and last rescue. Those onboard the *Kearsarge* could follow events on the ground thanks to surveillance aircraft invisible from the ground. The British military contractor, having escaped the roof, was patched through to the Americans to request their help. He described the neighborhood and requested an airstrike against an RUF command post targeting the

Mammy Yoko from a few hundred yards away. A few minutes after the U.S. commander politely explained that Operation Noble Obelisk's rules of engagement prohibited such strikes, the sobel nest was vaporized by a laser-guided missile.

It didn't take long, however, for a new wave of sobels to resume their attack. The British high commissioner, as its ambassador is termed, was in regular communication with the American chargé d'affaires as she went about reassuring frightened civilians. (The U.S. ambassador was meeting evacuees in Conakry when the Mammy Yoko was attacked.) The high commissioner also made contact with his compatriot within the hotel, who informed him that the Nigerians had run out of ammo. A sobel coup seems not to have been on ECOMOG's radar just then. Its commanders in Abuja and Monrovia were likely distracted by the looming prospect of Charles Taylor in the Liberian presidential palace.

Awaiting reinforcements, the dispirited Nigerians within the Mammy Yoko faced hundreds of heavily armed sobels as they surrounded the hotel. Many of the civilians still trapped inside were panicked. It wasn't clear who was in charge of either Sierra Leone or the defense of the Mammy Yoko. Several of the Lebanese businessmen within were cutting deals for their own safe conduct through sobel lines. The high commissioner traded threats with the sobels in order to convince them to hold their fire long enough to evacuate the civilians, but the rebels' initial response was neither heartening nor diplomatic: Let the Americans dare to come ashore! They'd already taught the Nigerians a lesson, or were about to!

The high commissioner knew how to throw shade right back. Signaling an invisible but clearly lethal aircraft carrier offshore to sobels uninformed about U.S. rules of engagement during civilian rescues, the British diplomat threatened to "call in a U.S. bombardment from nearby American naval units if they did not stop the attack on the hotel."[48] The envoy's threat, and the mysteriously smart bombing of the rebel nest, worked long enough for foreign nationals within to escape—although there was bitter debate when the Briton with serious firearm skills refused to follow the International Committee of the Red Cross out the front door. He led the majority of the

Mammy Yoko refugees to relative safety via the back door to a hotel farther down the beach. The next morning, the gallant high commissioner joined 1,261 other civilians boarding helicopters to the *Kearsarge*. As the carrier lumbered north of White Man's Bay into the open Atlantic and north toward Conakry, the U.S. State Department announced the ship would not be returning.

The Nigerian contingent inside the Mammy Yoko was trapped and outgunned, and most of their white-human shields were now on the *Kearsarge*. As ECOMOG troops stationed in Monrovia began reaching Freetown by helicopter, sobel forces took many of them hostage. Detained peacekeepers wouldn't be storming any hotels. The Nigerians had scrambled their alpha jets and proceeded to bomb what they claimed were sobel positions. But airstrikes weren't likely to free the men defending the hotel, either: the sobel alliance had taken the trouble to mount an antiaircraft gun on top of the nearby Freetown Golf Club. Although many hotel staff escaped under an RUF banner hastily crafted from bed sheets, most soldiers trapped inside did not. Those still alive surrendered to rebel forces, who proceeded to enter and pillage the Mammy Yoko.

There's little doubt that some of the Nigerians who fell during the siege of the Mammy Yoko and elsewhere in the city were killed by ammunition and ordnance from countries contributing troops to ECOMOG. But much of the ammo was reserved for civilians. Bailor Barrie was still with a group of students demonstrating around Family Kingdom—probably the only amusement park in Sierra Leone, by then the least fun place on Earth:

> I was standing there with a friend from my neighborhood—he was a
> student at Fourah Bay—chanting, "We want peace, we want peace."
> I saw him fall down, and then everyone scattered. I took a quick
> look, saw the blood oozing, and ran away. I couldn't help him. I don't
> know where the gunfire came from. I later learned he died.

The Mammy Yoko remained standing, unlike many other structures—and unlike many civilians who found no refuge in the weeks during which the battle for Freetown raged. Arson and looting remained the order of the day.

Government buildings, the Treasury and Central Bank among them, were pillaged, then set afire. So were many commercial banks, retail businesses, and the homes of officials in the Kabbah government.

In the heart of Freetown, the Cotton Tree stood watch over the smoking city.

The month of June 1997 saw daily clashes between embittered ECOMOG forces (sometimes in the company of the Kamajors and other militias) and sobels. As diplomats and heads of state called for more peace talks, civilians with no recourse to airlifts fled the city—on foot, by boat, and in *poda podas*—by the tens of thousands. Looting continued as Major Koroma demanded that Foday Sankoh, still detained in Nigeria, be installed as his regime's number two.

The pillage hadn't been all big-ticket: the chief justice's wigs and Koran were stolen on June 9; Koroma was sworn in as head of state on June 17. There couldn't have been many foreign delegations in attendance, since most embassies in Freetown were shuttered in protest. ECOWAS, the West African equivalent of the European Union and the mother of ECOMOG, condemned the coup, of course. So did American, British, and UN authorities. Within Sierra Leone, Koroma was vocally opposed by prodemocracy civilians and threatened by rival factions and wannabe warlords. But several African nations—Burkina Faso, Libya, and the Ivory Coast were most often named, along with Taylor's chunk of Liberia—were widely thought complicit in deposing Kabbah. In spite of near-universal condemnation of the coup, the junta proved difficult to dislodge. What was left of Sierra Leone was stuck with a government in exile and a dyed-in-the-wool sobel claiming to be head of state.

Although soldiers and rebels had morphed into sobels to overthrow Kabbah, ECOMOG remained pledged to beat back the RUF. Neither the Nigerians nor the reconfigured Kamajors let up because a bewiggèd judge swore in a sobel president with a stolen Koran. Some portion of the army remained loyal to democratic rule, but no one knew how large that portion was. Though often less well-armed than the insurgents, civilian militias—who likely outnumbered the combined strength of the army and the RUF—bested the sobels in pitched battles in Kenema, Bo, and other towns to the south and east. But it was the Nigerians who expelled RUF looters from Freetown. Their scorched-earth tactics helped reduce the battered capital "to a smoking, corpse-filled hull of a city," as Greg Campbell observed, "but they did chase the RUF back to the bush to defend their diamond mines."[49]

These efforts did not, however, restore constitutional rule in the person of the deposed Tejan Kabbah. That would require unilateral military action from Nigeria, after months of fruitless parley. In the interim, and from east to west, the country was in a parlous way. Freetown was without electricity for close to a month after the coup, and other cities for longer. Nor did the government put in place by the army's sobel and lumpen elements place a high priority on either public health or clinical services. A year before the first sobel attack on Freetown, an estimated 16 percent of Sierra Leone's health centers were functioning, although many had been reopened after Kabbah's election. They were almost all shuttered after the coup. The public hospitals in Koidu and Kenema had been reduced to burned-out husks, as had several other district hospitals.

Attempts to repair the wounds of war, or the afflictions to which all flesh is heir, faltered, then failed. Unlike the Mammy Yoko, the injured could not often be patched up and given a second life, since operating rooms and blood banks had been closed or pillaged or torched. So had labs. On June 26, 1997, health authorities in Makeni reported that over three hundred children had died of cholera or typhoid in the previous two days, but it was impossible to know either numbers or culprit pathogens. By then, the collapse of most of Sierra Leone's social, political, and economic institutions was complete. Marx and company said it best: all that is solid melts into air; all that is holy, profaned.

As factions and militias proliferated on both sides of the Mano, the young men (and women) who populated them easily shifted allegiances and bases of operations. After all, they needed to go where the jobs were, and the tools required for the work of war continued to flow into Upper West Africa. By July 1997, U.S. intelligence agencies estimated that there were up to eight million firearms in the region—more or less one for every man, woman, and child still drawing breath within the boundaries of Sierra Leone and Liberia. How else could tiny and ragtag forces like the nascent RUF and NPFL have come to control such a large and valuable piece of real estate? As the weapons of the weak came to include Kalashnikovs and RPGs, the dissolution of already strained social bonds between the young and those to whom they were once beholden ensued. How else could the warlords so rapidly pollute long-standing social institutions, such as the region's secret societies? How else could they force the collapse of social norms that long regulated land tenure, marriage, kinship, and age-grade hierarchies? How else, in the absence of rapid and radical transformation of an economy, does all that is solid melt into air?

Then again, the economy of Upper West Africa, moral and material, *had* been radically transformed by war. Patronage had always been part of the local political formula. But access to rifles, automatic weapons, grenade launchers, and the like helped to transform patronage politics into warlord politics. On July 19, to the astonishment of many following events in West Africa, Charles Taylor intimidated Liberian voters into electing him to the post he'd long sought by force of arms. (His chief opponent was Ellen Johnson Sirleaf, the finance minister who narrowly escaped the fate of most in William Tolbert's cabinet.) If Liberians didn't elect him, Taylor warned a war-weary electorate, they'd get no peace. He did not discourage the campaign slogan chanted by young supporters beholden to him: "He killed my ma, he killed my pa, I'll vote for him!" And they did.

It didn't seem that the conflict could be stopped, even after a modicum of calm returned to Freetown's streets and Taylor was finally in his palace. By 1997, war had become too profitable to those able to control the extractive trades to be stopped by accords struck ceremoniously in Guinea, Togo, the Ivory Coast, or Nigeria. These palavers led nowhere as long as back-room deals made in these same cities, and in Freetown and Monrovia, continued to offer the promise of handsome profits to big men able to goad expendable youth into fighting, and there were still, in the eyes of sobels and warlords, plenty of those. As larger factions fissioned into dozens more, just keeping up with the new acronyms, to say nothing of shifting allegiances, proved challenging. These splinter groups may have been short-lived, and long forgotten by most. But that doesn't mean they were small or of little consequence.

Nor did their evanescence mean these factions had no history deeper than that unearthed by journalists allotted neither the time nor space to cover anything other than the most spectacular mayhem. A group called Ulimo-K (not to be confused with its rival, Ulimo-J) established training camps, ran its own customs and immigration service, and counted more than five thousand under arms by the mid-1990s. Based in northern Liberia, an island of resistance to Taylor, Ulimo-K consisted heavily of "Mandingo traders"— most reports made it sound as if all Mandingos were traders—with recent memories of mistreatment at Taylor's hands and the older grievance of being considered foreigners within a country they'd inhabited prior to its founding.[50] Their alliance with Guinean army officers claiming similar ethnic roots facilitated access to a mother lode of weapons and allowed Ulimo-K to take revenge on those whose birtherism had pushed said Mandingos out of Liberia in previous years, and to take over towns where they had no historical rights of residence.

The biggest Liberian faction was the NPFL, and Charles Taylor was the biggest profiteer. Harbel may have been restored to Firestone, but Taylor no longer needed it once he'd seized the necessary infrastructure elsewhere, which occurred well before his election. During the years the Nigerians kept him out of the palace, Taylor saw himself the leader of what he called Greater Liberia, which apparently included the diamond fields of Sierra Leone. He knew an army of indentured porters and diamond mules couldn't replace ships, planes, and trucks, which required deepwater ports, airfields, and some semblance of roads. Taylorland came to include all of these, as well as its own central bank, into which flowed cash from multinational commercial concerns.

These weren't small sums, as the U.S. ambassador to Liberia reported in congressional testimony: "Between 1990 and 1994, Liberia's diamond exports averaged $300 million per year; timber exports $53 million; rubber exports $27 million; and gold exports $1 million." Doing the tally, the envoy reckoned that Taylor "could have upwards of $75 million a year passing through his hands as a result of taxes levied on these trades."[51] This total included Firestone's contributions, which some back at headquarters worried might violate the U.S. Foreign Corrupt Practices Act. But it didn't count a brisk international trade in marijuana and other drugs, which were also for local consumption by combatants with slender confidence in amulets, invisibility cloaks, and protective spells.

As for the administrative skills required to keep up the looting—since warriors, thralls, and other laborers couldn't very well eat hardwoods, rubber, or diamonds—and to keep the looters in weapons and ammo, the American ambassador had this to say to Congress:

> Most of the Liberian faction leaders and their associates have spent
> many years in the U.S., often as students, temporary workers, even as
> permanent residents. They own property, own or operate businesses,
> and more importantly, they know how the U.S. system works and
> how to make it work for them.[52]

The warlords also knew how the Liberian system worked, the better to strip it bare. The factions' day-to-day operations were assured, concluded the diplomat, by "members of the same relatively small group of politicians and technocrats who have dominated public life in Liberia since the 1970s, and who tasted power for the first time under Samuel Doe."[53]

Once Taylor was Liberia's duly elected head of state, the NPFL had vowed to lay down its arms. But elections couldn't end the war. By the time it was finally over, NPFL leaders could claim that more than two hundred thousand had carried arms for Taylor's faction. Hyperbole aside, not bad for a millenarian fugitive who invaded his country with a hundred or so fighters.

Meanwhile, back in Sierra Leone, the imperial powers successfully rebranded as Western democracies began to enforce an ECOWAS embargo on petroleum and weapons, as well as trade sanctions, against Koroma and the gang. The RUF's amputation campaign, rather than coups and postcoup purges and the general misery, had finally led to an international outcry about blood diamonds; even blinkered executives of the diamond cartel had scrambled their PR teams. But international clamor from West Africa's former colonial powers is not what restored civilian rule in Freetown.

The high command in Abuja was outraged and humiliated by the setbacks of 1997, and their officers and troops based in Sierra Leone were stricken by the heavy casualties among their ranks. Their official pronouncements about negotiations may have sounded gung-ho, but ECOMOG's force commanders had zero faith in the value of diplomacy with the Freetown sobels. Although Major Koroma sought to fill what remained of the capital's administrative apparatus, there was no way the Nigerians would tolerate them for long. Within a few months of the coup, Abuja had trebled its force to ten thousand; with Taylor in his palace, more troops were redeployed from Liberia to Sierra Leone. So why should they back down before the uniformed allies of the cross-dressing insurgents who'd killed or captured their comrades, including members of Kabbah's presidential guard and the Mammy Yoko martyrs? When, during the course of November parleys in Abidjan between the exiled Kabbah and Foday Sankoh, Koroma declared his intention to hand over power sometime in 2001, the Nigerians replied by bombing the junta's headquarters.

By January 1998, Major-President Koroma and his pariah junta had been largely deprived of the RUF wildlings, at least in Freetown, and had failed to win either popular support or diplomatic recognition. It was then that Nigeria decided to strike, launching a nine-day blitz from the east to unseat Koroma and restore Kabbah. The force met little resistance in the city, but an estimated five hundred thousand civilians were pushed west toward the sea, and left without food, water, or shelter. The Pottery Barn rule—you break it, you own it—did not prevail: the Nigerians were unable or unwilling to prevent widespread looting and revenge killings. As Kamajor and other militias harried the sobels to the east, Koroma was rumored to be seeking asylum in Liberia, and fled for parts unknown in mid-February. On March 10, the weary Nigerians, having wrenched the ruined capital from the sobels and their treasonous leaders, summoned Tejan Kabbah back to the presidential palace.

President Kabbah's restoration led promptly to the arrest of about two thousand for alleged collaboration with the sobel junta. Some of them, including twenty-four officers from the army's high command, were executed for treason. With Freetown deemed sobel-free, Foday Sankoh was extradited for trial there. "If ever the sordid tale of Sierra Leone should have ended," Greg Campbell wrote, "it should have ended there."[54] But it was not to be, even after October 23, when Sankoh was sentenced to death for treason. War crimes did not figure in the charges against the original sobel gangster; neither did his collusion with Charles Taylor in supplying the RUF. This may have come as a relief to some in the diamond cartel, and other extractive industries, and within certain West African governments. But in Freetown and beyond, many were spooked by Sankoh's presence, even behind bars. No earthly prison, these citizens reasoned, was secure enough for human leopards like him and Taylor.

A rotating parade of diplomats, peace brokers, and relief workers—likely oblivious to at least some of the previous failed attempts to bring to book the oft-jailed and oft-sprung pair—dismissed such fears as native superstition. Native or not, civilians and refugees across the region had ample reason for fear, while confident claims from international peace brokers might more reasonably be dismissed as superstition. As 1998 waned, peace certainly hadn't yet been brokered. Freetown was quiet, and progovernment forces controlled Kabala and Koinadugu (Kamajor strongholds), all of Kambia and Tonkolili Districts, and parts of Port Loko. But five large towns in the north, including Lunsar and Makeni, were in sobel hands, as were Koidu and its nearby diamond fields. Rebel forces were again moving west, as the people of Bantoro learned in October, when that village was added to the long list of those destroyed by rebels and sobels.

The Kabbah administration tried to reassure fearful citizens that at least Freetown and most of the western parts of the country were firmly under ECOMOG control. Thousands of civilians took Kabbah and the force commanders at their word and abandoned disputed districts in favor of the war-swollen capital. Yabom Koroma and other Bantoro survivors were among them. Their dispersal—to the city and elsewhere in Sierra Leone, to Guinea, and later back to rebuild Bantoro—would subsequently constitute pathways for Ebola's spread. But Yabom and her family then feared fevers less than feuds. In spite of coup the third and ECOMOG's collateral damage, many in Freetown believed Nigeria could protect them. After all, almost a quarter of its armed forces had invested Sierra Leone by New Year's, when ECOMOG forces counted close to twenty thousand troops. The Kamajors and sundry antisobel militias, regrouped in the south and east and increasingly armed with modern munitions, were said to number thirty thousand.

What could go wrong?

Quite a lot, it turns out. In contrast to many of its victims, the RUF had a couple more tricks up its sleeves. West African standing armies from Niger to Burkina Faso—and by some reports rogue units in Guinea and Nigeria—continued to sell and smuggle arms and ammo to various factions in Sierra Leone and Liberia after ECOWAS and Western powers tightened the arms embargo. As usual, one trick up RUF sleeves was Charles Taylor, his election certified legit by Jimmy Carter and others concerning themselves with the proper conduct of elections in strife-torn nations. That meant Taylor had a presidential plane, one of several ways the quartermaster of conflict skirted the embargo. In addition to his assistance with procurement, an area of expertise since the Doe days, Liberia's head of state helped the RUF, once locked and loaded, to orchestrate Operation No Living Thing.

This was the bush-Freetown alliance's big push to seize the ship of state by replacing the elected captain and crew (native and imported) with their own, and killing anyone in their way. In official chronologies as in popular memory, this second sack of Freetown began on the morning of January 6, 1999, with an assault on Freetown's East End neighborhoods. But Operation No Living Thing was in fact the culmination of a month of attacks on ECOMOG positions in Port Loko and other towns along the overland route to Guinea, and on government posts on the eastern and northern fringes of the capital. One of the most reliably targeted sites was the international airport in Lungi, but on December 31 the rebels also attacked the Hastings airfield, the heart of the old colony and only fifteen miles from central Freetown. ECOMOG spokesmen claimed the insurgents had been swiftly beaten back, if not so swiftly they couldn't try to torch the newly rebuilt Hastings Police Academy and nine other government buildings.

At 3:00 a.m. on January 4, sobel forces again targeted the Hastings airfield and other government structures still standing. The assault on the city's fringes occurred even as the ranking ECOMOG commander claimed, on national radio, to have "effectively thrown a security dragnet around the capital." Freetown's residents, he added over the roar of alpha jets, "need not have any fear."[55] Similar assertions, including those claiming the barbarians had been routed outside the city gates, were soon revealed to be wishful thinking. As thousands of insurgents reached the feebly beating heart of Sierra Leone's central administration, they set fire to the Nigerian embassy, naturally, and to police headquarters. The sobels then headed to Pademba Road Prison, where they freed political detainees—largely mutinous soldiers—and common criminals alike. Foday Sankoh wasn't there, having been spirited to an undisclosed location. The next targets, announced the RUF, would be the State House, Wilberforce Barracks (another ECOMOG keep), and—of course—the Lungi airfield. In popular memory, at least, the rebels and sobels tried to seize Lungi no fewer than twenty-three times during the course of the war.

President Kabbah, claiming the rebels had also burned down Fourah Bay College and the former State House, called for a cease-fire and parley. But the assault continued. According to Sebastian Junger, veteran of many battle zones, "War does not get worse than January 6, 1999."[56] I'll leave it to historians— and to Junger and other credible observers of Operation No Living Thing—to back up this claim, as well as to describe in detail the indiscriminate horror of the campaign. It was again straight out of Taylor's doomsday playbook, and of colonial ones, but the RUF and sobels were by then plenty practiced in these methods. Medical care remained pretty much absent by the time the battle for Freetown was once again joined. (Public-health measures, even unwelcome ones, were a distant memory.) With the exception of ECOMOG losses, the body count among combatants was difficult to know. But more than six thousand civilians were killed during the course of Operation No Living Thing and in quelling it.

The second battle for Freetown had no certain outcome when it began, even though Nigerian-led forces had the numerical and tactical advantage. But they'd long ago started down the path of demoralization that follows the diagnosis of a quagmire. By January 1999, they were clearly in one. The Sierra Leonean operation was costing Abuja about a million dollars a day and was increasingly unpopular at home. Many Nigerian troops, from poor families and pursuing the only path out of poverty available to them, were exhausted by long deployments and short supplies; even their boots and uniforms were falling apart. Poor morale was also evident among officers, who made fatal errors in planning and communication during the battle. These led not only to a failure to protect the city but also to major losses among the ranks under their command: almost a thousand Nigerians were killed in the course of Operation No Living Thing.[57]

Such sacrifice hadn't endeared ECOMOG to the citizenry, in part because of its heavy-handed tactics. No Living Thing left many Nigerian troops resentful of the people they were protecting. Then again, "ECOMOG" was the one-acronym answer, unlovely as it may sound, as to why Charles Taylor couldn't take Liberia's executive mansion by force during five years of no-holds-barred fighting and in spite of much public torture and murder of civilians. "Nigerians" would be the best one-word answer to the question of how sobels controlling much of Sierra Leone were twice repulsed from Freetown. ECOMOG had served as a bulwark against the anarchy of the warlords, but it wasn't even clear (some Nigerians seethed) that civilians preferred their protection to rule by self-appointed and violent homegrown juntas. A number of vocal Sierra Leoneans had the effrontery to note that Nigeria was itself ruled by one of those.

The second sobel invasion of Freetown found Bailor Barrie in his second year of oft-interrupted medical training. Like most city residents unable to flee—his hometown, Makeni, was then in rebel hands—Barrie cowered inside until necessity drove him and two of his cousins into civilian-free streets to forage. "We went out looking for rice in the third week of January, and you could still see dead bodies everywhere," he told me. "The center of town reeked of death and houses were smoking ruins. But we were so hungry." On their way home with a few cups of rice, Barrie and his cousins passed by still-standing Connaught Hospital, which was of course also Barrie's classroom.

Nigerians on full alert were deployed there, and across the city. Most were angry about their losses, many were frightened, and some were trigger-happy. A goodly number were all three.

Since the sobels could be anyone, and because the Nigerians knew they were unpopular in many quarters, they looked for any evidence of affiliation with the RUF, including scars like the ones mentioned by Ishmael Beah. Aside from standing next to a friend felled by an unknown sniper during the first battle for Freetown, or his perilous escape to Guinea by boat, the closest Barrie came to dying during the war was when a notorious Nigerian officer patrolling the area around Connaught saw the mark left by Barrie scalding himself making coffee in an effort to stay awake to study:

> People out in the streets would be stripped by the Nigerians to look
> for scars, especially fresh scars. "You're RUF! Give me six feet!"
> And then they'd fire. When this happened to me, my cousins started
> to plead with the soldier, but if they didn't shut up, they would also
> get shot. I was saved by the guy working at the morgue where we
> did dissection—he came running out yelling my name. "Do you
> know him?" the Nigerian asked. "Yes! He's a medical student!" The
> Nigerian kicked me in the butt and told me to bugger off.

Other students weren't so lucky, but ECOMOG wasn't often to blame. Njala University College lay in ruins, having been sacked twice by the RUF in 1995. During Operation No Living Thing, Fourah Bay College was pillaged by sobels. In this instance, Kabbah's claim was mostly true: the red-brick buildings of the old campus were put to the torch. Its wooden floors and rafters burned better than concrete boxes like the Mammy Yoko.

Arthur Abraham, Fourah Bay's director of African studies and one of the world's foremost historians of Mende-speakers like Sengbe Pieh and the real Kamajor hunting societies, had already fled to a green and stately American university. But many students and lecturers from both Njala and Fourah Bay had been raped or killed, or both. For years, the charred remains of both institutions were inhabited by squatters and ghosts. Higher education, like health care, had been snuffed out in the former Athens of West Africa.

Throughout these years of profound insecurity, many affected by it—and who wasn't?—continued to speak anxiously of raids, bombs, deadly cross fire, and machetes. Weapons, and tools turned into them, worked in the traditional ways: the ability to end lives in a second, the threat of death ever-present, fear oozing into everyday life like latex sap. Those with weapons and those without them kept open a second front. Muslim or Christian, partisan or neutral, civilian or militia or army (or all three), people on both sides of the Mano River bemoaned spirit attacks, swears, sorcery, and witchcraft. Amulets, charms, and cowrie scapulars complemented less visible protectives.

As with Samuel Doe, and the Convivial Cannibal before him, Charles Taylor publicly cultivated connections to the spirit world. He sought to co-opt secret societies, including those banned or subjected to intense antisuperstition campaigns earlier in the century but openly embraced by Supreme Zo William Tubman and by Samuel Doe. (The latter's ultimately ineffective amulets were evident in his final filmed appearance.) Americo-Liberian Taylor—who was part Gola, though his only Liberian language was English—cultivated the leaders of these societies for political support but also for what most anthropologists regard as their primary portfolio: healing, concealment from one's enemies, and ritual protection through spells, elixirs, talismans, and the like. This was largely to embolden foot soldiers. Of course, an abundance of mind-altering drugs and the invincibility of youth helped. But these were temporary palliatives in the face of abundant evidence of youth vincibility.

Journalists from Europe and North America watched these proceedings, and elicited local commentary, with a mix of bemusement and fascinated revulsion. When reporting on Taylor, it was impossible for journalists to ignore the dark, supernatural world he so regularly invoked. "This gave him access to a world of unseen power and allowed him to project an aura of mystery and invincibility," wrote one Liberia-experienced *New York Times* correspondent. "Rumors that he practiced cannibalism, human sacrifice and blood atonement rituals merely added to his mystique."[58] Foday Sankoh tended to follow the Taylor playbook, if not in personal appearance (by 1999, in contrast to the natty Liberian, he sported a white beard and tangled dreadlocks), then in obscurantism.

If Sankoh was captured without visible talismans, some of his shock troops, like irregulars from Taylor's and other factions, were as lavishly festooned as the bush devils of yore. Bits of bone and shards of mirror and glass pleated into wigs and hair, fright masks, bizarre fashion accoutrements, layers of looted lingerie—it was hard not to stare in uncomprehending horror at the spectacle of the rebels. Antisobel forces were equally picturesque. Sebastian Junger described the Kamajors for the readers of *Vanity Fair*:

> They had come from the bush, these men, and they'd brought with them their protective magic and their claims of special powers. They wore sackcloth tunics and fishnet shirts studded with crocheted pouches that were supposed to stop bullets. They sewed cowrie shells onto their clothing and wore bone necklaces that hung down over their ammo belts and clacked against their guns. One guy had nothing on but shorts and a pink ski-parka hood.[59]

Other journalists still referred to these Kamajors, most of whom had not come from the bush and few of whom could be classed as hunters prior to the war, as the witchcraft battalion. It was a hard term to beat, even after anthropologists who'd spent years among the Mende in less disrupted times pointed out that many of the heavily armed and scantily clad boys and men were too young (and too high) to have learned the protective arts used to conceal hunters, homes, and entire settlements from witches and corporeal foes alike.

What did all this juju mean in the context of a war where someone in such a get-up might chop off hands or suddenly hoist a traditional grenade launcher? Rambo iconography and platinum wigs aside, there was much talk of the "ancient hatreds" of this progress-resistant and conflict-besotted part of West Africa. The violence was extreme enough, and to most eyes macabre enough, to trigger a wide echo of essentialist claims about the obvious deficiencies of an irrational and barbaric culture. Related doomsday claims focused on depletion of natural resources as the cause of the mayhem, and the shape of things to come in other parts of the world. In an influential 1994 essay in *The Atlantic Monthly*, faxed to U.S. embassies across Africa, the American commentator Robert Kaplan pinned much of the blame for allegedly tribal conflicts on overpopulation in the face of growing resource scarcity: depleted mineral wealth, shrinking forests, vanishing fauna, exhausted and overfarmed land. Past greed fed new grievance in Sierra Leone—which Kaplan deemed beyond salvage—and offered a foretaste of the "new barbarism" coming soon to a theater of war near you.[60]

Anthropologists and historians with experience or origins in West Africa disputed that the violence was a reflection of largely local struggles over scarce resources.[61] The region's natural bounty—flora, fauna, mineral—may have been shrinking, but it was also unsafe to hunt or gather and ever more unevenly shared. Bushmeat aside, most of it was for nonlocal consumption. Nor was barbarism new or native to Sierra Leone and Liberia. Unlike the Mende uprising or Hut Tax War a century earlier, however, the modern equivalent of Maxim guns were now in the hands of those who had once relied on spears, muskets, nets, and amulets. New trappings of battle dress were added to the old, just as automatic weapons and drugs were added to older arms and inducements to fight. But was this war really a rebellion or rather a war of theft, a trade war like the banditry associated with the slave trades? The battle to control the region's wealth engendered familiar claims of causality about premature death and sickness. Across the region, much misfortune was attributed to sorcery and witchcraft—native business—but even in war supernatural claims of causality were not without pointed reference to greed and theft, especially when part of the thievery involved the theft of labor.

As with accusations of ritual murder, allegations of illicit enrichment during the war were pointed as regards the unnatural means by which the greedy acquired the objects of their desire. These no longer included glass beads or shiny ribbons, but rather the same luxury items and services desired on either side of the Atlantic and equator. Writing at the height of the war, the anthropologist Rosalind Shaw reported that many of her Temne hosts

> described a prosperous city where skyscrapers adjoin houses of gold and diamonds; Mercedes-Benzes are driven down fine roads; street vendors roast "beefsticks" (kebabs) of human meat; boutiques sell stylish "witch gowns" that transform their wearers into animal predators in the human world; electronics stores sell tape recorders and televisions (and, more recently, VCRs and computers); and witch airports despatch witch planes—planes so fast, I was once told, that "they can fly to London and back within an hour"—to destinations all around the globe.[62]

In previous generations, such fanciful notions were portrayed or dismissed as native superstition. They're now often termed fabulist holdovers from a by-gone era. But even on the face of it, they're complex images, dense with local referents while global in sweep, and decidedly up to date.

The early ethnographers of West Africa (and many colonial officials) sought to explain the natives' commentaries and claims about the unseen world as "local beliefs." Back then, there were few attempts to tie responses to a ubiquitous question—Why do some people meet with misfortune while others are spared?—to the empirical and historically informed study of questions that were more than just quaintly local. There were too few attempts, in other words, to link the exotic to the mundane suffering that was the lot of so many, then as now. Much commentary on the war, and on the postwar Ebola epidemic, fits neatly into a similar template. In both cases, this suffering was often generated or amplified by forces that were anything but local. An anthropology focused exclusively on the local, and on tribal affiliations as the bedrock of social life, was at a loss to illuminate the workings of structural violence—and the causes of war.

That's what Shaw tries to remedy in considering her informants' elaborate confections, including the witch-city with its supersonic aircraft and other high-tech wizardry, in the context of the current misery. "It is common knowledge," she observed toward the end of the war, that

> the nation's mineral wealth has hemorrhaged into the overseas
> bank accounts of politicians and of local and foreign business
> tycoons, who have indeed built houses in foreign cities out of
> Sierra Leone's diamonds. And the juxtaposition of images of
> mobility, luxury, consumption, and predation on the witch city's
> streets speaks eloquently of the interconnections between two
> striking statistics: even before the rebel war, Sierra Leone had both
> one of the highest rates of infant mortality and one of the highest
> percentages of per capita ownership of Mercedes-Benz cars in
> the world.[63]

The conflict in Sierra Leone did not end with a whimper, and many laid the blame for ongoing bangs on in-house greed and grievance, both fanned by the extractive trades. Others blamed Charles Taylor. As the millennium ended, however, he was increasingly busy fighting off warlords seeking his removal in a second Liberian civil war—the latest installment, in many eyes, of one long Mano River war.

Taylor's travails didn't mean, however, that he had no time to think about his neighbors. Greg Campbell details one instance among many of how Freetown sobels and bush combatants came to be armed with the military-grade munitions in evidence well over a year after an international arms embargo had been applied on both sides of the Mano:

> On May 13, 1999, 68 tons of weapons arrived in Ouagadougou, the
> capital of Burkina Faso. The manifest listed 715 crates of small arms
> and ammunition, antitank weapons, surface-to-air missiles, and RPG
> tubes and warheads. The shipment was part of a contract between a

Gibraltar-based acquisitions company acting on behalf of the Burkina Faso Ministry of Defense and a Ukrainian arms manufacturer.[64]

The shipment didn't remain in Burkina Faso for long. A jetliner, formerly Taylor's presidential ride, made eight runs between Ouagadougou and Monrovia in the month after the delivery. The weapons were destined for Sierra Leone, the more portable ones to be ferried by the human mules who moved blood diamonds in the opposite direction. As this traffic violated terms of various peace agreements, Sierra Leoneans in the know were quick to underline their deficiencies.

The most notoriously failed peace accords were struck in the capital of Togo on July 7, 1999. The Lomé treaty was signed by President Kabbah and Foday Sankoh, the latter's death sentence having been overlooked or commuted. Togo's president was then chair of ECOWAS, but it was less well known that his son was married to Sankoh's daughter. ("Personal relations, always a crucial element in West African diplomacy," Ismail Rashid noted of the Lomé negotiations, "had intersected deftly with high politics." What the sobel alliance "could not gain through violence and terror it now sought through aggressive negotiating tactics.")[65] As Taylor and the presidents of Nigeria and Burkina Faso shuttled back and forth to Lomé, teams of negotiators—the RUF's was headed by an abductee with a serious case of Stockholm syndrome—haggled over a power-sharing agreement between the elected and the unelected, and over the treaty's enforcement. The most heated debates thus also centered on the fates of Sankoh and ECOMOG.

The accords again protected the RUF from prosecution, but this time the rebels received an added bonus: none other than Sankoh himself was placed in charge of mines and minerals. (The appointment, observed Sebastian Junger, was tantamount to naming the warlord the "diamond czar of Sierra Leone.")[66] Lomé counted other deficiencies. Not only did it fail to afford incentives for peace, but the treaty gave war a chance by low-balling the size of a proposed UN peacekeeping force, especially if a newly elected civilian government in Abuja chose to bring home the troops. It soon did. The Nigerian drawdown meant that the UN math unveiled after Lomé didn't add up. On October 22, 1999, the UN Security Council passed Resolution 1270, authorizing the deployment of six thousand peacekeepers under the acronym UNAMSIL—short for the United Nations Mission in Sierra Leone—to disarm some thirty-two thousand combatants who had about as much interest in the Geneva Conventions as in singing "Kumbaya."

As usual, the majority of the rainbow coalition in blue helmets hailed not from the well-heeled armies of Europe, North America, or East Asia, but from India, Pakistan, Nepal, Croatia, Ghana, Guinea, Kenya, Kyrgyzstan, Bangladesh, Zambia, the Gambia, and (of course) Nigeria. With the dispatch of UNAMSIL, "variously disciplined forces that had never operated in concert were thrust into what was at the time the hottest military zone on Earth next to Kosovo."[67] Disaster ensued. In May 2000, disarmament forces were disarmed by the sobels, who killed seven peacekeepers and relieved fifty more not only of their weapons and vehicles but also of their liberty, launching a fresh campaign of hostage taking. After hundreds of Zambian soldiers received similar treatment, that country's president blasted the force commander, an Indian major general who'd taken a dim view of his new Nigerian colleagues and said as much in a report leaked to a retreating ECOMOG.

When Abuja called for the commander's dismissal, Delhi querulously withdrew its three thousand troops. "Only months into the mission," reported Campbell, "the UN was having an embarrassingly public debate about command-and-control issues while a twelfth of its force was held prisoner."[68] The UN contingent was further humiliated when British special forces were asked to intervene to free British hostages and the blue helmets. The Brits made short work of these tasks, but London made it clear they weren't in their savaged former colony to serve as peacekeepers; they were there to protect U.K. citizens and (as ever) U.K. investments. Nor, evidently, were they or other foreign troops there to stop Sankoh and Taylor from looting what was left of the country's diamond wealth.

Heartened by successes against a UN force halved by Indian defection, Sankoh's irregulars continued to harry UN troops in order to keep prying eyes away from the diamond fields. In one clash, the entire Kenyan contingent at a new UN base in Makeni was taken hostage. Unnamed "progovernment forces" back in Freetown staged a retaliatory raid on Sankoh's compound there, uncovering detailed plans for an imminent coup as well as clear evidence of the diamond trafficking by then familiar to all parties. (The names of sobel officers, politician-warlords, vendors, and other middlemen, and even prices paid per carat, were laid out in childlike scrawl in school-kid notebooks.) The ensuing street fight shook the capital, prompting fears of escalation beyond his neighborhood.

On May 17, 2000, with assistance from the United Kingdom, Sankoh was arrested yet again. British officers reported the warlord was apprehended, in the words of an embedded English correspondent, "along with a witch-doctor, his personal guide to the dark arts of West African spiritualism."[69] The master of coin and mayhem was himself spirited to the old slaving way station on Bunce Island. (Its golf course had fallen into disuse in recent centuries, but its dungeons were apparently still serviceable.) And there Sankoh sat, under bristling guard and far away from rescue by either the RUF or Liberia's president—even if few on either side of the Mano River believed that either man could be held in even the deepest dungeon.

Even fewer believed that the two men were unable to cause trouble from Bunce and Monrovia, respectively. The RUF continued to violate the Lomé accords as its comrades and serfs in the diamond fields stepped up their pace during the early months of 2001. Douglas Farah, *The Washington Post*'s bureau chief in West Africa, was the first to allege that this frenzied extraction was to sell the rough, with Taylor's help, to an obscure outfit called al-Qaeda.[70] The allegation earned the journalist credible death threats from Taylor associates, which Farah—seasoned veteran of Colombia's drug wars and other boiling cauldrons—quite sensibly heeded by leaving West Africa with his family.

Fewer still believed in the promise of parley, but various parties limped to another one to sign a new sheaf of peace accords. This time, in contrast to cease-fires inked in Abidjan and Lomé, the Security Council weighed in. This time, the RUF and its leaders, as well as Taylor, were named the primary sponsors of the war in Sierra Leone. The treaty established a Special Court—still a thing—to prosecute them and a handful of the conflict's chief architects as war criminals. Confusingly, in the eyes of a war-dazed population, the treaty also established a Truth and Reconciliation Commission. This was an increasingly common manifestation of a widely propagated ideology of repair: victims and perpetrators alike would promote social healing by sharing their war stories.[71] Although the idea was feared by many and derided by some, both Court and Commission limped forward.

The removal of Sankoh and Taylor from these palavers was probably what made them matter—that and what would eventually be the world's largest deployment of UN peacekeepers.

Toward the end of 2001, Freetown began to feel like a city after war. Tejan Kabbah was back in the presidential palace; his Praetorian guard was now an international force. The city, its older quarters half-burnt and new neighborhoods thrown up weekly, was full of the halt and the maimed. Also, and everywhere, were powder-blue helmets topping standard camo uniforms. Along the coast, the thrum of UN helicopters drowned out the surf, but the deadly little Nigerian alpha jets were gone, and so, for the most part, was the clatter of automatic weapons.

By this time, the American journalist Greg Campbell had been covering the trail of blood diamonds for years. He was finishing up his book, sometimes using the lounge of the Mammy Yoko, which, once cleared of looting and lounging rebels, had been patched up and reopened. Even he discerned a glimmer of hope. "If there ever seemed a time in the past ten years when peace may have a lasting chance in Sierra Leone, it was the latter half of 2001," he wrote, "even though every previous peace attempt had been a dramatic and bloody disaster." Forays to the east and north led Campbell and other astute journalists to wonder if another one might be just around the corner. In this regard, they joined millions of Sierra Leoneans socialized to expect unending conflict amid other bloody disasters.

Homegrown peace skeptics included many of the young men and women massing in disarmament camps. When Campbell visited Port Loko at the close of the war, he passed by the one established in Maforki. To the Partners In Health team a dozen years later, Maforki was a run-down chiefdom with an abandoned complex of makeshift sheds designated as an ETU at the height of an explosive Ebola epidemic. It took us a while to learn that the bakery-turned-triage area of 2014 had been slapped together as a bakery in 2001 to knead combatants into placid tradesmen, but it didn't take Campbell long to judge the prospect of such transformation unlikely. With three thousand RUF and Kamajors crammed into it, the camp looked, he wrote, "more like a POW compound than the first stage in a reintegration process."[72] This was the inauspicious launch of the DDR, the UN-sponsored program to disarm, demobilize, and reintegrate tens of thousands of young (or youngish) people who'd known only the work of war and payment in spoils during their brief time on earth.

As on the eve of the 1919 food riots that protested the hoarding of food and medicine after the world's worst pandemic, the threat of imminent violence was palpable in the DDR camp. Whether or not he knew about the previous century's riots, Campbell could see that residents of the Port Loko camp were restive, and that their UN guards were skittish. There were many more guns in the vicinity than at the close of the Great War, and many more factions. There were drugs or, in the eyes of the recently disarmed, a severe and sudden shortage of them. There were also many more young men, and some young women, crammed into lousy barracks and manifesting scant interest in baking. When the disarmed and demobilized spied a white journalist in the company of a photographer, several young men began declaiming loudly.

As in 1919, the most acrid complaints were about social conditions. Across Sierra Leone, life expectancy at birth was likely not much greater in 2001—when it was pegged at 34.5 years—than it was when the Spanish flu struck. And it could always get shorter thanks to new hardware and new hard-heartedness. The disarmed but not yet reintegrated had, however, more diverse grievances than had the hungry peasants of yore. In return for laying down arms, complained the rebels, they'd been promised money, jobs, and schooling. Where were they? One teenager Campbell talked to began ticking off these and other demands, which did not include new baking skills. Among the boy's grievances: no soccer balls, no video entertainment, no medical care, poor-quality food and flip-flops, and none of the promised money. He tacked a bicycle onto the list of unkept promises made by the architects of the DDR.

"What makes you think you're getting a bike?" asked Campbell. To which the teen responded, "It's in Lomé!"[73] The disastrous treaty had of course been superseded by a new one, but neither included bicycles.

The Kamajors, who seemed to have shed their war-boy getups and dropped their blood feud with the RUF in order to stake similar claims, were just as disgruntled.[74] But spelling out these demands to foreign correspondents did not ease camp tensions. Concluding their presence was "inciting unrest that lacked only the spark to transform it into a riot," the correspondents quickly took their leave of Maforki.[75] Amazingly enough, however, the latest batch of peace accords held, once backed with an adequate number of peacekeepers. In spite of unpromising conditions in Freetown and Port Loko, and downright apocalyptic ones in the east, the civil war was declared over, and more than seventy thousand fighters disarmed. The last disarmament camp in Kailahun District was closed on January 11, 2002.[76]

On May 14, close to two million voted in elections that reelected Tejan Kabbah president. Ten months after that, the Special Court for Sierra Leone indicted Foday Sankoh on seventeen criminal counts, this time including war crimes. Also this time around, Charles Taylor was indicted on identical charges. When later found guilty, Taylor became the first elected head of state convicted of war crimes and crimes against humanity since the Nuremberg trials. But to stand trial, the Liberian president had to be apprehended. Taylor was attending more peace palavers—these ones in Ghana—when the Special Court unsealed its indictment and warrant. His blindsided hosts in Accra let him slip back to the palace in which William Tolbert met his end at the hands of Samuel Doe, and not far from where Doe met his end at the hands of another future (and current) statesman.

Many again voiced doubts about whether or not Taylor would or could be detained. But if he and the founder of the RUF were believed to have been granted immunity by higher powers, Sankoh didn't live up to his supernatural reputation. Stashed in a Bunce Island oubliette, he suffered a stroke in 2002 and died in a Freetown hospital the following year. And if Taylor had nine lives, he'd surely run through most of them. As something like peace settled over Sierra Leone, the Mano River war moved south. As the arms embargo against Liberia finally began to bite, Taylor faced a substantial rebellion. By the time Sankoh left the capital for parts unknown, but readily divined, a couple of factions had besieged Monrovia. Ulimo-J stalwarts—not to be confused with those from Ulimo-K—had reassembled as a new rebel group "formed in Sierra Leone but structured in Guinea," its declared mission to end Taylor's "cancerous influence on the stability of the entire sub-region."[77]

As the Special Court brandished its arrest warrant, and as Monrovia was encircled, the administration of George W. Bush—aware of the links between blood diamonds and al-Qaeda—voiced inhabitual support for a UN ruling. Later that year, Bush even placed a bounty on Taylor's head. This meant the game was up. The warlord-president resigned in 2003 and fled to Nigeria— "an attractive dumping ground," in the words of one informed anthropologist, "for African elites in need of isolation."[78] Backed by the great powers of the day, the Special Court pressed Abuja to extradite Taylor to Sierra Leone, but it was not until 2006—when Ellen Johnson Sirleaf, who had somehow survived previous transitions to become the first woman to be elected president of an African country, requested his extradition—that he was arrested by Nigerian forces and remanded to a Freetown prison. Many there vocally wished for his removal to a more secure one.

Eventually Charles Taylor was safely stowed in The Hague, allowing West Africa's peace skeptics perhaps to breathe a sigh of relief. More and more of those socialized for violence and privation began imagining a future of farming, studying, playing soccer, riding bikes—and perhaps even a bit of baking. For a long time after the cease-fires, however, imagining a peaceful future wasn't easy along the Upper Guinea Coast or across its savaged hinterland. War's tragic aftermath continued to unfold long after Sankoh and Taylor were removed, whether by the long and fickle arm of the law or by the hand of God. One tragedy of the conflict was that it allowed so many to grow the calluses required for turning away from the suffering of others. But a significant fraction of the citizens of Sierra Leone and Liberia had done a lot more than turn away from violent partisan struggle during fifteen years of it. A UN spokesperson in

Freetown alleged that making peace might be hampered by vigorous attempts to prosecute war crimes: "Everyone's guilty," she proclaimed.[79]

Such relativism fails us, however, in assessing blame for these disasters. Even among killers, not all were equally guilty, as advocates for former child soldiers invariably noted. Neither were other towns and cities in both countries. If by the rockets' red glare—or in dancing shadows cast as all of Bantoro and parts of Harper, Koidu, Kailahun, Port Loko, Freetown, and Monrovia went up in flames—we were able to make out the features of the architects of this destruction, we'd not see the faces of children or rural farmers. We wouldn't see the ritual specialists responsible for hiding masks, amulets, and talismans in sacred groves, thinned as these were by the dry rot of complicity. This conflict and ruin were the work of the era's real heartmen and of their unseen sponsors and business associates.

It's unlikely Bentley College, Charles Taylor's alma mater, will be awarding him an honorary degree anytime soon.

THE CRISIS CARAVAN

The war in Sierra Leone ruined the productive capacity of its
economy, which relied mostly on the exportation of the country's
mineral resources. Thus, economic recovery, a major concern
for the government in its postwar reconstruction effort, focused
on rebuilding infrastructure damaged during the war to attract
investors.

—Tamba E. M'bayo, "Ebola, Poverty, Economic Inequity and Social Injustice
in Sierra Leone," *Journal of West African History*, 2018

Ebola was not simply a deadly viral disease; it was the manifestation
of neoliberalism as an affliction, which wreaks havoc in the world's
most vulnerable societies.

—Ibrahim Abdullah and Ismail Rashid, *Understanding West Africa's Ebola
Epidemic: Towards a Political Economy*, 2017

AS THOSE WHO'VE TENDED TO THE SEEN AND UNSEEN WOUNDS OF WAR
know, it's easier to declare peace than to forge it. The strife of the 1990s drew
the entire region and then the world police into the fray—and still proved difficult to end. Still, the biggest warlords were at last removed. As reconstruction efforts began, might medicine and a new vision of public health have
something to offer?

Like Sierra Leone and Liberia, Rwanda as of late 1994 had been desert-
ified by genocide and war, and by their antecedents. The preexisting conditions included not only endemic corruption but also exported corruption of a

different sort: policies calling for radical reductions in already anemic public funding for health care and other social services. Rwanda's new leaders insisted on responding to widespread demands for health care and education; it was a central part of their peacemaking strategy. They showed it to be possible, and within fairly short order, to assemble the staff, stuff, space, and systems required to deliver basic clinical services to those who'd previously been denied them. This required substantial investments from Rwanda's tiny treasury, which meant bucking neoliberal trends calling for austerity—as if anything termed "austerity" could be deemed a virtue after what had just happened there.

Responding to demands for life-saving and life-enhancing social services also meant aligning the priorities of humanitarian and development agencies with new priorities—a hard task in Rwanda, and an even more challenging one on the other side of the continent. A hangdog minimalism, and pervasive clinical nihilism, retained an iron grip on Upper West Africa despite the arrival, right after the cessation of hostilities, of what some have termed the "crisis caravan."[1] That caravan counted UN peacekeepers, of course, but also representatives of the alphabet soup of UN agencies and humanitarian and nongovernmental organizations such as the Red Cross, MSF, and a raft of smaller institutions concerned with addressing war's varied wounds, including those of a social, political, and economic nature.

You might think that this caravan came to set right the imbalances that had begotten conflict. But the imported humanitarian logic dominant in West Africa after war was undergirded by the neoliberal one that triumphed in the decade before it began. Although structural adjustment had by then been widely discredited within Africa, the austerity virus once again spread from development banks and UN agencies to nongovernmental organizations, shattered or shuttered public institutions, and even (for heaven's sake!) missionary groups. Efforts to address complex illness and injury among the war-dazed poor, many of them massed in slums and refugee camps, were widely dismissed by international health experts as low-priority, unfeasible, unsustainable, and—the gravest insult of today's public-health lexicon—not cost-effective.

Neoliberal logic—with security as offered by police and soldiers rarely encompassing much-needed *social* security—had the advantage. The crisis caravan had the money; the national institutions required to weave a safety net were stony broke. Instead of tapping the wellspring of utopian visions bubbling up after the war, influential leaders of the crisis caravan drank from their own wells, even when they considered them poisoned by others. The heavies of that diverse group everywhere and uncritically termed "the international community" invested most of their resources in a narrow vision of security that left little for rebuilding health facilities—and less than a little for training a new health workforce.

Medical education wasn't even on the imposed agenda, although Liberia—down to about fifty practicing physicians at the time of Charles Taylor's arrest—graduated only a handful of doctors during the following years. In shell-shocked Sierra Leone dwelt a single psychiatrist, and the institution still known as the Kissy Lunatic Asylum, still without basic medications, continued to hold its inmates in chains. Sparse health care in both countries and in Guinea's refugee-packed forest districts meant that structural violence determined the fates of many well after the guns had fallen silent.

The narrow vision of the humanitarian organizations privileged a control-over-care approach to postconflict epidemics of cholera, typhoid, Lassa fever, malaria, and several outbreaks of measles, pertussis, and diphtheria. But it didn't have to be this way. The illness and injury taking the greatest toll over the decade prior to Ebola's eruption was in large measure preventable. When prevention failed, as it so often did, care and often cure were still possible. Training clinicians and administrators, establishing supply chains for medical supplies and lab reagents, and building new clinics, hospitals, and labs were all within reach, at the cost of investing the money and effort. The short-term thinking of peacekeeping and emergency assistantialism left little room, however, for building "resilient" (already a buzzword in these circles) national health systems.

Working conditions certainly did not favor the return of physicians and nurses who fled the conflict. Nor did many recent graduates wish to stay. On the eve of the Ebola epidemic, years later, there were still only about fifty Liberian doctors actually practicing clinical medicine—the equivalent of having a half dozen or so physicians for the entire city of Boston. Many Liberian clinicians had snapped up well-paid jobs within the caravan, which meant they were diverted from the disconcerting and hard job of providing care to those stranded in the desert. These were the consequences of policies deliberately or thoughtlessly applied.

Damning critiques of the humanitarian response to the suffering engendered by the Mano River war have been leveled by several of the scholars and other commentators cited approvingly in these chapters. On the other hand, investments in the Special Court helped bring some of the war's architects to account, and medical and social services were offered to surviving amputees and many other victims of conflict. International peacekeepers permitted the machinery of humanitarian assistance to operate in both countries—slowing camp epidemics ranging from cholera to Lassa fever, restarting vaccination and family-planning programs, and launching efforts seeking to prevent and, later, treat AIDS, tuberculosis, and malaria. But spending for health care was a small fraction of that going to peacekeeping operations. A failure to build or rebuild public institutions meant that there wasn't a safety net for the impoverished majority in either country, or sufficient civic engagement in the project of building back better.

The lamentably inadequate postwar response came to pass in part because those with control over the funds for health care allocated much of them to narrowly defined "vertical" projects with clearly marked beginning and end dates. Work to address certain pathologies was pitted against efforts to address others. The dull and vital chore of strengthening health systems after war couldn't withstand the dynamic of competing vertical interventions. Narrowly targeted initiatives promised to deliver desperately needed services, and often did. But the implementers of vertical programs found themselves obliged to provide their funders and overseers "clear metrics" of success, and even proof of "exit plans" and "sustainability," in settings of desolation and utter privation. In places where everything was needed, the relentless stovepiping was frustrating and worse.

As the proceduralism of fuzzy or irrelevant metrics and rigid work plans triumphed, so did the tyranny of the either-or. Some of the humanitarian groups, and a few of the larger nongovernmental organizations, committed themselves to address the epidemics that had earned the region its febrile colonial epithets. Many showing up after the cessation of hostilities focused on AIDS. They did so because resources designated to address that disease—resources absent before and during the war, and desperately needed after it—were, if not abundant, at least greater than those targeted to address more common illnesses and injuries. But the effort was misdirected. HIV, held by UN guesstimates to infect fewer than 2 percent of Sierra Leoneans, was likely less prevalent in eastern Sierra Leone than Lassa fever, about to consume Humarr Khan's time in Kenema, or the surgical disease that Martin Salia was learning to confront without the tools of the trade. But since priorities in the crisis caravan are set to follow the money, AIDS programs were elevated above the project of building health systems able to tackle the disease along with more common causes of suffering and early death.

Adia Benton's *HIV Exceptionalism*, based on research conducted in postwar Sierra Leone, serves up a withering critique of "the carving up of spaces and distribution of resources to people according to the presence or absence of HIV antigen or antibodies in the blood." This, the anthropologist explains, is an "ideological verticality," which holds that "HIV is exceptional and requires separate funding, programs, and personnel." Such exceptionalism "reproduces and reflects global hierarchies in relationships between the various donors, NGOs, and government agencies and community-based organizations that comprise the AIDS industry." These agencies and organizations, many of them new to Sierra Leone, further complicated the relationship between citizens in dire straits and a frail state with almost nothing to offer in the way of health care. Adia Benton describes the resulting dilemma: "On one hand, Sierra Leoneans lament the inadequacy of the state to provide care for its citizens. On the other, they uphold its indispensability as the embodiment of sovereignty and social order and see the state as an entity capable of providing care through its policies."[2] Dependence on a failed state was especially perilous in a wrecked country partly run by its own wreckers.

Although the emphasis on AIDS care may have been misplaced, there were lessons to learn from the response to that epidemic. More than 70 percent of the world's people living with HIV in 2010 lived in Africa. AIDS treatment has saved millions of African lives while preventing tens of millions of new infections. In some settings, including Rwanda, mother-to-child transmission of HIV is becoming rare, meaning pediatric AIDS is disappearing. It's not clear that any other recent humanitarian efforts have been anywhere near as effective as comprehensive AIDS programs. But the effectiveness of comprehensive AIDS programs is explained by their comprehensiveness.

It's easy to forget that *treatment* of AIDS in Africa was until recently dismissed as not sustainable, not cost-effective, not feasible. For more than two decades, as HIV spiraled out of control on the continent, only *prevention* programs received much in the way of public funding. Control-over-care dismissals were flung at those seeking to address, among the impoverished, pretty much all afflictions and injuries deemed difficult or costly to attack: surgical disease, diabetes, cancers of any sort, major mental illness, obstructed labor, and so forth.

Even taken together, however, favored and funded projects (almost all of them narrowly focused) could not rebuild war-wrecked health systems or war-wrecked lives. Some of these projects did address the visible wounds of war—the thousands of maimed and injured—while others sought to help the more numerous who'd sustained less visible wounds, such as post-traumatic stress disorder (PTSD), a label coined in the United States in the years following the Vietnam War. But verticality was even more painfully inadequate when social suffering and psychological distress were the primary problems at hand. There isn't some straightforward laboratory test to diagnose PTSD and related ills. How many, in either Sierra Leone or Liberia or on their borders—or among, say, the young men of ECOMOG—hadn't been traumatized or stressed by the events recounted in the previous chapter?

As funding became available for narrowly defined sequelae of war, the social traumas of the West African conflicts, to say nothing of their historical roots, were collapsed into the category of the "psychosocial." The adjective was soon trending across both countries, where it referred to the psychological far more than the social. The order of the day was to forget the past—public exhortations to do so were loudly repeated there, even though these contradicted equally emphatic exhortations regarding truth and reconciliation—and to focus on such ineffables as psychological and cultural resilience. Resilience is an undoubtedly worthy goal, but it's not entirely clear how it's best cultivated and on what (or whose) time line. It's not even clear what resilience means. What were the relevant metrics or "key performance indicators" by which to gauge the success or failure of such a project? How could the implementers of these efforts—diviners and seers aside—offer the required "exit plans"?

People who might reasonably be regarded as endowed with Olympic-class psychological and cultural resilience were still finding their own earthly exit plans advanced by the usual pathogens and pathogenic forces. Time ran out for many who survived the war but faced a peacetime graveyard.[3] Just as it was hard to find any family that hadn't suffered emotional trauma of some sort during the conflict, it was abundantly clear that cancers and obstructed labor and trauma caused by road accidents—conditions often requiring surgical intervention—weren't going away just because peace had been decreed. The ability to provide surgical care had, however, gone away. Even cesarean sections remained unavailable in most provincial towns and cities of Upper West Africa; they'd never been available in the rural areas where most poor women lived prior to the war. Well before Ebola made them afraid to go to hospitals or clinics for prenatal care or skilled delivery or contraceptives, the women of Sierra Leone faced the highest maternity-mortality ratio in the world, a report card on the country's lack of a functioning health-care system. In the past few years, thanks to Ebola, maternal mortality rose yet higher. Liberia can't be far behind.[4] Ebola hit less than a decade after the Mano River conflict ended, and the perils now facing pregnant women in the most Ebola-affected nations aren't much different from those faced by their female forebears centuries earlier.

Obstructed labor and other third-trimester catastrophes, like major trauma and surgical conditions in general, call for functioning and readily accessible hospitals embedded in a health system. Several nongovernmental and UN-affiliated organizations claimed to "hand off" rebuilt hospitals to local health authorities. But these public institutions didn't have the staff, stuff, and systems to run them; they didn't have the cash to acquire or pay for these ingredients, either. The public facilities in Zwedru, Harper, Koidu, Kenema, and Port Loko couldn't really function as rudimentary hospitals because, once rebuilt or renovated, they didn't have the personnel or supplies required to do so. Neither did referral centers. As Ebola exploded across Upper West Africa, there wasn't a single well-equipped referral hospital in Freetown or Monrovia. The face-saving fiction that humanitarian groups had reopened hospitals (they'd done that) in order to hand them over to local health authorities (they hadn't really managed that part) further deepened West Africans' distrust of their own national institutions. The story within the education sector was similar.

The proliferation of civil-society organizations with varied and partisan agendas continued apace in Sierra Leone and Liberia even as public-sector efforts in health and education remained pathetically understaffed and anemically funded. Jobs and services came and went. In Rwanda, it was fear of this trap that had prompted postgenocide leaders to request that many nongovernmental organizations and humanitarian groups commit to building *local* capacity—or else to amble off with the crisis caravan. Its provisional government even expelled, briefly and shockingly, the United Nations delegation. Rwanda's rapid recovery from genocide and war has been unprecedented.[5] But with most of Sierra Leone's and Liberia's security in UN hands, there was little room for such bold gestures. People clamored for medical care and social assistance, and for patronage and protection, from whoever could get it to them. Nongovernmental organizations and sundry contractors continued to demand, in turn, their slice of the pie. They were often the only ones throwing lifelines to those unable to get by in resilient fashion.

By the time billions of dollars had been allocated to emergency assistance, it was clear that efforts to build resilient national health systems had failed. Proof of this failure, which contradicted rosy reports and clear exit plans, stretched as far as the eye could see when the postwar crisis caravan withdrew from what remained West Africa's clinical and public-health desert. Anyone who paused to read about centuries of crises in West Africa, or who bothered to plumb recent medical archives, could have found plenty of evidence in the decade after war's end that Ebola—and other pestilence—was likely to come back with a vengeance.

Greg Campbell returned to Sierra Leone in July 2011, almost a decade after the armistice and not long before the unrecognized return of Ebola. Happy as he was to not hear the clatter of automatic gunfire or the thud of mortars, the journalist saw little progress. In 2011, there was still scant electricity in Freetown, to say nothing of cities to the east (forget about towns and villages); the roads were vile; and some of the scars of war looked as fresh as if forming over wounds just inflicted. The sick and maimed were still everywhere. Disarmed combatants, robbed of their childhoods and bored or disgruntled, loitered around such public edifices as were still standing or rebuilt. These young men, many of them caught up in the war on the losing side, hadn't always been welcomed home. The same was true for many young women, abducted as girls and later rejected or feared by surviving kin as wild and dangerous after life in the bush. Most of these abducted women had dependent children, and few had benefited from vocational training beyond a few short courses in hairdressing, soap making, batik production, or weaving.[6]

If batik futures were down and soap markets tanking, Sierra Leone's diamond trade was booming. The nature of the boom had, however, changed. Although artisanal mining had drawn thousands east since war's end, the yield of the shake-shakes had dwindled while the take from Kono's kimberlite pipes, by then exposed in monstrous, funneled Mordor pits, had soared. Exports of rough diamonds had reached $142 million by 2007, and huge piles of tailings and slag towered over everything but Koidu's ornate mosques—the only things of beauty still standing besides the rocky outcroppings emerging from a shrinking forest. The biggest industrial operation, again run by a South African company, was rumored to boast a high-end medical facility. Bailor Barrie and our other Sierra Leonean colleagues often speak of it, though they say little about baking or batik.

The resurgence of the legitimate diamond trade and the proliferation of nongovernmental organizations following the crisis caravan were no doubt two of the reasons Greg Campbell couldn't find a jeep to rent in order to visit Koidu. The reporter, who ended up going by bus, tried to take his mind off the pain of being pretzeled into a cramped seat, each pothole and knocked head leading him to commiserate with those always forced to take the bus. As his bus lurched eastward toward the source of much public suffering and private gain, the journalist became aware of an indignant voice raised above the ambient noise he was trying to ignore. "You have all the diamonds coming from Kono," someone was griping, "but look at the schools, look at the hospital, look at the road! There is no power, there is no transportation. Where's the money going?"

After extracting himself from entangled limbs and bags, Campbell did look at Koidu Government Hospital. The sole public hospital serving more than half a million souls didn't seem to be a good place for the critically ill or injured. The rebuilt facility still looked as if it had been nuked by a neutron bomb—again, if that's the one that kills the living but leaves buildings intact. Not that there was much in the way of infrastructure, beyond resurrected walls. It was "too risky to give surgery patients general anesthesia," an American working in the hospital reported, "because they can't intubate patients who stop breathing." This, she explained, was because the hospital lacked pulse oximeters to monitor blood levels of oxygen. The instrument is portable and costs under $100. Walmart offers one for $13.50: a bargain, especially compared to diamonds.

Even were the monitors on hand, there wasn't much electricity to power them. Nor was there running water. "Instruments were sanitized in an industrial pressure cooker heated on a propane burner," Campbell continued. "Because the plumbing didn't work, the water came from a hand pump in the courtyard via bucket brigade, as did the water for flushing toilets and washing surgeons' hands." In the diamond fields, many of the shake-shakes, and some of the dangerous dredge diving, had been replaced by industrial washing stations; remarkably, their plumbing worked just fine. "The excuse for all this deficiency," added the journalist, "is that the government has no money to pay for improvements and modern equipment, an argument that's hard to buy with round-the-clock diamond production happening fewer than five miles away." In theory, at least, any of the hospital's poor-to-mediocre services were free to all who needed them. In most cases, an out-of-pocket expenditure was required.

Greg Campbell knew this well, but he had an unwelcome reminder during his trip to Koidu. One of the reasons the journalist paid a visit to the hospital was that his fixer, who'd been fine when they boarded the bus in Freetown, "was shivering from chills and throwing up bright green bile the consistency of paint." It was malaria. As Campbell spoke to the young doctor in Koidu, he recognized him as the indignant fellow passenger on the bus. It was none other than Bailor Barrie, who'd finally completed the medical training that war had so often interrupted. "My own personal view," he told the journalist with some heat, "is that the government is corrupt. The money from the diamond revenues meant for communities goes into their pockets or their bank accounts. Kono is the wealthiest district in the country, but we don't even have a college."[7] The thud of mortars may have been replaced by the boom of more carefully planned explosions deep in the diamond pits, but Koidu didn't look like it was on the short list of likely sites for a new university, public or private.

We're back, in closing Part II of this book, to its central question. Why did Ebola devastate these three countries and not others? It's important but insufficient to blame weak health systems. Of course they're weak.

Even before we look at the strikingly similar experience of Liberia, Sierra Leone, and Guinea during the past few years, it's easy to see that many forces beyond contiguity and war had pushed them into the structurally similar circumstances here termed medical impoverishment. These are medical deserts even by West African standards. All three nations had very poor indices of health and well-being in the face of rapid growth of GDP per capita; low levels of public investment in health (when compared to, say, Rwanda or Cuba, but also to Ghana or Senegal); high levels of premature and preventable morbidity and mortality (compared to most countries, regardless of GDP); weak laboratory infrastructure and disease surveillance; and thus high levels of risk for the rapid spread of unidentified epidemic disease. Upper West Africa is a *public-health desert*, where a diagnosis is more likely to come from a diviner or traditional healer than from an accredited laboratory or health professional. It's also a *clinical desert*, where to be injured or sick means more or less what it did a century ago.

There can be no understanding of this medical wasteland, and its vulnerability to Ebola, without knowledge of the shared and distinct histories laid out in the preceding chapters. Their shared history has long involved rapacious extraction and forced labor regimes. Rapacity on this scale requires and foments violence, resulting in more illness and injury. In the health-care arena, many of the terms of current debates about what's possible and what's not were set in the era of colonial rule. That's where control-over-care strategies originated, and yet another reason recent calls to restore colonialism are even more disturbing than the preposterous success of imperial propaganda. The rural poor, the great majority in all three Ebola-afflicted nations until war drove them into towns and cities, were rarely viewed as deserving of medical care under colonial rule—even as a therapeutic revolution gathered force in Europe and North America.

How could it be otherwise? In the first part of the twentieth century, at least, black doctors were shunted aside or formally excluded from the colonial medical services. (Doctors of any hue remained pretty much absent from Liberia.) Many West Africans still harbor memories of campaigns to isolate (and sometimes destroy) settlements afflicted by smallpox, cholera, and vector-borne diseases such as plague, malaria, and trypanosomiasis.[8] In the course of many of these epidemics, and for a century and more, funerals and wakes were banned, travel restrictions imposed, and punitive measures (from fines to incarceration) routine. Medical care was not. After independence, tardy efforts to link disease control to care were nonetheless under way in Guinea and Sierra Leone and, to a lesser extent, Liberia. But health expenditures of any sort remained a tiny fraction of postcolonial national budgets.

That fraction shrank further when their governments signed on to structural adjustment programs—and geared up for war.[9] There was never, in other words, a golden era of medicine in West Africa, a heyday of public health.

Between the early twentieth century's explosive outbreaks of yellow fever, smallpox, plague, cholera, influenza, and trypanosomiasis and the twenty-first century's westward march of Ebola across West Africa stretched decades of neglect of the destitute sick. Neglectful policies first written by the sanitarians of fading colonial governments have left a disastrous imprint, but other disastrous policies were advanced by development institutions claiming to represent the poor, or frail or failed states. Few of these ventriloquists were natives of West Africa.

Externally imposed austerity meant that governments lost much of their scant capacity to engage in anything resembling caregiving. They did, however, retain their ability to hector and blame, discipline and punish. Across the region, and prior to the warlords' savage campaigns, such scolding was sometimes the only aspect of health authorities' attention that became visible to those most at risk of Ebola—the rural poor and their kin who'd sought refuge, employment, or education in Freetown, Monrovia, or Conakry. And that's before any consideration of acute violence, perpetrated in part by the authorities of these countries during the course of the conflict that led millions to flee—and that brought down public institutions charged with protecting health and providing care. It was, we Ebola responders heard repeatedly, the perfect storm.

A more critical reflection on the abuse of the perfect-storm metaphor reveals its unsuitability (and overuse) in describing epidemics of Ebola and of several other pathogens. The links in the chain—a more apt and sadder metaphor—may be seen by anyone with an interest in history. Slavery and extraction. Murderous and enduring conflict. Formal colonial rule and more extraction. Contested independence. More conflict, much of it over diamonds and other commodities. Structural adjustment. Outright war, usually over whatever's being extracted, and massive dislocations. Discovery of an epidemic, followed by solemn declarations about the perfect storm.

But if storms like the one in West Africa are perfect, they've long been brewing. To paraphrase Camus, epidemics, like war, are seen to crash down upon us from a cloudless sky in part because we aren't attentive to storms of our own making.

Commentary on most epidemics sends history down the drain. That's no accident. Surely the successful rebranding of European empires as "Western democracies" and the inevitable focus on "local" disasters of African politics or epidemiology stand as impressive examples of willed amnesia. This entire process of shrugging off human agency—a.k.a. history—lets external actors and forces off the hook, allowing expatriate pundits and self-dealing global bureaucrats to argue that local greed and tribal grievance are the primary cause of independent Africa's woes, including its poor economic, political, social, and physical health. But those without shelter are of course obliged to pay closer attention to the clouds above.

Members of the crisis caravan could see everywhere the effects of West Africa's history, without knowing that history itself. As a participant in the caravan, I've tried to track back to the causes of the devastation we witnessed. Knowing what I know now, it's plain to me what we need to do, and how we can and must avoid repeating the same mistakes—and crimes.

DEATH AND LIFE AFTER EBOLA

He has

    sent hither swarms of Officers to harass our people.

He has plundered our—

      ravaged our—

       destroyed the lives of our—

taking away our—

     abolishing our most valuable—

and altering fundamentally the Forms of our—

In every stage of these Oppressions We have Petitioned for Redress in the most humble terms:
       Our repeated
Petitions have been answered only by repeated injury.

We have reminded them of the circumstances of our emigration and settlement here.

    —taken Captive
      on the high Seas
        to bear—

—Tracy K. Smith, "Declaration," 2018

9.

How Ebola Kills

AN EXERCISE IN SOCIAL MEDICINE

An understanding of the definition of a pathogen is not required when a clinician is faced with an infected patient who needs treatment. However, if we are to understand disease-associated microbes and discover effective therapies, we will also need to appreciate their fundamental biology and the ecological setting in which they secure a niche . . . So-called emerging infectious diseases reflect various aspects of imbalance in the relationships between host, pathogen, and environment. Many of the most serious and feared infectious diseases occur when humans are infected by microorganisms that prefer, and are better adapted to, another mammalian host. In fact, most emerging infectious diseases in humans are of zoonotic origin.

—David Relman and Stanley Falkow, "A Molecular Perspective of Microbial Pathogenicity," in *Principles and Practice of Infectious Diseases*, 2010

Le microbe n'est rien, le terrain est tout.

—Louis Pasteur, September 28, 1895

EBOLA WAS FIRST IDENTIFIED IN OCTOBER 1976, IN A MISSION HOSPITAL IN the village of Yambuku, in the northern reaches of Zaire, which today is known as the Democratic Republic of the Congo. But there's no reason to believe that the pathogen was new to the clinical desert. It took time for the virus to be recognized as a novel species, a process that required staff, stuff, space, and systems.

This process of discovery began after blood samples from infected patients were collected in Kinshasa, the capital of Zaire, some seven hundred miles from Yambuku. Some were sent thousands of miles away, to Antwerp, Belgium, where, with the help of an electron microscope, they were classified as "a Marburg-like virus." Other samples were dispatched to the U.S. Centers for Disease Control and Prevention, in Atlanta, and to the Army High Security Laboratory in Porton Down, England. Soon the virus would be declared a new member of the filovirus family, along with Marburg, and given the name Ebola, after a river that runs close to Yambuku. By the time that happened, however, the virus had already killed many of those seeking and giving care in or around the village.

One of several people credited with the discovery of Ebola is Peter Piot, a Belgian infectious-disease doctor who was among those dispatched from Antwerp to Yambuku to conduct an investigation of the outbreak, which claimed the lives of several Flemish nuns. Piot was a junior partner in the investigation, especially after the arrival of seasoned smallpox hands and other heavies from the Centers for Disease Control, but he did speak Flemish. He has since worked, over a forty-five-year career, in places as varied (and connected) as Kinshasa, Antwerp, London, and Geneva. From the early days of his training, Piot loved the work of microbe hunting and its therapeutic promise. As he has written in his memoir, "You came in and figured out what the problem was. And if you managed to figure it out quickly enough—before the patient died, basically—then you could almost always solve it, because, just like my medical school professor of social medicine had said, solutions had by this time been found for almost every kind of infectious illness."[1]

For clinical practitioners of social medicine, the problem beyond scientific discovery—whether of microbes or vaccines or therapies—was one of delivery. How do you deliver solutions old and new to those in greatest need? Under colonial rule, at least across much of Africa, the question was rarely posed and never answered. While "extractive science"—evaluating afflicted villagers and then shipping samples to labs in Europe—may uncover previously unknown pathogens and lead to the discovery of new therapies, these will be offered mostly to those who are deemed more worthy than others. This was a problem that had bedeviled even the most well-meaning colonial health officers, regardless of their empires of origin. It had bedeviled even missionaries, including Flemish ones laboring in their former colony. Medical historians working in the social-medicine tradition have shown as much in study after study.

If nothing else, Ebola teaches us the importance of social medicine, which focuses attention not only on why plagues afflict some and spare others but also on how inevitable mutations—social and biological, among pathogen and host—are related to differential risks for infection and death. As Peter Piot and all who ventured from cities like Antwerp to villages like Yambuku discovered, if you want to address the delivery problem, you need a social medicine incorporating staff, stuff, space, and systems. But West Africa, like the northern Congo, has not known this sort of social medicine, because of the extractive arrangements that I've described in the previous four chapters: slavery, racism, colonialism, and war. Its medical and public-health systems have failed repeatedly to deliver on the promise of discovery.

Social medicine includes the study of how pathogens—and pathogenic forces—get in the body, how they take their toll, and how and why these processes vary so radically from time to time, place to place, and person to person. Practitioners of social medicine pay attention to pathogenesis, which medical dictionaries define as "the development of morbid conditions or of disease; more specifically, the cellular events and reactions and other pathologic mechanisms occurring in the development of disease."[2] By any criterion, more has been learned about the pathogenesis of serious Ebola infections in the past few years than in all of the years since 1976.

That's not saying much. Ebola, like Marburg, has received scant attention from the best basic scientists and clinical researchers, and from the world's largest research-based pharmaceutical concerns, for a simple reason: there's not much money in it. Valiant exceptions aside, few well-equipped researchers have focused on how these viruses cause human disease, and even fewer have focused on treating it by taking up the clinical battle against the pathogens. If social medicine is a field suggesting that clinical endeavors should be informed by context—looking *around* (at what's going on outside the hospital) and looking *back* (in time)—then the social medicine of filoviruses is nascent at best.

The West African Ebola epidemic made this clear. There was more focus on looking around (at the mistrustful locals) than at looking back (at the events and processes that made them so mistrustful). Disturbingly, what we've learned in its aftermath is that some of our post-2013 discoveries about these viruses are better termed rediscoveries—or, in harsher terms, a failure to recall lessons from the not-so-distant past, including those learned and forgotten in towns and villages from the Sudan to Angola, and in European cities like Marburg, Frankfurt, and Belgrade.[3] But unforeseen developments can lead to rapid and positive change.

There's been stunning progress, for example, in our understanding of the structures of these viruses. Molecular biology and phylogenetics have permitted not only the publication of Ebola's genome but also the construction of its family tree, with many of its ramifying branches limned by large teams of laboratory scientists and computational geneticists, including Humarr Khan and Pardis Sabeti and their colleagues. This achievement did not come to pass because of some long-standing and exceptional focus on a pathogen afflicting primarily the rural poor in Africa, although that's what motivated Sabeti et al. The achievement occurred in part because much research on lethal viruses has been propelled by fear-based funding.

Nor was this scientific achievement linked to robust efforts to match it with clinical ones. The desire to identify "the molecular basis of human disease"—the name, or something like it, of one of the massive textbooks I tried to digest in medical school more than thirty years ago—is above reproach. We all live in bodies, composed of tissues and organs and fluids; these components of our bodies in turn are made up of cells, they of molecules, and molecules of atoms. And we all, alas, become diseased or injured, or both, on the way to a universally shared destination.

Infectious-disease clinicians (mostly doctors and nurses) recognize typical and atypical presentations of disease caused by viruses that sicken humans; they're usually also informed about other matters relevant to clinical practice. It's a lot to know, since that practice requires familiarity with a host of diagnostic tests of varied accuracy; specific therapies (antiviral drugs, for example) and some notion of how they are best dosed and for how long; their complications and side effects; nonspecific therapies (such as fluid resuscitation, correction of acid-base imbalances, and replenishment of lost electrolytes, as well as therapies to counter symptoms ranging from diarrhea to vomiting); common complications of viral infections (for example, the secondary or opportunistic infections seen in the course of afflictions ranging from influenza to measles, as well as HIV); and late complications of viral infections capable of persistence among human hosts who survive acute infection.

Clinicians and public-health practitioners alike also learn about preventive measures, including vaccines, postexposure prophylaxis (for rabies, say, or HIV), and respiratory or contact precautions (such as barrier nursing and infection control) needed to prevent a pathogen's spread within crowded settings such as hospitals, nursing homes, and schools. (For those working in the sorts of places described in these chapters, "crowded settings" include mines, military barracks, prisons, refugee camps, and a host of informal settlements and precarious slums.) But there's a lot that even the most seasoned clinicians don't know, much of which, embarrassingly enough, is termed "basic science."

Most clinicians, including nurses and doctors who treat viral diseases on a daily basis, will admit that the basic science of virology and immunology is wondrously and devastatingly complex. We know that these pathogens are classed as either DNA viruses—herpes viruses, for example—or RNA viruses, like measles, coronaviruses, and filoviruses. We learn that mutations can confer increased virulence, as the influenza pandemic of 1918 suggested even before the causative pathogen was identified, or increased resistance to proven therapies. But the clinical and epidemiological implications of specific mutations are usually contested or unclear.

The same might be said of the basics of viral pathogenesis, even though they are easy enough to master. In the straightforward reviews read by medical students and trainees in infectious disease, there's usually mention of seven steps in the interaction between virus and host: entry into the host (in this case, us); primary replication in infected cells; spread within the host; "tropism," or preference, for specific host cells or tissues, such as liver, lungs, or brain; secondary replication in these preferred tissues and cells; cell injury and death; and the host's immune response in tandem with the clearance or persistence of virus. These steps have been studied—during the course of acute illness, through autopsies, and after experimental infection of living animals—for many years.

Some of these seven steps are also studied in laboratory models using human or animal cells and tissues. In the case of the filoviruses, our familiarity with the unfolding of viral pathogenesis has been limited by more than a lack of adequate funding: Ebola and Marburg are classed as pathogens to be studied only in biosafety-level-four, or BSL-4, laboratories. Few such labs exist. (One proposed for Boston was approved, funded, and built only to see its opening delayed for years because of objections from frightened neighbors.) Since the discovery of Ebola, much filovirus research has relied on studies using primates. The course of Ebola caused by the Zaire species is thought to be fairly similar in humans and rhesus macaques, the most common unwilling volunteer. So, too, with Marburg.

But not all steps in filovirus pathogenesis are readily studied in animal models—even in the right labs and even when the intent is to develop specific therapies and vaccines. It's too dangerous. During the West African outbreak, researchers like Pardis Sabeti, who lacked ready access to BSL-4 laboratories, were obliged to develop "fake viruses" in order to study Ebola mutations.

To understand the complexities of real-world epidemics, you need a firm grasp of social medicine.

The towering mortality seen in African outbreaks of Ebola and Marburg—and within the families of Ibrahim and Yabom—occurs in part because these outbreaks have occurred in the absence of basic supportive care. Starting not long after the middle of the twentieth century, most Europeans afflicted with any serious viral infection might reasonably assume that basic supportive care would be part of what's quaintly referred to as "the natural history" of their diseases. It was natural, in other words, for them to receive such care—which is why most of them survived. In that same period, however, it was almost unheard of for rural Africans to receive supportive care during severe viral infections, which is one reason that many did not survive them.

Disturbingly, the pattern has persisted in the twenty-first century. Why? How? Variants of these questions are the oldest in social medicine, and likely in medicine tout court. One key to a full understanding of pathogenesis—for our purposes, how Ebola sickens and kills—is pathology, the study of diseased human tissue. Autopsies are considered routine in seeking to understand pathogenesis. But they're almost never undertaken when the disease in question is caused by a filovirus. In settings where autopsies are performed, this is out of concern that they might afford another setting for spread of these pathogens.

Among those at risk for such afflictions, the residents of rural villages and small towns in Africa, autopsies aren't performed at all. The French filovirus expert Pierre Rollin and his colleagues recently reviewed all of the existing pathologic evidence of filovirus disease in human tissue. It proved worse than scant. Their exhaustive study, published in 2015, "identified only 30 fatal cases where an autopsy or post-mortem biopsies were performed and pathological descriptions were reported." They were referring not to recently performed studies but rather to *all* studies performed since Marburg was identified in 1967. Since most of these weren't full autopsies, and since Rollin knows a thing or two about social medicine, he cautioned that "efforts to explain the pathogenesis of Ebola and Marburg haemorrhagic fevers must consider a multitude of factors, including clinicopathological and epidemiological data."[4]

This multitude of factors does not come into view, indeed cannot come into view, as long as we're peering solely through the lens of a microscope. What if failure to treat, rather than treatment failure, is central to Ebola's pathogenicity? The handful of American Ebola victims who received ventilatory support or renal dialysis and lived to tell about it know that their lives were saved first by supportive and critical care, and then by their own immune systems. West Africans have vigorous immune defenses, too. But people living in extreme poverty are denied most or all of the critical-care interventions that give patients the time required for a robust immune response. This applies to patients who, prior to infection with a filovirus, struggle with acquired immune deficiency caused by diverse pathogens that often include HIV, malaria, tuberculosis, hookworm, and the long list of ailments laid out elegantly in the works of Graham Greene and by the Harvard expedition to Liberia. All of these afflictions cause and are worsened by malnutrition and anemia.

What about West Africans who do not suffer from poor nutrition? The three countries in which the great majority of Ebola cases have been counted constitute one of the most medically underserved regions of the world, so even the well-nourished and healthy lack access to the sort of medical care available to those living in more fortunate parts of urban Africa, which isn't markedly different from how it's practiced in affluent cities in Europe and the Americas. During the West Africa epidemic, even well-nourished and healthy doctors and nurses had only slim chances of survival. If they remained in the clinical desert, getting out was their best hope.

Understanding how viruses kill humans—that is, understanding microbial pathogenicity in the human host—requires understanding the social context. And in West Africa, that social context includes chronic failures to deliver effective therapies available elsewhere in the world. *The* critical step in preventing future epidemics will be finding ways of delivering vaccines and therapies to those who need them—and who need them in part because they live in a clinical desert that was created when their predecessors were enslaved and subjugated so that people and nations in other parts of the world could amass great wealth and prosperity.

Additionally, we have to stop telling ourselves horror stories about an unstoppable mutant virus, because those stories often legitimate our inaction. In Richard Preston's *The Hot Zone*, the Centers for Disease Control's Joe McCormick is singled out for praise during the Reston virus outbreak in monkeys, having predicted, correctly, that the culprit species would not prove highly infectious or pathogenic to human hosts. He also led an investigation of an outbreak of Ebola in Sudan after being dropped off in the countryside by a rickety plane in order to collect samples from people sick and dying in several remote villages. McCormick was of course collecting samples—that was his primary mission—but it felt wrong to him to leave these suffering villagers alone to their fates. He was, after all, a doctor.

When Joe McCormick missed his ride out of the clinical desert, he watered it a bit by tending to critically ill and dying patients in their miserable huts, by the light of a headlamp. In the course of his ministrations, the CDC doctor jabbed himself in the thumb with a bloody needle. And then Preston credits him with "another Joe McCormick discovery, one of the few breakthroughs in the treatment of the Ebola virus. In Sudan, thinking he was going to die of Ebola, he had discovered that a bottle of Scotch is the only good treatment for exposure to a filovirus."[5] Fortunately, this is poetic license. There are several more effective means of treating Ebola than therapeutic doses of whiskey. But the story says a lot about both the control-over-care paradigm and its twin, therapeutic nihilism: both led to or reinforced or excused poor-quality care for natives of the regions that have long known these and related outbreaks. The historically inclined could have guessed that, during the West African outbreak, getting to zero new Ebola cases through containment would trump efforts to achieve zero mortality among the afflicted.

Joe McCormick, who survived his unplanned evening in rural Sudan and went on to become the head of the Special Pathogens Branch at the Centers for Disease Control, knew this well. But so did the majority of expatriate clinicians—doctors, nurses, physician assistants—who showed up to help in West Africa two decades later: taking care of sick people was why they had volunteered. The voices and opinions of professional caregivers providing supportive and critical care on the ground revealed this. At the height of the western surge, one response team laid out the dilemma starkly, months after the Ebola-containment gurus had declared matters well under control. Acknowledging "a certain unease about treating a highly transmissible infection for which there is no vaccine, no specific therapy, and a high mortality rate," the team went on to note that *most* viral illnesses, and most critical illnesses, actually fall into this category, but we don't consider them "untreatable." There is plenty one can do, they wrote, to treat Ebola. "After spending much of the past five months treating patients with Ebola virus disease," they wrote, "we are convinced that it's possible to save many more patients. Our optimism is fueled by the observation that *supportive care is also specific care for EVD*—and in all likelihood reduces mortality. Unfortunately, many patients in West Africa continue to die for lack of the opportunity to receive such basic care."[6]

Unfortunately, when the epidemic was raging in Upper West Africa, such views were drowned out by the din created by pundits, politicians, and members of fearful international health bureaucracies obsessed with containment and mitigation—right until a sudden surge of cases took out what was left of the region's health-care systems. With regard to Ebola, professional caregivers had something important to add to the diagnosis of delivery failure: honest acknowledgment of our collective failure to even *try* to provide high-quality care. This failure clearly troubled the handful of specialists in critical care and emergency medicine (both physicians and nurses) who arrived fairly early on the scene. But they couldn't show up in the sense of putting their clinical skills to use. They didn't have the requisite staff, stuff, space, or systems.

Those intensive-care specialists, whether physicians or nurses, further encountered a distinct lack of ambition to get these tools, and the care they enable, to Upper West Africa. It wasn't just the disease-control enthusiasts. Such basic and "nonspecific" treatments, had they been available in Yambuku—a 120-bed "hospital" without a single doctor and zilch in the way of infection control—would surely have lessened the horrific mortality described by Peter Piot and others in 1976. But a delivery failure in 1976, when the viral culprit was unknown, is not the same as a delivery failure in 2014. By the time of Upper West Africa's western surge, we had more tools and fewer excuses not to deploy them. Even in 1976, Piot and his colleagues in Yambuku were clear that alternatives to bad and dangerous care should be offered.[7] Taking care of the Ebola sick was never, in other words, a fool's errand.

In the intervening decades, however, contrary conclusions have been advanced as based on sound evidence when they in fact rested on slender data. Animal models of pathogenesis furnish much of this basis. But even when the goal of such experiments is to study candidate therapies, rather than the "natural history" of untreated disease, the impact of nonspecific therapies has never been explored among nonhuman primates. Never, as far as I could ascertain, have these studies included any notion of testing the impact of supportive and critical care—or even therapeutic doses of whiskey—on the clinical outcomes among the unfortunate monkeys and macaques who gave their all to generate such understanding.

The critical-care specialists François Lamontagne and Robert Fowler were among those who felt that "certain unease" on the ground in West Africa in 2014. Lamontagne, a clinician-researcher at Quebec's Sherbrook University Hospital, investigates renal replacement therapy, mechanical ventilation, and the use of vasopressors in the treatment of shock. All of these, he observed, were absent in the clinical desert but proved useful or lifesaving in caring for many of the two dozen or so patients rescued from it.

Robert Fowler, also a Canadian intensivist, was spending his sabbatical at the World Health Organization when Guinea reported its first confirmed Ebola cases in March 2014. While in Geneva (and well before the onset of the West African epidemic), he had mulled "over the high mortality rate in Ebola outbreaks, and how a clinical response team focused on treating the syndrome of Ebola—dehydration, organ dysfunction and shock—might help to drive this mortality down." Fowler was one of the first ICU doctors deployed to West Africa—initially in Guinea and then in Sierra Leone and Liberia—helping to treat Ebola patients (including Conakry's first confirmed cases), training international teams as they arrived, and advising beleaguered public-health authorities. But as soon as he arrived, he ran smack into the wall of therapeutic nihilism. *These people are likely doomed*, he heard public-health experts worry. *There's little to be done once prevention fails.*

Clinical skills like Fowler's are inevitably poorly used in the face of such nihilism. As grueling months passed, and as the surge swelled, advocating for better patient care became his personal and professional mission. In an interview with the WHO in December 2014, he offered the following reflection:

> The clinical care of patients is a tiny piece of the response. However, I think it is a very, very important one. When mortality is very high, and Ebola treatment centers function more to isolate people than to provide care to patients, the population is reluctant to voluntarily seek care due to fear . . . Despite its image, there is nothing magical about the syndrome of Ebola: it causes a severe, febrile, gastrointestinal illness with lots of diarrhea and vomiting—lots of dehydration. We need to prevent this dehydration, prevent and treat the organ failure and severe metabolic and electrolyte abnormalities that develop.[8]

When the clinical care of patients is apologetically reduced to "a tiny piece of the response," you can bet that therapeutic nihilism has already infected many responders.

Signs and symptoms of such nihilism flourished from the beginning of West Africa's Ebola epidemic to the very end. Supportive and critical care were described as imprudent, dangerous, and not cost-effective; they were held to divert attention from disease control. Not only were autopsies forbidden, basic laboratory tests were deemed unnecessary or impossible—even though, as the Canadians and their colleagues noted, "we are routinely measuring Ebola viral loads in some of the world's most logistically challenged medical care environments using advanced assays that are unavailable in most tertiary care centers."[9] Most clinicians didn't even have the ability to measure basic vital signs. No hospital in the United States, Canada, or Europe would be credentialed without the capacity for such measurements. But most of West Africa is a public-health desert, which is why Ebola (like many other pathogens) spreads there, and it is a clinical desert, which is why it kills there.

The reasons that this is so are not natural at all.

Filoviruses can have wildly variable case-fatality rates, ranging from nobody dead in some cohorts to everybody in others. Disease-control experts, public-health authorities, and the popular press often explain this by talking about *differential virulence* among different species and strains. But to pose once more obvious if contentious questions: How do we explain why two humans the same age stricken by the same species may have such different outcomes? How do we learn where and how a divergence of this sort can be lessened in the face of medical and scientific progress?

Although important biological variations between strains surely account for some of these embodied disparities, it's the social and economic *terrain*, as Louis Pasteur observed, that accounts for many of them. Ebola in West Africa offers plenty of support for his point. When humans stricken by identical strains of the same pathogen have vastly different fates, as happened when an Ebola mutant first identified during the outbreak became its dominant driver, the most salient variable is the economic and social terrain. Those who work in settings in which social determinants of exposure risk and access to care are thrown into relief—settings of poverty, war, or famine, or during natural or manmade disasters—know this to be true.

Laboratory scientists and epidemiologists often know it, too. But many of them lack the ability to link their precious expertise to an understanding of the social drivers of epidemics; others tack on such social perspectives tardily, usually in the aftermath of a significant outbreak. Most leave such exercises to behavioral scientists, medical anthropologists, and historians.[10] If context or terrain is as important as Pasteur insisted, however, these complementary ways of understanding and responding to epidemics are as important to integrate as are prevention and care.

As for variations between strains: What do we know about these differences and about the strength of these claims? As of early 2018, Ebola was held to comprise five genetically and serologically distinct species: Zaire, Sudan, Bundibugyo, Taï Forest (the virus formerly known as Côte d'Ivoire), and Reston. Claims about the correlation between clinical outcomes and species variation are reliably pat. I cite a June 2015 review in the *Journal of Clinical and Diagnostic Research* only because it is typical: "Five different species of *Ebolavirus* are established, of which four are known to cause disease in humans. These, in their decreasing order of virulence and lethality, are Zaire virus . . . , Sudan virus . . . , Bundibugyo virus . . . , Taï Forest virus . . . , and Reston virus."[11] But as Joe McCormick learned, there have been outbreaks of Sudan virus with case-fatality rates of 65 percent or higher, and only a single case of Taï Forest virus has been documented in humans—or rather, a human.

There are also various clades, or families, within these species. The West African epidemic, as Pardis Sabeti and her colleagues have shown, was caused by one of several Zaire clades. The Makona variant is named after a river that cuts through the trizone area; it's the one that caused the West African epidemic.[12] Sabeti and others have offered in vitro evidence of a mutation in the Makona genome, first documented in March 2014, that was held to confer increased infectivity for primates, including the human sort. Some working with real-world primates of the nonhuman variety, and with mice, disagreed.[13] But within human primates infected by this mutant, case-fatality rates varied widely between those plucked from the clinical desert and those who received what passed as care within it.

Here, Louis Pasteur's famous aphorism, cited on the first page of this chapter, remains important more than a century after his death. The virus is never the only protagonist of the story. The view that the pathogen itself determines everything—and that the host and his or her social conditions are irrelevant, unworthy of serious scrutiny—legitimates therapeutic nihilism. But are we sure these variants are more virulent than other Zaire strains? Did they become so by acquiring new virulence factors? If so, why did Americans and most Europeans stricken with these mutants mostly survive, while the majority of West Africans did not?

Confident claims about predictable levels of lethality and virulence would seem overstated even as regards all the filoviruses, including the four species known (as of this writing) to cause human disease.[14] The previously cited 2015 review by Pierre Rollin and others—well written and helpful regarding the structure of the virus and the pathophysiology of acute infection, if less instructive regarding the reasons for such varied clinical outcomes— reminds us that claims of causality regarding how Ebola kills aren't credible unless they're informed by an understanding of a complex web of causation. This web is as invariably social (in the broadest sense, encompassing variables often classed as economic, cultural, and psychological) as it is pathophysiological (encompassing not only comorbid disease and variables such as age of the host but also mutations in the pathogen).

The best clinicians and researchers—Rollin among them—know that their own disciplinary training shouldn't prejudge the answers to questions posed about Ebola's clinical course any more than it should limit questions about its distribution and spread within human populations. Rollin and his coauthors conclude their review by pointing back to factors located squarely in the realm of social medicine: "The highly virulent and infectious nature of filoviruses, increasingly porous geographic borders, breakdown of public health measures, poverty challenges and social inequity create significant and daunting challenges ahead."[15] These social challenges become clinical ones if the primary goal is to stop these viruses from killing.

For these reasons and for others explored below, a weak and disputed understanding of filovirus pathogenesis, and how to halt or reverse it, has persisted even after the genome and structure of these agents became known, and even as significant mutations were described. Ongoing mutations may alter the virulence and infectivity of such pathogens—investigating this topic was of great interest to Humarr Khan and his Sierra Leonean and American coworkers—but evidence of this was lacking at the outset of the Ebola epidemic.[16] (That's one reason why, had fate been kinder, Khan was to join Pardis Sabeti and her Boston-based team in the fall of 2014.) The strains that spread from the eastern trizone forests to the cities on the Atlantic coast may one day be found to cause a different clinical course when the playing field is level as regards the capacity for supportive or critical care. But this has yet to be proved, since the playing field has yet to be leveled.

If anything, it keeps getting more uneven.

Claims about who lives and who dies during filovirus outbreaks, and why, are sometimes made with an unreflective abandon that should make medical editors blush. Virologists, pathologists, and many others working in the basic sciences often make these claims, but this is to be expected. Their training and expertise don't position them to know much about *le terrain*.

Less understandably, epidemiologists and clinicians also make thoroughly desocialized or decontextualized claims about epidemics. (When their reports refer to the social, it's usually to individual behavior, local culture, and traditional beliefs and practices, rather than to the historical events, processes, and policies discussed in previous chapters.) And because so many in the scientific community make these claims, science writers and journalists naturally make them, too, echoing a confidently laid-out hierarchy of virulence that ranges from 90 percent in the case of the Zaire species, to zero percent in the case of Reston.

The Reston virus may not be regarded by most experts to be pathogenic for humans, but it did spark an outbreak of fear among our species. It's the star, after all, of *The Hot Zone*, a book that echoed and amplified a number of myths and mystifications about how Ebola kills, or doesn't. Consider this passage:

> The Ebolas were named Ebola Zaire and Ebola Sudan. Marburg was the mildest of the three filovirus sisters. The worst of them was Ebola Zaire. The kill rate in humans infected with Ebola Zaire is nine out of ten. Ninety percent of the people who come down with Ebola Zaire die of it. Ebola Zaire is a slate wiper in humans.[17]

The fates of a dozen survivors introduced in this book's pages—Ibrahim, Yabom, Momoh ("the linebacker"), Mariatu, the Chairman and his family, the kids in the Port Loko pediatric ward—put the lie to such claims, as do the fates of those airlifted to safety, or the West Africans who received care in Nigeria or in Hastings, once more aggressive treatment regimes were implemented. Since the West African epidemic and its global tendrils were all caused by the Makona variant of Ebola Zaire, one wonders what happened to take away its slate-wiping sting since Preston wrote. By the spring of 2015, Partners In Health had already hired more than seven hundred survivors in Sierra Leone alone, all of them infected after the Makona mutant had become dominant. What doom awaits them is unknown, but right now they are deeply engaged in helping their fellow sufferers and in recovering from their losses.

Historians of epidemic disease will recognize familiar patterns here. Social, economic, and geographic factors, including those shaping access to quality health care, can make all the difference for people stricken with a disease like Ebola. Early accounts of the West African epidemic scanted these factors and instead focused most of the available attention on exaggerated genetic and other biological factors, and allegedly local and cultural ones—a blind spot compounded by a lopsided control-over-care response that widened a sinister outcome gap. And that gap was widened by the differential availability of therapies both old (remedies for shock and sepsis) and new (promising if still-unproven Ebola-specific preventives and treatments). Those with ready access to prompt and effective interventions, of course, did much better than those without them. This is yet another way of saying there's no longer such a thing as the natural history of disease, since disparities of access are anything but natural.

There have been flashes of clarity among those who struggled with data coming from the lab and the field—the real world of outbreaks. When the field includes both the clinical desert and the oases of the day, those flashes illuminate how outdated the notion of a natural history is in our unequal and interconnected world. Some recent reviews of Marburg's history have sought to revise unthinking repetition of its lesser virulence, when compared to its evil stepsisters.[18] The next step in such a reevaluation is to ask *why* outbreaks caused by the same or similar strains of Marburg display the same dramatic variation in case-fatality rate registered in outbreaks caused by Ebola. Pasteur's aphorism should steer all such exercises, which have to include an understanding of the terrain.

Pasteur's protégés, the colonial sanitarians who arrived in West Africa in the late nineteenth century and after, were too little interested in shaping the terrain by extending clinical services to the forest villages from which these pathogens emerged. The sequence of events laid out in chapter 6 suggests that therapeutic nihilism as policy comes from influential sanitarians and their heirs, not from the research laboratory. Nor can it be shown that such policies were favored by a majority of clinical practitioners, a difficult topic to study since there were so few of them around during and shortly after colonial rule. By the time twenty-first-century Marburg epidemics were described, the control-over-care paradigm had long shaped most public-health responses to the disease. High case-fatality rates were read as a sign not that improved clinical care could make a difference but rather that a strict implementation of the control-over-care paradigm was necessary. A contagious disease with a 90 percent fatality rate would seem to leave little choice in the matter.

Experience of the disease in the city that gave Marburg its name, or in other European cities, had disappeared down the memory hole. It's pretty clear that some of those who responded to the Marburg outbreak that began in northern Angola in 2004 were already convinced that the virus was not Ebola's "gentle" little sister but rather its implacable twin. According to the Médecins Sans Frontières website, their work in Angola had "one, clear priority in mind: to contain the epidemic and save lives by isolating contagious persons and bodies as fast as possible." Local responses to this priority were not unlike those registered more recently in Guinea, Sierra Leone, and Liberia, as the MSF authors themselves reported:

> The backlash was that fear-inspired rumors quickly spread among
> the inhabitants of Uíge—the town in northern Angola that was the
> focal point of the epidemic. Some of the inhabitants said the new
> foreigners were "stealing the dead"—a serious charge given
> the local belief that people who are not properly buried will turn

into bad spirits and take revenge on the living. Others claimed the "astronauts" (aid workers in full-body safety suits) were "demons" who were "confiscating the sick" or even worse, "killers" who had "come to exterminate us" by spreading the Marburg virus.[19]

This report—titled, apparently without irony, "Marburg Outbreak, Angola: When Saving Lives Seems Cruel"—starts by noting that the first question the MSF team received was, "You're doctors, why don't you treat us?" The coordinator of the Marburg response, who would later shape MSF's interventions in West Africa and the eastern Congo, replied as follows: "There isn't much you can do against Marburg."[20]

The fact that gentle Marburg killed 90 percent of those afflicted living in the war-torn region of Uíge, Angola, while sparing over three-quarters of infected Europeans in 1967, or that case-fatality rates in outbreaks of the Sudan Ebola virus were all over the map—depending more on where on the map they occurred, and thus where on the social ladder one was standing—has thus far done little to change the standard approach to outbreaks of these pathogens: namely, identify the culprit using high-end lab equipment brought in by expert teams, surround contaminated villages, and close down the hospitals and clinics until the outbreaks "burn themselves out." As during past outbreaks of smallpox and sleeping sickness, some hamlets were put to the torch along with clothes, sheets, linens, mattresses, and sleeping mats.

But the resonances between martial disease-control efforts under Portuguese rule and after independence have deeper roots in Angola, of course. So do the accusations and rumors of foreigners coming to steal bodies during the Uíge outbreak in 2004. Between 1514 and 1867, Portuguese and other slavers shipped close to six million people in chains from ports on the Angolan coast and surrounding region; the majority were landed in Brazil.[21]

Before 2013, many outbreaks of Ebola or Marburg "burned themselves out" before anybody outside of the medical desert noticed them. But the Ebola outbreak that began in West Africa was different. The control-over-care approach—long the cornerstone of colonial officialdom's response to malaria, plague, sleeping sickness, smallpox, Lassa, and even influenza—didn't work. The outbreak didn't go away with standard containment measures and didn't spare capital cities. But this was not solely because of an unprecedentedly virulent new Ebola mutant. It was that the terrain itself was so virulent.

One manifestation of this virulence was the delivery of poor-quality medical care. Since it was well known that the remedy didn't match the ailment, the mismatch would have been termed malpractice on a less virulent terrain. Dr. Dan Chertow and colleagues diplomatically summed things up in *The New England Journal of Medicine* when discussing the control-over-care approach. "Although this strategy by itself may be effective in controlling small outbreaks in remote settings," they wrote, "it has offered little hope to infected people and their families in the absence of medical care. In the current West African outbreak, infection control and clinical management efforts are necessarily being implemented on a larger scale than in any previous outbreak, and it is therefore appropriate to reassess traditional efforts at disease management."[22]

By October 2014, when we visited the giant Monrovia ETU introduced in the preface to this book—the ETU from which Chertow was writing—it was clear that a substantial fraction of patients weren't living long enough for a protective immune response to kick in—or even to display late hemorrhagic manifestations of the disease. This was in part because the *T* in these ETUs did not often include aggressive supportive care, and never included critical care. By the time the intensivists and trauma and emergency-care specialists weighed in, clinicians of all stripes—especially experienced nurses—were bumping up against the clinical nihilism then seeping into most discussions of how best to respond to the West African epidemic. Some of them learned that deploring a lack of focus on improving care in the clinical desert sparked controversy and resentment.

Robert Fowler was willing to go on record in a *New York Times* investigation of the debate about intravenous therapy for Ebola patients in or approaching hypovolemic shock. He called for hospitals and Ebola treatment units in West Africa to begin treatment of Ebola with "early, liberal use of intravenous fluid and electrolyte replacement." Anything less, he concluded, is "not medically justified and will result in continued high case-fatality rates."[23] Fowler, Chertow, François Lamontagne, and other intensivists all made such claims, but they were rebutted by MSF's filovirus gurus, whose views about Ebola were pretty much the same as those earlier proffered about Marburg. As regards supportive care and mortality, one of them allowed that aggressive intravenous therapy "would probably push it down some, but I'd be surprised if it were dramatic."[24]

In the end, this wasn't largely a clinical dispute, although it sounded like one. It was mostly a control-over-care dispute about protecting clinicians. As *The New York Times* put it, "Some argue that more aggressive treatment with IV fluids is medically possible and a moral obligation. But others counsel caution, saying that pushing too hard would put overworked doctors and nurses in danger and that the treatment, if given carelessly, could even kill patients."[25] As the outbreak took off, the MSF Ebola experts made their opinions very clear: aggressive treatment was reckless and potentially lethal. But some of those experts began to change their minds—or to openly express internal disagreement—as it became clear the control-over-care approach wasn't working. In December 2014, a group of MSF veterans wrote an open letter to their colleagues. It was a wrenching critique of their own Ebola response. "For any physician it's a disaster to lose a single patient in hypovolemic shock," they wrote. "We lost hundreds."[26]

Early in the course of Ebola's western surge, a surgical colleague from the Brigham and Women's Hospital passed on a historical review of "The Mystery of Shock."[27] Since our previous exchanges had consisted of clinical recommendations for patients we shared in Boston, I wasn't sure why he'd send me this work, which explores the efforts of Walter B. Cannon, who worked at Harvard Medical School a century before us, pushing forward the boundaries of the still-young fields of physiology and pathophysiology. It didn't take more than a few minutes of reading to make the connection to a passing discussion of Ebola.

Walter Cannon, who began his medical studies in 1896, focused his attention on shock, whether due to blood loss, infection, or causes unknown. He was motivated in particular by how little was known about the pathophysiology of these varied conditions. This was at the time when some of his British and French peers were launching their Pasteurian revolution. Although that revolution didn't include much interest in the treatment of shock among their African subjects, the great bloodletting of the Great War made this an urgent topic among surgeons and microbiologists alike. When Cannon was called up to serve as a medic on the front lines, Allied commanders were made aware of his clinical interests and assigned him the urgent task of reducing mortality among the wounded in field hospitals. It was in such MASH units, which were sometimes under fire from German artillery, that Cannon and others came to develop what would come to be known as replacement therapy.

The reason my Brigham colleague passed along this historical review of Cannon's work was that I'd been complaining publicly, during the summer of 2014, about the mismatch between the most striking symptoms of severe Ebola—massive fluid loss due to vomiting and diarrhea—and the treatment most often prescribed that summer: oral rehydration salts. We'd all seen ORS work wonders among babies dehydrated by diarrheal disease of various etiologies, and didn't hesitate to prescribe this elixir for just about anyone with fever, diarrhea, the flu, a bad cold, or even a debilitating hangover. Even before Partners In Health began obtaining packets of these miraculous salts in bulk, about thirty years ago, we shared strong opinions about ORS. If you can keep it down, the stuff usually works wonders. Never leave home without it. In fact, we'd taught ourselves and thousands of rural Haitian moms how to brew a similar remedy at home in case their kids needed it, which was often.

Then there was the heartening impact of rapidly administered ORS in the midst of a medical emergency, which I'd seen not once but twice before the West African Ebola epidemic. These salts revived thousands of postwar cholera patients in Peru in the early 1990s, and even more of them in 2010, when post-earthquake Haiti became home to the world's largest cholera epidemic.[28] But that's a bacterial illness that kills through radically different mechanisms than those seen in viral hemorrhagic fevers. Cholera secretes a toxin, long known down to the molecule, that triggers a chain reaction. The toxin causes the gut lining to stop absorbing sodium and chloride at the same time that it causes the secretion of water and chloride. The "rice-water stool" that spurts out has the consistency of plasma, and much the same content: it's as if your lifeblood is pouring out of your anus.

That's why cholera wards are full of cots with holes permitting free passage of liquid stool into ten-gallon buckets below. Severe cholera is regarded as one of the true infectious-disease emergencies, because of both the volume and speed at which fluids and electrolytes are lost: the buckets under the cots have been known to fill up with rice-water stools within hours. In one instance at a hilltop cholera tent in rural Haiti, I laid eyes on a young woman whom I mistook for dead. (I was, alas, fairly well schooled in that diagnosis.) Her eyes were sunken and rolled back in her head; her skin was papery; her lips, thin and pale, were drawn back from her teeth in a frightening rictus. Even her teeth looked as dry as bleached bone. As ominously, I heard no sound of liquid trickling into the bucket under her cot. She was, I concluded, shriveled and gone. But one of my more astute Haitian colleagues, a nursing assistant, saw signs of life and started tipping ORS between her parted teeth. The moribund woman gagged but kept it down.

I moved on to other patients soon after that, but three hours later, when I returned to check on the young woman, she had her eyes trained on the cup as the aide kept tipping the solution patiently into her mouth. I never thought I'd be so happy to hear the sound of liquid "stool"—it really had no solid matter in it—hitting the bottom of a bucket. After fewer than six hours of this therapy, the young woman was able to sit up and thank the nursing assistant. (She tried to thank me, too, unaware that I'd almost written her off.) Shortly thereafter, for the first time in three days, she felt the need to urinate, and did. She improved rapidly. With the help of her son, who looked to be about ten, she walked out of the tent the following day, looking downright healthy. Hers was the quickest turnaround I'd seen in years, but turnarounds can be rapid when the remedy matches the pathophysiology of the disease and is delivered in time—in her case, barely. Just thinking about it now, several years later, and after thousands of needless deaths to cholera in Haiti, makes me smile with gratitude.

Cholera, like most infections causing illness in humans, causes a wide spectrum of disease severity. In both Haiti and Peru, we saw that some had mild cholera—a bit of diarrhea, no fever—while others died within hours. Once teams get good at diagnosing and treating cholera promptly, usually with ORS alone, almost no one dies. But in the early days of the Haitian epidemic, up to 20 percent of all cholera patients perished. In rural regions, and among those vomiting, some village health workers reported that up to half of those afflicted died in those horrible first weeks. This wasn't much different from outcomes in the nineteenth century, and thus another twenty-first-century example of malpractice rather than one of the "natural history" of cholera. A year into the epidemic, case-fatality rates had dropped in places like central Haiti—where I was lucky enough to witness this young woman's recovery, and many others—to less than 2 percent. Within two years, it had been halved again.

Untreated severe cholera can, in other words, have a case-fatality rate as high as Ebola's and is more rapidly fatal. But lucky patients walk away without any lasting damage. That is, their affected organs—the gut lining, the kidneys, the heart, the blood vessels, the brain—are not left with permanent lesions. Some of the lessons we learned in the course of treating thousands of cholera patients raised questions that weren't altogether irrelevant in the face of a large Ebola epidemic. Was it possible that there was a wide spectrum of Ebola virus disease? Was it possible that there were, at least early in the course of the viral illness, few irreversible changes? Or did Ebola boast a set of virulence factors or toxins far worse than cholera's that might account for the exceptionally high mortality seen in West Africa? If so, why such wild variation in the course of disease caused by the same strain of the Zaire species of Ebola? Were survivors diagnosed earlier and cared for better?

It wasn't necessary to pose, even just rhetorically, the question heard in discussions within West Africa's ETUs: Was ORS sufficient for all or even most patients?

Anyone who has seen as many cholera patients as I have knows plenty of people—some vomiting, some delirious, some unresponsive—who were saved with intravenous solution, sometimes administered directly into the bone when patients were so dehydrated that it was impossible to find a vein to stick. The same can be said about patients severely ill from meningococcal or pneumococcal disease, both of which kill through very different mechanisms. Many infections can be lethal without replacement therapy, with cholera at the top of the list. But MSF's leading Ebola specialist thought such comparisons misleading. "In cholera, you can get fatalities down from 50 percent to 1 percent," he told reporters from *The New York Times*. "We've been putting people on IVs for Ebola for 14 years. If just tanking them up worked, we'd be doing it."[29]

"Tanking them up" is a term used in hospitals across the United States. It implies an ability to fill a receptacle. But when patients are vomiting or already unresponsive, their receptacles sealed, it's difficult or impossible to administer ORS: the young woman in central Haiti survived by the skin of her bone-dry teeth. Failure to provide such care was my error and almost killed her. Had she died, her death might have been deemed medical malpractice in a hospital in the United States—her heart was still beating, after all. At the Brigham and Women's Hospital, she would have received fluids through large-bore intravenous lines or, had it proved difficult to find a vein, an intraosseous needle passing through bone. In central Haiti, it took a nurse's aide hours of full-time attention to get as much fluid and electrolytes in this shriveled-up woman as could have been done in thirty minutes through other means, and the cholera unit was packed with sick patients needing care.

This dilemma was familiar to many working in the big Ebola units in West African cities. In the big ETU we'd visited in Monrovia, it was estimated that most patients received about one or two minutes of skilled medical attention per shift. What did this mean for patients who, as Dan Chertow and his colleagues put it, were "in shock with evidence of organ failure whose outcome would not be altered by any available medical intervention"?[30] They were, to put it a little less clinically, shit out of luck.

That oral rehydration salts are no panacea for severe disease due to Ebola, Marburg, or Lassa had been obvious from every previously documented outbreak. The presenting symptoms of the Ebola in West Africa's 2014 epidemic included nausea and vomiting almost as often as diarrhea and fever; in many early reports, gastrointestinal symptoms were about ten times more frequent than the famous hemorrhagic symptoms. (I never saw a patient bleeding out of his eyes.) So my heart sank when, in the first weeks of Ebola's explosion in urban Liberia, MSF, the world's largest and most influential health NGO, decided to halt intravenous fluid resuscitation and lab tests in its centers and instead recommended oral rehydration salts as the *sole* treatment of choice for all patients, regardless of clinical presentation.

MSF justified its decision on various grounds, among them, as one colleague put it, "massive caseloads, limited number of health care workers, and limited time in personal protective equipment."[31] Its spokespersons often also mentioned the risk of hemorrhage around venipuncture sites, in spite of a lack of evidence that it had much clinical significance. Much more significant, and entirely reasonable, was fear of occupational exposure. Because oral therapies involve no "sharps"—as needles, catheters, scalpels, and the like are termed in clinical settings—they are naturally safer to administer than intravenous therapy. Safer for caregivers, that is.

Sharps have always been associated with the transmission of blood-borne pathogens to health professionals. But it should go without saying that exclusively oral and largely self-administered therapies are never likely to save those too sick to sip them. Even for those who could, oral therapies were clearly inadequate for some of the sentient but nauseated. During the outbreak, ORS were often served warm to patients, who, exhorted to chug them, complained that the taste was unpleasant. In addition, the standard formulation contains certain electrolytes and not others, or some in insufficient quantities. We didn't know the best recipe for severe Ebola, even for those who could keep it down, since there was often little interest in performing the basic laboratory tests that might have informed that recipe.

Wouldn't it have been better to just admit we were all afraid of contagion, rather than to argue that ORS was the treatment of choice for all West Africans with Ebola?

West Africa's improvised ETUs were, admittedly, scary places. Kenema in the months that eastern Sierra Leone was swamped and Maforki and Monrovia at the height of the western surge were about as bad as it gets. But fear was only one of many emotions there, and it wasn't always at the top of the list. Defeatist attitudes and low-ball clinical aspirations of the summer and fall of 2014 bred resentment and discouragement among the medical professionals called to rely on safer oral therapies—and to observe a no-touch policy even when gloved and gowned.

Most of the time, defeatist and nihilistic recommendations came from expatriate experts, whose low aspirations were on behalf of unknown others. Turning back to a previous century and its field hospitals, where Walter Cannon served a short distance from the front lines of the mother of all wars, offers a striking contrast. "The laboratories can have anything that is desired," he wrote elatedly to his wife in 1917, "men detailed from any unit, materials at whatever cost, and transportation of the most effective sort."[32] The young Peter Piot, in thinking about setting up what would be the world's first ETU near the shuttered Yambuku Mission Hospital, had a similarly can-do attitude in 1976. "Naturally the very ill would need to be transported from their villages," he wrote, "and that meant a helicopter would have to be available on a daily basis."[33] Naturally.

In West Africa's first big Ebola epidemic, can-do attitudes were largely reserved for infection control rather than driving down case-fatality rates among those already infected. When the control-over-care paradigm failed to contain Ebola in isolated villages to the east, the containment discussion also turned to requesting helicopters, but for transporting troops and disease controllers, not patients. If the sky was literally the limit for containment, clinical discussions were all about "making hard choices" between one necessary thing and another, and being "realistic" about what was possible in a clinical desert.[34] These were painful discussions in the middle of an epidemic that was taking out the very people—skilled nurses—who made use of things like infusion pumps, intraosseous needles, ventilators, and the like.

Dr. Moses Massaquoi, a hospital administrator and the director of the Clinton Foundation in Liberia, was one of the handful of Liberians I knew well prior to the epidemic. Of course he signed up to serve in the fight against Ebola. During our first and tardy trip to Liberia, at what proved to be the height of its western surge, I had meals with him regularly. I never saw him look downcast, much less haggard, until one day when I found him looking defeated. In private, at least, he complained about the double standard then playing out within the country's handful of Ebola treatment units, including the big one in Monrovia. "I can't manage the unhappiness of the Liberians working in the ETUs," he said late one night, "because some of them are nurses or medical students, and they all know we can't save these patients without intravenous fluids."

One night, Massaquoi missed a meal with me and the chief medical officer of Partners In Health. After three hours went by, we started to worry. We kept calling his cell phone. No answer. So the two of us kept vigil, sitting in the tiny lobby of our hotel, thumbing through e-mail and looking up anxiously whenever anyone came through the doors. The hotel, like others in the city, was packed with public-health teams, journalists covering Ebola, and no small number of members of the U.S. Army, its engineers and logisticians dispatched in response to the Liberian president's appeal for their help. Shortly before midnight, Massaquoi appeared, apologizing even as he strode through the door. One of the French volunteers working in the big Monrovia unit had just been diagnosed with Ebola. He'd received this news along with an urgent request for an infusion pump—one of the tools he'd been asking international nongovernmental organizations to supply for weeks. "I couldn't be sarcastic," he said without guile. "That wouldn't be correct or humane."

Dr. Massaquoi, who'd just spent hours searching for the pump, apolo-

gized for missing dinner. The nurse was airlifted to her native country before
he succeeded in finding it.

This double standard of imagination was evident exactly a century earlier,
when colonial Pasteurians across the Mano River in Sierra Leone worked
from the same minimalist playbook in confronting the plagues of that era. But
much more was expected back in the metropole during the Great War.

The idea that hardworking clinicians in sweltering bioprotective gear might
aspire to have (in Walter Cannon's 1917 formulation) "anything that is desired"
was pretty much absent on the front lines of the war against Ebola in West Africa. It's worth noting that some local health authorities also disparaged the quest
for more aggressive therapy—the sort administered through infusion pumps—
usually because other priorities (case finding, isolation, and contact tracing)
were held to be more urgent. Urgent they surely were, but those priorities were
almost always presented as competing for the same scarce resources, including those allocated for care. So it was more than a little confusing when the
82nd Airborne, a sharp-looking group with handy helicopters, materialized
in Monrovia in the midst of the crisis.

MSF had called the world's attention to the epidemic, and for logistical help
from its armies, but some of its leaders continued to disparage the tools and skills
of critical care—"Dialysis machines? Ventilators? Infusion pumps?"—even
well after some of their own volunteers had been saved by them. As the sociologist Renée Fox has noted, MSF has a reputation for "a culture of debate," so
it was no surprise to later learn of a deep internal divide in the organization,
with several senior MSF leaders deploring an Ebola response characterized by
"no medical tools, no ambition to try." Among this group were the cosigners
of the open letter I cited earlier in this chapter, which concluded in this way:

Those of us who witnessed the emergence of the HIV/AIDS
pandemic in the nineties and the widespread reluctance within
MSF to address patient care can find identical features in the way

MSF is dealing with the Ebola epidemic. A bundle of ill-founded suppositions leads to the conviction that little can be done. The resulting institutional conservatism prevents access to quality care for our patients, but is also a major obstacle to development of innovative care strategies. This is an uncomfortable repetition of history that we need to urgently address as a movement.[35]

A copy of this letter, dated December 4, 2014, reached me a couple of months after our own public dust-up with MSF, which was trifling compared to its internal feuds.

Besides, the failure of imagination on display in West Africa was standard among humanitarian groups, and MSF was far from the most culpable among us. At least the MSFers had shown up early in the clinical desert, where many have been socialized to accept that scarcity is the norm for the poor. Yet in the ETUs established in 2014 in West Africa, usually only a single lab test per patient was performed: a diagnostic test for the Zaire species of Ebola. This was simply inadequate. When someone in the recovery phase of Ebola suddenly dropped dead, it might be due to electrolyte abnormalities, or it might not. Who could know without basic lab tests? A patient who looked like he or she might have metabolic acidosis due to hypovolemic shock might or might not. Again, who was to know? Even blood pressures and temperatures were seldom taken.

Laboratory support on the front lines of the Great War were more robust than those found in most Ebola treatment units a century later. After a brief stint working with colleagues in London, Walter Cannon returned to the French front line, where he used a battlefront field hospital to unravel "the mystery of shock" while taking care of critically ill and injured soldiers:

First, he hoped that determining the blood sugar level of patients in shock might reveal whether the inception of acidosis in the wounded was a "starvation acidosis" brought on by a carbohydrate-deficient diet or a lack of food and water before and after action on the battlefield. Second, he examined the possibility that providing the badly-wounded with a reserve of material in the blood would fortify them during operations against dangerous drops in blood pressure and increase in acidosis. And third, he tried to develop efficient methods to prevent the onset of secondary shock in wounded patients during their transit from the trenches to the rear.[36]

It surely took both courage and imagination for Cannon and others to conduct research while delivering care in field hospitals well within the strike zone of German artillery, and the courage of the MSF staff sent as first responders in 2014 to contend with Ebola in West Africa was not in doubt. MSF doctors, we knew, also regularly worked in war zones, and several of them paid the ultimate price for their bravery. But a bit of Cannon's can-do spirit would have gone a long way toward helping patients in the war zone that was Ebola-stricken West Africa. The aggressive treatment of shock syndromes, even as primitively as Cannon had done it, would likely have saved many lives.

The mystery of shock wasn't so confounding a century after Walter Cannon's work. There were, however, other mysteries to unravel concerning Ebola, including its potential complications.

During the height of Ebola's western surge, it might not have seemed the right moment to discuss complications, which were seen in a minority of survivors. But as 2014 wore on, and as my colleagues and I became more experienced, we learned it was a substantial minority. As we saw more and more patients with ongoing complications, we began to worry deeply (and publicly) about three, in particular: ocular inflammation leading to blindness, seizure disorders, and sanctuary sites in which the virus might persist.[37] To give one example from Sierra Leone in 2015: among 643 survivors screened by our colleagues at the Port Loko survivor clinic, 96 were diagnosed with uveitis, a potentially blinding inflammation of the eye.[38] (Yabom Koroma was one of them.) Was this inflammation, which also seemed, on exam, to affect other parts of the eye, a postinfectious complication? Or was the virus still alive and replicating in the eye?[39]

We had good reason to ask how such patients—with visual or hearing loss or seizure disorders—should best be cared for over time. Think of Isatu and Little Ibrahim, the children I introduced in chapter 3. Ibrahim was blind, and Isatu was having seizures. If Ibrahim had a dense inflammatory reaction in his eyes, shouldn't he have been treated right away with steroids, which were readily available or could be made so, even in Port Loko? If Isatu had already experienced seizures in Maforki, shouldn't she already have been on antiepileptic medications, which could be easily procured and were, hours after her dramatic fall to the floor during a grand mal seizure? To anybody who plumbed the medical archives, the answers were yes and yes.[40]

On the ground in West Africa in 2014, we were never sure how much of what we were learning was actually old news. Sequelae were declared "surprising" or "unprecedented" and attributed to increased virulence or to novel spread in an immunologically naïve population. This too was false. Then again, serological surveys conducted in the same region in the years before and after the war suggested that Ebola wasn't new to this part of West Africa.[41] But these surveys, like studies of Marburg's complications, had been forgotten. Throughout the latter months of 2014 and well into the next year, many commentators, including some from the World Health Organization, continued to insist that Ebola was "completely new" to West Africa.

Among the questions circulating at the outset of the West African epidemic, many were clinical and concerned differential mortality and long-term sequelae. Was the former attributable to age? Were the elderly and frail likely to die even if they received supportive and critical care? Did those who died have comorbid conditions, such as malnutrition or anemia or concurrent infections—or HIV or tuberculosis or malaria? Were infants too young to mount a rapid and effective immune response? Was it true that most immunologically naïve, otherwise ill, elderly, young, and pregnant patients were flat-out doomed? (We heard repeatedly that saving pregnant women with Ebola was pretty much a lost cause, and that their infants never, ever survived.)[42] Had partial immunity been conferred by previous infections with closely related viruses, or even previous infections with a different clade of Ebola? Were some complications predictable and treatable, such as the seeping of gut bacteria into the bloodstream, causing secondary and sometimes fatal infections even as blood levels of Ebola were dropping thanks to an adaptive immune response?

The list of clinical questions went on. Were we missing cases of renal failure due to failure to test for it? There were unconfirmed rumors of deaths from acute renal failure more than a year after survivors were classed as Ebola-free, and reports of chronic joint pain.[43] A number of our patients had irregular heart rhythms, which they sometimes diagnosed themselves, since they were so rarely examined by overworked, harried, hot, and fearful professional caregivers. Were renal failure and arrhythmias signs of complications of immune response, of direct viral damage to kidneys and hearts, or both? Were these new and unrelated afflictions, or tardy Ebola sequelae? Without hospitals equipped with decent labs—or with, as in Kenema, a decent lab but no decent hospital—there was no way of knowing.

Although not everyone involved in the response was interested in such clinical questions, many were. It was Tony Fauci who said it best, when I called him from Monrovia in September 2014. I wanted to get his thoughts on a couple of new therapeutics about to go into clinical trials, and on an old one (transfusion of convalescent plasma) that hadn't yet undergone formal evaluation. "Shame on us," he said, "if we don't learn anything in the course of these next few months." But the amount of learning that took place during those next few months was modest when compared to both the need and the scope of opportunities for it. During the course of the plague year, few field trials of new diagnostics, therapeutics, or preventives were conducted and completed.

The majority of academic articles published during the course of that year were reviews, editorials, or descriptive studies of large cohorts of patients that covered both presenting symptoms and outcomes: namely, survival, death, or transfer (the last outcome usually representing a missed opportunity for follow-up). ZMapp (and a less well-known combination of antibodies) and antiviral agents were not subjected to rigorous evaluation during the western surge, although many observational studies were conducted in all three countries and in the first-world ICUs to which expatriates were airlifted.[44] In Sierra Leone, the handful of field trials conducted inside an Ebola treatment unit included a Partners In Health–sponsored study that compared the cumbersome and slow "gold standard"—a polymerase chain reaction, or PCR, assay—with a new rapid point-of-care diagnostic. The main reason my coworkers conducted the trial was to lessen the time between blood draws and the return of a reliable result: a matter of minutes with the rapid test versus hours to days when confirmation required sending samples to Freetown. A head-to-head comparison, published in *The Lancet*, suggested that the rapid diagnostic was at least as good as, and perhaps better than, PCR—at least among patients with high viral loads.[45] Rapid tests promised to be far cheaper, too, as had similar assays used to diagnose HIV infection, malaria, and other common infections.

The studies mentioned above were all fairly inexpensive. Several costly vaccine trials were also set in motion, but most were delayed or canceled altogether. Only one, perhaps the saving grace of the epidemic, was completed. A Canadian vaccine was assayed in Guinea using a ring-vaccination approach modeled on the one found effective in eradicating smallpox. The vaccine—a recombinant, replication-competent vesicular stomatitis virus-based vaccine expressing a surface glycoprotein of Zaire Ebola virus, which only somewhat helpfully went by the acronym rVSV-ZEBOV—was offered to contacts of patients with confirmed Ebola either immediately or twenty-one days later. Among the 4,123 people vaccinated immediately after exposure, there were no new infections; among the 3,528 people vaccinated after a three-week delay, there were 16 of them. The conclusion, unlike the name of the vaccine, was mercifully straightforward: according to the scientists who conducted the assay, the vaccine "might be highly efficacious and safe in preventing Ebola virus disease, and is most likely effective at the population level when delivered during an Ebola virus disease outbreak via a ring vaccination strategy."[46]

What about supportive and critical care for Ebola in its advanced stages? Shouldn't basic care be subjected to a similar process of evaluation? A good number of people felt so. But choosing the right study design posed serious ethical challenges, in that it would be impossible to justify a study comparing a treatment group receiving such care with a control group that did not. Besides, that grim study of unnatural history had been going on for years: evidence had piled up in favor of replacement therapy in the treatment of hypovolemic shock, but none for new Ebola treatments among the severely hy-povolemic in the absence of replacement therapy. Fortunately, instructive information arrived in early 2015 in the form of a letter from Hastings, the largest Ebola treatment unit in Sierra Leone, where both Ibrahim and Yabom and many hundreds more were treated.

The letter, published in *The New England Journal of Medicine* on February 5 of that year, reported a steady reduction in the case-fatality rate over the first three months of operations. During the first couple of weeks, case-fatality rates exceeded 60 percent. A couple of weeks later, among the first 151 patients, the average mortality was reported as 48 percent. By month four, it had been halved again. The chief therapeutic changes in the course of these months had been the institution of "the Hastings protocol," which included aggressive fluid resuscitation (several liters of Ringer's lactate and dextrose saline given intravenously each day for the first three days as well as ORS), broad-spectrum antibiotics, vitamin K injections to decrease risk of bleeding, antimalarial treatment, antidiarrheals and antiemetics, and nutritional supplements. Its implementers admitted frankly that they weren't exactly sure why their efforts had been so successful. "It is unclear why the case fatality rate is decreasing at Hastings," they wrote. "We are unable to assess any individual component of the treatments we used, since we applied a package of interventions."[47]

What the Hastings staff were doing in applying this package of interventions, of course, was supportive care—and it's what we should have been doing in our first chaotic month in Maforki. But it's hard to implement a Hastings-style protocol without reliable electricity, running water, more prompt referrals from remote villages, and rigorous clinical triage. These were usually available within the commandeered policy academy but largely absent within the abandoned, rotting, and weed-covered vocational school on the outskirts of Port Loko.

One troubling question kept coming to mind during the height of the surge, and after. How could we know so much about the molecular structure of

Ebola but so little about the key steps in the pathogenesis of the disease in humans, and even less about how to arrest or reverse them? At least 109 full-length Zaire virus genomes were published in 2014 alone. Yet many basic questions about filoviruses—from pathogenesis in the human host to likelihood of viral persistence and late sequelae—remained unanswered.

Why was this so? In large part because the primary victims of Ebola were poor people living in remote villages.[48] The mechanisms by which tuberculosis or cholera or HIV kill, or don't kill, will vary significantly with time and circumstances, with conditions on *le terrain* determining events and outcomes as much, and often more, than microbial mutations. The few who have fallen ill with a filovirus infection in a place with modern medical care—in the course of a laboratory accident in Germany, say—have had a far greater chance of survival than those infected in the course of caregiving or burial in West Africa. An even smaller number saw the terrain shift under them as they were airlifted to safety and hope.

A properly biosocial analysis of how Ebola kills us, its accidental human host, will someday come to honor the memories of those lost to the disease. In the meantime, some of the basic issues worth addressing in a rudimentary exercise are straightforward. In such analyses, an understanding of the terrain can be linked to an even cellular-level pathogenesis—the seven steps required for Ebola to sicken and kill, as described at the beginning of this chapter. These steps are really processes that involve a series of feedback loops, occasionally altered by serendipity or (perhaps more often) bad luck. Since humans, unlike macaques, can fight back with more than innate and acquired immunity, there are or could be actions taken to block and reverse each of these processes. And so we must reconsider these seven steps from the perspective of social medicine, bearing in mind that, from this perspective, the steps differ in some significant ways.

The first step is obvious. *The Ebola virus must enter a human host*—a process discussed at the molecular level in virology, and at broader levels in social medicine. The human body is often an unexplored terrain for viruses adapted to nonhuman hosts. But age and concurrent illnesses (especially those associated with immune deficiency), and breaches in human-engineered defense mechanisms, are also likely to influence the rate at which viral load peaks, and the rate at which an effective immune response to viral invaders is mounted. Humans have evolved barriers to viral entry that no other primate has—gloves, gowns, masks, hoods, face shields, and other protective gear.[49]

The entry of a virus into a human host is never merely a molecular event. As with all things human, inequality plays a noxious role. This kit was part of *my* social integument, but it was just the sort of stuff that professional caregivers in West Africa did not have, and often don't to this day. I can say from sorry personal experience that advancing age may adversely affect the dexterity and diligence required to don and doff personal protective equipment, while lessening the stamina needed to spend more than an hour within a steamy Ebola treatment unit. But how often are "air-conditioned clinical space" or "running water" found on lists of factors diminishing the chances of viral entry?

In the medical desert, a more important question may be posed: What about family caregivers, especially those living in rough and rural conditions? During the crisis, many observers made the bushmeat connection, but how many of those who did then took the step of providing the personal protective equipment called gloves and soap to anybody who hunted, dressed, transported, or sold it? Precious few, I'd bet, despite the fact that much latex—like the palm oil referenced in the name of Palmolive soaps—originated in West Africa. How many villagers conducting burials in the region have received help from well-protected professionals? Until recently, the answer was almost none.

Step two involves *the infection establishing itself in the host*. Ebola has seven genes encoding eight proteins, some of which are crucial to this process. But there's a broad array of innate and acquired immune responses, and these, too, are shaped by social conditions. In fact, the immune response in a host—the recognition of the nonself—traces one history of lived experience and the experience and exposures of one's forebears. In humans, as in other mammals, the immune system evolved primarily to prevent infection and death caused by microbes, including viruses. Infectious-disease textbooks contain whole chapters listing the many factors associated with the variable course of disease caused by these pathogens. These include, for starters, the impact on host immune response of diet and nutritional status, age, concurrent disease, certain hormones, stress (as defined physiologically and colloquially), previous infections, and the presence or absence of indigenous microbial flora—these days termed the microbiome.

The list of mitigating factors, as far as the course of illness goes, also includes "natural antibodies." These are less specific than those generated in the course of the humoral immune response triggered by microbial invasion, but healthy hosts are able to call them forth earlier in the course of serious infections. Whether natural antibodies and other first-line defenses are robust is not merely a question of their presence or absence; it's also a question of their effectiveness, always a matter of microbes and terrain, with the terrain including the social and economic and ecological conditions of the host. All of these change, sometimes rapidly. This is true even without considering the potentially revolutionary change that ensues when another human adaptation, the vaccine, is rolled out where it is needed most—typically in settings where it is least likely to be deemed affordable as a commodity.

Step three: *the virus, once established in the human host, must acquire nutrients in order to survive.* Although this might reasonably be said of any living thing, viruses, unlike many bacteria, fungal pathogens, and parasites, can't live for long outside of their hosts' cells. A virus acquires nutrients by hijacking the machinery of the cells it invades. Even though Ebola virus has no trouble taking over human cells to acquire what it needs to survive and replicate, disease severity is altered by ambient conditions within its hosts. The extent to which host conditions, ranging from nutritional status to concurrent disease, enhance Ebola's rate of replication is unknown, but there's clear overlap, in West Africa, among epidemics of tuberculosis, HIV, blood- and nutrient-sapping intestinal parasites, and recurrent malaria—all of which, like Ebola, cause chronic anemia, and all of which may cause malabsorption of nutrients and malnutrition through varied mechanisms. At play, too, are pathogenic forces and events, which might include unfair trade arrangements or wild fluctuations in the cost of rice or flight into receding rain forests during civil conflict. Subject somebody to enough of these pathogens and pathogenic forces, as often happens in remote villages, and they *have* to consume game to survive. Which suggests that instead of blaming those who eat bushmeat for their own misfortunes, we should be helping them figure out a way to eat it more safely.

To cause a human host's death, the virus must take a fourth step, *circumventing innate defenses*. These defenses include nonspecific innate immunity, which, though less targeted than acquired ones, is complex and formidable among healthy adults—one of the reasons why so few families of viruses cause serious or lethal illness among humans. The strength of these defenses depends on a list of factors that arise so often in social medicine: age, years of schooling, nutritional status, concurrent disease or its absence, history of previous immunogenic infections and vaccines, hygienic and otherwise healthy comportments, availability of clean drinking water, access to trusted professional caregivers who can diagnose and treat their ailments, and several others. It's a long list.

Fifth, *the virus must replicate rapidly*. The size of the inoculum—the amount of virus introduced—determines how much virus is around to replicate in the hours after exposure. Many lethal infections, including those acquired by otherwise well-protected nurses and physicians, have likely involved small amounts of virus acquired during the process of doffing gowns and other personal protective equipment. But studies of Ebola suggest, unsurprisingly, that the higher the viral load, the higher the mortality—and the higher the chances of transmission to a new host.[50] These are features common to many, if not most, infections causing human disease. Inocula can be significant in the case of puncture wounds from large-bore needles, and massive in the course of caring for patients with heavy bleeding during, say, a delivery. Like traditional birth attendants, family members who nurse patients who are incontinent or vomiting uncontrollably, or for those charged with preparing the dead for burial, face exposure to astronomical numbers of infectious viral particles.

Sixth, *the virus must invade and replicate in those tissues and organs for which it exhibits tropism*. Here again, Ebola may be reliably drawn to certain early targets. But the result of such affinity is not written in stone, nor does

Ebola invariably inflict lethal damage on its chief targets. Some of this variation is best examined through the lens of social medicine, which includes—or
should—microbial genomics *and* political economy. We have collectively
shaped a global economy in which blood diamonds move out of Sierra Leone,
for example, but supportive and critical care don't move in. Nor do ophthal-
mology, neurology, psychiatry, surgery, or even basic primary care. The specialists who tend to the organs that Ebola attacks—nephrologists for the
kidneys, immunologists for fixed and mobile immune cells, ophthalmologists
for the eyes, and neurologists for seizures—are almost as entirely lacking in
Upper West Africa as are resolute and well-protected obstetricians.

Such care could and should be among the human responses, innate and
acquired, to Ebola. Kidney failure can be treated by dialysis, and it was when
needed by Americans and Europeans who received care in the United States
and Europe. Ian Crozier was on dialysis for weeks, and the Port Loko volunteer from Texas was on the brink of it. Respiratory failure, whether from
direct viral attack on lung tissue or from rare cases of fluid overload, can be
addressed by ventilatory support. Crozier was mechanically ventilated for
the better part of a month; the Texan, for about ten days.

In the twenty-first century, when our defenses against disease are imagined to include a health-care system worthy of the name, Ebola does its
work by evading not just biological but also *social* defenses. This is how
Ebola kills. The virus keeps at this work even among those who have survived the disease. The gravity of its sequelae depend on how well it evades
social defenses—such as the prompt follow-up care that Yabom should have
received after reporting seeing smoke in her eye. This is how Ebola blinds.

Seventh, *the virus must be transmitted to new and susceptible hosts.* As
regards Ebola in West Africa, this happened in the ways explored in previous chapters: human-to-human transmission in the course of caring for the
sick or burying the dead. Both kinds of transmission can be interrupted by
professional and material assistance with both of these forms of caregiving,
through barrier nursing (and its equivalent in last rites and interment) and
other forms of infection control.[51] It's less clear they can be interrupted by
banning caregiving altogether. The questions raised by the experiences of

both Ibrahim and Yabom, and by any thoughtful review of the history of epidemic disease in West Africa, is whether banning caregiving and funerals without respectful professional assistance is effective in stopping transmission. The answer may well be yes, but it was a rocky and anguished process.

The verdict is in on the control-over-care approach that was used to address the Ebola crisis in the villages, towns, and cities of West Africa in 2014. It didn't work during the height of the surge. During the first months of the epidemic, frightened families wanted professional and social assistance with caregiving, but what they got were martial, legal, and prejudicial approaches to Ebola, often downright disrespectful of cultural norms that could have been made safer. Such approaches were not and could not be consistently applied because of brisk resistance from historically minded and thus distrustful locals—and because of clumsy and often contradictory messages from long-resented authorities. Nor would these approaches prove effective until linked, however tardily and imperfectly, to goodwill efforts to take care of the sick and to bury the dead with dignity.

Precisely such compassionate integration—and the respectful deployment of new vaccines and therapeutics—could be the foundation of the next Ebola response.

During the Ebola crisis, one intensive-care specialist cited the above termed medical care as just "a tiny piece" of the overall response. That's wrongheaded thinking, tantamount to suggesting that strain variation alone accounts for massive differential mortality among those infected by the same strain.

This opens the well-oiled trapdoor to suggestions that because of intrinsic factors, medical intervention cannot change the outcomes. Therapeutic nihilism again, which often leads into the dank dungeon into which black bodies, more than white ones, fall. Opening this trapdoor to consider how Ebola kills, or blinds, is a perilous exercise. Certainly, no white medical professor from Harvard is well placed to play the race card, or to suggest that his friends and colleagues who'd shown up in dangerous conditions were all subject to unconscious bias. But future historians attuned to social medicine will have much to say about how, during the Ebola crisis, strains of racial essentialism worked their ways into the care of those who were at greatest risk of being killed by Ebola. Racialized inferences and convictions, unlike their historical roots, have never disappeared down into the oubliette. The control-over-care policies of colonial Pasteurians set the stage for today's aftermath. Racialized readings have, however, been transformed and multiplied. In a previous era, racial differences were reliably invoked to explain differential mortality along the Upper Guinea Coast. Terms like "heredity," "unfitness," and "racial susceptibility" abound in colonial reports from both sides of the Atlantic during the slave trades and long after. For centuries, race—and, later, tribe—served as a handy all-purpose explanation for difference in general. Difference in capability, difference in circumstance, difference in destiny.

In recent decades, "culture" has surged to the fore as an explanatory variable. Health officials, epidemiologists, writers, sundry journalists, Internet trolls, and more than a few academic commentators alleged that strange rituals and habits native to the regions in which epidemics killed so many were the cause of differential attack and mortality rates. The folk theories of these armchair anthropologists have enjoyed a renaissance in the Ebola era. And though culturalist in nature, folk theories were often flavored by the racist stew in which they marinated. When white folk fell in harm's way, it was not *their* cultures that were invoked to explain ensuing deaths and disability.

In the spirit of turnabout, however, one could point to specific, socially constructed values that had brought Belgian nuns to Yambuku, a village in what was once part of the Belgian Congo. It's not hard to identify many Western cultural concepts and behaviors that were proximate causes of the 1976 epidemic. Without the socialization for scarcity and thrift celebrated among missionaries who'd taken vows of poverty, which paled in the face of the involuntary poverty of their Congolese neighbors, the nuns might not have reused unsterilized needles. (They might not have used needles at all during the course of routine prenatal care, which seldom calls for them.) Socialization for scarcity might not seem to fall readily under the rubric of racism, but it's one of the unintended consequences of low aspirations on behalf of those both poor and black. This was true in Zaire in 1976, and it's true today.

While racial differences in immunity to Ebola (whether innate or acquired) have never been demonstrated, racism has much to do with its varied outcomes. For example, vaccines and drugs required to treat many emerging infectious diseases are rarely developed. "When a disease's victims are both poor and not very numerous," *The New Yorker*'s James Surowiecki has observed, "that's a double whammy. On both scores, a drug for Ebola looks like a bad investment."[52] Fear of Ebola as a bioweapon may have made a vaccine against it a more appealing investment, which is a good thing for future caregivers in the regions in which Ebola erupts. But some couldn't resist observing that vaccine development was hastened by Ebola's spread to expatriate clinicians and missionaries. When headlines in the satirical weekly *The Onion* reported the Ebola vaccine to be "at least 50 white people" away, they weren't far off.[53]

I will close this grim review of how hemorrhagic fevers kill by detailing how they took out two of West Africa's experts on hemorrhagic fevers: Humarr Khan and his predecessor at the Kenema Government Hospital, Aniru Conteh.

Beginning in the late 1970s, Dr. Conteh contributed to the study of Lassa fever in Sierra Leone and helped found the world's only dedicated Lassa ward, in Kailahun District, under the eaves of the Gola Forest. Then came the civil war that led Conteh and his team to reestablish the ward at the government hospital in Kenema, which they believed to be a safer city. The war's approach meant that Conteh never had even a tiny fraction of the staff, stuff, and space needed to fight Lassa and the region's many other ills. It also meant that he and the rest of the staff at the hospital were always in harm's way. As often as not, they had to struggle to keep the ward open. Then Kenema became ground zero of the conflict, the hospital was attacked, and the work ground to a halt. But Conteh remained at his post throughout the war.

When peace was declared, Aniru Conteh permitted himself some optimism and helped to rebuild the hospital. He believed, at least for a while, the promises made by what is termed "the international community." But over time he grew disillusioned, and in 2003, shortly before he died, Conteh predicted that none of the internationals flocking to Sierra Leone at the war's end as part of the crisis caravan would pay sustained attention to Lassa or other viral hemorrhagic fevers. They were drawn, he said, to short-term fixes rather than to building robust—now termed "resilient"—health systems.

In 2004, Aniru Conteh was infected by his viral foe through an accidental needle stick during the care of a pregnant patient. He died a couple of weeks later. This tragedy was followed by renewed commitments from some of the partners absent during the war: the World Health Organization, the U.S. Centers for Disease Control and Prevention, and Tulane and other universities, including my own. But research funds from such partners are notoriously hard to steer toward the upgrade of public infrastructure that's ostensibly there to take care of the sick. So instead, just as Conteh had predicted, came a series of short-term fixes, advanced by private contractors, humanitarian organizations, and international nongovernmental organizations. Although some of these outfits worked with public institutions, among them the hospital in Kenema, others built parallel systems of health care and education and were often deemed "unsustainable"—a grave insult, as noted, in the development lexicon.

Certainly, these projects were not sustained during the aftermath of war, since the influx of reconstruction funds from abroad was largely targeted to the project of keeping a fragile peace. But the billions spent on peacekeeping are only part of the story of transnational capital flows in and out of Kenema District. Most of the portable wealth expropriated from the nearby diamond fields didn't end up in the coffers of Kenema's hospital before, during, or after the war that those same diamonds fueled for well over a decade. Blood diamonds could, it seems, sustain a long and brutal war, but not a research and teaching hospital.

That didn't stop Aniru Conteh's successor from trying to improve the place, though. Sheik Humarr Khan—"Umarr" to his family—was one of ten children born to the wife of a schoolteacher. They lived in Lungi, not far from the rickety dock from which ferries and smaller boats crossed the estuary to Freetown. Childhood friends report that Khan knew he wanted to be a physician early on. He also knew about Lassa, informing schoolmates, "I want to cure Lassa fever."[54] Apocryphal or not, the story rings true. The young Khan applied for Conteh's post upon hearing of his death, in spite of misgivings on the part of Khan's family. Tulane's Dan Bausch and Robert Garry were impressed, and recruited him to run the Lassa ward while initiating him into the rarefied and insulated world of academic research. When named physician-in-charge, Khan followed in Conteh's footsteps in more ways than one.

Rounding on patients every day, Khan adopted the staff, especially the nurses, as his new family. Some of them, like the midwife Mbalu Fonnie, had worked in Ward A, as the Lassa unit was called, since its founding; before that, she'd worked on Lassa in Kailahun District with Conteh. She initially regarded Khan as overeager, but he won her over. The two of them delivered clinical care in Kenema for years and recruited new staff to Ward A. With far-flung and local colleagues, they helped to re-initiate research interrupted during the war. The team in Kenema was able to kickstart and then expand these studies in part because of renewed U.S. interest in hemorrhagic fevers as potential "agents of bioterrorism." Although Sierra Leone is surely one of the world's least likely settings for intentional bioterrorism, the work there generated a great deal of knowledge about Lassa and other causes of febrile illness.[55]

In spite of this upsurge in research funding and resumed collaboration with the U.S. Centers for Disease Control and the World Health Organization, Khan and his team knew there was too little investment in the staff, stuff, space, and systems required to diagnose and *treat* these fevers, to say nothing of all the other sickness and calamity facing those who'd survived the war and were returning to the ruined town and its ruined hospital. This irony was not lost on him, especially in light of his wry sense of humor. But he loved the research and counted several of his international colleagues, perhaps especially Bausch and Garry and Pardis Sabeti, as dear friends.

A new laboratory went up, thanks to narrowly allocated research funds, but the hospital, including Ward A, continued to decline. The effects on this imbalance were made clear by the terrible events of the summer of 2014, when Ward A suddenly became Sierra Leone's first Ebola ward. Dan Bausch offers the first real insider's account of these months:

I always felt bad when comparing the shiny new research and
diagnostics laboratory at Kenema Government Hospital with the
dilapidated, cramped, and poorly resourced Lassa ward only some
50 meters away. Considerations of building a new Lassa ward have
been ongoing for over a decade and have even led to ground breaking
and initial phases of construction promoted and sponsored at times
by the European Union, the WHO, and the U.S. Department of
Defense. However, each time, some logistical demon raised its
head—contractors had insufficient capital, budgets were frozen,
funds were lost, and key personnel changed.[56]

The basic outlines of what occurred in Kenema that year became widely
known, because it was Khan and colleagues who identified Sierra Leone's
first confirmed Ebola cases—a diagnosis that, thanks to the new lab, could
be confirmed right there in Kenema. But if the imbalance between funding
for research and funding for care had disturbed Bausch and rankled Khan
(and many of their coworkers) for years, the summer of 2014 was about to
transform anxiety into dread, regret into grief, fear into prophecy, and lopsid-
edness into full-blown tragedy.

Humarr Khan and his colleagues—including those at Tulane and Harvard and in Geneva, Atlanta, and Freetown—were well aware of an outbreak
of a lethal and contagious illness in Guinea and Liberia, identified as Ebola in
March 2014. Although Sierra Leone was then said to have been spared, Khan
and his team were not surprised by what came next. On May 23, a pregnant
woman with fever and fetal distress reached Kenema from Kailahun, on the
Guinean border. When her Lassa test was negative, according to several of
Khan's colleagues, his response was straightforward: "Then she has got Ebola."[57] On May 25, Kenema's lab director confirmed Khan's hunch, and two
other Ebola diagnoses were made that day. Khan immediately informed national authorities and the World Health Organization. But he knew this was
just the beginning.

The Kenema team had learned that the pregnant patient and many others had attended the funeral of a famous traditional healer from Kailahun—the one later branded a "superspreader." Khan told his staff, mostly nurses and aides, to brace themselves, predicting that others who'd administered her last rites would fall ill. He was right on that score, too: Team Kenema soon discovered that fourteen of the hundreds who'd attended the funeral were already sick. Tulane's Robert Garry flew immediately to Sierra Leone with as much protective gear as he could carry. He and Pardis Sabeti and others had already sent crates full of supplies to Sierra Leone and had testified before the U.S. Congress about the need for urgent assistance to the team in Kenema.

Suddenly, Humarr Khan was seen as *the* national Ebola expert, and patients sick with the disease flocked to Kenema, often simply to die, some of them before the hospital gates. Infection control was revealed to be poor even in Ward A, which initially had only a dozen beds. The unit was soon overflowing, as were buckets under cholera cots and at the bedside. "Ward A consisted of eight small rooms lining a dingy corridor of exposed wiring, peeling paint, and grimy cement floors," wrote one American journalist. "It was narrow and stiflingly hot, crowded with as many as 30 patients. Nurses squeezed between the beds, injecting antibiotics, emptying buckets of diarrhea, and hosing down vomit with chlorine."[58] Ward A had never smelled good, but now it was swimming with shit and vomit and urine and chlorine. Nobody bothered to chart I's and O's, but the O's were soon all over the patients, their clothes, the beds, the floors, and even the walls.

Wasn't this the singular and famous Lassa ward, affiliate of some of the world's leading institutions conducting or supporting research on viral hemorrhagic fevers? It was, and its important work was set up to fail in the face of Ebola: a research-over-care paradigm proved as dangerous as its control-over-care cousin. Khan and others, including Bausch and Garry, had clamored for a new Lassa ward for years. Several of the agencies that had funded their research made pledges, and so had beleaguered health authorities and a few nongovernmental organizations. Even the U.S. Navy had pledged to help. There were a few false starts, and a foundation was half-laid and a wall or two were thrown up. But as Aniru Conteh had predicted, humanitarians had short attention spans, and universities and foreign militaries were inconstant patrons of care delivery in Africa. Even when the world's attention was focused on Kenema in the summer of 2014, the stalled project remained stalled.[59]

People sick and dying from Ebola soon filled Ward A, then the general hospital, and finally a makeshift Ebola treatment unit fashioned from a tent. (Initial attempts to erect one a month earlier were thwarted when the roof collapsed.) Within weeks, the dead lay unattended in their beds or (in the words of one investigative journalist) "stacked like cordwood" in an unrefrigerated shed.[60] Others died in the courtyard of the hospital. As in previous Ebola outbreaks, the hospital served to amplify the epidemic through nosocomial transmission. The hospital was overwhelmed and overrun, and some staff refused to report to work. But many of the nurses, including stalwarts like Mbalu Fonnie, did show up, and Khan's American friends had arrived almost immediately with personal protective equipment. However, donning and doffing this gear took time (and collegial supervision) that the beleaguered and thinned out Kenema nurses didn't have.

As in previously documented Ebola outbreaks, nurses and their assistants were the first of the professional caregivers to sicken and die, since they're the professional caregivers who give most care. Dan Bausch describes what happened next. "It was in June in Kenema that the outbreak started to become increasingly personal," he recalled.

It seemed that almost every day another healthcare worker who was part of our Kenema Lassa (now Ebola) team who I had been working with for decades, some who I had even recruited, including the now sadly famous Dr. Sheik Humarr Khan, was coming down with a fever, testing positive for Ebola, and becoming a case rather than a caregiver. It was like some surrealistic nightmare—"I dreamt that an Ebola outbreak hit Kenema, and everyone I knew was getting infected and dying." A few months later, the dream-like quality extended to the United States, with imported cases, occasional secondary transmission, and much public panic.[61]

Most of those who later evaluated the evidence regarding the fates of Kenema's health professionals believe that Mbalu Fonnie and three other nurses were infected while trying to save a pregnant coworker. (She was, after all, a midwife.) Khan soldiered on as many of Kenema's nurses, some of them his closest friends, fell ill in the course of late June and early July. When the senior nurses fell ill, more nurses refused to show up for work. Bausch was there in mid-July, entering one ward with fifty patients, but not a single nurse or doctor. Writing in *The New Yorker*, Richard Preston described Khan as "a general in a battle where many of his troops were dead or fleeing."[62]

I was following these grim developments with dismay and shame from Rwanda. Less than a month after leaving Freetown in late June, I learned that Khan, our admired colleague and Sierra Leone's best-known physician, had fallen ill with fever and malaise. It was July 19. It must be malaria, Khan told his closest friend, another of the Kenema nurses, as sick professionals tended to do throughout those weeks and months. (This friend was already sick, and shortly thereafter succumbed to Ebola.) Khan's first Ebola test was negative, but the second one confirmed his fears and the fears of his scattered family and friends—in Kenema, Freetown, Philadelphia, New Orleans, Boston, Geneva, and Kigali. As in Liberia, the disease was picking off health professionals in a country that had so few of them to begin with. And now one of the continent's most respected experts on hemorrhagic fevers had, like Aniru Conteh, fallen ill with one.

Humarr Khan's illness stoked local dread, confusion, and anger, provoking something of an international crisis. This news was understood to be the death knell of Ward A and the hospital by many, if not most, of the staff. Khan confided to friends and family that he feared that if he were to die in Kenema, the entire effort, everything he and others had built over the previous decade, would collapse as quickly as the roof on the first makeshift Ebola unit. He had other reasons not to remain in Kenema. Chief among them was that Khan would likely not receive supportive or critical care there. He needed to fly west—not to medically bereft Freetown, but to Atlanta or Boston or New Orleans—or north, to Geneva or London. He had, after all, strong ties in the medical communities in each of these cities. But he didn't yet have a means of flying to any well-equipped locale. Everyone knew he had Ebola, and a bio-secure plane would take time and a lot of money to charter.

So Humarr Khan first headed east, transported by rough roads to the Ebola treatment unit recently opened by MSF, and supported by the World Health Organization, in the godforsaken town of Kailahun. The newly opened facility was about five hours away by unpaved road. "It's the shittiest road I've seen in my life," observed a medical colleague with experience else-where in rural Sierra Leone—and in the rural reaches of South Sudan, Leso-tho, Malawi, and Tanzania. "I'd rather cross the River Styx with Charon at the helm." But it was the dearth of supportive care in the MSF unit that most rankled my colleague. "When we were in our pre-deployment training in Amsterdam," he told me, "the clinicians were asking about lines and intraos-seous needles. We asked about them again in Kailahun, but 'they weren't in the protocol.' That was the mantra."[63]

What happened next, according to an investigation by the journalist Joshua Hammer and to several involved in Humarr Khan's care, was what was happening within the Monrovia ETU we visited two months later. "The doctors immediately placed Khan on a standard regimen of oral treatments—paracetamol for pain relief, antibiotics for diarrhea, and rehydration salts," wrote Hammer. "Doctors Without Borders seldom use intravenous fluids with Ebola," he explained, "believing that the risks of death from bleeding are greater than the potential benefits."[64] But the Kailahun team's own study of all patients cared for there suggested that hemorrhage was rarely seen. Among 255 survivors of confirmed Ebola, only one had evidence of bleeding; among 270 who died, only 10 were deemed to suffer significant hemorrhage.[65] So it was no surprise that Khan's signs and symptoms didn't include it. They did include, however, fever, profuse diarrhea, and vomiting, and it became difficult for him to keep up with losses of fluids and electrolytes by drinking coconut water. What Khan needed, and would have received in a first-world hospital, was replacement of lost fluids and electrolytes delivered through a large-bore intravenous line threaded into the heart or, at the very least, into the upper arm.

Placement of a central venous line was, in many ways, the chief therapeutic intervention in the American hospitals that received Ebola patients via bio-secure planes. Here's what the doctors in Omaha, Nebraska, had to say about intravenous access when they received their first two American patients, both of whom survived: "Patients arrived with peripheral IV catheters in the upper extremity. Because of an anticipated need for ongoing fluid resuscitation and frequent laboratory sampling, central venous access was deemed necessary." In the United States, line placement is a procedure every physician learns to do in the first year after medical school, if not before. But Team Omaha didn't need to rely on interns. Without counting senior physicians, of whom there were more than a dozen, it consisted of "40 registered nurses, respiratory therapists, and patient care technicians with members on-call" twenty-four hours a day. It was the same story in Bethesda, Atlanta, and New York.

It was, of course, a different story in Kailahun, for reasons already discussed in each of the previous chapters. But there were physicians and nurses present, most of them expatriates. They were in conflict over MSF's treatment protocols even back in late July. And as Moses Massaquoi would note in Monrovia in October, it was well known among West African and expatriate clinicians alike that deficient protocols were unlikely to save the majority of patients critically ill with Ebola. Reluctance to use intravenous therapy in Kailahun certainly spelled trouble for that subset of patients with severe gastrointestinal symptoms.

Humarr Khan was in trouble, and everyone seemed to be watching. That's why, on July 22, the president of Sierra Leone directed his health minister, in spite of her recent intemperate remarks about two Kailahun health professionals dead of Ebola, to search high and low for two things. The first was a course of ZMapp, which had by then been shown to prevent death in rhesus monkeys experimentally infected with Ebola but had yet to undergo clinical trials in humans. The minister's second assignment was to medevac Khan to a first-world hospital, an appeal echoed by his far-flung family and friends.

As for the first task, there were precious few doses of ZMapp in the entire world. But a few of them, providentially, were in a refrigerator not more than a few hundred paces from Humarr Khan's cot. There was brisk disagreement regarding ZMapp's use in Khan's case. Accounts vary as to the contours of the debate, but no small fraction of it concerned "reputational risk." The risk in question was not to ZMapp or the company that manufactured it, nor to Sierra Leonean health authorities, nor to the notion of trying experimental therapies in desperate cases. It was the reputational risk to the world's top health authority and its largest medical charity, which had (however ambivalently) been pushing ORS as the standard of care and no-touch policies, even for women in labor. On July 25, according to Joshua Hammer, "the international groups finally informed Khan that they had decided against treating him with ZMapp."[66] The patient himself was not really consulted on the matter.

As for the minister's second objective, medevacking Dr. Khan, it was by then clear to officials in Freetown that Kenema was not equipped to provide basic care for patients with copious fluid loss from both vomiting and diarrhea. Neither was Connaught Hospital. (The holding unit there was still sending patients east to Kenema and Kailahun.) As Khan's family and friends pleaded for a transfer to a European or American hospital, the government of Sierra Leone engaged the services of a private air ambulance, which flew to Freetown's international airfield, and waited. But the doctors in Kailahun deemed Khan too sick for transport to Lungi, and (by some reports) the pilots weren't keen on flying him, either. Khan was incontinent, unable to keep down food, and had a low white-blood-cell count. (Even in a unit in which laboratory tests were discouraged, his blood count was documented almost daily.) The air ambulance left empty.

Khan's decline continued. One of his close friends went to visit him as he lay dying. This sparked more internal debate. Visits were also not in the protocol; he was denied entry to the unit. Finally, when it seemed clear that Khan was near death, the MSF-WHO team relented, and he was able to see one last familiar face a few hours before he died. The Kailahun doses of ZMapp went by private plane to two American missionaries in Liberia, crossing flight paths with a UN helicopter sent from Liberia to collect the precious vials for the Americans.

One of them was Dr. Kent Brantly, who'd been stricken at about the same time as Khan and was by then desperately ill. The physician who took

the decision to give Brantly ZMapp, also an American, watched a gowned-
and-gloved nurse administer it. He stood outside, peering through an open
window as the first infusion took place. "Kent is about halfway into the first
dose," he texted a colleague who'd helped obtain the experimental therapy.
"Honestly he looks distinctly better already. Is that possible?"[67] The answer
to that question is still unclear, although many West Africans following the
events of that week closely were sure that ZMapp made the difference.

Most who cared for Brantly believe it was probably the proper supportive care he received at Emory, rather than the experimental treatment with
ZMapp, that saved him and most other expatriates airlifted to similar units.
One of my former Harvard trainees in infectious disease was among those
caregivers. His chief take-home message during subsequent conferences and
presentations was also a mantra: "Supportive care, supportive care, supportive care." But part of the ZMapp story—that it was given to the white expatriates rather than to Khan—struck a deep chord among many in Sierra Leone
and elsewhere on the continent.

Humarr Khan died in Kailahun on July 29, the day after Ramadan ended, the
same day that Ibrahim's sick kinsman reached his mother's house in Lumley,
and that Yabom's husband felt the onset of his malaise. But while our patients'
family members suffered and died in anonymity, Khan's death was major
news, and it had a predictably powerful social impact. It seemed to confirm
what many local health professionals working in the region suspected: that
Africans infected with Ebola would receive inferior care.

Ebola had by then invaded cities and towns in Sierra Leone, Liberia, and
Guinea. In all three countries, health professionals threatened to go on strike
in protest. Many did, and others, spooked by the high numbers of health-care
workers who were dead or dying, fled their posts. These doctors and nurses
had ample reason to believe that inferior care was being delivered to their
colleagues, but this wasn't a surprise, nor was it what really rankled. They
were angered by the fact that a lower standard of care was *fixed as policy*, or
was felt to have been fixed as policy, through treatment protocols elaborated

by humanitarian organizations and by public-health experts. As Moses Massaquoi would later tell me, the few physicians and nurses still practicing in Upper West Africa "read the same textbooks you did."

Acrimony mounted. While Sierra Leonean health professionals complained openly that influential nongovernmental organizations and global standard-setting bodies were recommending inadequate care, perceived double standards caused significant distress among the expatriate doctors, too. The American colleague cited previously, who arrived in Kailahun after Khan died, reported that the debate was ongoing in the Kailahun unit:

> Almost as soon as I got off the plane, one of the first things I heard was "we're not doctors or nurses; we're all medics. We don't have the manpower to do intravenous therapy because it takes too much time to change the bags." The day before I got there, an IV pole fell over, and some blood backed up in the line. No one was exposed, nor was it of clinical significance—it was just a few c.c.s of venous return. The next day, the medical director banned all IVs.

Across this part of West Africa, the T in ETU too rarely included supportive care for diarrhea, nausea, delirium, and severe fluid and electrolyte imbalances, or for shock, opportunistic infections, or bleeding disorders. Of course, these were precisely the interventions and therapies unavailable in that clinical desert. The same was true of critical care and of laboratory capacity. But could they be made available? This question was at the heart of many of the most acrimonious debates during the plague year.

After Khan's death, the ZMapp debate was more about equity than efficacy or safety. On August 11, as a result of the Khan controversy, the World Health Organization convened yet another meeting of experts, this time bioethicists, among others, to reconsider the decisions being made about access to experimental therapies for Ebola. "Circumstances warrant the use of unproven interventions with as yet unknown efficacy and adverse effects both for treatment and for prevention," they concluded. "Deciding which treatments should be used and how to distribute them equitably were matters that needed further discussion."[68] There was much more palaver, but if too few West African health professionals received ZMapp or other experimental therapies, far too few received enough in the way of supportive care. Most of them died.

When the dust settled on the first months of the Sierra Leonean epidemic, it was reported that, in Kenema District, an estimated 15 percent of Ebola victims had been health-care professionals—the highest percentage in the nation. Those who, like Khan, sought care in Kailahun fared poorly. Of thirty-one professional caregivers admitted with a positive Ebola test, twenty died, nine survived, and two were "transferred to another health facility," their fates unrecorded. That meant (according to MSF) that "the overall mortality rate for healthcare workers with a known outcome was 69 percent."[69] With socialization for scarcity blanketing the region, it is perhaps understandable that the unit's mortality rate for all confirmed Ebola cases—just over half died—was deemed "favorable" by the MSF doctors (and colleagues) who later published these figures.

We didn't do much better in Maforki, but certainly did not regard these results as favorable. Joanne Liu, the international president of MSF and a specialist in emergency medicine, also viewed such outcomes as dismal. In a speech delivered in Brussels on March 3, 2015, about the same time her Kailahun coworkers were working on the final version of their report, Dr. Liu's assessment was withering: "At a time when Ebola case numbers are notably lower, we—collectively—continue to fail patients and those who remain at risk of contracting the virus. The mortality rate in our treatment units is at a staggering 50 percent. This is unacceptable."[70]

Dan Bausch, one of Humarr Khan's closest friends and, like him, an advocate for robust clinical trials, has gone on record saying that Khan should have received the ZMapp. So did Pardis Sabeti and Robert Garry. They all mourned the failure of the Lassa ward and Kenema Government Hospital, its condition squaring all too well with Professor T. B. Kamara's assessment of surgical care in such hospitals: if Kenema's research laboratory was of the twenty-first century, its clinical care was stuck somewhere in the nineteenth. Bausch concludes his own doleful reflection by reporting "periodic discussions with MSF-Belgium, which had a malaria project in a neighboring district, about taking over the running of the Kenema Lassa ward, but nothing ever materialized. How much better and safer might Ebola care have been in Kenema if these projects were seen through to completion?"[71] He likely didn't take even a shred of comfort in learning that clinical outcomes in Kenema weren't much different from those registered in Kailahun.

MSF's internal critique—of fixing low standards rather than failing to aim for higher ones—was devastating. The aforementioned letter to the broader MSF community, written in the last month of 2014, includes the following: "The reduction of mortality in an outbreak of a deadly disease should be a prime objective of our interventions—something that we should have strived for right from the beginning. However the focus was and still is mainly on containment through isolation." The letter suggests that Moses Massaquoi's and other Liberians' complaints had resonated across the Liberian islands of MSF's complex archipelago:

> In Liberia, the government implored MSF repeatedly to improve
> patient care (through IV hydration and transfusion of convalescent
> whole blood). It is true that the situation in Liberia was extremely
> difficult over the summer (high caseload, limited number of
> competent staff, few other actors), which may explain parts of MSF's
> intervention strategy aiming at containment. However, even when
> the situation stabilized MSF did not adequately react to rapidly
> raise standards of care. Persistent calls by MSF medical doctors
> for better patient care remain unheard. As we invested time and
> energy to rightfully ensure security and safety of our health staff, we
> paradoxically invested too little resources in our patients—the very
> people whom we were asking our staff to take risks for.[72]

The letter's signatories, including longtime MSFers, invoked the La Mancha agreement, which was crafted by the organization in 2006 with a nod to the quixotic efforts, and risks, undertaken by its members.[73] The chief point of this cri de cœur was made unstintingly: "In the opinion of the authors MSF failed to abide to the La Mancha agreement throughout the first nine months of our Ebola intervention in West Africa. MSF collectively failed to demonstrate that—even in an Ebola outbreak—the survival of every individual patient is a battle worth fighting."[74]

What lessons may be drawn from Humarr Khan's death and from so many others? Recrimination and finger-pointing are futile. But clear acknowledgment of widely shared failures with an eye toward improvement is not. Even the most basic supportive and critical care would have likely saved colleagues and unknown others who entered, but did not exit, what they hoped were treatment facilities. Once interned within isolation centers extravagantly billed as Ebola treatment units, many were cut off from expert mercy and modern medical therapy. Some never had much more of a chance to survive than those who died at home.

I won't be surprised, of course, if this assessment triggers defensiveness and rancor among those who gave their all to respond bravely during the course of the plague year. Such sentiments have indeed already constituted a significant social response to Ebola among my peers and friends, so I wish to underline a shift in pronouns: I know *they* gave their all. The world has reason to know it, and to thank them for it. I cheered when, at the close of 2014, Ebola responders were named *Time*'s "Person of the Year," and when MSF was awarded the prestigious Lasker Award for bringing Ebola to the world's attention. But the point of this chapter—a review of the mechanisms by which Ebola kills or does not kill—is to say, echoing Joanne Liu, that collectively, as experts or professionals or just plain humans, *we* did not give *our* all.

10.

The Silly Things and
the Fever Next Time

Our people are stubborn. Until they stop doing what I call the silly things we
will have cases popping up here and there.

—Major Palo Conteh, director of Sierra Leone's National Ebola Response Centre,
September 8, 2015

THIS BOOK BEGINS IN ONE PATCH OF THE CLINICAL DESERT, MONROVIA, and ends in another, Freetown. It's a study of the causes and consequences of an Ebola epidemic widely believed, at this writing and in this place, to be behind us. But is the West African Ebola epidemic truly over? It certainly isn't over for those still suffering from its late-stage consequences, which have included blindness, seizures, and ongoing psychological distress. Nor is it over for the bereaved families and traumatized communities who bear the invisible scars of social suffering.

Ebola also lives on for the ill and injured unattended during the surge and after the collapse of the region's health system. That collapse has given rise to a brutal tsunami of problems that is sweeping away young women and their infants during childbirth; causing outbreaks of vaccine-preventable illnesses such as measles and whooping cough; leading to a spike in deaths from AIDS, tuberculosis, and new infections, while fanning the rise of drug-resistant strains of pathogens that cause them; increasing deaths and disability due to minor trauma in the absence of surgical care; and leaving those struggling with less visible trauma and other mental-health problems on their own or in the care of family and traditional healers.

There are other reasons not to consider the West African epidemic over. After the western surge of 2014, viable Ebola virus persisted in the bodies of thousands of survivors who'd received laminated certificates declaring them Ebola-free. We don't really know what implications this persistence will have. Even if Ebola is unlikely to become endemic in the way that HIV and other pathogens with zoonotic roots have done, it was transmitted between sexual partners, and from mothers to children, causing symptomatic disease among some.[1] This, in turn, sporadically gave rise to new outbreaks and re-minded concerned parties that it's not easy to mark the beginning or end of an epidemic in a clinical desert.

That's one reason the epidemic held to begin in eastern Guinea in 2013 was declared over many times in the three years that followed. Sporadic outbreaks emerged among those not immune—who, as far as we know, make up the great majority of the population, even after tens of thousands in the region were exposed to natural infection, and after thousands received the world's first effective Ebola vaccine. In spite of these and other reasons for modesty regarding beginnings and endings, pat origin stories still abound in narratives about Ebola's triumphant march across Upper West Africa, and in equally common if less convincing ones about triumphant human efforts to stop it.

Consider Ebola's West African spillover event. The dominant origin story alleges that a toddler from the Guinean village of Meliandou was first in line among humans as a virus new to West Africa made its cross-species jump from fruit-eating bats. (Early iterations of the story usually left aside the fact that the felled tree was said to be home to insect-eating bats, and that Meliandou's tested bats, regardless of dietary preferences, did not show evidence of Ebola infection.) Most with even passing interest in the place or the pathogen have heard and read about this epidemic's alleged Patient Zero and his last known address on this earth. But was Ebola really new to the people of this region?

Do we really have much reason to believe that the cause of so much devastation was the result of his handling of bats in a hollow tree trunk, or of ingesting a mango or a plum, ripened on one tree to be gnawed by Ebola-infected bats resident in another? Although such speculations were recent imports to southeastern Guinea, at least one bat-infested tree in Meliandou was felled two days after Guinean health officials reported that the forest region's sudden rush of febrile deaths was caused by Ebola. (This was the day before the authorities banned bat soup.) But there were always reasons to interrogate confident claims of causality about what was crisply decreed the world's twenty-fifth Ebola outbreak. What we do know with some confidence is that the virus, however and whenever it was introduced to the human family, spread rapidly from person to person.

As for Ebola's alleged novelty in West Africa, if our appetite for historical understanding were commensurate with that for stories about Patient Zero—or about bushmeat, pet monkeys, secret societies, and all manner of native superstition—the outbreak clock might be set ticking at any point during or after the civil conflict that gutted the region during the course of fifteen long years. After all, postwar research had revealed Ebola's presence in the area around Kenema close to a decade before Meliandou was invaded—first by the virus and then by journalists, research teams, and the diverse personnel of the control-over-care apparatus. But by the time the capacity to diagnose Ebola was introduced to Kenema, everyone seems to have forgotten studies suggesting its presence in West Africa prior to the outbreak of war.

As for the finales, it isn't straightforward in the clinical desert to mark the end of one, either—even after the arrival of a crisis caravan focused on the control of a single disease in a region where diverse epidemics abound. Ebola, having survived multiple countdowns to zero, retreated into distrustful populations. In Liberia, for instance, in June 2015—after the epidemic had already twice been declared contained—the health authorities had to interrupt their countdown to zero to announce that Ebola had just killed a teenage boy.[2] Six more cases were linked to this tragedy.

Nor was that the end of Ebola and the social suffering it engendered. Health officials initiated a third countdown in late July, after a survivor of this outbreak was discharged from an ETU.[3] The ritual began yet again in November, when another teenage boy, and then his father and brother, fell ill with Ebola. The boy also went on to die, but not without occasioning public rebuke, much of it postmortem, for having evaded the public-health dragnet. The episode brought intense scrutiny to his neighborhood, and soon the default measure of blaming the sick and their local caregivers, including family and traditional healers, kicked in. Some blame was leveled at professional clinicians, too, but by that point there weren't many of them left in Liberia.

It was a similar story in Sierra Leone, where on August 28, 2015, in the northern village of Sella Kafta, a sixty-seven-year-old woman died of Ebola. The government quickly dispatched its recently reconstituted armed forces to the area, where, in a classic control-over-care move, they decided to ring-fence the entire settlement—consisting of close to a thousand people—for twenty-one days. Few in the public-health apparatus raised any objection. According to the head of the National Ebola Response Centre, a retired army major named Palo Conteh, the villagers themselves were to blame. "Until they stop doing what I call 'the silly things,'" he said on September 8, "we will have cases popping up here and there."[4] The "silly things" included nursing sick family members and performing last rites, which were by then proscribed by law.

There's evidence that some families were relieved by the new rules, since many of them freed kin of the sacred duty to nurse the sick and to bury the dead in the midst of a very real—and very experience-near—epidemic. Major Conteh's remarks were consistent with others made more than a year earlier.

He knew these laws would be resisted by some, but he wagered that a frightened citizenry would largely obey. (The same wager is now being made in the course of the COVID-19 pandemic.) "I am now using the 'carrot and stick approach,'" Conteh said at the time, in a speech delivered at the height of Sierra Leone's western surge. "I have been giving out the carrot since I took over, but our people still do the wrong things. When I start using the stick, I will see all kinds of headlines in papers and radio programmes but will not be deterred by them."[5]

That's pretty much what came to pass in Sella Kafta, where the military made goodwill efforts to provide the villagers with food and water.

There's nothing easy about social distancing in West African villages; sheltering in place is nearly impossible in such places. According a report by the World Health Organization the quarantine had the problematic effect of "keeping them from their fields in the middle of the growing season."[6] Army medics and platoons of public-health workers supplemented ring-fencing with ring vaccination, an intervention that had worked—social scars aside—to end smallpox. It worked to end Ebola, too, but that didn't mean everyone fell into line. "While soldiers and police had been brought in to ensure that over 1,000 villagers remain in their homes during a quarantine period," Reuters reported, "one individual who had been in contact with the dead woman was still missing."[7]

The pattern repeated itself a couple of months later, not far over the border, in Guinea. After Ebola surfaced in the hamlet of Tana, and the village was subsequently proclaimed by international authorities to be the last place on earth in which the person-to-person transmission of Ebola was still occurring, residents were hectored by officials from Conakry for their backward beliefs and practices. These again included caregiving, burial of the dead, and refusal to comply with reporting and surveillance requirements. And once again there was the mystery of a missing woman—in this case one who had cared for a friend who'd recently died of Ebola. "I demand the cooperation of the population," exhorted Guinea's prime minister, who showed up in the village shortly thereafter. "A woman is missing, and I can't understand why."[8]

The prime minister may have expressed bewilderment, but everybody else understood why the woman had disappeared: to avoid punishment. Unable to find her, the government turned its attention to her next of kin. "No one offered any clues after she went into hiding," reported *The New York Times*, "so the authorities jailed her husband, a heavy-handed approach meant to convey the seriousness of the problem."[9] The prime minister further threatened to strip the village chief of his title if the woman and, it turned out, others who had gone missing weren't flushed out of hiding. All "suspects" (as presumed victims of Ebola were termed) and their contacts were expected to identify themselves and stay put in the area for at least three weeks—a confinement that's hard to imagine for anyone who has visited, much less lived in, a village anywhere in Africa. There's no room service, home delivery, or Amazon Prime.

The control-over-care paradigm, with its faulty moral arithmetic, leaves open many avenues for Ebola's persistence or return. As previous chapters have shown, the origins of this paradigm, and the wellspring of its flawed math, lie in the late nineteenth-century colonial experiment in Africa as much as anywhere else.

If most colonial-era conflict stemmed from the fundamentally extractive nature and increasingly racist tenor of European rule, Pasteurian priorities made it difficult to credit their reports of public-health success in West Africa. From the time that Europeans laid claim to the continent until independence, boasts of local, national, and regional disease control—and even eradication—were made for plague, yellow fever, trypanosomiasis, cholera, rinderpest, schistosomiasis, yaws, polio, anthrax, malaria, and many of the vaccine-preventable illnesses of childhood. But most such claims were shown, usually in short order, to have been premature. More than a century later, rinderpest and smallpox aside, only polio and Guinea worm eradication are nearing their endgames.[10]

Then as now, such boasts were often based on faulty reasoning, incomplete understanding, poor-quality data, and no small amount of wishful thinking, political exigency, and propaganda of varied purpose. Throughout the vaccine era, the dramas of disease control have been muddled by persistent conflict and by the world's growing inequalities. (It's no accident that transmission of poliovirus is thought to occur on this continent only in strife-torn northern Nigeria.) Contact tracing, quarantine, and isolation—necessary components of an effective response to many epidemics—are rendered more difficult and less effective by both conflict and inequality, also indissociably linked. But the ranking obstacle to success has often been the refusal to recognize that what the sick-poor seek is *care*.

As anybody would, the victims of varied epidemics—from Ebola to COVID-19—need care, empathy, and expert mercy. All too rarely did West Africans receive such things beyond the confines of close family and friends. Among the affluent, it would be scandalous to promote disease control without care. Within an affluent and inegalitarian nation, like my own, the idea of walling off afflicted towns and cities without attempting to treat the sick with therapies existing anywhere in the global economy would be dismissed as a nonstarter. Public-health nihilism and its control-over-care variant retain their force largely among the poor living in what are now called low-income countries. These countries are, of course, the former colonies; strains of the paradigm run rampant within them, and in the field now widely known as global health.

For the poor in poor countries—those seen to be dragging down the incomes of entire nations—even vaccines may be dismissed as neither cost-effective nor sustainable. Consider the frightening example of plague due to *Yersinia pestis*, famous for taking out at least a quarter of Europe's population in the Middle Ages.[11] A vaccine against *Yersinia* was developed at the close of the nineteenth century, and it was long licensed in the United States, where sporadic plague cases still occur each year. But its manufacture ceased two decades ago, again on grounds that it was neither needed nor cost-effective. The likelihood of kick-starting vaccine production was never substantial. But it's a colossal and ubiquitous error to blame such inattention to a sudden focus on providing curative care to those most at risk of falling ill with the disease.

That never happened. If attention to *care* for the poor—the chief victims of plague—had displaced *prevention* as a priority, then the case-fatality rate would have dropped as new infections did. That did not occur, as we've seen in Senegal, where the antibiotic era began for white settlers well before it began for the natives. Nor was it only in Senegal and elsewhere in West Africa that colonial Pasteurians rejected offers of curative therapy for the natives while availing themselves of it. If plague is still famous as the Black Death, it's less often remembered for its twentieth-century devastation, killing untold millions in Africa, Asia, and the Americas. That includes more than ten million souls in India in the first half of that century alone, the last decades under British rule.

When we can't blame colonialism for the most recent developments, we can blame its successor regimes. The postcolonial world still suffers from control-over-care logic, and from the plague. In the Indian state of Gujarat, population forty-five million, plague killed hundreds in the 1990s—with the diamond-polishing city of Surat the epicenter of a major outbreak in 1994.[12] Roughly a quarter of Surat's residents fled, airlines shut down, and Bombay's stock market crashed. Plague outbreaks occur regularly, too, in Africa's clinical deserts. The disease recently exploded in the clinical desert between India and Africa, when Madagascar faced its largest epidemic in years.

The control-over-care paradigm is now caught up in a broader neoliberal one: when everything is for sale and public goods are few, both prevention and care are at risk of becoming commodities. That's why the plague story is unnervingly similar to that of cholera, which has enjoyed a recent resurgence from Sierra Leone to Sudan—to say nothing of its catastrophic 2010 introduction to Haiti and subsequent spread across the Caribbean and parts of Latin America. Oral vaccines had gone through trials showing them to be safe and to confer substantial protection by the time Haiti was afflicted. They were not supplied or even recommended to Haitians in immediate danger of contagion.

Worse still, I know from bitter personal experience that objections to their use came chiefly from international public-health authorities who argued that the vaccines were too expensive, and moreover an unproven and unnecessary distraction from the long-term mission of improving sanitation.[13]

This even though the most influential of these authorities were from the top health agency of the United Nations, whose peacekeepers inadvertently introduced the bacillus to Haiti seven months after the 2010 earthquake.[14] In the next eight years, cholera sickened more than eight hundred thousand Haitians; ten thousand of them perished.[15]

Until the insidious control-over-care paradigm is broken, the response to those epidemics will be continued mistrust and recalcitrance on the part of populations already scarred by the insults and injuries of colonialism, war, and a public-health approach that fails to prioritize effective caregiving.

Ebola is a virus, but it shares some things in common with the bacteria that cause plague and cholera. All three pathogens cause a broad spectrum of illness, including minimally symptomatic disease, and have nonhuman hosts and reservoirs. (The cholera bacillus may live on in tiny crustaceans called copepods, and in other aquatic reservoirs.) And now there are vaccines against all three of them.

One of the few happy aftermaths of the West African Ebola epidemic has been the development of what appears to be a safe and protective vaccine. Folks who received it promptly in places like Sella Kafta and Tana did not fall ill, and this was bigger news—in the sense of being new—than the social churn inevitably triggered by the control-over-care paradigm. But we can expect the usual debates about whether further and different clinical trials are needed, which regulatory hurdles must be cleared before it and other vaccines are licensed, and by which agencies. As noted in chapter 2, Ebolanomics is sure to influence these discussions, since the disease's victims, like those sickened by cholera and plague, are mostly poor people of color, as are their primary caregivers.[16]

What's equally sure is that discussion of the mundane, including the cost and effectiveness of new Ebola vaccines, will be complemented by much commentary on the exotic. This is often couched in terms of the "behavior" and "beliefs" and "culture" of those who've long received the short end of

the stick. Throughout the West African epidemic, we heard confused stories about the people who believed in the existence and force of an unseen
world—not that of invisible filoviruses but of superstition, sorcery, and the
like. The significance of these tales varied with the intent and station of those
who peddled them. When shared by authorities of one sort or another, they
were usually parables about the alleged intransigence or lack of trust among
villagers held to be at once superstitious and prime targets for informational
campaigns; credulous and stubbornly tied to their unchanging beliefs; silly
and violent; communitarian and inhospitable. But all of us, including anthropologists and physicians, have our reasons for invoking the exotic.

As Port Loko and Freetown emerged as the epicenter of Sierra Leone's
Ebola epidemic, it became clear that events recent and remote would shape
social responses to what was termed an unprecedented affliction. They did
just that in the third week of November 2014, when a just-bereaved family
from the village of Matweng threw stones at the "burial vehicle" sent to collect yet another young, anonymous body. Alex Jalloh—a driver newly hired
by Partners In Health who before becoming a colleague had spent many years
as a war refugee—put the rock-throwing in context for me. "It's true that people are superstitious," he said, alluding to the way national and international
authorities continued to assign local superstition an outsize role in Ebola's
spread. "That's why they didn't want to put the body in the burial car. The
authorities," he added, "disappear the body, and you don't know where to,
maybe a city far away. No one can recognize them behind their masks. It *is*
like witchcraft."

This book seeks to explore how economic and social forces—which
might reasonably be glossed as "history"—shape both epidemics and the lived
experience of them. For centuries, sickness and premature death have been
commonplace in this part of West Africa. So, too, have forced labor, the extractive trades, conflict, and outright war. That's why the everyday here is
saturated by discretion, concealment, and fear. Why else would the region's
ubiquitous secret societies, which almost everyone joins, be secret? How else
does an ambulance become a "burial vehicle," or a morgue the portal to a

witch city? By whose logic are such things more fantastic than my own tribe's conviction that a virus never seen by the unaided eye can rip apart a family or a village almost as quickly as ordnance from a flying gunship hovering just above the forest canopy, or from an aircraft carrier that's stationed invisibly a mile off the coast?[17]

The idea of writing about superstitions and witchcraft in this book gave me pause. I was not, after all, an expert on the region, spoke only the languages of the colonizers, and was staying in hotels or guest houses rather than in villages. I was there as a physician, not an anthropologist, and could almost hear the embarrassed clucking of medical colleagues native to these countries, or the perplexed questions of clinical coworkers new to the region. *Really?* Ritual cannibalism and human leopards and swears and witch cities? Surely thinking about these things in the midst of a deadly epidemic was silly? In fact, no. In the light of both the ethnographic and historical records, these tales of the occult were the opposite of silly.[18] Indeed, those records raise questions of grave importance. Was the runaway Ebola epidemic the result of such beliefs and understandings, as many seemed to suggest? Or were they, like the dimensions of the epidemic, the result of material privation and a long history of predation?

I've suggested throughout this book that the commonly registered responses to a presumed diagnosis of Ebola—concealment, flight, and low expectations of weak health-care systems previously inaccessible to the poor—had less to do with superstition, intransigence, and "the silly things" than with fairly realistic assessment of people's chances within that system. The same holds true, more generally, for the responses one often encounters to contact tracing, isolation, and quarantine, not just in villages but also in cities and towns. The anthropologist Mariane Ferme spelled this out in a commentary posted in October 2014:

> Early coverage of the Ebola epidemic in Guinea, Sierra Leone, and Liberia highlighted the public health risks presented by widespread lack of trust in government health workers, who in some cases were suspected of spreading the disease. Given that now the Centers for

Disease Control website recommends avoidance of hospitals as a key preventive measure, the fact that citizens of the region stay away from their countries' ill-equipped and poorly sanitized hospitals seems a rational decision, rather than one informed by superstition and baseless rumors.[19]

Whether or not such avoidance is judged rational or reasoned, those confronted by control-over-care tactics will likely remain mistrustful as long as they're considered "vectors" or "superspreaders," or regarded as recalcitrant, superstitious, obstructionist, backward, and ignorant—as obstacles to progress, in other words, rather than victims of all-too-related and largely extractive regimes of colonialism, neocolonialism, and neoliberalism.

This nexus of -isms and ideologies excludes many from the marketplace of medicine and even of public-health services once considered public goods. As long as health care remains largely a commodity rather than a right, it's likely that the strengthening of health systems will continue to spark only transient enthusiasm among history's victors—and only when calamity strikes.

As apocalyptic as it seemed, and was, the world's worst Ebola epidemic isn't a patch on some of the plagues that previously afflicted West Africa. I've evoked many of them in these pages, as an explanatory move and as a measure of scale.

Assessing the significance of any particular epidemic requires attention to the lived experience of the afflicted, of course, but also to the less visible social forces that shape that experience. In the medical desert, these are often the same forces shaping risk for infection *and* of finding little in the way of expert mercy once stricken, with poverty and exclusion at the top of the list. Structural violence of varied stripe has always shaped Ebola outbreaks and responses to them, and continues to do so. In April 2018, a Zaire strain of Ebola erupted in a couple of villages in Équateur Province of the Democratic Republic of the Congo. These villages are hundreds of miles from Yambuku, the site of the first documented Ebola outbreak. Yambuku is a small village near a small river, but Équateur is traversed by the vast, flowing highway that is the Congo River, across which lies (on the confusing postcolonial map) the Republic of the Congo.

This epidemic was said to be the ninth to hit the Congo since 1976, but there's evidence from serological surveys that Ebola viruses have long circulated in parts of the country—now immodestly labeled "non-outbreak settings"—without sparking official recognition.[20] In the absence of European missionaries, it's when these pathogens move from tiny villages to towns or to cities that they're apt to be recognized. The outbreak soon sickened fifty-four and killed more than half of them, soon reached the city of Mbandaka, with a population about as large as Freetown's or Monrovia's. Kinshasa and its twin city of Brazzaville, the nations' capitals, are five hundred miles downstream. That's about as far from Équateur's first confirmed Ebola cases as the Kissi Triangle is from the capital cities of Sierra Leone, Liberia, and Guinea. In West Africa, Ebola made that overland trek in weeks.

In the medical desert, the more people present, the more chances of viral transmission—viruses can't replicate outside of a host organism. So it's worth noting that, together, Kinshasa and Brazzaville count close to fifteen million residents. The dramas and conflicts detailed in this book played again in this particular Congolese epidemic. Professional caregivers stricken. Patients fleeing hospitals and isolation wards that didn't have enough in the way of staff, stuff, space, or systems. Attribution of these escapes, and other rumblings of *réticence*, to superstition and exotic beliefs. Difficulty reaching rural areas, and thousands of contacts to track down. But there have been new and heartening developments, and at least two of them stem directly from hard experience during the West African epidemic.

The first is that there's now an effective vaccine, and likely more than one. This is promising, because it means that ring vaccination might limit the spread of the virus. For it to work, however, health professionals in the country needed to clear the medical desert's difficult logistical hurdles—among them, poor cell-phone coverage, few all-weather roads beyond the Congo's broad back, and the need to refrigerate the vaccine at eighty degrees Celsius below zero. Within a month of confirmation that Ebola was the outbreak's culprit, seven hundred people had received the vaccine in Mbandaka, which was also the beneficiary of a new cellular tower. (It's hard to regard either vaccination or tower erection as stunning achievements when one considers the Congo's role in supplying fissile materials for the nuclear age.)

A second development involved the pace of the response and the amount of hubris informing it. The response was more brisk this time. Anthropologists and religious leaders, and varied other interpreters and influencers of opinion, were called up early to help address mistrust within, and miscommunication with, a population that—much like the population in Upper West Africa—is well aware of the deficiencies of its care-delivery system. Even more significantly, disease controllers, chastened by recent experience, strove to learn from their errors. As *The New York Times* reported on June 1, 2018, "The WHO's emergency committee gathered 10 days after the Congolese government notified the organization of an Ebola case"—an event, the paper continued, that stood in "stark contrast to the West African epidemic in 2014, when the group did not convene until almost 1,000 people had died."[21]

As I've tried to make clear in this book, Ebola and other public-health calamities strike most often in places from which human capital and raw materials have been extracted for centuries. From the rural reaches of Haiti and Rwanda, from the prisons of Siberia, and from the slums of urban Peru: for thirty years, I've been pointing out how the epidemics that people have suffered in these places have arisen because of the inequalities—political, economic, and medical—that such extraction invariably worsens.

The same holds true in all of the world's overlappingly scorched clinical and public-health deserts. On this score, however, Upper West Africa brooks few rivals.[22] Brimming in towns and cities is a young and battered population that, in the aftermath of war, plagues, and other catastrophes, has little in the way of access to health care and education, to say nothing of meaningful employment. This part of the world still lacks the sort of tranquility and opportunities that families dream of after war, plagues, and other catastrophes.

These hurts have left social scars of the obvious and the most discreet kind. But past afflictions are not the most striking thing about working in the region. What's more striking is just how much can be achieved in the way of irrigating the desert.

Take the government hospital in Koidu, a city in the heart of Sierra Leone's diamond district. The hospital was pretty much shut down by Ebola's western surge, but by the close of 2014, Partners In Health and Wellbody Alliance together employed at least three hundred staff working in and around the facility, which finally boasted general anesthesia, a digital X-ray machine, and 24/7 electricity; there was blood for transfusion on hand. The hospital had ready access to an inelegant but reliable Ebola lab, fashioned from a shipping container parked on the grounds of Wellbody's clinic. The lab had been stood up by a group of briskly efficient Dutch technicians, who spent much of their time training local lab techs.

The hospital and clinic dropped all charges for these and related services, despite the costs of making them available. It's hard to imagine any other means of providing them to a population facing both poverty and disease. To serve a desperate and destitute population during the Ebola crisis, Koidu and other public hospitals had to stop charging because the neoliberal curse of "user fees" served largely to keep patients away and generated next to no resources. Even at the height of the Ebola crisis, this raised the question of sustainability, of course. But the improvements in Koidu *were* sustained after the crisis subsided, in part because the crisis had exposed an important truth: there is a significant cost to not having a health system. The returns on having one were apparent a year after we helped reopen Koidu's hospital at the height of the western surge.

In December 2015, as Sierra Leone prematurely marked the end of the epidemic, the government hospital was being repainted, from dark brown to titanium dioxide bright white; medical teams were rounding on patients; and the pharmacy and warehouse were fairly well provisioned. There were over a dozen doctors and nurses present, a goodly number of them Sierra Leoneans, as were almost all the nonclinical employees. The staff based there were working full tilt. One evening that month, the on-call team—led by two young Sierra Leonean physicians more versatile than their expatriate colleagues—patched up the victim of a gunshot wound and successfully delivered two babies by emergency cesarean section. It was, said these medics, a night like any other.

An American emergency physician with whom we'd worked for years in central Haiti described the changes she'd seen in Koidu during the previous year:

> For so long, the hospital had been "desolate," people told me.
> It wasn't Ebola. For years prior to Ebola, the community didn't
> trust the hospital. Few, if any, of the staff, stuff, space, or systems
> necessary for quality health care existed at Koidu. And then the
> Ebola epidemic finished it off, coupling a real lack of trust with well-
> founded fear: If you went to the hospital, "you wouldn't come out."
> You'd get sick with Ebola, or really anything else, inside the hospital,
> and die. Over the past nine months, we've worked to address these
> deficiencies and to rebuild—or just build for the first time—that
> trust between us and the community. That started by taking on the
> also well-founded belief that if you go to the hospital, you might find
> help for your illness or injury and then have to pay exorbitant fees.
> Patients are now being screened at triage, vital signs are obtained
> with electronic monitors, and they're lining up outside clinic rooms
> and the operating theater.[23]

During many of my subsequent visits to Koidu Government Hospital, I had a similar impression: the hospital had become a beehive of purposeful, trustworthy activity. I saw the same transformation when I visited the district hospital in Harper, Liberia. With staff on hand, the biggest problem was—and still is—financial: how to pay the staff, buy the needed stuff, and maintain the space and equipment.

The environs of both Koidu and Harper remain vulnerable to outbreaks of Ebola, Lassa, and other similar pathogens—and to the kind of widespread mistrust that arose during efforts to contain the spread of the 2014 epidemic. But the time I've spent in their public hospitals has led me to believe that we might be able to detect and address the coming plague—and it *is* coming—more quickly and humanely. "Might" is a necessary qualifier, of course, as the lessons of Ebola start to fade. But I'm not the only one to have felt satisfaction during recent visits to Port Loko, Kono, Harper, Freetown, and Monrovia.

Seeing the uplifting engagement of hundreds of new coworkers cleaning, rebuilding, tending to the sick, reclaiming buildings destroyed by war, learning from each other, sharing meals, and building new friendships—and sometimes rebuilding damaged ones—brings some semblance of happiness to many involved in life after Ebola.[24] Scratch that surface of fellowship, however, and a deeper layer of suspicion is still there. As a newcomer to West Africa, I found it painful to witness the degree of distrust accorded national and local health authorities.

Although a recent history of armed conflict may be largely to blame, the control-over-care paradigm launched by the colonial Pasteurians has played an unrecognized and corrosive role in stoking the region's deep distrust of outsiders and authority. Local news reports spew tale after tale of politicians, thieves, witches, and other alleged malefactors spiriting away vast sums earmarked to improve health services, and the local population finds itself caught in a web of suspicion.[25] In the clinical desert, where populations have been abandoned for so long, trust is unlikely to flourish without long years of service. Keeping promises to protect health and dignity for all by improving the delivery of care might help release the trap in which this part of West Africa is now ensnared.

This oft-mentioned epidemic of distrust had transmission chains of its own, and they traveled up and down gradients of inequality. National and international health authorities complained about each other, and about intransigent and superstitious natives, and this carping became the background noise for ongoing debates about what sorts of medical care are possible, advisable, sustainable, cost-effective, reasonable, or (even) prudent in the clinical desert of Upper West Africa. No such debates accompanied the prosecution of the wars that rolled out the red carpet for Ebola. These were generously financed by the extractive trades, their lethality amplified by all the modern weaponry that diamonds could buy—from AK-47s almost light enough for a child to heft to flying gunships right out of a witchcraft legend.

Caught up in caring for the sick during the first months of the Ebola crisis, I was unaware (in 2014) of the extractive economy's inner workings. So were most of my expatriate colleagues. But the clues were all there: occupational injuries from accidents in mines or diamond pits, traffic accidents involving trucks full of ore, the sound of muffled explosions from under the earth, people crushed by rocks or falling timber, and the occasional story of someone swallowing diamonds in the rough in order to make off with a stone or two. This, too, served as the largely unacknowledged backdrop of the crisis.

As war has ravaged the region in recent decades, many of those who sifted through its red soil for diamonds or other trafficked treasures were laborers who did so under coercion. Traffickers included modernizing chiefs, the always-trading Mandingo, Lebanese diamond dealers, warlords, politicians, and others held to have a heavy hand in the extractive trades—or who simply hoped to profit from war. But the more we learn about the shadowy dealings of these big men, the more it becomes clear that some of their patrons and many of their clients are us. Where do the peddlers of diamonds from Upper West Africa find most of their customers today? In the United States, where people from many different tribes practice exotic marriage rituals that involve a powerful superstitious belief in the symbolic power of diamonds.

The glittering gems weren't forgotten during the crises. Take, for example, a conversation that the CEO of Partners In Health and I had in the summer of 2015 with a UN official from Belgium who'd helped us to procure and transport supplies for clinics, hospitals, and several Ebola treatment units during months in which it had been almost impossible to get such things in and out of Sierra Leone. During the worst month of the crisis, the official told us, he'd expressed his own grateful admiration to a couple of the Belgian pilots who had continued to fly to the region after many commercial carriers had halted their service. Matter-of-factly, the pilots had responded, "Well, we can't halt these important flights. There are thirty or so folks from De Beers going back and forth each week." They may have been mistaken when they singled out the world's largest diamond-trading company, which had closed its offices in Sierra Leone. What they likely got right was that international diamond merchants retain a keen interest in Kono's mines.

I don't mention this to argue that we should conflate war, serfdom, and epidemic disease with trade in diamonds—or in minerals, timber, and rubber. But seldom if ever has such a small patch of our planet had to endure so much extraction for so long. That injury, illness, and death has ensued was the entirely predictable result of a centuries-long chain of injustices. Breaking these chains will require more than symbolic justice or public denunciations of the guilty, more than truth and reconciliation. It will require material reparations.

Writing at the close of the war, the anthropologist Michael Jackson got to the heart of the matter. "Although people had suffered humiliation, bereavement, mutilation, and grievous loss," he wrote,

> few spoke of unhinged minds, broken spirits, or troubled souls. Rather, suffering was seen as something shared, and healing was sought not through therapy but in things. Not through words, but deeds. Fees to send children to school. Cement and roofing iron to rebuild houses. Grain. Micro-credit. Food. Medicines. It may well be that a diagnostic label like post-traumatic stress disorder is empirically justified, but it is imperative that we acknowledge that psychic wounds and national reconciliation are, for many Sierra Leoneans, not the burning issue. Rather it is the material means that are needed to sustain life, and ensure a future for one's children.[26]

Most of the people I've met in Liberia and Sierra Leone, and almost all those who survived Ebola there, say they need precisely those items listed by Jackson.

Tin roofs and cement foundations, schools (including universities) and school fees, books, computers, smartphones, medicine and medical care, paved roads, motorcycles, electricity. Decent salaries and jobs other than baking or making baskets or batik. These are what's demanded in the aftermath of war, epidemics, and catastrophes of all sorts. Those who take the trouble to listen know, which is why another anthropologist cited in these pages, an American, worried more during the Ebola crisis about getting a truck full of rice to a hungry community in central Sierra Leone than she did about what sort of contribution she might make qua anthropologist. They later informed her that hers was the only aid that reached the quarantined village where she'd worked prior to Ebola.[27] She and her colleagues should be proud of such gestures, and of their scholarly work.

Public-health practitioners and humanitarians, whether homegrown or foreign, clearly need the sort of knowledge compiled by anthropologists—especially those alive to the pleas of their friends, hosts, and informants. Disease controllers also need the perspectives of social historians. But honest looks back over even the past decades are rare in public health, whose practitioners—and I speak as one of them—generally evince little awareness of even recent history, and still less of ethnographic studies. As books and print journals are replaced by digital databases, the prestige of the new, the peer-reviewed, and the brief has eclipsed in-depth research and reflection of relevance to the task of irrigating clinical and public-health deserts. Yet in-depth knowledge about these deserts is surely needed, regardless of initial claims of causality (eating bushmeat versus caregiving versus structural violence), of how widely one's analytic net is cast (village, district, nation, region, the Atlantic world), or of how historically deep one probes (from the actions and policies of postwar humanitarians and the civil war, to structural adjustment programs after independence, to extractive colonialism and its control-over-care paradigm, and all the way back to the slave trades).

Just as clinicians and public-health authorities need to learn from anthropologists and historians, social scientists need to be interested in—and more militant about—the staff, stuff, space, and systems needed to slow or stop epidemics once loosed *and* in the care of the afflicted. During the Ebola crisis, experts in the region's local social worlds too often neglected the hard, material surfaces of life, and of lives foreshortened. Some of these experts were as territorial as leopards, taking umbrage when not consulted by short-term do-gooders about Ebola and social responses to it, and even at times taking umbrage when they were consulted.[28] None of this was umbrage underpinned by misanthropy or guile. It's just a reminder that, as the epidemic spread and social responses to it changed rapidly, there was one pervasive constant: conflict.

The good news is that it's hard to point to a single ailment in West Africa for which there's no remedy. The bad news is that new ones keep emerging and the situation in this part of Africa is worse than a decade ago, when the historian Emmanuel Akyeampong offered the following prescient summary:

> Most of the diseases that were present in 1900 have resurfaced, with the notable exception of smallpox. Major environmental changes, such as global warming and changes in land use, have transformed higher and cooler areas in Africa that were previously malaria-free into malaria zones. In 2000, malaria, and not AIDS, remained the number-one killer in Africa, accounting for between 20 and 30 per cent mortality in school-age children and for the whole population. New diseases such as HIV/AIDS and Ebola have complicated disease patterns.[29]

Since Akyeampong wrote, Sierra Leone, Liberia, and Guinea has each lost a substantial fraction of its doctors and nurses to Ebola.

Sierra Leone is weaker today in its fight against Lassa because of the deaths of Humarr Khan and his nursing colleagues. The nation is less able to address traumatic injuries, still among the nation's top killers of youth and young adults, because of the death of Martin Salia, who helped shape our report on access to safe and affordable surgical care. Many others who were able and willing to provide such care died during the epidemic, too, so our dismal estimates of the availability of surgical care in West Africa were out-of-date by the time they were published. These are grim developments and must be tallied along with the professional outmigration that occurred during war and its aftermath. Ebola and its losses are part of that aftermath, as is the less visible trauma faced by each of the survivors—caregivers all—introduced in these pages.

In the face of such pressing need, and with so many pragmatic tasks undone, it's fitting to ask why I have chosen to dedicate so much of a book about a twenty-first-century epidemic to the events of previous ones. The American writer Saidiya Hartman has posed that question in concentrated form. "To what end," she asked in 2002, "is the ghost of slavery conjured up?"[30] To this end, I would say: the slave trades were a motor force of the great reversal of fortunes registered on the two sides of the Atlantic. Extractive trades, even when declared legitimate, are global trades. The biggest markets for many of the commodities extracted, and the biggest sink for profits, have been Europe and North America. By evoking the ghost of slavery in the face of current miseries in West Africa, I mean to point out that the injuries of the trades, legitimate or not, have been peculiarly concentrated on one side of the traffic.

Perfect storms strike in perfect conditions, but, as Albert Camus said, they are long in the making. The long history of injury and injustice and extraction in West Africa made the Ebola crisis feel inevitable. What is *not* inevitable, however, is the cynical notion that misery and privation will continue unabated in the region. With a modicum of investment, a larger dose of social justice, and attention to the needs of those already sick or injured, the disastrous health conditions of this region can be reversed. Stalled development, long-standing antagonisms, and pervasive institutional debility—especially those of weak or disabled or distrusted *national* institutions—need not stand in the way of this rebuilding. There's deep mistrust here, it's true, but also goodwill and evidence of a commitment to move forward without forgetting to look back.

Both were on display on November 7, 2015, when Sierra Leone marked forty-two days without a new case of Ebola, thereby meeting the World Health Organization's criterion for being declared Ebola-free. Such a designation wasn't quite correct, given the virus's ability to persist for months or longer in sanctuary sites within the human body. The natural reservoir of the virus is still out there somewhere. But only a grim critic would disparage as indulgent the national celebrations declared that day. Informal celebrations broke out the night before, after the muezzins' last call to prayer rose and fell. A vigil commemorated the 221 Sierra Leonean nurses, doctors, and other health professionals who had perished during the epidemic. It was held under Freetown's great Cotton Tree, Sierra Leone's national symbol, where their names were read aloud.

Several friends and colleagues, including the Ebola survivors cited in these pages, were there. As the sun set, the tree's massive canopy glowed red-green, at least to those far away and high enough up to see it. Many, including Ibrahim Kamara and Yabom Koroma, didn't feel much like celebrating. But that didn't mean they didn't appreciate the symbolism of marking the date at the foot of the iconic tree. Like many, Ibrahim is awed by it, even though massive specimens aren't rare in Sierra Leone. "It has stood so long," he once told me. "It sees much that we no longer see."

Across West Africa, giant silk-cotton trees often point to ruined, rotting settlements and suggest the presence of graves somewhere nearby. But there's another way to see the tree. In Freetown, it towers over the cramped public square, no longer really a green space unless one looks up, rather than down. Looking back, the tree is a memorial. Looking forward, it's a sign not only of new life budding from old branches and ancient roots, but of the possibility, verdant and elusive, of something more than mere endurance.

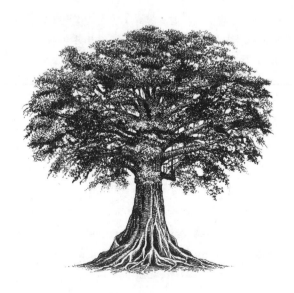

Epilogue:
The Color of COVID

"THE ONLY MEANS OF FIGHTING A PLAGUE," OBSERVES DR. RIEUX, THE protagonist of Albert Camus's novel set in a fictional Algerian city, is "common decency."[1] Refusing to pass under the crossed beams of fear and loathing, Dr. Rieux looks for decency and fellow feeling among the citizens, and strives, usually successfully, to cultivate it in himself. Decency, he says at one point, looks like just doing his job. Eventually, through a mix of caregiving and containment, the plague disappears from the city, the real protagonist of

The Plague. But not without great loss and not without revealing deep social fissures in colonial North Africa.

These social fissures were anything but fictional in 1947, when Camus's novel was published, and they're not fictional today, as a novel coronavirus strain sweeps the globe. If Europe's former African colonies aren't yet scenes of dislocation and despair, it may be because COVID-19 has not yet settled on them. But it's starting to, and my friends and colleagues in West Africa, at least, are preparing as best they can. Most of them tally the number of ICU beds in the region on one or two hands. (According to *The New York Times*, ten countries in Africa have no ventilators at all.) Even after all that transpired in West Africa, as recounted in these pages, the COVID-19 response there is operating, so far, on a wing and a prayer.

Today is April 10, 2020, and some here in Boston are celebrating Passover; for others, it's Good Friday. (Ramadan, creeping in early with the next waxing moon, will begin soon.) But no one is able to go to synagogue, church, or mosque. When this book about Ebola in West Africa was declared finished a few months ago, there was no hint that New England's largest city would soon be under curfew. Even those who have long and often predicted that a pandemic would strike North America seem surprised by the waste laid by a newly described coronavirus. That's because it's been more than a century since the continent was so thoroughly paralyzed: the last Boston shutdown occurred during the course of the last great pandemic due to a respiratory pathogen, the Spanish influenza crisis that emerged at the close of World War I.

With the advent of COVID-19, caused by a virus first identified in the Chinese city of Wuhan, another long-prophesied Big One may be upon us. Despite the pandemic preparedness folks who've been warning against such scenarios for years, the crisis caught us unprepared. ("Nobody knew there would be a pandemic or epidemic of this proportion," said President Donald Trump, weeks after it had taken hold of the U.S. mainland. *Except me*, Anthony Fauci might have added.) Few in Boston's famous hospitals, including the one I know like the palm of my hand, anticipated prepping this week for an imminent surge in cases of a plague unknown only a few months back by converting their dozens of operating rooms into ICUs. The hospital campus, which abuts the white marble grandeur of Harvard Medical School, has been transformed. Friendly colleagues recognize one another over and around masks, and by the sound of familiar voices muffled faintly by PPE.

Things aren't getting real, they're getting surreal: it's pandemic time. Four months ago, the acronym COVID-19 had not been coined. Now, the once-obscure medical terms and abbreviations used in these pages—PPE, social distancing, isolation, contact tracing, viral load, PCR, nosocomial spread, mechanical ventilation, dialysis, supportive and critical care, specific and nonspecific therapies, minimally symptomatic infection—no longer trouble my editor. Concepts like flattening the curve, diminishing the surge, and (more irritatingly) superspreaders are suddenly everyday parlance.

Several characters figuring prominently in these pages certainly stand to become better known as the COVID-19 crisis widens. Anthony Fauci is now a household name. A couple of days ago, I saw my friend and mentor's face on the cover of a Boston newspaper, on a "COVID cake," and on a half-dozen doughnuts.

At the core of this book is an argument for why it's wrong and invariably self-defeating for public authorities to put controlling an epidemic before caring for its victims. That's not what expert mercy looks like. When people do not expect that they or their loved ones will receive the best treatment available, they're unlikely to take well to containment measures such as quarantines or contact tracing. This point is now likely to be understood readily by a public torn between the desire to be protected from infection and the anxiety of wondering whether care will be adequate when protection fails.

Nor is the story this book tells really over. The Ebola epidemic recently declared finished in the eastern reaches of the Congo was today revealed to stutter on in the city of Beni: a new case must now be added to the 3,455 confirmed or probable ones already registered in the region, where two-thirds of the afflicted have died—another blow to trust among those on either or both sides of the control-over-care equation. Indeed, the physician-anthropologist

Eugene Richardson, a trusted colleague in West Africa and during the course of other epidemics, wonders if the term "eluding depredation" might not be an apposite way of describing the mistrust encountered in efforts to roll out a new Ebola vaccine in the eastern Congo.[2]

The affluent reaches of the world have long been spared the most draconian incarnations of the control-over-care paradigm. But today's empty streets must surprise many who predicted widespread resistance to containment orders within the United States. Unlike the restive populations eager to mark the end of war in 1918, now it's only a restive fraction that bemoans the shutdown of commercial air travel, cruise lines, and spring break. Yes, heedless youth have recently frolicked on Florida's beaches, but they weren't much slower than others to adopt something approaching the difficult recommendations of public-health authorities. Writing about a 2009 influenza pandemic that raised widespread concern but did not turn out to be the Big One—several thousand died in the United States, but there were only seven hundred school closings—the historian Nancy Tomes observed that "it may be easier for people to understand the rationale for social-distancing measures now than it was in 1918."[3] Well, we'll see.

The current COVID-19 crisis, should it deepen, may well force us to straddle both control and care—and to do some soul-searching about how to achieve the "social cohesion" and "resilience" we're told we need when tens of millions of jobs disappear in a matter of days. As of today, the majority of the world's population is under some sort of lockdown. In the meantime, we ask: Why has South Korea avoided, so far at least, the catastrophic tolls seen in Italy? What accounts for the astonishingly low fatality rates in Taiwan? Why has Germany fared better than its close European neighbors? The temptation to refer to slippery concepts like trust and resilience has again proved irresistible, and these, too, have been limned as national characteristics. "Maybe our biggest strength in Germany," observed an eminent German virologist as Chancellor Angela Merkel returned to office from two weeks of isolation, "is the rational decision-making at the highest level of government combined with the trust the government enjoys in the population."[4]

Well, again, maybe. It would be nice if such philosophical and cultural wherewithal were sufficient to address viral pathogens, but as in the Ebola case, it seems somehow safer to return to more material matters, such as the inventory of staff and stuff and spaces and systems. How many COVID-19 tests are being done in Germany? How many within its borders have health and unemployment insurance? What is the quality of supportive and critical care? Germany has far more ICU beds than its neighbors, and has far out-paced them in testing, already reaching close to 350,000 coronavirus tests a week at a time when its hard-hit neighbors on the continent and across the Channel have been conducting a small fraction as many. As a result, Germany has been able to find and isolate not only contacts like Angela Merkel—the doctor who'd administered her a pneumococcal vaccine, not the chancellor, later tested positive—but also asymptomatic, possibly infectious persons. These interventions have helped to flatten the curve in Germany, just as an extensive network of critical-care beds has kept mortality low.

If there's anything to be learned from a big Ebola outbreak that might be applied to our current (and truly global) predicament, it's that material con-straints, more than cultural differences, will shape the COVID-19 pandemic. It's important to understand how calls for social and physical distancing will remain unheeded by those who will find it materially impossible to heed them. Imagine being torn between orders to shelter in place and orders to provide essential services. Or imagine living in a slum, a tenement, a refugee camp, or a prison. Or just imagine living in a cramped apartment that's too small to keep restive inhabitants apart. Who suffers most when tempers flare in crowded confines? Imagine, finally, how hard it must be for so many to fill prescriptions for antihypertensive medications, or insulin.

Just as "the perfect storm" has become the most tired metaphor of catastro-phe, so too is the erroneous banality that a pandemic afflicts all people alike. Here comes coronavirus, the great leveler: none of us is immune, we're all at risk. But the quaint notion that respiratory pathogens do not discriminate—because we all draw breath—is almost never true, and it's already proven false as regards this new coronavirus. In some corners of the United States, the racialization of the COVID-19 outbreak has already shriveled trust to the size of a sour lemon. As the material difficulty of social distancing becomes apparent, so do racial disparities in both risk of infection and—even worse—risk of death after infection. Seven of ten who died of COVID-19 in Chicago last week were black. Today, as a Cook County prison outbreak caused hundreds to fall ill, the governor of Illinois began commuting prison sentences across the state. In Louisiana, where African Americans account for 33 percent of the population, they have accounted for 70 percent of COVID-19 deaths.

One of my medical colleagues here in Boston just announced a talk on this topic: "Is COVID-19 Becoming a Black Disease?"[5]

The story this book tells will seem more familiar to readers who are now experiencing, and for the first time, the pangs of social distancing, or worse. But we're now all living the strange temporality of a pandemic. The suspense and the lack of our typical pastimes afford abundant room to the quest for origin stories, heroes and villains, Cassandras and denialists.

The outbreak narratives now being written rely, as does jazz, on theme and variation. The export of pestilence remains a staple theme, with xenophobia as the main line in many origin stories. In this week's *New Yorker*, the Haitian American writer Edwidge Danticat explores the impact of COVID-19 on immigrant communities in the United States. She notes that when her family moved to the Miami neighborhood known as Little Haiti in 2002, she sometimes heard her neighbors say, "Whenever Haiti sneezes, Miami catches a cold."[6] Danticat knows that a variant of this aphorism was invoked by Haiti's nemesis, Napoleon. His version, however, concerned not his Haitian foes but a perceived danger from the east. "When China sneezes," he's alleged to have said, "the world catches a cold."

Blaming the neighbors is an eternally popular sport, and so is mocking their food. The Ebola-era obsession with bushmeat is neatly enough reflected in commentary about Wuhan's wet markets, where (one imagines) caged civets pace, eels and strange fish squirm and flop, and pangolins shed scales like golden tears. But let's not pretend that this is a uniquely Chinese problem: we all mess with Mother Nature. Human history is one long messing with the natural world, which is one reason zoonoses so often figure in Her basket of deplorables. For the moment, She seems not at all displeased that sharp downturns in air travel and manufacturing have cleared the air (and have dropped the price of fossil fuels) over much of the world. The lagoons of Venice are now as pellucid as the skies over Mumbai. But this brief truce will end.

If I aver this with Olympian assurance, it's less because infectious-disease specialists are now in high demand as the people who might start the machines of the world economy back up and more because we've seen already how quickly we forget pestilence. But it's better to confess that we don't have crystal balls, even though we know that zoonoses come in all the flavors described in this book—viral, bacterial, parasitic, fungal—and that the worst of them for humans are usually caused by viruses. The worst of those are often RNA viruses. Both Ebola and the novel coronavirus fit into this category, and both cause mayhem in human hosts, and much of it is familiar.

Many features of COVID-19 are familiar to infectious disease clinicians. When we describe "new" clinical presentations—cardiac involvement, encephalopathy, and anosmia (the loss of one's sense of smell)—we know the only new thing about them is their link to a newly described virus. Most of these novelties are simply a few more unsurprising features of systemic viral pathogens. Familiar, as well, is the idea that a walloping or sustained dose of this coronavirus, like any other poison, is more likely to cause serious disease than a smaller one. This was, after all, the idea behind the centuries-old practice of variolation for smallpox, and it's why we need to remain militant about PPE, and to protect those unable to shelter in place—and all those suddenly deemed "essential workers." Some have already become our sacrificial lambs.

Clinicians are also newly valued because people need care, perhaps especially in the case of a caregivers' disease such as Ebola or COVID-19. Most of my colleagues in the medical and scientific community have turned from their usual clinical and research activities to responding to COVID-19. That, too, is something I've never witnessed before—even back when Anthony Fauci called on members of a similarly broad community to turn our efforts to the new syndrome, AIDS, that he helped to describe. It may have been easier back then to believe that HIV was a pathogen narrowly afflicting the four-H club (homosexuals, heroin addicts, hemophiliacs, and Haitians). But little such cold (and again erroneous) comfort can be taken with COVID-19. It may not be the great leveler, but it has leapt across neatly defined social categories more nimbly than any blood-borne virus could.

My colleagues who are historians of epidemics like Ebola and pandemics like the Spanish flu are cautious about drawing lessons relevant to today, and that's in part because the causative pathogens have different nodes of spread. But who, in the end, can resist?

Other features of the global spectacle of COVID-19 will be familiar to close readers of this book about Ebola: pharaonic field hospitals are assembled in days; cavernous convention centers are repurposed, and so, more grimly, are refrigerated trucks and trailers; cataclysmic waves of contagion strike aircraft carriers and cruise ships alike. The influenza-exporting *Mantua*, the giant merchant ship converted to an armed cruiser that inadvertently introduced Spanish flu to Freetown on a memorably sultry day in August 1918, recalls the current dilemma of the USS *Theodore Roosevelt*. When the *TR*'s skipper pleaded for help with a brisk onboard COVID-19 epidemic, his appeal was leaked to the press. (There are so far no American censors in the war against this virus.) Then, as the captain fell sick with the disease, he was unceremoniously fired. Thousands of sailors cheered him after he was relieved of his command, reminding me of nothing so much as Italians singing praise for their caregivers from their balconies.

Donald Trump's cheering the captain's cancellation reminded me of no one so much as Donald Trump. He has remained true to form as a longtime xenophobe and germophobe, but his bully pulpit has ballooned to unimaginable proportions since 2014, when he first started tweeting about Ebola. As for missing the COVID-19 boat, some have argued that Trump deserves no special scorn for his denialism. He wasn't the only one, not at all. But Trump *is* the president of the world's most powerful nation, and so his decisions and public statements deserve special scrutiny. These arrive in daily and meandering press briefings—in the company of a stone-faced Dr. Fauci, who has thus far managed his usual balancing act of speaking truth even when he must contradict the boss.

President Trump brags about closing the doors to Chinese visitors, but genomic studies suggest that New York is being ravaged by viral strains introduced from Europe.[7] This suggests to many that any head start offered by their late arrival was squandered. Global spread was surely bound to occur, but some of the same *New York Times* reporters who described similar setbacks in West Africa during the spring of 2014 are now able to use more or less the same term—"a lost month"—to describe Trump's dithering in the early months of 2020.[8] Whether or not he's held to account will be known at about the time this book appears between hard covers. His current play seems to be to try to blame the Chinese, and even to suggest a nefarious plot to spread a virus manufactured or mishandled in a Wuhan laboratory.

Even if there are few villains in the COVID-19 drama, there have been heroes. These are people like Camus's Dr. Rieux, who survives the outbreak he was able to foretell from the sudden profusion of dead rats in the streets—a bad sign, for those who study zoonoses like the plague.

Dr. Rieux survives, but too many of our flesh-and-blood heroes had to die before getting recognition. Like Humarr Khan announcing the arrival of Ebola to Kenema, Li Wenliang was quick to observe that something disastrous was afoot in Wuhan in December 2019. Dr. Li, a young ophthalmologist, had the eyes to see a new illness with severe but otherwise unremarkable signs and symptoms. There was nothing pathognomonic, no vivid rash or other stigmata, to announce that this was a new disease. All he heard was the sound of previously comfortable patients—many old, like most of his patients, and some young—gasping for breath. And that, alas, is how Li Wenliang died. We can only hope that he was blessedly unaware of his air hunger because he was ventilated and sedated when he passed. That mercy was never accorded Humarr Khan, who died, as they say, with his eyes wide open.

With the exception of heroes like Humarr Khan and Martin Salia, the non-fictional people who populate this book are all engaged in responding to COVID-19 or are enduring its effects. Sheila Davis, who led Partners In Health's Ebola Response, is now the executive director of the organization, which has grown substantially through its efforts in West Africa and which she has turned toward COVID-19. Jon Lascher, oft-cited in these pages, is now the director of Partners In Health–Sierra Leone, and, in a lucky turn of events that seemed inevitable, Dr. Marta Lado has become its medical director. Lado has also become a continent-wide hero by traveling along with other Partners In Health clinicians, including Eugene Richardson, to places like Beni in the eastern Congo. She's now grounded in Sierra Leone and unable to travel to the eastern Congo to help attend to any outbreaks there.

Although they wouldn't likely want to know it, I've sometimes worried about these friends, and members of my family, caught in the nonheroic pose of gasping for breath. It's the way my mind works in pandemic time. *Would my friends and loved ones be okay? Would they have help breathing, if they needed it?* But here we are, alive and well and desperate to do something, anything, that might help. It's that sentiment, and really no other, that impelled us to work to rein in Ebola in West Arica. And that fellow feeling continues to lead us to other exotic locales.

Joia Mukherjee remains the chief medical officer of Partners In Health, and a week ago today we were in another unfamiliar setting, an empty state capitol, and in unusual company. Having worked together to confront AIDS, Zika, cholera, and Ebola, the two of us now joined the governor of Massachusetts to announce a new COVID-19 contact-tracing endeavor to be led by Partners In Health. After witnessing decades of clinical nihilism proffered on behalf of others—nothing can be done for "those people"—we now faced a species of containment nihilism. Why bother now with contact tracing and isolation when the coronavirus has already spread so widely? "I'm so sick of people saying it's too late to flatten the curve," the governor said, if in more colorful language.

None of us believed it would be acceptable to give up publicly on trying to save the afflicted in spite of the disturbing and familiar patterns of racial disparities that have already emerged. But less than a dozen years after the last big threat of pandemic influenza, Joia and I stood next to the exceedingly tall governor and his diminutive but tough secretary of health, trying to avoid a retreat into *containment* nihilism by announcing a new "Contact Tracing Collaborative" between Partners In Health and state health authorities.[9] It's not surprising that, in the United States at least, clinical nihilism—a political and social impossibility, at least as public policy—was not so prominent as containment nihilism. But the litmus test for advocating specific prevention *and* care efforts should be a simple one: Might this help?

Writing in 1919, Colonel George Soper, who ran the U.S. Army's public health corps, made a similar point. "If doubt arises as to the probable efficacy of measures which seem so lacking in specificity," he wrote at the close of the last Big One, "it must be remembered that it is better for the public morale to be doing something than nothing and the general health will not suffer for the additional care which is given it."[10]

Friends who are medical historians may be right that it's perilous to draw too many lessons from past epidemics, but that's not what struck me this past week. If there's indeed a lesson to be learned from Ebola, it may be this one: for everything we do, or say, in pandemic time, let's keep asking the same question. *Might this help?* So much that might have helped was never even tried in Upper West Africa. There, at least, the curve was not flattened— not until the western surge of 2014 crashed into the Atlantic Ocean—and so the collapse of rickety health systems ensued with terrifying rapidity. We shouldn't let this happen again.

So back to the Massachusetts State House, where I nervously looked around elegant rooms laid down at the close of the eighteenth century. Beautiful murals adorned floor after floor. We walked through marble halls behind the governor and his secretary of health, a state ranger and I bringing up the rear. I was trying (and failing) to stay six feet apart from Joia Mukherjee. As we silently descended three flights of resounding marble, I looked at the murals and their bewigged cast of all-white characters. In a mural depicting the drafting of the Massachusetts Constitution or some such, there were some Adamses, of course, including Samuel and John. (Were the two related? It didn't seem a good time to ask.) I looked in vain for John Quincy Adams, feeling that the *Amistad* drama should have been portrayed on those walls. Since my thoughts were on Ebola—I knew I would have to say something during the press conference about what it's like to see a health system swept away—they turned suddenly to Sierra Leone, and to former patients like Ibrahim Kamara and Yabom Koroma.

Here we were, with the entire nation and the world, called to shelter in place. Here we were, caught in the rotten trap of nationalism, with countries shutting people within arbitrary borders. The idea of imposing social distancing on those living in slums, refugee camps, or—like Yabom and God knows how many others—in crowded multigenerational homes. Unequal access to the Internet, or none at all. No running water to wash one's hands for a second, much less twenty seconds. And worst of all, at least to me, walking in the beautiful Massachusetts State House, the grotesquely differential rates of infection and death within the United States. Even without a visual reminder of Sengbe Pieh and John Quincy Adams, there it was, not so far from where we stood, the living hand of slavery, a stillborn Reconstruction, and Jim Crow already reflected in a pandemic scarce described. The true colors of COVID.

I am finishing this book not in a clinical desert, but in the richest nation in the world. Its subtitle—"Ebola and the Ravages of History"—was chosen by my editor. I like it but don't want to feel those ravages. What I most don't want to see, or feel myself, is the horror of knowing what's in store for those sickened with a respiratory illness and with not enough respirators and oxygen available. Because I know we might all gasp for breath at the end.

Boston, Massachusetts
April 10, 2020

PREFACE: THE CAREGIVERS' DISEASE

1. Médecins Sans Frontières (MSF), the humanitarian organization running this particular Ebola treatment unit, learned the hard way that the green zones (which included staff offices, pharmacies, latrines, meeting spaces, and changing areas) were low-risk areas, rather than no-risk ones. A French nurse, whose repatriation took fifty hours, was thought to have been infected while working in the triage area of the Monrovia facility we were visiting, but most who fell ill while working with MSF were likely infected beyond the confines of an ETU. By the time this organization folded up its tents and decommissioned its treatment units in West Africa, twenty-eight members of its staff had been infected. Half of them died.

See Médecins Sans Frontières, *An Unprecedented Year: Médecins Sans Frontières' Response to the Largest Ever Ebola Outbreak* (Geneva: Médecins Sans Frontières, 2015), p. 19.

2. Previous Ebola outbreaks in Africa, including the first one documented, in 1976, offered ample evidence that the virus (once introduced into a human population) is spread primarily from person to person. In contrast, uncertainty about Ebola's natural reservoir persists. But policies that discouraged or forbade the consumption of bushmeat sprang up in West Africa as soon as the virus was detected in March 2014. Just days after receiving confirmation of an Ebola outbreak within its borders, for example, the Guinean government banned "bat soup." Its health minister went on record to justify the directive, telling Bloomberg News, "We discovered the vector agent of the Ebola virus is the bat. We sent messages everywhere to announce the ban. People must even avoid consumption of rats and monkeys. They are very dangerous animals." Such measures were further discredited after the publication, in August 2014, of an analysis of Ebola virus genomes derived from seventy-eight patients in eastern Sierra Leone. Conducted by the Harvard computational geneticist Pardis Sabeti and her colleagues, the study demonstrated that human-to-human transmission had been responsible for sustaining the outbreak in the months prior. Sabeti understood the implications of these findings. "We're really concerned because a lot of the messaging going around is, 'Don't eat bushmeat; don't eat mango; don't eat anything that might be in contact with animals,'" she told National Public Radio. "When you see some of those fliers, you're like, 'Okay, you just told them not to eat all the main sources of food.'" A slew of similar studies ensued, all confirming the same point. A sampling of the relevant publications: Stephen K. Gire et al., "Genomic Surveillance Elucidates Ebola Virus Origin and Transmission During the 2014 Outbreak," *Science* 345, no. 6202 (2014): pp. 1369–72; Daniel J. Park et al., "Ebola Virus Epidemiology, Transmission, and Evolution During Seven Months in Sierra Leone," *Cell* 161, no. 7 (2015): pp. 1516–26; Jason T. Ladner et al., "Evolution and Spread of Ebola Virus in Liberia, 2014–2015," *Cell Host and Microbe* 18, no. 6 (2015): pp. 659–69; Miles W. Carroll et al., "Temporal and Spatial Analysis of the 2014–2015 Ebola Virus Outbreak in West Africa," *Nature* 524, no. 7563 (2015): pp. 97–101; Jeffrey R. Kugelman et al., "Monitoring of Ebola Virus Makona Evolution Through Establishment of Advanced Genomic Capability in Liberia," *Emerging Infectious Diseases* 21, no. 7 (2015): pp. 1135–43; Etienne Simon-Lorière et al., "Distinct Lineages of Ebola Virus in Guinea During the 2014 West African Epidemic," *Nature* 524, no. 7563 (2015): pp. 102–104; Yi-Gang Tong et al., "Genetic Diversity and Evolutionary Dynamics of Ebola Virus in Sierra Leone," *Nature* 524, no. 7563 (2015): pp. 93–96; Joshua Quick et al., "Real-Time, Portable Genome Sequencing for Ebola Surveillance," *Nature* 530, no. 7589 (2016): pp. 228–32; Armando Arias et al., "Rapid Outbreak Sequencing of Ebola Virus in Sierra Leone Identifies Transmission Chains Linked to Sporadic Cases," *Virus Evolution* 2, no. 1 (2016): p. vew016; Gytis Dudas et

al., "Virus Genomes Reveal Factors That Spread and Sustained the Ebola Epidemic," *Nature* 544, no. 7650 (2017): pp. 309–15.

3. Mike McGovern, "Bushmeat and the Politics of Disgust," *Cultural Anthropology*, October 7, 2014, culanth.org/fieldsights/bushmeat-and-the-politics-of-disgust.

4. Jessica Mitford, *The American Way of Death* (New York: Simon and Schuster, 1963), p. 17.

5. Hence the book's title, which I'll admit is inspired in part by the geographer, physiologist, and ornithologist Jared Diamond's *Guns, Germs, and Steel*. Unlike some event-focused historians, looking for the causes of the causes of why today some have so much and others so little, Diamond doesn't neglect the role of highly infectious pathogens, including smallpox, measles, yellow fever, and influenza. The conquistadors' and colonists' relative resistance to these pathogens—"Europe's sinister gift to other continents"—was a result, he claims, of a "long intimacy with domestic animals" lacking among the conquered. But pathogens and immunity were only part of it; guns and steel contributed their share, as did the grim conditions endured by those living in the Americas, and much of the world, at the time of the Columbian exchange. See *Guns, Germs, and Steel: The Fates of Human Societies* (New York: W. W. Norton, 1997), p. 214.

6. Richard Preston, *The Hot Zone* (New York: Random House, 1994), pp. 46–47.

7. During the West African epidemic, eleven patients with confirmed Ebola virus disease—nine Americans, one Liberian, and one Sierra Leonean—were cared for in U.S. hospitals; every American survived. European hospitals saw an additional sixteen Ebola patients, thirteen of whom survived. The clinical interventions that sustained and saved over 80 percent of patients treated outside of West Africa are reviewed in Timothy M. Uyeki et al., "Clinical Management of Ebola Virus Disease in the United States and Europe," *The New England Journal of Medicine* 374, no. 7 (2016): pp. 636–46; Aleksandra Leligdowicz et al., "Ebola Virus Disease and Critical Illness," *Critical Care* 20, no. 1 (2016): p. 217. This topic—who lives, who dies?—will be revisited in every chapter. It's a staple of social medicine.

1. THE TWENTY-FIFTH EPIDEMIC?

1. Liberia and Sierra Leone consistently recorded much higher annual growth in GDP per capita than Europe and the United States during the decade prior to Ebola; Guinea, less consistently so. In Sierra Leone, GDP per capita grew by 18.1 percent in 2013, the world's largest such increase. Within two years, this figure had plummeted to negative 22.3 percent, the world's second lowest, above only war-torn (and cholera-riven) Yemen. The economic impact of Ebola was uniformly disastrous in the most affected countries and negative across West Africa—and in parts of the continent far from any Ebola transmission. See "GDP Per Capita Growth," World Bank Group, 2020, data.worldbank.org/indicator/NY.GDP.PCAP.KD.ZG.

2. One compelling variation of this tale was laid out by virologists Sylvain Baize, Delphine Pannetier, and their colleagues in "Emergence of Zaire Ebola Virus

Disease in Guinea," *The New England Journal of Medicine* 371, no. 15 (2014): pp. 1418–25. This report—which draws on analysis of blood samples flown to laboratories in France and Germany, as well as conventional and molecular epidemiology—reconstructed early chains of transmission and traced the outbreak back to the death of a toddler in Meliandou. Speculation about the means by which the virus made its jump from an unknown natural host to humans also abounded in the popular press. One plausible enough version was laid out by journalists and researchers working with the television program *Frontline*, which in May 2015 released a documentary about Ebola in West Africa: *Outbreak*, directed by Dan Edge (Boston: WGBH Educational Foundation, 2015), pbs.org/wgbh /frontline/film/outbreak.

3. History graduate student Chernoh Alpha M. Bah disputes several details of the dominant outbreak narrative and comes up with theories of his own. His exploration of the role of "Eurocentric epistemology" in dominant Ebola origin stories will strike some readers—even those taking pains to avoid being Eurocentric—as accusatorial in tone. But it's worth noting, in part because Bah's tenor is common among West African critics of extractive science and in part because he adds important information that he took the trouble to collect himself. See "Eurocentric Epistemology: Questioning the Narrative on the Epidemic's Origin," in *Understanding West Africa's Ebola Epidemic: Towards a Political Economy*, edited by Ibrahim Abdullah and Ismail Rashid (London: Zed Books, 2017), pp. 47–65.

4. Laurie Garrett, "Ebola's Lessons: How the WHO Mishandled the Crisis," *Foreign Affairs*, August 18, 2015, foreignaffairs.com/articles/west-africa/2015-08 -18/ebolas-lessons. (Formatting altered.) Previous Ebola epidemics in Zaire and Sudan are detailed in Garrett's book, *The Coming Plague: Newly Emerging Diseases in a World Out of Balance* (New York: Farrar, Straus and Giroux, 1994).

5. The details of the investigation were published in Almudena Marí Saéz et al., "Investigating the Zoonotic Origin of the West African Ebola Epidemic," *EMBO Molecular Medicine* 7, no. 1 (2015): pp. 17–23.

6. Etienne Ouamouno, Émile's father, is quoted in Misha Hussain, "Hunger and Frustration Grow at Ebola Ground Zero in Guinea," Reuters, March 3, 2015, reuters.com/article/us-health-ebola-guinea-village-idUSKBN0LZ1R220150303. As with many illnesses occurring among those lacking social safety nets, Ebola—and social obligations in response to it—stripped Ouamouno of more than just his family. Ebola left him an indebted pauper.

7. For a concise report on refugee settlements within this socially porous region, see Wim Van Damme, "How Liberian and Sierra Leonean Refugees Settled in the Forest Region of Guinea (1990–96)," *Journal of Refugee Studies* 12, no. 1 (1999): pp. 36–53. "The Liberia-Guinea-Sierra Leone tripoint," adds historian Guillaume Lachenal, "may be seen as a specific transborder 'pathocenosis': a bio-political environment producing rubber, diamonds, parasitic diseases, emerging viruses, and war injuries." See "Outbreak of Unknown Origin in the

Tripoint Zone," *Limn*, January 2015, limn.it/outbreak-of-unknown-origin-in
-the-tripoint-zone.

8. In 1967, attempts to save Germans and Yugoslavians from the unknown affliction later named Marburg saved close to 80 percent of them. When researchers, armed with new diagnostic tests, later looked for evidence of Marburg in the
course of lethal outbreaks of febrile disease in parts of Africa, they sometimes
found it. They also found that 80 percent or more of afflicted Africans died. This
high mortality was seen in all documented Marburg outbreaks in Africa for the
rest of the century and into this one; there were no more outbreaks documented
on other continents.

9. For prewar evidence of Ebola infection in Upper West Africa, see, for example,
J. Knobloch, E. J. Albiez, and H. Schmitz, "A Serological Survey on Viral Haemorrhagic Fevers in Liberia," *Annales de l'Institut Pasteur / Virologie* 133, no.
2 (1982): pp. 125–28; M. Hughes, W. Slenczaka, and J. Neppert, "Serologic
Evidence for the Occurrence of Human Infections with Marburg- and Ebola-
Virus in the Republic of Liberia," *Zentralblatt für Bakteriologie, Mikrobiologie,
und Hygiene A* 267, no. 1 (1987): p. 128; Fransje W. van der Waals et al., "Hemorrhagic Fever Virus Infections in an Isolated Rainforest Area of Central Liberia: Limitations of the Indirect Immunofluorescence Slide Test for Antibody
Screening in Africa," *Tropical and Geographical Medicine* 38, no. 3 (1986): pp.
209–214. See also the commentary on this evidence by Bernice Dahn, Vera Mus-
sah, and Cameron Nutt, "Yes, We Were Warned About Ebola," *The New York
Times*, April 7, 2015, nytimes.com/2015/04/08/opinion/yes-we-were-warned
-about-ebola.html.

10. In August 2014, Air France stopped flying to Freetown but maintained its flights
to Conakry. When France's president hosted Guinea's the following month, he
lauded the airline's continued service to the former French colony, calling it an
expression of his country's "solidarity" with the Ebola-afflicted. Nevertheless,
there were reports throughout the fall of Air France crews threatening to refuse
to board flights destined for Conakry and other West African cities. In mid-
October, when temperature checks were introduced at French airports for passengers arriving from Guinea, Air France unions issued a joint statement calling
for services between Paris and Conakry to be suspended until the epidemic was
brought to a halt. The flights, they argued à la Donald Trump, carried "a serious risk of spreading the epidemic, particularly in our country." See David
Chazan, "France Introduces Ebola Screening at Airport," *The Telegraph*, October
18, 2014, telegraph.co.uk/news/worldnews/ebola/11171620/France-introduces
-Ebola-screening-at-airport.html. The numbers contradict both Trump and the
French unions. Two patients who contracted the disease in West Africa—a
French nurse working with MSF and a UN employee whose nationality was
undisclosed—were evacuated to a hospital near Paris, but no one was infected
while caring for them. Both survived.

11. Adam Nossiter, "Fear of Ebola Breeds a Terror of Physicians," *The New York Times*, July 27, 2014, nytimes.com/2014/07/28/world/africa/ebola-epidemic -west-africa-guinea.html.

12. Kevin Sack et al., "How Ebola Roared Back," *The New York Times*, December 29, 2014, nytimes.com/2014/12/30/health/how-ebola-roared-back.html.

13. The Soviet quest during the 1980s to build a filovirus arsenal to complement their nuclear one is summarized—with less frenzy and perhaps less fiction than is common in such accounts—by Milton Leitenberg, Raymond Zilinskas, and Jens Kuhn in *The Soviet Biological Weapons Program: A History* (Cambridge: Harvard University Press, 2012). By the time the Soviet Union collapsed, a "dry formulation" of Marburg virus was alleged to have been developed, aerosolized, and tested in monkeys; the project of weaponizing Ebola appeared to be a more difficult one, if a scientist formerly based at the Vector Institute is to be believed. According to the same scientist, the Soviet military had estimated that a Marburg attack would "cause about 25 percent lethality if used in Europe and about 80 percent if used in Africa" (*The Soviet Biological Weapons Program*, pp. 219, 217.). The largest recorded African outbreaks of Marburg—which occurred in the Democratic Republic of Congo from 1998 to 2000 and in Angola from 2004 to 2005—hadn't yet occurred but would later suggest that the Soviets' forecast of disparate lethality wasn't far off.

14. Daniel Bausch has written a detailed account of the failure to enhance the region's laboratory capacity. "In 2004, the World Health Organization, Tulane University, the Mano River Union country (Guinea, Sierra Leone, and Liberia) governments, and various collaborators and funders established the Mano River Union Lassa Fever Network," he reports. "Although the initial focus was Kenema, the project was also to enhance capacity in existing laboratories in Monrovia, Liberia; Conakry, Guinea; and most pertinent now, N'Zérékoré, Guinea. The N'Zérékoré laboratory, just a few hours away from the Guéckédou region, where Ebola virus apparently was introduced into humans to start the terrible West African outbreak, was created during my time working on Lassa fever with the Centers for Disease Control and Prevention. We eventually discovered that the incidence of Lassa fever and thus the potential for research was much less in Guinea than in Sierra Leone. Enthusiasm for the project waned, and 2002 was the last year of the CDC funding." The rest of the paper deals humbly with the lethal failure to link research capacity to both improved clinical care and formal training. See "The Year That Ebola Virus Took Over West Africa: Missed Opportunities for Prevention," *The American Journal of Tropical Medicine and Hygiene* 92, no. 2 (2015): p. 229. (Formatting altered.) This is the most important such critique to appear in the specialist literature about the West African outbreak.

15. See Randal J. Schoepp et al., "Undiagnosed Acute Viral Febrile Illnesses, Sierra Leone," *Emerging Infectious Diseases* 20, no. 7 (2014): pp. 1176–82. This paper was held up for a year in reviews and initially rejected.

16. The timeline of the young woman's symptoms suggests that she may have been infected later in the course of her pregnancy. When she experienced signs of early labor, she sought care in a small public clinic and found herself in a bed next to another pregnant woman. This happened to be the granddaughter of the healer's sister, who died shortly thereafter. (Of note, the two pregnant women had been in the care of the same midwife, who would go on to die from Ebola at the end of May.) When the twenty-year-old's condition worsened, she traveled ninety miles to Kenema Government Hospital. Upon arrival, on May 23, she was documented to have a high fever, prompting her diagnosis. These and other details, meant to reconstruct formerly undetected transmission chains in Sierra Leone, are presented in Augustine Goba et al., "An Outbreak of Ebola Virus Disease in the Lassa Fever Zone," *The Journal of Infectious Diseases* 214, supplement 3 (2016): pp. S110–S121.

17. Sinead Walsh and Oliver Johnson, *Getting to Zero: A Doctor and a Diplomat on the Ebola Frontline* (London: Zed Books, 2018), p. 96.

18. Tim O'Dempsey, "Failing Dr. Khan," in *The Politics of Fear: Médecins Sans Frontières and the West African Ebola Epidemic*, edited by Michiel Hofman and Sokhieng Au (New York: Oxford University Press, 2017), p. 175.

19. These were just a few of the startling figures presented by Daniel Bausch and a district health task force in an investigation of health worker infections in and around Kenema Government Hospital. The 92 cases ultimately accounted for 15 percent of the total number of infections registered in the district. The peak of this trend came during the harrowing summer of 2014, when health workers represented up to a quarter of Kenema's Ebola-afflicted—a proportion commensurate with that recorded 20 years earlier in Kikwit, Zaire, where 80 of the outbreak's 315 documented cases were registered among health workers of one description or another. The Kikwit story, like others before it, laid bare Ebola's affinity for overburdened caregivers in poorly equipped hospitals and clinics. But even in such comparisons, Kenema's district hospital—the largest in Sierra Leone's Eastern Province—deserves special mention. According to staff rosters, approximately 145 clinical personnel worked in the 350-bed facility during the outbreak. That so many of them were diagnosed with the infection—18 were staffing the Ebola wards and 48 were working elsewhere in the hospital—suggests the virus had little difficulty dodging weak infection-control measures. It's important to add that high levels of Ebola transmission beyond hospital walls meant that some employees were likely infected in the course of caregiving at home. See Mikiko Senga et al., "Factors Underlying Ebola Virus Infection Among Health Workers, Kenema, Sierra Leone, 2014–2015," *Clinical Infectious Diseases* 63, no. 4 (2016): pp. 454–59. For a review of what transpired in Kikwit, see Ali S. Khan et al., "The Reemergence of Ebola Hemorrhagic Fever, Democratic Republic of the Congo, 1995," *The Journal of Infectious Diseases* 179, supplement 1 (1999): pp. S76–S86.

20. "Experts: Ebola Vaccine at Least 50 White People Away," *The Onion*, July 30, 2014, theonion.com/experts-ebola-vaccine-at-least-50-white-people-away-1819576750.

21. No small part of the polio-eradication campaign in Nigeria has been supported by the Bill and Melinda Gates Foundation. The couple who founded and funded it is well aware that integrating prevention and care for one epidemic was likely to prove helpful in the event of others—as long as rigidly narrow focus on one pathogen can be shifted to others when circumstances require it. Making his debut in *The New England Journal of Medicine* as the epidemic was ongoing, Bill Gates observed that "Ebola has spread much faster and more widely in countries whose health systems—and especially whose primary care systems—were severely weakened by years of armed conflict and neglect." His diagnosis is followed by a prescription: "Strengthening health care systems not only improves our ability to deal with epidemics, but it also promotes health more broadly. Without a functioning health system, it is very hard for a country to end the cycle of disease and poverty." See "The Next Epidemic—Lessons from Ebola," *The New England Journal of Medicine* 372, no. 15 (2015): p. 1382.

22. That team, which included a couple of local journalists, had the misfortune to arrive in the company of high-ranking government officials with political baggage. Guinean sociologist Alpha Barry has recently alleged that some regional authorities, echoing the practices of colonial Pasteurians, had fanned the *forestiers'* long-standing mistrust of authority in general. He reports that "certain territorial administrators made threats such as: 'if you don't come out we'll gas you.' In addition to giving the impression that spraying houses with chlorine to disinfect them was a punishment, such statements reminded the people of the harsh colonial practices of the French that were marked by abuses and harassment of all kinds." See "Interpreting the Health, Social, and Political Dimensions of the Ebola Crisis in Guinea," in *Understanding West Africa's Ebola Epidemic*, p. 78.

23. Barack Obama, quoted in Mark Landler and Somini Sengupta, "Global Response to Ebola Is Too Slow, Obama Warns," *The New York Times*, September 25, 2014, nytimes.com/2014/09/26/world/africa/obama-warns-of-slow-response-to-ebola-crisis.html. The *Times* article used a different HR calculus to describe the recent deployment of U.S. forces, referring to "3,000 doctors and other personnel." Some fraction of these military personnel had medical or nursing degrees, certainly, but the majority were soldiers. Ban Ki-moon, then the UN's secretary-general and the convener of the special session at which President Obama spoke, made subtle note of this incongruity. "Just as our troops in blue helmets help keep people safe," Ban said, referring to UN peacekeepers' headwear, "a corps in white coats could help keep people safe." Across West Africa, editorials, cartoons, and radio broadcasts made the point less subtly, as did abundant local commentary shared on social media and in casual conversation.

24. Donald Trump, Twitter post, October 9, 2014, 4:49 p.m., twitter.com/realdonaldtrump.

25. See Martin I. Meltzer et al., "Estimating the Future Number of Cases in the Ebola Epidemic—Liberia and Sierra Leone, 2014–2015," *Morbidity and Mortality Weekly Report* 63, supplement 3 (2014): pp. 1–14.

26. Michael Winter, "Timeline Details Missteps with Ebola Patient Who Died," *USA Today*, October 17, 2014, usatoday.com/story/news/nation/2014/10/17/ebola-duncan-congress-timeline/17456825.

27. Donald Trump, Twitter post, October 4, 2014, 11:35 a.m., twitter.com/realdonaldtrump.

28. Jared Owens, "Ebola Migration Ban Best for Nation, Peter Dutton Says," *The Australian*, November 6, 2014, theaustralian.com.au/in-depth/ebola-crisis/ebola-migration-ban-best-for-nation-peter-dutton-says/news-story/83f9053fb4612287573e53f699824135.

29. Paul Richards, *Ebola: How a People's Science Helped End an Epidemic* (London: Zed Books, 2016), pp. 54–55.

30. Donald Trump, Twitter posts, October 23, 2014, 7:38 p.m., 7:24 p.m., 5:31 a.m., 10:31 p.m., twitter.com/realdonaldtrump.

31. Perry Stein, "After the Ebola Outbreak, the World Moved On. One Family Didn't," *The Washington Post*, July 14, 2016, washingtonpost.com/lifestyle/magazine/after-the-ebola-outbreak-the-world-moved-on-one-family-didnt/2016/07/13/125786fa-0e29-11e6-a6b6-2e6de3695b0e_story.html.

32. Paul Wafer, "Access Criteria for Kerry Town 12-Bed Facility," Department for International Development (DFID) Sierra Leone. These criteria were published as an appendix to Miriam Shuchman, "Sierra Leone Doctors Call for Better Ebola Care for Colleagues," *The Lancet* 384, no. 9961 (2014): p. e67.

33. When Salia was admitted to the Omaha biocontainment unit, his heart was racing, his respiratory rate was fast, and he was somnolent. Blood tests revealed significant electrolyte abnormalities, and an echocardiogram was consistent with persistent, severe hypovolemia. Blood cultures drawn at time of admission did not reveal bacteria in the bloodstream, but cultures drawn the following day were found to be positive for *Escherichia coli*, a common gut organism. Antibiotics were started for presumed secondary bacterial sepsis. (Salia had by report received a similar regimen at Hastings but boarded the plane without much in the way of medical records.) In the hours prior to his death, in the early hours of his second day in Omaha, Salia's heart rate slowed dramatically, his blood pressure plummeted, the level of lactic acid in his blood shot up, and his abdomen became rigid. This suggested to the team caring for him that "death was hastened by a perforated viscus or some other abdominal catastrophe." See Viranuj Sueblinvong et al., "Critical Care for Multiple Organ Failure Secondary to Ebola Virus Disease in the United States," *Critical Care Medicine* 43, no. 10 (2015): p. 2070.

34. Some of the largest sign-and-symptomatology data sets, including information about thousands of Ebola patients, were published in *The New England Journal of Medicine*. According to these summaries, the most common early signs and symptoms reported among confirmed Ebola cases were fever (86 percent), fatigue

(82 percent), loss of appetite (78 percent), headache (66 percent), vomiting (63 percent), diarrhea (60 percent), joint pain (58 percent), and abdominal pain (57 percent). Hemorrhagic manifestations were seen less frequently than in previous outbreaks, including those due to the Zaire species: most reviews peg evidence of bleeding disorders among West African patients at fewer than 10 percent. See the supplement to WHO Ebola Response Team, "Ebola Virus Disease Among Male and Female Persons in West Africa," *The New England Journal of Medicine* 374, no. 1 (2016): pp. 96–98. Humarr Khan and coworkers in Kenema found a similar ranking of top signs and symptoms and the same rarity of hemorrhagic ones. During the month following their diagnosis of Sierra Leone's first confirmed cases, only 1 of 106 Ebola-positive patients showed evidence of bleeding at presentation, and few hemorrhagic signs were observed during other stages of disease, as patients progressed toward recovery or, more commonly, death. See John S. Schieffelin et al., "Clinical Illness and Outcomes in Patients with Ebola in Sierra Leone," *The New England Journal of Medicine* 371, no. 22 (2014): pp. 2092–2100. Many more cohort reports and clinical summaries would be published throughout the remainder of 2014 and in the years that followed, further suggesting Ebola caused a clinical syndrome characterized predominantly by gastrointestinal illness. See, for example, the study of 464 Ebola patients admitted to Connaught Hospital's holding unit, conducted by the heroic Dr. Marta Lado and her colleagues, who are introduced the next chapter: "Clinical Features of Patients Isolated for Suspected Ebola Virus Disease at Connaught Hospital, Freetown, Sierra Leone: A Retrospective Cohort Study," *The Lancet Infectious Diseases* 15, no. 9 (2015): pp. 1024–33.

35. See Stephen K. Gire et al., "Genomic Surveillance Elucidates Ebola Virus Origin and Transmission During the 2014 Outbreak," *Science* 345, no. 6202 (2014): pp. 1369–72. The journal, its editors faced with what was in all likelihood an unprecedented situation, ran an obituary of the fallen authors to accompany the article when it was published online. A sixth coauthor died of other causes while the study was in press. See Gretchen Vogel, "Ebola's Heavy Toll on Study Authors," *Science*, August 28, 2014, sciencemag.org/news/2014/08 /ebolas-heavy-toll-study-authors.

2. TOUGH CALLS

1. See Joseph Crompton et al., "Comparison of Surgical Care Deficiencies Between U.S. Civil War Hospitals and Present-Day Hospitals in Sierra Leone," *World Journal of Surgery* 34, no. 8 (2010): pp. 1743–47.

2. For more on these inequities in health-care financing, see Anirudh Krishna, *One Illness Away: Why People Become Poor and How They Escape Poverty* (New York: Oxford University Press, 2010); Paul Farmer, "Who Lives and Who Dies," *London Review of Books* 37, no. 3 (2015): pp. 17–20; Rob Yates, "Universal Health Care and the Removal of User Fees," *The Lancet* 373, no. 9680 (2009): pp. 2078–81; Adam Wagstaff et al., "Progress on Catastrophic Health Spending in 133 Countries: A Retrospective Observational Study," *The Lancet Global Health* 6, no. 2 (2018): pp. e169–e179.

3. Vicious hardware has a way of lingering long after war is over: even a decade after war and genocide had ended in Rwanda, we'd cared for a few kids newly maimed by land mines. In the interest of deepening the discussion of neo-liberalism presented in the chapters that follow, let me cite the conclusion of Gino Strada's book *Green Parrots*, titled after a nickname for small, bright green plastic land mines, designed to look like toys. "We had thought that war was an old, primitive instrument, a cancer that mankind did not know how to eradicate; on this point we were mistaken," he writes. "Tragically, we—and not only we—had failed to see that war, rather than being a burdensome inheritance from the past, was becoming a fearful prospect for our future and for generations to come. In the operating theatre we saw the devastation produced in human bodies by bombs and mines, by projectiles and rockets. Yet we did not succeed in grasping the effects of other weapons, 'unconventional' ones: finance and international loans, trade agreements, the 'structural adjustments' imposed on the policies of many poor countries, the new arms races in richer countries." See *Green Parrots: A War Surgeon's Diary* (Milan: Charta, 2004), p. 132.

4. I've explored this in a hastily written book meant to serve as a record of those grim times (and to exorcise some of their hold over me) in *Haiti After the Earthquake* (New York: PublicAffairs, 2011).

5. Jim Kim couldn't believe that there wasn't some sort of insurance against the devastating impact of such epidemics. Why wasn't there a "pandemic emergency fund," with access to it triggered by an outbreak? Kim proceeded to launch one, but such innovations take time, as would the implementation of any Ebola-related projects that might be funded by World Bank dollars. For more on this effort, see "World Bank Launches 'Pandemic Bond' to Tackle Major Outbreaks," Reuters, June 28, 2017, reuters.com/article/us-global-pandemic-insurance/world-bank-launches-pandemic-bond-to-tackle-major-outbreaks-idUSKBN19J2JJ.

6. "Culture is epiphenomenal," Paul Richards credibly asserts. "It is a symptom, not a cause. Burials create pathways for virus spread, but so do several other, more mundane activities, not least practices of caring for the sick. So it is not helpful to distinguish ritual from practical aspects, and to invest the former with the sense of something exotic or bizarre." See *Ebola: How a People's Science Helped End an Epidemic* (London: Zed Books, 2016), pp. 66–67.

7. As Richards explains, "The government of Sierra Leone made the washing of corpses a criminal offence, punishable by two years in jail. Liberia imposed cremation. But draconian approaches only added to social disquiet. Perhaps unsurprisingly, it was after the law against washing bodies was passed that response agencies began to refer to 'hidden bodies' and 'secret funerals.' People were taking the law into their own hands. Death laid upon them a higher moral imperative. The problem, as the anthropologists tried to convey, was that staying safe in an Ebola epidemic cannot be attained without also addressing the social challenges of death" (*Ebola*, p. 52). Such "social challenges of death" are brought

into vivid relief by the accounts offered by Ibrahim Kamara and Yabom Koroma in the next two chapters. For other anthropological perspectives on the impact of such punitive measures, see Mary H. Moran, "Missing Bodies and Secret Funerals: The Production of 'Safe and Dignified Burials' in the Liberian Ebola Crisis," *Anthropology Quarterly* 90, no. 2 (2017): pp. 399–421; Umberto Pellecchia et al., "Social Consequences of Ebola Containment Measures in Liberia," *PLOS ONE* 10, no. 12 (2015): p. e0143036; Raphael Frankfurter, "'Safe Burials' and the 2014–2015 Ebola Outbreak in Sierra Leone," in *The Routledge Handbook of Medical Anthropology*, edited by Lenore Manderson, Elizabeth Cartwright, and Anita Hardon (New York: Routledge, 2016), pp. 355–58; Annie Wilkinson and Melissa Leach, "Briefing: Ebola—Myths, Realities, and Structural Violence," *African Affairs* 114, no. 454 (2015): pp. 136–48.

8. "President Obama to the International Community: We Must Do More to Fight Ebola," The White House, September 25, 2014, obamawhitehouse.archives.gov /blog/2014/09/25/president-obama-international-community-we-must-do-more -fight-ebola.

9. Joanne Liu, quoted in Médecins Sans Frontières, "Global Bio-Disaster Response Urgently Needed in Ebola Fight," press release, September 2, 2014, msf.org/global -bio-disaster-response-urgently-needed-ebola-fight.

10. Sinead Walsh and Oliver Johnson, *Getting to Zero: A Doctor and a Diplomat on the Ebola Frontline* (London: Zed Books, 2018), p. 169.

11. Albert Camus, *The Plague*, translated by Stuart Gilbert (New York: Alfred A. Knopf, 1948), p. 122.

12. Anne Atai-Omoruto, veteran of several Ebola outbreaks in her native Uganda, survived this big one but has since passed away. See the obituary by Clair MacDougall, "Anne Deborah Atai-Omoruto, 59, a Leader in the Ebola Fight in Liberia, Dies," *The New York Times*, May 10, 2016, nytimes.com/2016/05/11/world/africa /anne-deborah-atai-omoruto.html. Dr. Atai-Omoruto will be missed.

13. Clinical nihilism was certainly evident in MSF guidelines for the care of pregnant women with Ebola. Mothers had, asserted their authors, a 93 percent case-fatality rate, while babies were certain to die; care was, in this view, both dangerous and futile. These guidelines are still available online. See Médecins Sans Frontières, "Guidance Paper—Ebola Treatment Centre: Pregnant & Lactating Women," 2014, rcog.org.uk/globalassets/documents/news/etc-preg -guidance-paper.pdf. This guidance is compared to that offered for "a Western context" by Benjamin Black, "Principles of Management for Pregnant Women with Ebola: A Western Context," Royal College of Obstetricians and Gynaecologists, 2014, rcog.org.uk/globalasscts/documents/news/ebola-and-pregnancy -western.pdf. Since Sierra Leone is located in similar longitude as the Royal College, Black is referring not to "a western context" but to a medically impoverished and postcolonial one. Admittedly, the country and its former colonizer might as well be on different planets.

14. Frederick William Hugh Migeod, *A View of Sierra Leone* (London: Kegan Paul, Trench, Trubner & Co., 1926), p. 19. Migeod regarded the Temne to "have been very fully worked up," and "passed through their country quickly." He dedicated the majority of this book, and others, to the Mende, the colony's most numerous tribe after the British traced Sierra Leone's boundaries at the close of the nineteenth century. Colonel Migeod didn't much care for the Temne. "The want of politeness in the people is very striking," he wrote, "and I found it much the same through all Temne country. There seemed to be a generally tacit agreement to show neither marks of respect to Europeans nor even to be reasonably well behaved when near them" (*A View of Sierra Leone*, pp. xi, 21). Our own experience, brief as it has been, hasn't borne out this or other much-commented-upon "tribal" essentialisms. We never found our Temne-speaking hosts to be impolite. Then again, we didn't spend three decades putting down revolts in and around Port Loko.

15. Migeod, *A View of Sierra Leone*, pp. 20–21, 16.

16. Donald Trump, Twitter post, October 26, 2014, 7:20 a.m., twitter.com /realdonaldtrump.

17. See Eugene T. Richardson et al., "Biosocial Approaches to the 2013–2016 Ebola Pandemic," *Health and Human Rights* 18, no. 1 (2016): pp. 115–28.

18. See Eugene T. Richardson et al., "Minimally Symptomatic Infection in an Ebola 'Hotspot': A Cross-Sectional Serosurvey," *PLOS Neglected Tropical Diseases* 10, no. 11 (2016): p. e0005087.

19. One of the Cuban physicians, Felix Báez, fell ill with Ebola while working near Freetown. He was airlifted to Geneva, where his boss—Jorge Pérez, a fellow infectious-disease specialist and good friend of mine—flew from Havana to meet him. One of the first things the sick doctor said to Pérez was that he couldn't wait to get back to Sierra Leone. Sure enough, I first met Báez when he came to visit his colleagues in Maforki. For a profile of both Cubans and their contributions to fighting the epidemic, see Gail Reed, "Meet Cuban Ebola Fighters: Interview with Félix Báez and Jorge Pérez," *MEDICC Review* 17, no. 1 (2015): pp. 6–10.

20. The Ebola Recovery Tracking Initiative has monitored pledges made by donors at a UN conference held in July 2015, when substantially fewer Ebola cases were being recorded than during the fall of 2014. Estimates as of January 2018 suggest that of the roughly $9.1 billion requested to finance the national and regional recovery plans presented by the presidents of Liberia, Guinea, and Sierra Leone at the conference, $4.5 billion was pledged. Seventy percent of pledges were undisbursed two and half years later. And disbursement is only the prelude to implementation, which is what really matters if the goal is to prevent the next catastrophe. It's also evident that disbursed funds have not been primarily channeled through public institutions, and that donors and implementing partners haven't permitted recipient governments the flexibility to deploy the funds as needed. See "Ebola Recovery— Financial Tracking of Ebola Recovery Funding," accessed January 22, 2018, ebolarecovery.org, as well as journalist Betsy McKay's report on these findings,

"Ebola Funds Pledged for Recovery Are Slow to Come," *The Wall Street Journal*, March 20, 2018, wsj.com/articles/ebola-funds-pledged-for-recovery-are-slow-to-come-1521547201. This hard (and often thankless) work of tracking pledges has been led by Jehane Sedky, Abbey Gardner, and Jennie Weiss Block. Thanks, too, to David Lambert and others who contributed, and to a small group of funders, including Darren Walker of the Ford Foundation, who made it possible.

21. As of April 2015, the Ebola treatment units built by U.S. military and contractors in Liberia had cared for just twenty-eight Ebola patients. Most opened in late December 2014 or January 2015, when the number of new weekly cases in Liberia had fallen from the peak numbers recorded in September. See Norimitsu Onishi, "Empty Ebola Clinics in Liberia Are Seen as Misstep in U.S. Relief Effort," *The New York Times*, April 11, 2015, nytimes.com/2015/04/12/world/africa/idle-ebola-clinics-in-liberia-are-seen-as-misstep-in-us-relief-effort.html. For more on the British unit in Kerry Town, see Walsh and Johnson, *Getting to Zero*, pp. 256–89.

22. Jon Lascher put it well, as ever: "It wasn't enough, and it wasn't fast enough. But Maforki was the only treatment facility in the district for weeks, and it remained a trusted one until the day it was closed."

23. See David von Drehle and Aryn Baker, "The Ebola Fighters: The Ones Who Answered the Call," *Time*, December 10, 2014, time.com/time-person-of-the-year-ebola-fighters.

24. American volunteer clinicians detained against their will, or mocked and derided in tweets, surely had good reason for umbrage. Although U.S. health authorities were largely united against making political fray of Ebola, there were warnings that intrusive monitoring would prove expensive and unnecessary: "Between July 31 and mid-September, New York City's health department received 57 calls reporting suspected infections based on fevers. Of these, only six merited further testing. Three cases were caused by malaria and one by anaplasmosis; two were of unknown causes. Ebola was not found in any of the cases." See Siddhartha Mukherjee, "How to Quarantine Against Ebola," *The New York Times*, October 12, 2014, nytimes.com/2014/10/13/opinion/how-to-quarantine-against-ebola.html. This wasteful and unsettling approach was repeated nationwide and throughout the rest of the epidemic.

25. Adia Benton and Kim Yi Dionne, "Pundits Panicking About Ebola Hurt Cause They Mean to Help," *The Washington Post*, September 1, 2014, washingtonpost.com/news/monkey-cage/wp/2014/09/01/pundits-panicking-about-ebola-hurt-cause-they-mean-to-help.

26. James Surowiecki, "Ebolanomics," *The New Yorker*, August 18, 2014, newyorker.com/magazine/2014/08/25/ebolanomics.

27. See Steven M. Jones et al., "Live Attenuated Recombinant Vaccine Protects Nonhuman Primates Against Ebola and Marburg Viruses," *Nature Medicine* 11, no. 7 (2005): pp. 786–90; Denise Grady, "Ebola Vaccine, Ready for Test, Sat on the

Shelf," *The New York Times*, October 23, 2014, nytimes.com/2014/10/24/health /without-lucrative-market-potential-ebola-vaccine-was-shelved-for-years.html.

28. The patient from Dallas underwent MRIs and what was likely one of the first lumbar punctures performed on an Ebola patient. See Daniel S. Chertow et al., "Severe Meningoencephalitis in a Case of Ebola Virus Disease," *Annals of Internal Medicine* 165, no. 4 (2016): pp. 301–304; Daniel S. Chertow et al., "Cardiac MRI Findings Suggest Myocarditis in Severe Ebola Virus Disease," *JACC: Cardiovascular Imaging* 10, no. 6 (2017): pp. 711–13.

3. IBRAHIM'S SECOND CHANCE

1. Most of these early interviews were conducted along with Bec Rollins, who launched Partners In Health's "Survivors Count" campaign (Partners In Health, November 7, 2014, youtube.com/watch?v=fji-iVo3C7Q). A similar effort was launched by the American actor Jeffrey Wright: "Ebola Survival Fund," ebola-survivalfund.org.

2. The term's origins refer to the rail lines that used to lead north and southeast. These were ripped up during the one-party rule of Siaka Stevens and sold as scrap to a Chinese firm, and the word's meanings changed over time. Ishmael Beah, who first saw Freetown after years as a child soldier in the south and east, adds: "*Upline* is a Krio word mostly used in Freetown to refer to the backwardness of the inner country, its inhabitants, and their mannerisms." See *A Long Way Gone: Memoirs of a Boy Soldier* (New York: Sarah Crichton Books, 2007), p. 184.

3. It's worth noting that religious strife has remained rare in Sierra Leone, and Islamic fundamentalism is almost unheard of. For more on the topic, see Kevin A. O'Brien and Ismail Rashid, "Islamist Militancy in Sierra Leone," *Conflict, Security and Development* 13, no. 2 (2013): pp. 169–90.

4. This was true not only in Freetown but also in schools across the country. Ishmael Beah's haunting memoir of his years as a child soldier, *A Long Way Gone*, includes many references to American popular culture and more high-brow fare. By the time he was twelve, Beah could recite from memory parts of *Julius Caesar* and *Macbeth*, and did so at village gatherings. But Beah and his friends had also formed a hip-hop group, inspired by African American classics from the 1980s. After his informal conscription into Sierra Leone's army, he and other boys regularly watched testosterone-infused movies starring Arnold Schwarzenegger. Paul Richards includes a thoughtful explanation of the significance of these movies to young rebel conscripts and youth in general. "West African urban youth," he writes, "are probably better informed about international trends than many of their young American or British contemporaries . . . Video and film are invitations to the sociological imagination and a stimulus to the power of positive thinking. We should think twice before too hastily concluding that rebels feed Rambo films to their young conscripts as an incitement to mindless violence. It seems more likely that such films are intended to support a political analysis about

the wider society's neglect of the creative potential of the young." See *Fighting for the Rain Forest: War, Youth & Resources in Sierra Leone* (Oxford: James Currey, 1996), p. 114.

5. Richards, *Fighting for the Rain Forest*, p. 51.

6. Michael Jackson continues: "As for the new sources of power that preoccupy them—diamonds, commerce, education, Islam, and the military—these seem to belong to a world apart, where justice is subject to no known laws." See *In Sierra Leone* (Durham, N.C.: Duke University Press, 2004), p. 147.

7. Freetown, as Paul Richards notes, "is an outward-looking city. If at times it appears somewhat cut-off, mentally, from the realities of provincial life, appearances can be deceptive. The city has long been a destination for young migrants from the provinces, seeking employment and social freedom. Backed by the forests of the peninsula mountains Freetown is more easily penetrated by 'bush' issues than some other West African coastal capitals" (*Fighting for the Rain Forest*, p. 106).

8. Internal household discord is related to complexities beyond my skill to unravel. In Sierra Leone, such conflict is related not only to blood ties but also to birth order of children, age, and, especially, gender. As a largely agricultural society became increasingly urban, the importance of wage labor in determining who was deemed the ricewinner altered, but did not erase, these traditions. The traditions vary from group to group and of course from family to family. No one explores these complexities, and how they've changed over time, with more social and psychological nuance than Michael Jackson. I would recommend all of his books. Start with *Life Within Limits: Well-Being in a World of Want* (Durham, N.C.: Duke University Press, 2011), and work backward. See also the work of Marian Ferme, Chris Coulter, Adia Benton, Danny Hoffman, and other anthropologists referenced throughout this book.

9. Michael Jackson, *Paths Toward a Clearing: Radical Empiricism and Ethnographic Inquiry* (Bloomington: Indiana University Press, 1989), p. 99.

10. English writer Roy Lewis called kola nuts "West Africa's stimulant and sedative in one—aspirin, nicotine and caffein [*sic*] together." The nuts, he wrote, "have social significance throughout West Africa: kola that is the symbol of friendship, proper offerings at meetings and departings and religious occasions—kola whose quinine-bitter taste accompanies a power to keep hungry porters on the march beneath their 80-pound head loads, to nourish sick men unable to take or keep down food, to underpin the jaded bridegroom's prowess, to prolong the Bundu dancer's strength from midnight till dawn and on into high noon again." See *Sierra Leone: A Modern Portrait* (London: Her Majesty's Stationery Office, 1954), pp. 15, 21. As for funerals, one Christian theologian teaching at Sierra Leone's (and West Africa's) oldest university presented a paper at a 1966 academic conference about Freetown. He cites a certain Canon Harry Sawyerr, who had "collected some of the prayers offered at gravesides in or near Freetown on special Christian festivals." One Christian prayer was directed more toward ancestors than to God—indeed, the theologian felt that mention of God was likely

prompted by the presence of Sawyerr—and sounds a lot like what Ibrahim described as his Muslim family's plans for the funerary rituals for his grandmother and others lost to Ebola. Prays Sawyerr: "You all, please, help us to pray to God to bless all of us—the children and the grandchildren, your son-in-law and all who are joining us and so joining the family . . . Here is your water . . . Cool your hearts. See that your hearts are cool towards us. We who are here, whatever wrong we commit, please reveal the same to us in a dream . . . Here is your kola. May whatever we may say or do to you, make your hearts cool." He is quoted in Reverend E. W. Fashole-Luke, "Religion in Freetown," in *Freetown: A Symposium*, edited by Christopher Fyfe and Eldred Jones (Freetown: Sierra Leone University Press, 1968), p. 136. See also Michael Jackson's extended discussion of funerals among the Kuranko in *Paths Toward a Clearing*.

11. See Rashid Ansumana et al., "Ebola in Freetown Area, Sierra Leone—A Case Study of 581 Patients," *The New England Journal of Medicine* 372, no. 6 (2015): pp. 587–88.

12. In Frederick Migeod's view, there was little of note beyond "a stone mosque in the course of construction, but it struck me the architect seemed to be more acquainted with building churches or chapels than mosques." See *A View of Sierra Leone* (London: Kegan Paul, Trench, Trubner & Co., 1926), p. 21.

13. This was a point we tried to make months earlier, at the outset of Sierra Leone's western surge. See Paul Farmer and Joia Mukherjee, "Ebola's Front Lines," *The Boston Globe*, September 24, 2014, bostonglobe.com/opinion/2014/09/23/responding-ebola-countries-need-staff-stuff-space-and-systems/ugSFKkOw9S7Ser0p8PGeOK/story.html.

14. Abu Bakar Kamara, quoted in Jeffrey Gettleman, "Despite Aid Push, Ebola Is Raging in Sierra Leone," *The New York Times*, November 27, 2014, nytimes.com/2014/11/28/world/africa/despite-aid-push-ebola-is-raging-in-sierra-leone.html.

15. Gettleman, "Despite Aid Push, Ebola Is Raging in Sierra Leone."

16. Paul Richards and colleagues recount how Ebola reached the village of Fogbo, population about five hundred, in early August, and how it then spread. From Fogbo, on the border with Guinea, where the epidemic began, the virus spread west toward Daru, a military outpost in Kailahun District. It's worth citing at length, since the towns mentioned have deep historical significance and will be discussed in part 2 of this book: "Ebola had reached Daru when a wife of the Paramount chief visited her sick sister, the wife of the Paramount Chief of Kissi Teng, the chiefdom including Koindu market on the Guinea border. A boy infected in the town of Daru came to Kenema, to visit his father. During the visit the young man began to develop symptoms, was taken to hospital, tested positive, and died." (This was of course the hospital where Humarr Khan and his nursing colleagues worked.) "The father had also become infected," continues Richard. "Apparently not wanting to be hospitalized, he left Kenema by night, evading the curfew, and traveled to his home town Fogbo, where he was cared for by his sister, a Sowei (an elder of the women's secret society—known for her medical

knowledge)." After the *sowei*-sister fell ill and died, "prominent women in the community insisted a Sowei respected by her society should be given a fitting burial, so they washed and buried the body." Soon, the chief's wife was dead, and by September, "somebody in the village was dying every day, and there was nobody to bury the corpses. Local officials sent a message that if the villagers buried the dead without the consent of the government the people would be fined or imprisoned. The Fogbo people waited for the burial team to come. The team had still to reach the village three weeks later." See "Social Pathways for Ebola Virus Disease in Rural Sierra Leone, and Some Implications for Containment," *PLOS Neglected Tropical Diseases* 9, no. 4 (2015): p. e0003567.

17. This e-mail was from Michael Drasher, who, along with Gabriel Warren and Gibrilla Sheriff, built the PIH survivors' program, and the friendships it nurtured, into something enduring. Their contributions to the early months of the program, and to morale in general, are not forgotten. I also have Drasher, a budding anthropologist and (I hope) future physician, to thank for much help with translation and for his friendship and collegiality with Ibrahim.

4. THE TWO ORDEALS OF YABOM

1. "In Sierra Leone," notes historian Stephen Riley in comparing the first post-coup government to various Liberian administrations, "the regime has had far closer and warmer relations with international financial institutions in recent years. The latest of many partially-implemented IMF and World Bank approved structural adjustment programmes started" just after the 1992 coup that overthrew the sitting Sierra Leonean president. Riley continues by noting that Valentine Strasser, who led the coup, "initially implemented it in full, although the costs of the rebel war have undermined its objectives. As the RUF became more active, coffee and cocoa production dropped by 50 per cent. In Sierra Leone, the costs of adjustment must be compared with the effects of long-term economic decline and the strength of the informal economy. Among the continuing difficulties of the central state have been its inability to control economic production leading to periodic fiscal crises and inadequate service provision, especially outside Freetown." See *Liberia and Sierra Leone: Anarchy or Peace in West Africa?* (London: Research Institute for the Study of Conflict and Terrorism, 1996), pp. 10–11. These economic policies, and their relation to war, are discussed more fully in part 2.

2. Carol P. MacCormack, "Health, Fertility and Birth in Moyamba District, Sierra Leone," in *Ethnography of Fertility and Birth*, edited by Carol P. MacCormack (London: Academic Press, 1982), p. 119.

3. Carol P. Hoffer, "Bundu: Political Implications of Female Solidarity in a Secret Society," in *Being Female: Reproduction, Power, and Change*, edited by Dana Raphael (The Hague: Mouton Publishers, 1975), p. 158. Note that Hoffer and MacCormack are the same person, who passed away in 1997. Kris Heggenhougen offered an obituary in *Anthropology and Medicine* 4, no. 3 (1997): pp. 327–28.

4. Andrew Buncombe, "Rebels in Battle for Control of Freetown," *The Independent*, January 7, 1999, independent.co.uk/news/rebels-in-battle-for-control-of -freetown-1045497.html.

5. Two anthropologists with experience in northern Sierra Leone later offered a concise enough explanation, which didn't vary much from Yabom's: "A swear is a vengeful curse unleashed on someone who has caused a rupture in the body politic through unfair dealings with another, and it is a common understanding of how deviations from pro-social conduct return to strike an individual, thus regulating social conduct." See Adam Goguen and Catherine Bolten, "Ebola Through a Glass, Darkly: Ways of Knowing the State and Each Other," *Anthropology Quarterly* 90, no. 2 (2017): pp. 437–38.

INTERLUDE I: DOWN THE RABBIT HOLE

1. The Matweng standoff did, however, make the DERC's weekly newsletter, where it was discussed with respect and sympathy for the bereaved family: "On the 19th of November, one of the DERC's burial teams (AG627) was attacked by the family of one Ebola victim at Matweng. The reason for the attack was an unfortunate misunderstanding regarding where the family could perform their prayers. The family wanted to pray at the house while the burial team told them that they could carry out their prayers at the community cemetery. The family did not agree with this option and started to throw stones at the burial vehicle. The attack has been reported to the paramount chief and the police who are taking care of the matter. Families have been informed by the SocMob teams that they can pray at their houses before they are moved as long as they do so from a safe distance."

2. For a review of social responses to Ebola during the course of previous epidemics, see the book-length study by anthropologists Barry S. Hewlett and Bonnie L. Hewlett, *Ebola, Culture, and Politics: The Anthropology of an Emerging Disease* (Belmont, Calif.: Thomson Wadsworth, 2008).

3. The anthropologist Mariane Ferme has written, similarly, of "history from underneath." Scratch the surface of stories and events and social exchanges in contemporary Sierra Leone, she suggests, and learn darker and deeper tales: "Local histories are bound up with matter, which carries sometimes eloquent and explicit, sometimes concealed clues to this region's entanglements with slavery and institutionalized inequality, with warfare, and with the precarious balance between economies characterized by the mobile exploitation of natural resources (hunting, alluvial diamond mining) and economies based on more stationary cultivation of those resources (farming of staple and cash crops)." See *The Underneath of Things: Violence, History, and the Everyday in Sierra Leone* (Berkeley: University of California Press, 2001), p. 6. The historian Ismail Rashid has dedicated much of his research—which has focused on Sierra Leone under British rule and on more recent events (from armed conflict, and attempts to end it, to Ebola)—on subaltern perspectives scanted in much scholarship on Sierra Leone. His work is cited throughout, but for an overview of the importance of restoring

these perspectives, see his essay "Rebellious Subjects and Citizens: Writing Sub-alterns into the History of Sierra Leone," in *Paradoxes of History and Memory in Post-Colonial Sierra Leone*, edited by Sylvia Ojukutu-Macauley and Ismail Rashid (Lanham, Md.: Lexington Books, 2013), pp. 13–36.

4. Paul Richards et al., "Social Pathways for Ebola Virus Disease in Rural Sierra Leone, and Some Implications for Containment," *PLOS Neglected Tropical Diseases* 9, no. 4 (2015): p. e0003567. Richards's book *Ebola: How a People's Science Helped End an Epidemic* (London: Zed Books, 2016) was instructive to someone who first came to Sierra Leone in 2014.

5. THE UPPER GUINEA COAST AND THE WORLD THE SLAVES MADE

1. Walter Rodney, "A Reconsideration of the Mane Invasions of Sierra Leone," *The Journal of African History* 8, no. 2 (1967): pp. 219–46. One recently published narrative history of Sierra Leone avers that the "most significant influence of the Mane was the emergence of Mende as the largest ethnic group in Sierra Leone." See Joseph Kaifala, *Free Slaves, Freetown, and the Sierra Leonean Civil War* (New York: Palgrave Macmillan, 2010), p. 10. Arthur Abraham, who is from the small but historically important town of Daru in Kailahun District, became an expert on his own Mende-speaking people by studying colonial archives (and anything else he could find) and by adopting some of anthropology's methods. Abraham went to Freetown before independence to study at Fourah Bay College and later completed doctoral studies in England. His slim volume, *Topics in Sierra Leone History: A Counter-Colonial Interpretation* (Freetown: Leone Publishers, 1976), offers an all-too-brief dip into some of the waters he has intentionally roiled.

2. João de Barros, *Décadas da Ásia*; translation from G. R. Crone, ed., *The Voyages of Cadamosto and Other Documents on Western Africa in the Second Half of the Fifteenth Century* (London: The Hakluyt Society, 1937), p. 147. Not until the Iberians settled along the coast of Ghana—then called the Gold Coast—did they find a way of breaking Muslim monopolies on gold and silver, since the bounty of New World mines had not yet been seized. When it was, it became a Spanish monopoly. Much of that bounty was invested in ramping up the triangular trade in which most European coastal states engaged.

3. Michael Crowder, *Colonial West Africa: Collected Essays* (London: Frank Cass, 1978), p. 2.

4. Alfred W. Crosby, *Ecological Imperialism: The Biological Expansion of Europe, 900–1900* (Cambridge, U.K.: Cambridge University Press, 1986), p. 138. For the historian William McNeill, similarly, the heavy burden of disease, "more than anything else, is why Africa remained backward in the development of civilization when compared to temperate lands." See *Plagues and Peoples* (Garden City, N.Y.: Anchor Books, 1976), p. 43. The historian Emmanuel Akyeampong distrusts such determinism. "This statement," he counters politely, "creates the erroneous impression that the only factor Africans have had to battle with in

the quest for their development is the environment, eliding the pivotal role that people—including outsiders—have played in the political economy of Africa." See "Disease in West African History," in *Themes in West Africa's History*, edited by Emmanuel Akyeampong (Athens: Ohio University Press, 2006), p. 187.

5. João de Barros, *Décadas da Ásia*; this translation is from C. R. Boxer, *Four Centuries of Portuguese Expansion, 1415–1825: A Succinct Survey* (Johannesburg: Witwatersrand University Press, 1961), p. 27. Although the watchword is water, the historian George Brooks puts it rather drily: "Climate, ecology, and human patterns of livelihood combine to create epidemiological conditions that are exceptionally challenging for the peoples of western Africa, particularly those living in the Upper Guinea Coast. High rainfall and high relative humidity, slowly flowing rivers and streams, large expanses of swampland, rice paddies, and pools of stagnant water following the rainy season create environments favorable to the prolific breeding of insects, many of which are vectors for diseases harmful to both humans and domestic animals. Endemic tropical diseases result in high morbidity and mortality rates, especially among infants and young children." See *Eurafricans in Western Africa: Commerce, Social Status, Gender, and Religious Observance from the Sixteenth to the Eighteenth Century* (Athens: Ohio University Press, 2003), p. 16.

6. Jared Diamond has famously argued that Europeans, having long lived in proximity to domesticated beasts absent from the New World, developed greater immunity to viruses and bacteria related to those common among their livestock, pets, and other animal familiars. Killers with likely zoonotic origins include measles (related to rinderpest, a disease of cattle and now held to be eradicated), smallpox (a cousin of cowpox), and influenza (derived from, and still partial to mixing with, similar pathogens afflicting pigs, ducks, and other birds). Diamond terms these pathogens "deadly gifts from our animal friends," and notes they were especially lethal in the Americas, where there were few domesticated animals, none of them beasts of burden or war. See *Guns, Germs, and Steel: The Fates of Human Societies* (New York: W. W. Norton, 1997), p. 207. It wasn't only viruses: some have recently argued that European strains of salmonella, leptospirosis, and other bacteria wreaked havoc once introduced to the Americas. See, for example, Ewen Callaway, "Salmonella Suspected in Aztec Decline: Ancient DNA Links Bacterium to Catastrophic Epidemics," *Nature* 542, no. 7642 (2017): p. 404; Åshild J. Vågene et al., "*Salmonella enterica* Genomes from Victims of a Major Sixteenth-Century Epidemic in Mexico," *Nature Ecology and Evolution* 2, no. 3 (2018): pp. 520–28; John S. Marr and John T. Cathey, "New Hypothesis for Cause of Epidemic Among Native Americans, New England, 1616–1619," *Emerging Infectious Diseases* 16, no. 2 (2010): pp. 281–86.

7. Diamond, *Guns, Germs, and Steel*, p. 158.

8. The physician-historian David Jones has compellingly debunked (in short articles and reviews, as well as in a monograph cited in this chapter and in others) facile claims of causality invoking epidemiological and immunological naïveté to

explain this precipitous mortality; see, for example, "Virgin Soils Revisited," *William and Mary Quarterly* 60, no. 4 (2003): pp. 703–742; "The Persistence of American Indian Health Disparities," *American Journal of Public Health* 96, no. 12 (2006): pp. 2122–34; "Death, Uncertainty, and Rhetoric," in *Beyond Germs: Native Depopulation in North America*, edited by Catherine M. Cameron, Paul Kelton, and Alan C. Swedlund (Tucson: University of Arizona Press, 2015), pp. 16–49. Outcomes of this native-newcomer encounter were, Jones also adds, varied and contingent. Some groups, such as the Navajo, benefited materially from the introduction of sheep and other livestock new to the region, and their numbers rose in the first centuries after contact. (The Navajos' trials at the hand of the white man would largely come later, from the U.S. armed forces or settlers under their protection.) But the Navajo were the exception. Two centuries before the founding of the United States, and well before the Pilgrims celebrated their first Thanksgiving, most societies of what would later be known as Latin America were hammered by pestilence, siege, attacks, open war, and loss of land. As regards the debate about the relative significance of epidemic disease in the long list of pathogens and pathogenic forces in the decline of New World populations, see also Suzanne Austin Alchon, *A Pest in the Land: New World Epidemics in a Global Perspective* (Albuquerque: University of New Mexico Press, 2003); Paul Kelton, *Epidemics and Enslavement: Biological Catastrophe in the Native Southeast, 1492–1715* (Lincoln: University of Nebraska Press, 2007).

9. Why then, asks David Jones, "is immunologic vulnerability singled out as the most relevant explanation, amidst a wealth of sophisticated alternatives?" Perhaps because if depopulation is rationalized as the unfortunate but inevitable result of a "unique historical-immunological moment," this great die-off "cannot be blamed on colonists or their descendants." By emphasizing the inherent susceptibility of American Indians, virgin-soil theories do valuable work for white and privileged Americans, absolving them "of responsibility for the disparity, and of responsibility to intervene." See *Rationalizing Epidemics: Meanings and Uses of American Indian Mortality Since 1600* (Cambridge, Mass.: Harvard University Press, 2004), p. 57.

10. Almost a century before the clock of American slavery is set ticking in most history books, "African actors enabled American colonies to survive, and they were equally able to destroy European colonial ventures," notes American historian Michael Guasco in "The Misguided Focus on 1619 as the Beginning of Slavery in the U.S. Damages Our Understanding of American History," *Smithsonian Magazine*, September 13, 2017, smithsonianmag.com/history/misguided-focus-1619-beginning-slavery-us-damages-our-understanding-american-history-180964873.

11. Patrick Manning, "Slavery and Slave Trade in West Africa, 1450–1930," in *Themes in West Africa's History*, p. 104.

12. See Kelton, *Epidemics and Enslavement*.

13. Walter Rodney, *A History of the Upper Guinea Coast, 1545–1800* (Oxford: Clarendon Press, 1970), pp. 17, 102.

14. Some early colonists of Massachusetts had slaves themselves. Cotton Mather, who "yearned for the days of the Puritan saints, when the hand of God swept the natives away," first heard of the African practice of smallpox inoculation from his African slave (Jones, *Rationalizing Epidemics*, p. 61).

15. Joseph E. Inikori, "Reversal of Fortune and Socioeconomic Development in the Atlantic World: A Comparative Examination of West Africa and the Americas, 1400–1850," in *Africa's Development in Historical Perspective*, edited by Emmanuel Akyeampong, Robert H. Bates, Nathan Nunn, and James A. Robinson (New York: Cambridge University Press, 2014), pp. 77, 73. See also Wendy Warren, *New England Bound: Slavery and Colonization in Early America* (New York: Liveright, 2016).

16. Even without sugar-cane plantations or gold or silver mines to exploit, early colonists in New England were inconvenienced and sometimes troubled by the rapid decline of the natives. But while the settlers witnessed "shocking mortality" among the tribes along the New England coast, they "struggled with devastating problems of their own. Half the Plymouth colonists died in their first winter." Survivors, adds David Jones, were pragmatists—"Needing land, colonists saw Massachusett depopulation as a gift of land"—and entertained varied outbreak narratives. Some fell back on providential explanations of their own good fortune. "If God were not pleased with our inheriting these parts," asked the governor of the Massachusetts Bay Colony in 1633, "why did he drive out the natives before us?" He responded to his own question with the claim that smallpox "cleered our title to this place" (Jones, *Rationalizing Epidemics*, pp. 46, 20, 37, 2). Later debates aside, the choice of the tropics was seldom a wise or safe one for European colonists. Had the Pilgrims gone to the tropics, rather than New England, asserts Alfred Crosby, they "would have left little more behind them than shallow graves in wet ground" (*Ecological Imperialism*, p. 144).

17. As the slave trade grew more profitable and drew in the major maritime powers of the day, no one, wrote Walter Rodney, "challenged the fact that the *Jihad* was the greatest recruiter of slaves in the latter part of the eighteenth century" (*A History of the Upper Guinea Coast*, pp. 116, 236, 102). His terse and passionate book was meant to demolish the claim that the Atlantic trade flourished by tapping into a preexisting internal slave trade propped up by religious conviction or more local cultural constructs. Rodney's underappreciated study is yet another reminder of what was lost when, on June 13, 1980, he was killed by a car bomb in Georgetown, Guyana. He was thirty-eight years old.

18. As "warfare expanded," Manning writes, "population declined across a substantial coastal belt, monarchy and elite families became heavily dependent on revenue from slave exports, government was transformed, residential patterns changed, and the holding as well as the selling of slaves expanded" ("Slavery and Slave Trade in West Africa," pp. 106–107).

19. The Bunce course may have boasted only two holes, but the slave-trading duffers, notes Adam Hochschild, kitted out their caddies with "loincloths of tartan wool woven near Glasgow." See *Bury the Chains: Prophets and Rebels in the Fight to Free an Empire's Slaves* (Boston: Houghton Mifflin, 2005), p. 25.

20. They observed that this traffic, unlike the trades that preceded them, "encouraged the creation of institutions that favored extraction rather than the creation of wealth." See Emmanuel Akyeampong et al., "Introduction: Africa—The Historical Roots of Its Underdevelopment," in *Africa's Development in Historical Perspective*, p. 15.

21. Captain John Newton, quoted in Hochschild, *Bury the Chains*, p. 71.

22. John Matthews, quoted in Rosalind Shaw, *Memories of the Slave Trade: Ritual and the Historical Imagination in Sierra Leone* (Chicago: University of Chicago Press, 2002), p. 215. See also Philip D. Curtin, ed., *Africa Remembered: Narratives by West Africans from the Era of the Slave Trade* (Madison: University of Wisconsin Press, 1967).

23. Michael Jackson, *Paths Toward a Clearing: Radical Empiricism and Ethnographic Inquiry* (Bloomington: Indiana University Press, 1989), p. 42.

24. Shaw, *Memories of the Slave Trade*, p. 211.

25. Rosalind Shaw, "The Production of Witchcraft/Witchcraft as Production: Memory, Modernity, and the Slave Trade in Sierra Leone," *American Ethnologist* 24, no. 4 (1997): p. 858.

26. Shaw, *Memories of the Slave Trade*, p. 223.

27. Susan Buck-Morss adds that the "exploitation of millions of colonial slave laborers was accepted as part of the given world by the very thinkers who proclaimed freedom to be man's natural state and inalienable right. Even when theoretical claims of freedom were transformed into revolutionary action on the political stage, it was possible for the slave-driven colonial economy that functioned behind the scenes to be kept in darkness." See "Hegel and Haiti," *Critical Inquiry* 26, no. 4 (2000): pp. 821, 822. Buck-Morss further wondered if Hegel, who had little to say about Europe's reliance on the slave trade or about the Haitian Revolution—which occurred during the height of his fame—might not be getting stupider with time. Here are Hegel's words on Africa and history: "Africa proper, as far as History goes back, has remained—for all purposes of connection with the rest of the World—shut up; it is the Gold-land compressed within itself—the land of childhood, which lying beyond the day of self-conscious history, is enveloped in the dark mantle of Night." See *The Philosophy of History*, translated by John Sibree, revised edition (New York: The Colonial Press, 1900), p. 91.

28. Hochschild, *Bury the Chains*, p. 87.

29. Buck-Morss, "Hegel and Haiti," p. 837.

30. Manning, "Slavery and Slave Trade in West Africa," p. 110.

31. Hochschild, *Bury the Chains*, p. 308.

32. Marcus Rediker, *The* Amistad *Rebellion: An Atlantic Odyssey of Slavery and Freedom* (New York: Viking, 2012), p. 41.

33. Michael Crowder, *West Africa Under Colonial Rule* (London: Hutchinson, 1968), p. 24.

34. R. J. Olu-Wright, "The Physical Growth of Freetown," in *Freetown: A Symposium*, edited by Christopher Fyfe and Eldred Jones (Freetown: Sierra Leone University Press, 1968), p. 25.

35. The twice-escaped slave was Boston King, who's quoted in Kaifala, *Free Slaves, Freetown, and the Sierra Leonean Civil War*, p. 54.

36. Hochshild, *Bury the Chains*, p. 199.

37. These women's engagement in sex work, observed historian Sheldon Harris, "had evidently conditioned them against racism—seemingly the only profession with the ability to transcend the color line—and they raised no objection to the forthcoming amalgamation of the races." See his biography, *Paul Cuffe: Black America and the African Return* (New York: Simon and Schuster, 1972), p. 44. It reads briskly.

38. The founders of Granville Town, notes Hochschild, didn't find "what they had been told awaited them in this tropical paradise: neither the supposedly plentiful oyster shells and limestone for making mortar nor the abundance of fruits, ripe for the picking" (*Bury the Chains*, pp. 151, 175).

39. Hochshild, *Bury the Chains*, p. 176.

40. Slaves from the Upper Guinea Coast were especially valued in the North American colonies. Nineteenth-century newspaper advertisements, auction posters, and correspondence suggest that plantation owners in South Carolina and Georgia were willing to pay more for slaves who came from Africa's Rice Coast because rice was what they were trying to grow. "The South Carolina and Georgia colonists had no experience with rice cultivation," notes the anthropologist Joseph Opala, "and they depended on African know-how and technology." See *Some Historical Connections Between Sierra Leone and the United States* (Freetown: Fourah Bay College, Institute of African Studies, 1985), p. 2. Opala has conducted ethnographic research on both sides of the Middle Passage—among Krio speakers in Sierra Leone and among Gullah speakers along South Carolina's and Georgia's coasts. Gullah and Krio, he asserts, share thousands of cognates.

41. Freetown's site was chosen, according to urban planner R. J. Olu-Wright, for three reasons: "The first was the deep-water channel of the fast-flowing Sierra Leone River on its left bank in preference to its right bank which is shallow and heavily silted. The second was the prevalence of good drinking water from the numerous streams, and the third was the height of the hills which afford strategic command of the river, as well as the protective shelter of the numerous bays" ("The Physical Growth of Freetown," p. 25). Both Ibrahim Kamara and Yabom Koroma, the subjects of the two previous chapters, live several hundred feet above sea level, while the poorer residents of Monrovia are doomed to stew, as are most

Sierra Leoneans and Liberians on the coast, in flat and humid mangrove swamps, or what is left of them. But Freetown's hills did not mean Ibrahim Kamara and his ravine-dwelling neighbors would be spared flash floods, as he learned in 2015 when heavy rains invaded his tiny house. It was even worse during the summer of 2017, when one of Freetown's hillsides crumbled under heavy rains, killing hundreds in a single day.

42. Harris, *Paul Cuffe*, p. 41.

43. Thomas Clarkson's *The History of the Rise, Progress, and Accomplishment of the Abolition of the African Slave-Trade by the British Parliament* (London: Longman, Hurst, Rees, and Orme, 1808) was published in two volumes. From Captain Cuffe's journal entry on February 13, 1811: "Gentle breezes, but fair southerly, SSE. Clear weather and pleasant smooth sea, but in the afternoon, a longfooted counterswell arose out of NW. My time employed in pursuing Clarkson's records on abolishing slavery, which account often battered my mind in the sin of his proceedings" (Harris, *Paul Cuffe*, p. 80).

44. Harris, *Paul Cuffe*, pp. 162, 194.

45. If Paul Cuffe "was not the father of black nationalism," observes his historian-biographer, he "became a leading contender for the distinction" (Harris, *Paul Cuffe*, pp. 58, 66).

46. Harris, *Paul Cuffe*, p. 244. To appreciate the depths of this hostility, read David Brion Davis's *The Problem of Slavery in the Age of Emancipation* (New York: Alfred A. Knopf, 2014).

47. Harris, *Paul Cuffe*, p. 205. (Formatting altered.)

48. Once one of the world's more prosperous regions, the Niger Bend has long had one of the highest burdens of malaria. "The fact that malaria bulked so large in the view of foreigners," notes economist David Weil, "may be attributable to their lack of immunity, which Africans acquired as children." But he, too, cautions against geographic determinism: "The theory that the health environment in Africa was particularly bad is not universally accepted. Premodern society was not healthy in any part of the world. People living in temperate zones, though freed from tropical parasites, faced many other health challenges brought on by climate, including nutritional deficiencies, diseases spread by being indoors, and diseases that made the jump from livestock with whom people were forced to share living quarters." See "The Impact of Malaria on African Development over the *Longue Durée*," in *Africa's Development in Historical Perspective*, pp. 123, 99.

49. Mary H. Kingsley, *Travels in West Africa: Congo Français, Corisco and Cameroons* (London: Macmillan, 1897), p. 681. Kingsley, who would become well known for her sympathies for Africans, was writing at the dawn of the bacteriological revolution, as the varied causes of serious febrile illness were first being identified. She herself died of typhoid while volunteering as a nurse in the Second Boer War. She was thirty-seven.

50. Crosby, *Ecological Imperialism*, p. 139.

51. Joseph Wright, quoted in Philip D. Curtin, "Joseph Wright of the Egba," in *Africa Remembered*, pp. 322, 331.

52. For more on Britain's naval interdiction of slave ships, see Christopher Lloyd, *The Navy and the Slave Trade: The Suppression of the African Slave Trade in the Nineteenth Century* (London: Longmans, Green and Company, 1949).

53. Abraham, *Topics in Sierra Leone History*, p. 13.

54. See Adam Jones, *From Slaves to Palm Kernels: A History of the Galinhas Country (West Africa), 1730–1890* (Wiesbaden: Franz Steiner Verlag, 1983), pp. 37–38.

55. Jones, *From Slaves to Palm Kernels*, p. 42.

56. Jones, *From Slaves to Palm Kernels*, pp. 49–50. The Amistads' origins and lives prior to capture is explored more thoroughly—and with the aid of new archives—by Marcus Rediker in *The Amistad Rebellion*.

57. Bruce A. Ragsdale, "'Incited by the Love of Liberty': The *Amistad* Captives and the Federal Courts," *Prologue*, Spring 2003, archives.gov/publications/prologue/2003/spring/amistad-1.html.

58. The original mural has gone missing, as the art historian Richard Powell explains in an article describing nineteenth-century portrayals of Sengbe Pieh: "During the spring of 1840, an exhibition of a 135-foot-long painting of the Amistad uprising toured New England. The broadside that publicized the exhibition exclaimed in bold, theatrical type: 'The Magnificent Painting of the Massacre on Board the Schooner Amistad!! by A. Hewins, Esq., of Boston.' A period wood engraving illustrating the death of the *Amistad*'s captain at the hands of the Africans may have been inspired by this now-lost painting, as suggested by the engraving's unusually long, bannerlike composition." See "Cinqué: Antislavery Portraiture and Patronage in Jacksonian America," *American Art* 11, no. 3 (1997): p. 55. (Formatting altered.)

59. Henry Clarke Wright, letter to the *Pennsylvania Freeman*, April 21, 1841, cited in Powell, "Cinqué," p. 66. (Formatting altered.)

60. John Q. Adams, reply to Roger S. Baldwin, November 11, 1840 (New York Historical Society Library Archive).

61. Kaifala, *Free Slaves, Freetown, and the Sierra Leonean Civil War*, pp. 155–56. The anthropologist Joseph Opala argues that it united the movement in the United States "as nothing before" (*Some Historical Connections*, p. 16).

62. Arthur Abraham, "Sengbe Pieh: A Neglected Hero?," *Journal of the Historical Society of Sierra Leone* 2, no. 2 (1978): p. 29.

63. Greg Campbell, *Blood Diamonds: Tracing the Deadly Path of the World's Most Precious Stones*, revised edition (New York: Basic Books, 2012), p. 27.

64. Mary H. Moran, *Liberia: The Violence of Democracy* (Philadelphia: University of Pennsylvania Press, 2006), p. 2.

65. Antonio McDaniel, "Extreme Mortality in Nineteenth-Century Africa: The Case of Liberian Immigrants," *Demography* 29, no. 4 (1992): p. 581.

66. A paper by Sir Harry Johnston claims (without citing sources) that, at the turn of the twentieth century, "the indigenous population of Liberia, not of extraneous origin, may be estimated with some correctness at a total of about 2,160,000."

See "Liberia," *Liberia: American Colonization Society*, no. 28 (1906): p. 24. Unless Sir Harry traces the borders of Liberia differently than do contemporary geographers, this is likely an overestimate. The World Bank, for example, estimated that Liberia counted only 1.12 million people in 1960. The historian-demographer Patrick Manning, who modeled the population sizes of various African countries from 1850 to 1960, posits yet another calculation in his 2014 study on the topic; for the year 1850, he approximated a population of about 500,000. See "African Population Totals, 1850–1960," Harvard Dataverse, December 6, 2014, doi.org/10.7910/DVN/28045.

67. Moran, *Liberia*, p. 72.

68. Moran, *Liberia*, p. 69.

69. Moran, *Liberia*, p. 71.

70. Richard L. Hall, *On Afric's Shore: A History of Maryland in Liberia, 1834–1857* (Baltimore: Maryland Historical Society, 2003), p. 94.

71. Hall, *On Afric's Shore*, pp. 95, 96.

72. Hall, *On Afric's Shore*, p. 47.

73. Hall, *On Afric's Shore*, p. 360.

74. Hall, *On Afric's Shore*, p. xv.

75. Hall, *On Afric's Shore*, p. 363.

76. Hall, *On Afric's Shore*, pp. 411, 412.

77. Hall, *On Afric's Shore*, pp. 425, 424.

78. Hall, *On Afric's Shore*, pp. 426, 429, 431. (Formatting altered.)

79. Hall, *On Afric's Shore*, p. 405.

80. On Fourah Bay College and its regional influence, see Daniel J. Paracka Jr., *The Athens of West Africa: A History of International Education at Fourah Bay College, Freetown, Sierra Leone* (New York: Routledge, 2003).

81. Thomas Pakenham, *The Scramble for Africa, 1876–1912* (London: Weidenfeld and Nicholson, 1991), p. 182.

82. The colonial roots of today's global health endeavors in Africa, including Livingstone's projects, are traced in a beautiful new book by Raymond Downing, who writes about its pioneers without romanticism. "What kind of doctors were these," he asks, who "were not very interested in seeing patients"? See *Such a Time of It They Had: Global Health Pioneers in Africa* (Nairobi: Manqa Books, 2018), p. 43.

83. Pakenham, *The Scramble for Africa*, p. xxiii.

6. THE GREAT SCRAMBLE AND THE RISE OF THE PASTEURIANS

1. Thomas Nelson Goddard, *The Handbook of Sierra Leone* (London: Grant Richards, 1925), p. 69.

2. The role of the telegraph as an enabler of "the new imperialism" is the subject of an instructive study by historian Daniel Headrick, *The Invisible Weapon: Telecommunications and International Politics, 1851–1945* (New York: Oxford University Press, 1991).

3. The historian Eugenia Herbert has compiled a review of the practice of variolation on the continent: "Smallpox Inoculation in Africa," *The Journal of African History* 16, no. 4 (1975): pp. 539–59. Another historian of anti-smallpox campaigns in Africa cites an elderly Hausa woman speaking about her childhood in the 1890s: "They used to scratch your arm until the blood came, then they got the fluid from someone who had the smallpox and rubbed it in. It all swelled up and you covered it until you healed. Some children used to die; your way of doing it is better." She is cited in William H. Schneider, "Smallpox in Africa During Colonial Rule," *Medical History* 53, no. 2 (2009): p. 198. For a richer account of this woman's reflections on life before and during colonial occupation, and of the Hausa, see the anthropologist Mary Smith's *Baba of Karo: A Woman of the Muslim Hausa*, reprint edition (London: Faber, 1954).

4. This is not to argue that resistance to vaccination campaigns was previously unknown in the colonies. It was encountered in new republics, too. The 1813 Vaccination Act, brainchild of Thomas Jefferson, was repealed in 1822 after a faulty batch of vaccine led instead to an epidemic of smallpox in small-town North Carolina. See Dorothy Long, "Early North Carolina Medicine: Smallpox in North Carolina," *North Carolina Medical Journal* 16, no. 10 (1955): pp. 496–99; Tess Lanzarotta and Marco A. Ramos, "Mistrust in Medicine: The Rise and Fall of America's First Vaccine Institute," *American Journal of Public Health* 108, no. 6 (2018): pp. 741–47; Atul Gawande, "Is Health Care a Right?," *The New Yorker*, October 2, 2017, newyorker.com/magazine/2017/10/02/is-health-care-a-right.

5. Joseph Conrad, *Heart of Darkness*, edited by Paul O'Prey (London: Penguin Books, 1989), p. 86.

6. In the words of the historian Richard Reid, "The European 'nation' was a military beast indeed, its roots in war, its outlook bellicose, its sense of self markedly martial; and it now intersected with not dissimilar, but nonetheless distinctive, processes of militarization further south." The Europeans almost invariably prevailed. "Industrial-era armaments swept aside an array of African armies and militias," he summarizes, "and dancing and painted warriors were thus consigned to distant and quaintly tribal memory." The African warriors who fought back weren't dancing and painted so much as outgunned. Reid argues that "guns had been present along the Atlantic coast, and in the Ethiopia Highlands, since the early sixteenth century, but their impact on tactics and organization was minimal for at least two hundred years. Across the West African savannah and in the deeper sub-Saharan interior, meanwhile, guns had little or no impact whatsoever." There were exceptions, however, and they grew rapidly in number during the years just after the Berlin Conference. See Richard Reid, "The Fragile Revolution: Rethinking War and Development in Africa's Violent Nineteenth Century," in *Africa's Development in Historical Perspective*, edited by Emmanuel Akyeampong, Robert H. Bates, Nathan Nunn, and James A. Robinson (New York: Cambridge University Press, 2014), pp. 407, 395, 399.

7. Michael Crowder, *West Africa Under Colonial Rule* (London: Hutchinson, 1968), p. 72.

8. Alice L. Conklin, *A Mission to Civilize: The Republican Idea of Empire in France and West Africa, 1895–1930* (Stanford: Stanford University Press, 1997), p. 34.

9. Crowder, *West Africa Under Colonial Rule*, p. 5. Crowder dedicated both his research and his teaching to West Africa, and was a professor at the University of Ibadan when it was (in the words of my own mentor) "a world-class center of learning." A similar level of commitment to cultivating West African scholars while contributing original scholarship is to be found in the life and work of Jean Suret-Canale. Both he and Crowder had to scrub through colonial whitewash, if of slightly different shades. Their books and essays may be profitably read as complementary, since one relied on English-language sources; the other, on ones written in French.

10. Jean Suret-Canale, "Découverte de Samori," *Cahiers d'Études Africaines* 17, no. 66/67 (1977): p. 386. (Translation mine.) This is from Suret-Canale's review of Yves Person's three-volume biography of Samory Touré: *Samori: Une Révolution Dyula* (Dakar: Institut Fondamental d'Afrique Noire, 1968–1975).

11. Thomas Pakenham, *The Scramble for Africa, 1876–1912* (London: Weidenfeld and Nicholson, 1991), p. 174.

12. Martin A. Klein, *Slavery and Colonial Rule in French West Africa* (Cambridge, U.K.: Cambridge University Press, 1998), p. 1.

13. Crowder, *West Africa Under Colonial Rule*, p. 87.

14. Fabrice Courtin et al., "Sleeping Sickness in West Africa (1906–2006): Changes in Spatial Repartition and Lessons from the Past," *Tropical Medicine and International Health* 13, no. 3 (2008): p. 336. Those on the margins of Samory's expanding-then-shrinking empire fared even worse during these conflicts. In his sweeping history of the African poor, John Iliffe observes that "the borders of Samori's Mande-speaking kingdom were wastelands of hunger and devastation." See *The African Poor: A History* (Cambridge, U.K.: Cambridge University Press, 1987), p. 36.

15. Crowder, *West Africa Under Colonial Rule*, pp. 87–88.

16. Walter Rodney disagreed heartily with such claims, arguing that "it was the Atlantic slave trade which spawned a variety of forms of slavery, serfdom, and subjection in this particular area." After the decline of the transatlantic trade, he adds, "one of the major problems facing the administration of the colony of Sierra Leone was the persistence of an internal slave trade, mainly supplying victims to the Mande and the Fulas," whom he terms "the great agents of the Atlantic slave trade." Although Rodney allowed that most societies in Upper West Africa were implicated in the traffic, "the Mandingas, Susus, and Fulas stood well to the fore— partly because of their own key role in slaving operations, and partly because they succeeded in reducing many littoral peoples and the inhabitants of Futa Djalon to a state of vassalage, under the banner of Islam." His conclusions continue to chafe today in Guinea and Sierra Leone, and across West Africa. See *A History of the Upper Guinea Coast, 1545–1800* (Oxford: Clarendon Press, 1970), pp. 261, 261, 264, 265. Arthur Abraham discusses this and other relevant matters in "The

Institution of 'Slavery,'" in *Topics in Sierra Leone History: A Counter-Colonial Interpretation* (Freetown: Leone Publishers, 1976), pp. 31–41.

17. Pakenham, *The Scramble for Africa*, p. 368.

18. The British governor at the time was one Sir James Shaw Hay. The French, according to Crowder, regarded Freetown as a "major thorn in their flesh in dealing with Samory, for it was from here that he gained most of his arms, albeit, as Hay pointed out, mainly from French shopkeepers" (*West Africa Under Colonial Rule*, p. 88). This would change when French forces cut off Samory's Freetown supply chain, which led him to look south to the Ivory Coast, the Cape Coast, Accra, and Porto Novo for both arms and gunpowder. For a detailed review, see Martin Legassick, "Firearms, Horses and Samorian Army Organization 1870–1898," *The Journal of African History* 7, no. 1 (1966): pp. 95–115.

19. Michal Tymowski, "Le développement de Sikasso, capitale du Kenedugu, en tant que siège du pouvoir politique et centre urbain," *Revue française d'histoire d'outre-mer* 68, no. 250–53 (1981): p. 437. (Translation mine.)

20. Babemba is quoted in Jean Suret-Canale, *Afrique noire occidentale et centrale: Géographie, Civilisations, Histoire* (Paris: Éditions Sociales, 1961), p. 237. (Translation mine.)

21. Alpha Oumar Konaré, *Sikasso Tata* (Bamako: Editions-Imprimeries du Mali, 1983), pp. 53, 58. (Translation mine.) Nine years after publishing this book, Konaré was elected president of Mali, serving two five-year terms.

22. "African Chieftain Captured: Samoray, the Soudan Warrior, Reported in French Hands," *The New York Times*, October 13, 1898, p. 7.

23. Téréba Togola, a Malian archaeologist, is quoted in Joan Baxter, "The Battle of Sikasso Revisited," *BBC Focus on Africa Magazine*, July–September 1998, joanbaxter.ca/wp-content/uploads/2016/04/1998-07-BBC-Focus-Mag-Battle-of-Sikasso-Revisited.pdf.

24. Baxter, "The Battle of Sikasso Revisited."

25. Among some rural Temne, at least, efforts to conceal and protect settlements from raids and other incursions did not cease with the British ban on ring fortification. Rather, they were focused on what Rosalind Shaw terms "the defensive containment of Closure," effected through charms and amulets and the counsel and spells of diviners and other ritual specialists. "In a striking parallel to the earlier construction of stockade towns," she explains, "diviners I knew from the 1970s to the 1990s erected ritual defenses through techniques of ritual Closure that encircled bodies, houses, and farms with invisible defensive barriers." See *Memories of the Slave Trade: Ritual and the Historical Imagination in Sierra Leone* (Chicago: University of Chicago Press, 2002), pp. 61, 60, 61.

26. Leland V. Bell, *Mental and Social Disorder in Sub-Saharan Africa: The Case of Sierra Leone, 1787–1990* (New York: Greenwood, 1991), p. ix.

27. British colonial officials may have been more ambivalent about such practices, abhorrent to many of its subjects back home, but its bureaucracies in West Africa

seemed to tolerate them. In Sierra Leone, abolitionist governors were under fierce pressure from native aristocrats, and from a surprisingly anti-abolitionist Creole elite. Within the protectorate at least, and for decades, Freetown would seek to defer to "customary law" on the matter of domestic slavery. "The colonial state lacked the money and the manpower necessary to end slavery, to transform labour relations, to economically exploit and to administer the colony without aid of the rural elite," explains Ismail Rashid. "The anti-slavery crusade gave way to pragmatic politics of accommodation." See "'Do dady nor lef me make dem carry me': Slave Resistance and Emancipation in Sierra Leone, 1894–1928," *Slavery and Abolition* 19, no. 2 (1998): p. 215.

28. John Desmond Hargreaves, "The Establishment of the Sierra Leone Protectorate and the Insurrection of 1898," *The Cambridge Historical Journal* 12, no. 1 (1956): p. 56.

29. Governor Frederic Cardew was initially commissioned in the Bengal Native Infantry and in 1879 was deployed in the Anglo-Zulu War in southern Africa, where he spent the next several years. He began his governorship in Sierra Leone in 1894 and served on and off until 1900. Ironically, perhaps, Cardew had previously been associated with efforts to bring down the internal slave trade by continuing Freetown's tradition of harboring escaped slaves. Although he was, in the words of Ismail Rashid, "an impatient imperialist," one of Cardew's primary gripes with the chiefs stemmed from their support of domestic slavery. For more on these complexities, see Rashid's "Slave Resistance and Emancipation in Sierra Leone," pp. 213–15.

30. Arthur Abraham, "Bai Bureh, the British, and the Hut Tax War," *International Journal of African Historical Studies* 7, no. 1 (1974): pp. 102, 106.

31. Edmund Dene Morel, *The Sierra Leone Hut-Tax Disturbances: A Reply to Mr. Stephen* (Liverpool: John & Sons, 1899), pp. 16, 12. The Hut Tax War was to long shape British policies in West Africa, as the archives of the Colonial Office reveal. J. D. Hargreaves summarized its lessons in a 1956 review: "The obvious explanation of the insurrection, accepted by the Royal Commissioner who inquired into it, was that the House Tax, with other features of the new administration, had been unacceptable." The uprising was, in the governor's dissenting opinion, "a deliberate rejection of progress, 'a reversion to the old order of things, such as fetish customs and slave-dealing and raiding.'" Hargreaves notes that "similar 'Whiggish' interpretations have been applied by many responsible officials to many other risings by Africans or Asians against European influences, from the Boxer rising to the Mau Mau. The sociologically minded observer tends to find the moral undertones of such statements too simply conceived; he prefers to talk of the disruptive effects of 'Western culture' on traditional beliefs and institutions, without trying to draw the moral implications too far" ("The Establishment of the Sierra Leone Protectorate," p. 57).

32. Sir David Chalmers, quoted in Morel, *The Sierra Leone Hut-Tax Disturbances*, p. 9.

33. "The Story of Bai Bureh," *Friends' Intelligencer*, January 7, 1899, p. 16.

34. Thomas Joshua Alldridge, *The Sherbro and Its Hinterland* (London: Macmillan, 1901), pp. 328, 333.

35. "These Frontier Police are loathed for the exactions and cruelties of which they have, for years past, been guilty towards their countrymen," complained journalist and peace activist Edmund Morel. "Between July, 1894, and February, 1898, no fewer than sixty-two convictions have been recorded against them for flogging, plundering, and generally maltreating the natives; and it is admitted that these 62 convictions can, by the very nature of the case, represent but an infinitesimal proportion of the offences actually committed" (*The Sierra Leone Hut-Tax Disturbances*, p. 18). These convictions did little to stanch the flow of blood, some of it shed by abusive policemen, imported troops from elsewhere in the empire, and white commanding officers.

36. Hargreaves, "The Establishment of the Sierra Leone Protectorate," p. 59.

37. As a leader in the Sande secret society, Mammy Yoko made political alliances and took younger initiates as wards, seeking to marry them into aristocratic lineages in an imitation of her own trajectory. In 1878, following her third husband's death, Mammy Yoko sought the post of paramount chief of Senehun. This was, as Arthur Abraham later observed, almost unheard of in Mende-speaking societies prior to the British introduction of the notion of inherited office. "Traditional" Sierra Leonean notions of meritocracy were often if not always, he explained, related to prowess in war. Since women were rarely invited to Poro war councils, they weren't often chiefs. Eager to delink chieftancy from war councils other than their own, the British proclaimed Yoko "Supreme Ruler of the Kpa Mendes" at the close of the Hut Tax War of 1898. For a critical discussion of Mende women chiefs, see "Women Chiefs: A Historical Reappraisal" in Abraham, *Topics in Sierra Leone History*, pp. 75–89.

38. Reverend Thomas Carthew, quoted in Christopher Fyfe, *Sierra Leone Inheritance* (London: Oxford University Press, 1964), p. 238.

39. Like other collaborationist leaders, Mammy Yoko grew unpopular with many of her subjects. She took her own life in 1906. For a favorable view of Yoko's contributions, see Carol P. Hoffer, "Madam Yoko: Ruler of the Kpa Mende Confederacy," in *Woman, Culture, and Society*, edited by Michelle Zimbalist Rosaldo and Louise Lamphere (Stanford: Stanford University Press, 1974), pp. 173–88.

40. Crowder, *West Africa Under Colonial Rule*, p. 191.

41. Conklin, *A Mission to Civilize*, pp. 11, 7, 6.

42. Alice Conklin adds further context to a reconsideration of French claims about their *mission civilatrice*: "However misguided, self-deluding, or underfunded—indeed, because they were all these things—these claims merit our attention. As an enduring tension of French republicanism, the civilizing ideal in whose name the nation of the 'rights of man' deprived so many people of their freedom deserves to be better understood." Conklin doesn't dismiss French racism as central to its colonial policies but seeks "to understand its particular course and

permutations before and after World War I, as well as its ability to coexist un-problematically—at least in the eyes of contemporaries—with republican values in the first place" (*A Mission to Civilize*, pp. 9–10). (Formatting altered.)

43. Crowder, *West Africa Under Colonial Rule*, p. 170.

44. Aspe Fleurimont, *L'organisation économique de l'Afrique occidentale française: Liberté, Réglementation*, Rapport Adressé à M. le Ministre du Commerce et de l'Industrie (Paris: Imprimerie F. Levé, 1901), p. 77. (Translation mine.)

45. The sums involved were far from trivial, as Conklin reports: "West Africa accounted for 11 percent of French export of rails, 15 percent of locomotives, and 19 percent of iron and steel structures between 1900 and 1904, and these figures would hold good until the war" (*A Mission to Civilize*, p. 56). Private profits were even more spectacular.

46. "Bassam's yellow fever epidemics occurred in 1899, 1902, and 1903, the last one killing nearly all of Bassam's European inhabitants," writes the physician-anthropologist Vinh-Kim Nguyen. "The later outbreaks led to near panic among the settlers, and a mounting rhetoric of epidemiological catastrophe produced by colonial administrators finally convinced metropolitan authorities that the ad-ministrative capital would have to be moved." Abidjan was born when colonial officials "conjured up a local capital from which rule could be exercised, and it materialized as a biopolitical fortress shaped by a double threat: a potentially rebellious population and tropical disease." See *The Republic of Therapy: Triage and Sovereignty in West Africa's Time of AIDS* (Durham, N.C.: Duke University Press, 2010), p. 115. For more on these epidemics of yellow fever, see Christophe Wondji, "La fièvre jaune à Grand-Bassam (1899–1903)," *Revue française d'histoire d'outre-mer* 59, no. 215 (1972): pp. 205–239. Although Conakry's drainage and sewage systems left much to be desired, even experts from the Liverpool School of Tropical Medicine had to admit, in 1905, that the new capital put Freetown to shame. "A visit to Conakry is a most instructive lesson," wrote a trio of (evidently Francophile) Liverpool professors after a brief tour of West African capitals. "One cannot fail to be impressed with the great skill and energy which in a few years has planned and constructed a modern town. Commerce was its *raison d'être*, nevertheless everything has been carried out true to the classic instincts of the French. Wide boulevards intersect at right angles equally wide avenues; there are fountains and public gardens, and, most striking of all in a West African town, a very fine statue in memory of the services rendered by Governor Ballay. A landing stage, a vast railway station, extensive waterworks of the most modern type, a new hospital, and a network of light rails, by means of which the goods landed from the ships on the wharf are conveyed expeditiously and directly into the various factories. The contrast to Freetown, only seventy-eight miles away, is striking." See Rubert Boyce, Arthur Evans, and H. Herbert Clarke, *Report on the Sanitation and Anti-Malarial Measures in Practice in Bathurst, Conakry, and Freetown* (London: University Press of Liverpool by Williams and Norgate, 1905), p. 11.

47. The colonial sanitarians and other Europeans weren't the only ones to turn a blind eye to the squalid conditions of the native majority. Writing about Dakar's 1914 epidemic of plague, and subsequent ones in the wake of the Great War, Myron Echenberg reports that African elites were largely unwilling to call out the postwar colonial administration for its failure to protect the health of the Senegalese poor. Another "potential source of criticism," he notes, "might have been the new class of petit bourgeois government clerks, schoolteachers, technicians in the health sector, and professional politicians at the municipal and state levels. But this group, able to afford improved living conditions within the racially mixed Plateau district of Dakar, for the most part made conscious choices not to criticize the insanitary conditions endured by their less privileged countrymen." French authorities were able to placate some middle-class Senegalese protesting health conditions during early plague outbreaks with political and economic reward. Notably, the "leading voice of protest on behalf of Africans during the 1914 epidemic, Blaise Diagne, joined the camp of Dakar boosters willing to overlook the city's insalubrity." Shortly after winning 1919 parliamentary elections, the flip-flopping Diagne not only overlooked insalubrity, but, like French authorities, spread stories of salubrious transformations engendered by their civilizing mission. A 1924 article in a newspaper Diagne had founded—its name had also flip-flopped, from *La Démocratie* to *L'Ouest Africain Français*—"boasted that Dakar had become the 'showpiece city of French West Africa,' with more dispensaries and clinics per capita than Lille." This, as Echenberg shows, was fake news. See *Black Death, White Medicine: Bubonic Plague and the Politics of Public Health in Colonial Senegal, 1914–1945* (Portsmouth, N.H.: Heinemann, 2002), pp. 197, 198.

48. André Marcandier, cited in Echenberg, *Black Death, White Medicine*, p. 108.

49. Raymond E. Dumett, "The Campaign Against Malaria and the Expansion of Scientific Medical and Sanitary Services in British West Africa, 1898–1910," *African Historical Studies* 1, no. 2 (1968): p. 166.

50. Festus Cole, "Sanitation, Disease and Public Health in Sierra Leone, West Africa, 1895–1922: Case Failure of British Colonial Health Policy," *The Journal of Imperial and Commonwealth History* 43, no. 2 (2015): p. 249.

51. M.C.F. Easmon, "Sierra Leone Doctors," *Sierra Leone Studies*, no. 6 (1956): pp. 85–86. (Formatting altered.)

52. For a description of the West African medical service formed in the wake of microbiology's allegedly golden age, see Ryan Johnson, "The West African Medical Staff and the Administration of Imperial Tropical Medicine, 1902–14," *The Journal of Imperial and Commonwealth History* 38, no. 3 (2010): pp. 419–39. A steady litany of complaints from British doctors in the service was published, largely anonymously, in *The British Medical Journal*. Most discontent was about pay, vacations and furloughs, housing conditions, and perceived unfairness regarding promotions. Only rarely were the health and well-being of the natives—or the demotion and exclusion of African medical peers from the service—mentioned.

The volumes of whinging became so large that, in 1908, the editors chose to print a summary of the rest. See "Medical Administrative Problems: The West African Medical Staff," *The British Medical Journal* 1, no. 2456 (1908): pp. 214–16. For a sample of the correspondence that made the cut before 1908, see "The Medical Services of West African Colonies and Protectorates," *The British Medical Journal* 1, no. 2153 (1902): p. 869; G. Rome Hall, "Some Grievances of the West African Medical Staff," *The British Medical Journal* 1, no. 2257 (1904): pp. 806–807; "Some Grievances of the West African Medical Staff," *The British Medical Journal* 1, no. 2374 (1906): p. 1572; "Medical Officers in Southern Nigeria," *The British Medical Journal* 2, no. 2387 (1906): p. 815; "The West African Medical Service," *The British Medical Journal* 1, no. 2404 (1907): p. 231; "West African Medical Service," *The British Medical Journal* 1, no. 2426 (1907): pp. 1579–80.

53. Emmanuel Akyeampong, "Disease in West African History," in *Themes in West Africa's History*, edited by Emmanuel Akyeampong (Athens: Ohio University Press, 2006), p. 197.

54. Thomas Winterbottom, *An Account of the Native Africans in the Neighbourhood of Sierra Leone*, volume 2 (London: C. Whittingham, 1803), pp. 29, 30. Winterbottom's description was detailed enough that infectious-disease specialists still refer to glandular tumors on the nape of the neck as "Winterbottom's sign," which calls into question subsequent assertions that trypanosomiasis was new to Sierra Leone. The same process of discovery and forgetting would later mark virgin-soil claims about trypanosomiasis elsewhere on the continent—and about Ebola in Upper West Africa.

55. For more on this epidemic—or epidemics, according to retrospective analyses revealing the presence of distinct trypanosome variants—and others in the region, see Daniel R. Headrick, "Sleeping Sickness Epidemics and Colonial Responses in East and Central Africa, 1900–1940," *PLOS Neglected Tropical Diseases* 8, no. 4 (2014): p. e2772; B. W. Langlands, *The Sleeping Sickness Epidemic of Uganda, 1900–1920: A Study in Historical Geography* (Kampala: Department of Geography, Makerere University College, 1967); Geoff Hide, "History of Sleeping Sickness in East Africa," *Clinical Microbiology Reviews* 12, no. 1 (1999): pp. 112–25; Harvey G. Soff, "Sleeping Sickness in the Lake Victoria Region of British East Africa, 1900–1915," *African Historical Studies* 2, no. 2 (1969): pp. 255–68; Maryinez Lyons, *The Colonial Disease: A Social History of Sleeping Sickness in Northern Zaire, 1900–1940* (Cambridge, U.K.: Cambridge University Press, 1992). Confidence about the causative subspecies during Uganda's massive epidemic—which was limited by colonial boundaries no more than other fly-borne plagues—is interrogated by Thorsten Koerner, Peter de Raadt, and Ian Maudlin in "The 1901 Uganda Sleeping Sickness Epidemic Revisited: A Case of Mistaken Identity?," *Parasitology Today* 11, no. 8 (1995): pp. 303–306; and by Eric M. Fèvre and colleagues in "Reanalyzing the 1900–1920 Sleeping Sickness Epidemic in Uganda," *Emerging Infectious Diseases* 10, no. 4 (2004): pp. 567–73.

56. See William A. Murray, "History of the Introduction and Spread of Human Try-panosomiasis (Sleeping Sickness) in British Nyasaland in 1908 and Following Years," *Transactions of the Royal Society of Tropical Medicine and Hygiene* 15, no. 4 (1921): pp. 121–28.

57. Inge Heiberg, quoted in Maryinez Lyons, "From 'Death Camps' to Cordon Sani-taire: The Development of Sleeping Sickness Policy in the Uele District of the Bel-gian Congo, 1903–1914," *The Journal of African History* 26, no. 1 (1985): p. 81.

58. Albert Schweitzer, *On the Edge of the Primeval Forest: Experiences and Obser-vations of a Doctor in Equatorial Africa* (London: A. & C. Black, 1922), pp. 85, 86. The answer to Schweitzer's question—"Shall we now conquer it?"—was no, we shan't. Many assessments suggest that sleeping sickness remained epidemic across vast swaths of West Africa until the 1960s, when it was said to have been brought under some semblance of control. But complacency hastened its come-back in the remaining decades of the twentieth century. For a schematic review of a century of trypanosomiasis and conflict in the region, see Courtin et al., "Sleep-ing Sickness in West Africa," pp. 334–44.

59. Charles Louis Alphonse Laveran, a French military veterinarian working in Al-geria, was awarded a Nobel in 1907 for his discovery of the parasite nearly three decades earlier; his work is described in L. J. Bruce-Chwatt, "Alphonse Laveran's Discovery 100 Years Ago and Today's Global Fight Against Malaria," *Journal of the Royal Society of Medicine* 74, no. 7 (1981): pp. 531–36. Writing in 2006, Diana Davis offers a brief history of the French military veterinarians in the nineteenth and early twentieth centuries, when they were obliged to care for both man and beast at a time when "the vast majority of power for all militaries came from animals." Although these were largely horses and mules, the conquest of north Africa introduced French veterinarians to camels, while the struggle to dominate Madagascar saw Zebu cattle called into service. "In every other colonial terri-tory conquered by the French in Africa," Davis notes, "military veterinarians accompanied the occupation forces and played pivotal roles in the success of the French war machine." See "Prescribing Progress: French Veterinary Medicine in the Service of Empire," *Veterinary Heritage* 29, no. 1 (2006): p. 2.

60. See John W. Cell, "Anglo-Indian Medical Theory and the Origins of Segregation in West Africa," *The American Historical Review* 91, no. 2 (1986): pp. 307–335.

61. Adds the unnamed correspondent: "The sickness is attributed to malaria; but, as the microscope is not generally employed for accurate diagnosis, it may at least be questioned whether there is not some other important disease factor." See "The Malaria Expedition to Sierra Leone," *The British Medical Journal* 2, no. 2019 (1899): p. 675. There's evidence that the correspondent was none other than Ross himself, incognito.

62. Day-biting mosquitoes that are the vectors of yellow and dengue fevers—and of Zika, chikungunya, and other afflictions not yet identified and named—also fed on residents as the humans went about their business in Freetown and elsewhere in the colony.

63. For an overview of jungle-doctor sensationalism, see Anna Crozier, "Sensational-ising Africa: British Medical Impressions of Sub-Saharan Africa, 1890–1939," *The Journal of Imperial and Commonwealth History* 35, no. 3 (2007): pp. 393–415. See also "Hippo Happenings: Jungle Doctors, Children and Animals" in Megan Vaughan, *Curing Their Ills: Colonial Power and African Illness* (Cambridge, U.K.: Polity Press, 1991), pp. 155–79.

64. From an 1899 Colonial Office report, cited in Stephen Frenkel and John Western, "Pretext or Prophylaxis? Racial Segregation and Malarial Mosquitos in a British Tropical Colony: Sierra Leone," *Annals of the Association of American Geographers* 78, no. 2 (1988): p. 215. The historian quoted parenthetically is John Cell, in "Anglo-Indian Medical Theory," p. 332.

65. Ronald Ross, "Sanitary Affairs in West Africa," in Edmund Dene Morel, *Affairs of West Africa* (London: William Heinemann, 1902), p. 163.

66. "This sanatorium is more or less a reproach to us," the military medics concluded. "With a wave of the hand, so to speak, crowded West African towns have been (we are told) rendered salubrious. Meantime health in these barracks is unchanged." See F. Smith and A. Pearse, "Fevers in Sierra Leone (Mount Aureol), Being a Preliminary Account of an Enquiry into the Causes of the Continued Prevalence of Ill-Health in an Apparently Favourably Situated Hill Station," *Journal of the Royal Army Medical Corps* 2, no. 3 (1904): p. 278. Contrary opinions were advanced by hard-line segregationists within the colonies and a few polite if misinformed visitors. The Liverpool tropical medicine experts who'd compared Freetown unfavorably to Conakry were, for example, taken by the promise of Hill Station—a shockingly modest campus—given the investments required and the fuss triggered. "A site for a cantonment was selected on a high ridge, nine hundred feet above sea level, far from native houses, and in 1904 some twenty-two model bungalows were finished," they wrote. "These have been occupied by the Government officials, and an adjacent area has been reserved for the erection of merchants' houses. A pure water supply is laid on to each house, and a most convenient highland railway, five and three-quarters miles long, carries the residents to and from Freetown to Hill Station" (Boyce, Evans, and Clarke, *Report on the Sanitation and Anti-Malarial Measures in Practice*, p. 25).

67. Emmanuel Akyeampong, who sees decisions made in order to protect the colonists from the natives as essential to the entrenchment of colonial racial hierarchies, reflects the views of most historians and scholars writing of these matters in recent decades. Festus Cole is withering ("Segregation," he asserts, "institutionalized a pernicious colour bar which excluded Africans from Hill Station Club and discriminated against blacks on the mountain railway"). So are Leo Spitzer (who writes of "the feelings of betrayal and bitterness with which Sierra Leoneans came to view the Hill Station"); Raymond Dumett (who describes segregation as just one of many manifestations of "the tendency to slight the welfare of Africans for the benefit of Europeans"); John Cell (who, commenting on an analogy drawn by the Royal Commission between cattle as reservoirs of trypanoso-

miasis and children as reservoirs of malaria, notes that the "implied strategy was the elimination, at least from proximity to the sleeping quarters of Europeans, of such wild species as African children"); Odile Goerg (who observes that as "fundamental changes in race theories were occurring," the opposition between "the Whites" and "the Natives" not only had "many legal consequences, such as new definitions for census purposes or the acquisition of citizenship," but further "served as a basis for actual spatial exclusion"); and the geographers Stephen Frenkel and John Western (who note that the attribution of malaria transmission to the *Anopheles* mosquito was "taken by Colonial Office medical authorities and reinterpreted in a racial context, that is, in order to promote and justify racial segregation"). See Cole, "Sanitation, Disease and Public Health," p. 242; Leo Spitzer, "The Mosquito and Segregation in Sierra Leone," *Canadian Journal of African Studies* 2, no. 1 (1968): p. 58; Dumett, "The Campaign Against Malaria," p. 170; Cell, "Anglo-Indian Medical Theory," p. 331; Odile Goerg, "From Hill Station (Freetown) to Downtown Conakry (First Ward): Comparing French and British Approaches to Segregation in Colonial Cities at the Beginning of the Twentieth Century," *Canadian Journal of African Studies* 32, no. 1 (1998): p. 5; Frenkel and Western, "Pretext or Prophylaxis?," p. 214.

68. Cell, "Anglo-Indian Medical Theory," p. 311. The physician-governor was Sir William MacGregor. Many colonial officials, MacGregor among them, "realized from the beginning the political dangers involved in a policy of housing segregation, but they were unable to resist the best medical advice of their day," adds historian Thomas Gale in "Segregation in British West Africa," *Cahiers d'Études Africaines* 20, no. 80 (1980): p. 495. The handful of Africans "represented in legislative councils, naturally agreed with MacGregor not least in regard to the use of their taxes" (Cell, "Anglo-Indian Medical Theory," p. 311). The great native majority must have been even more dismayed by such advice, but their views weren't solicited. MacGregor opposed segregation on paternalistic (or somewhat sardonic) grounds. "I do not see how the 'White-Man' can shirk any part of his 'Burden,'" he wrote. "Such segregation, if sufficiently marked to be of real benefit from the malarial point of view, will be followed by a terrible breach in the relations existing between the native and the European, who should be his teacher and friend" (Frenkel and Western, "Pretext or Prophylaxis?," p. 217). With more irony than paternalism—there are surely worse things than teachers and friends—Governor MacGregor argued that "if instead of being segregated Africans were cured of malaria, there would be no need to move." As for malaria, he found value in integrating prevention and care: the malaria program in Lagos (according to Thomas Gale) aspired to "the eradication of mosquitoes, free distribution of quinine to Africans, and for the first time in any tropical colony, the introduction of hygiene and sanitation courses in local schools." Such integration helped save European lives as well. "Between 1897 and 1900," summarizes Gale, "thirteen European officials died of malaria. In the five years after the anti-mosquito campaign and free quinine distribution were inaugurated in 1900, only three succumbed" ("Segregation in British West Africa," pp. 496, 497).

69. Governor Cardew was among the early cheerleaders of segregation. A separate residential settlement, he wrote the colonial secretary in the months before his departure, "could enable the European to live longer and to work better and more continuously by removing him from the heat and malarious influences of Freetown to the cooler and purer atmosphere on the summits of the adjacent hills." (Cardew is quoted in Goerg, "From Hill Station to Downtown Conakry," p. 8.) Cardew's previous revolt-suppressing tours of duty had been in other malarious and socially segregated outposts of the empire, including India and southern Africa, but this was before the parasite and the mosquito replaced miasma as malaria's presumed etiology and vector. The "medical justification for segregation as a protection against malaria emerged quite suddenly in 1900 in West Africa," notes John Cell. "Only afterward was the proposal made in India—as it happens by the very group from the Royal Society of London that first advanced the notion in Africa. In India the British had long maintained separate residential quarters, gymkhana clubs, churches, and so forth, all of which their town plans perpetuated. But the fad of justifying a doctrine of segregation primarily on medical grounds had an even shorter run there than it did in Africa—hardly, indeed, a run at all" ("Anglo-Indian Medical Theory," p. 312). Since Cardew returned to England in November of 1900, it fell to his successor to preside over the establishment and construction of the hill station.

70. Echenberg, *Black Death, White Medicine*, p. 262.

71. "Apartheid" is an Afrikaans word used to describe a series of policies held to mark a sharp departure from a kinder, gentler form of colonialism espoused in South Africa by the British when they ran the place—during roughly the same years as those in which they ruled over parts of West and East Africa. Even cursory scrutiny of pre-apartheid policies in South Africa and elsewhere in Britain's African colonies does not, however, lead to endorsement of British rule as significantly more benign than the policies later formalized by the Afrikaners. Nor is it clear that the experience of Africans under British rule varied radically from that registered in other reaches of the empire. In long-looted India, where protection of British soldiers and civilians remained the focus of most public-health interventions, less attention was paid to more numerous Indian troops, to say nothing of Indian subjects. "India's one hundred thousand villages," observes John Cell, undercounting, "remained untouched" by such campaigns. Once freed from colonial oversight, the Indian Medical Service fought to eradicate malaria by integrating prevention and care. The sanitarians of independent India were, on the first attempts at least, foiled by the vector and the parasite, both of which developed resistance to the agents used against them. But the historian gives them credit for trying. "Better undue optimism," Cell concludes, "than a deliberate and explicitly segregationist policy aimed only at protecting Europeans from the Indians among whom they served" ("Anglo-Indian Medical Theory," pp. 325, 335).

72. Paul Richards, "Chimpanzees as Political Animals in Sierra Leone," in *Natural Enemies: People-Wildlife Conflicts in Anthropological Perspective*, edited by John

Knight (London: Routledge, 2000), p. 89. "In the literature on modernity and the occult imaginary," adds Rosalind Shaw, "such creatures as Human Alligators, zombies, witches, and cannibals are usually located in an age of postcolonial states and structurally adjusted economies." Tales of these creatures erupted, she adds, "nearly seventy years after British authorities in the Crown Colony of Sierra Leone, based in Freetown, had replaced the Atlantic slave trade with a 'legitimate trade' in products such as palm oil, palm kernels, camwood, and timber. The stories entered the colonial record as rumours and reports of suspicious killings, as part of the correspondence between hinterland chiefs and colonial authorities, and as accusations and confessions in colonial court cases." See "Cannibal Transformations: Colonialism and Commodification in the Sierra Leone Hinterland," in *Magical Interpretations, Material Realities: Modernity, Witchcraft and the Occult in Postcolonial Africa*, edited by Henrietta L. Moore and Todd Sanders (London: Routledge, 2001), pp. 50, 55.

73. The anthropologist Paul Richards describes a "general class of beliefs, known to Mende-speakers as *bôni hinda* (somewhat misleadingly translated as 'cannibalism'), in which it is thought that power-seekers murder young people to obtain body parts for the manufacture of *hale nyamui* ('bad medicine') conferring special political or economic powers." These power-seekers "disguise themselves as leopards, crocodiles or chimpanzees (the only large animals in the Upper Guinean forest that kill humans other than in self-defence)." In noting the term *bôni hinda* is better glossed as "chimpanzee business" than "cannibalism," Richards is seeking to illuminate today's rumors of ritual murder, and the direction of accusations of guilt, in the societies of Upper West Africa. "Shape-shifted 'cannibals' freely crossed ethnic and linguistic boundaries in southern and eastern Sierra Leone through Liberia as far as the western Côte d'Ivoire," he writes. "For a time British colonial officers continued to accept 'cannibalism' cases on the assumption that cannibal secret societies might actually exist, and that 'cannibals' had perpetrated real crimes. Later colonial officials would become more circumspect about confessions beaten out of suspects in custody." Close to a century after colonial officials replaced Tongo players as the arbiters of guilt, Richards declines to weigh in as to whether or not such unlawful societies were guilty of ritual murder, taking care to enclose the words cannibals and cannibalism with quotation marks. "Whether such killing really occurs," he concludes, "is impossible for independent observers to decide. This is because, as Mende villagers today are quick to point out, the behaviour of real animals provides plausible cover for the alleged activity" ("Chimpanzees as Political Animals," pp. 78, 89, 93, 88). These comments are profitably considered in light of Arthur Abraham's devastating review of the Czech historian Milan Kalous's overview of the topic. Kalous claimed to collect an archive of over a thousand such accusations brought before colonial courts. But only a minority of them concerned human-leopard accusations. (See Abraham's "'Cannibalism' and African Historiography" in *Topics in Sierra Leone History*, pp. 120–30.) Those that involved claims of can-

nibalism were sometimes staked by surviving victims, which might imply that zombies can talk. Students of Haitian culture, or recent American television and film, would surely dispute this capacity.

74. If colonial officials argued about the very existence of cannibalism, it's in part because some of the disagreement was definitional. "Ritual murder, human sacrifice, and 'cannibalism,'" observes Arthur Abraham in reference to colonial archives, "are confusingly used as alternatives, sometimes in the same document . . . But the emotive term 'cannibalism' was well in accord with the whole concept of 'the civilizing mission'" (*Topics in Sierra Leone History*, p. 125). Nor was there colonial consensus regarding the relationship between human leopards—or alligators, crocodiles, chimpanzees, or baboons—and secret societies. The doyen of Sierra Leone's first generation of historians noted acidly that neither alligators nor baboons were present in the colony.

75. Thomas Winterbottom, *An Account of the Native Africans in the Neighbourhood of Sierra Leone*, volume 1 (London: C. Whittingham, 1803), p. 166.

76. Ernest Graham Ingham, *Sierra Leone After a Hundred Years* (London: Seeley, 1894), p. 272.

77. Sir William Brandford Griffith, in his preface to Kenneth James Beatty, *Human Leopards: An Account of the Trials of Human Leopards Before the Special Commission Court; with a Note on Sierra Leone, Past and Present* (London: Hugh Rees, 1915), p. viii.

78. Beatty, *Human Leopards*, p. 4.

79. Beatty, *Human Leopards*, p. 5.

80. Beatty, *Human Leopards*, p. 5.

81. Government of the Colony of Sierra Leone, quoted in Beatty, *Human Leopards*, p. 6.

82. Beatty, *Human Leopards*, pp. 7, 23, 9, 12; Alldridge, *The Sherbro and Its Hinterland*, p. 124. The ordinances sent by Governor E. M. Merewether to the colonial secretary on July 9, 1913, are reproduced as an appendix to *Human Leopards*. One wonders what the soon-to-be-besieged secretary in London made of this correspondence about supernatural savagery as German forces launched their materially savage attacks on Britain.

83. Beatty, *Human Leopards*, pp. 20, 25, 26. (Formatting altered.)

84. Beatty, *Human Leopards*, p. 9.

85. Beatty, *Human Leopards*, p. 28.

86. Beatty, *Human Leopards*, pp. 28, 29.

87. Beatty, *Human Leopards*, pp. 33, 34.

88. Sir William Griffith, preface to Beatty, *Human Leopards*, p. viii. Beatty's book featured an equally circumstantial case, also resulting in a death sentence. The hanging judge attributed this successful prosecution to "the chance overhearing by the District Commissioner's clerk that a boy had been killed by a leopard." Happily, this occurred before "all trace of evidence had vanished," which would have been "all the more difficult to disprove from the fact that in that neigh-

bourhood leopards abound" (p. 43). This, too, was hyperbole: human leopards wouldn't have to be plentiful to outnumber feline ones. The Mende term for cannibalism may be literally translated as "chimpanzee business," but the general notion of consuming others didn't require animals dangerous to young humans when there were plenty of dangerous (and fractious) humans about. In the early decades of British rule, authorities with power over life and death were among them. But there was, under colonial rule, no Innocence Project or Court of Appeals to prevent the execution of natives convicted of such crimes without adequate evidence. Sir William Griffith's conclusions about human leopards were of a more psychological nature. "To my mind," he notes "the chief factor in the uncanniness is the presence of numerous half-human chimpanzees with their maniacal shrieks and cries. The bush seemed to me pervaded with something supernatural, a spirit which was striving to bridge the animal and the human." Sir William continues his reverie with literal (or downright Freudian) observations: "All the principal offenders were men of mature age, past their prime," he added, suggesting the aggressors were out to enhance their virility through incorporation of younger body parts. Then again, the British magistrate allowed that the people of Sierra Leone *were* well endowed—"with the most marvellous faculty for keeping hidden what they did not wish to be known" (pp. viii, vii, viii).

89. Beatty, *Human Leopards*, p. 20. There's no evidence Kenneth Beatty wavered in the conviction that he should wield power over life and death. Then again, he might not have had much downtime to reflect on his time in Sierra Leone: Beatty was dispatched to fight in the Dardanelles, in what was then the Ottoman Empire, after it joined World War I on the side of Germany. This particular campaign, which ended in ignominious defeat of Allied forces, was engineered by a young military commander named Winston Churchill. Beatty survived the war (and Churchill).

90. Beatty, *Human Leopards*, p. 3.

7. A WORLD AT WAR

1. Jean Suret-Canale, *Afrique noire occidentale et centrale: L'ère coloniale (1900–1945)* (Paris: Éditions Sociales, 1964), p. 87. (Translation mine.)

2. This 1906 "Circular from the Governor of Sierra Leone to the District Commissioners" is cited in Ismail Rashid, "'Do dady nor lef me make dem carry me': Slave Resistance and Emancipation in Sierra Leone, 1894–1928," *Slavery and Abolition* 19, no. 2 (1998): p. 217.

3. "Significantly," adds Ismail Rashid, "these measures came at the peak of mass slave desertions from their masters in French colonies and Northern Nigeria" ("Slave Resistance and Emancipation in Sierra Leone," p. 218).

4. In Crowder's bilious assessment, the "achievements of French administration did not justify the near panegyrics" churned out by colonialism's propagandists and apologists, and even by some of his fellow academic historians. See *West Africa Under Colonial Rule* (London: Hutchinson, 1968), pp. 184, 175. Suret-Canale, an old-school Marxist, was decidedly not a member of any of these groups.

5. The promise of Reconstruction—the birth of participatory, multiracial democracy—remained only a promise. It nevertheless constituted, in the historian David Quigley's view, a veritable "second founding" of the United States: "Decided at this second founding were the rules of the democratic game. Though lasting only a few short years, Reconstruction involved countless Americans fighting over who would be able to play in that game, and on whose terms. A century and a quarter later, the democracy that emerged at Reconstruction's end remains our inheritance." See *Second Founding: New York City, Reconstruction, and the Making of American Democracy* (New York: Hill and Wang, 2004), p. ix.

6. Douglas A. Blackmon, *Slavery by Another Name: The Re-Enslavement of Black People in America from the Civil War to World War II* (New York: Doubleday, 2008), p. 148. To this day—and from Ferguson, Missouri, to the Deep South and on to Wisconsin—similar arrangements continue to "lock poor people into a cycle of fines, debts and jail." See Adam Liptak, "Charged a Fee for Getting Arrested, Whether Guilty or Not," *The New York Times*, December 26, 2016, nytimes.com /2016/12/26/us/politics/charged-a-fee-for-getting-arrested-whether-guilty-or -not.html. As of 2016, some 15 percent of black voting-age Alabamans, and a total of six million others across America, have been disenfranchised after conviction of a crime. Florida is even worse; the scale of disenfranchisement sparked change through a vote on a constitutional amendment in November 2018. See the editorial "The Movement to End Racist Voting Laws," *The New York Times*, October 5, 2016, nytimes.com/2016/10/05/opinion/the-movement-to-end-racist -voting-laws.html.

7. Patrick Phillips, *Blood at the Root: A Racial Cleansing in America* (New York: W. W. Norton, 2016), pp. 63–64. This long and shameful chapter of recent American history is finally acknowledged in a museum and national memorial built by the Equal Justice Initiative in Montgomery, Alabama. Their foundations were laid in a report—*Lynching in America: Confronting the Legacy of Racial Terror* (Montgomery: Equal Justice Initiative, 2015)—which documents over four thousand racial-terror lynchings in twelve states of the American South between 1877 and 1950. The origins and philosophical underpinnings of this monumental work are detailed in Bryan Stevenson's inspiring memoir, *Just Mercy: A Story of Justice and Redemption* (New York: Spiegel & Grau, 2014). For more on the memorial and museum, see Alexis Okeowo, "A Devastating, Overdue National Memorial to Lynching Victims," *The New Yorker*, April 26, 2018, newyorker.com /news/news-desk/a-devastating-overdue-national-memorial-to-lynching-victims; Jeffrey Toobin, "The Legacy of Lynching, on Death Row," *The New Yorker*, August 22, 2016, newyorker.com/magazine/2016/08/22/bryan-stevenson-and-the -legacy-of-lynching. Sherrilyn Ifill's book, *On the Courthouse Lawn: Confronting the Legacy of Lynching in the Twenty-first Century* (Boston: Beacon Press, 2007), offers a thoughtful examination of this period of racial terror and its legacies,

underlining the need for solemn commemoration of events currently crowded out by Confederate monuments.

8. This research revealed large parts of the American South to be (in the words of Du Bois) "an armed camp for intimidating black folk." See *The Souls of Black Folk: Essays and Sketches* (Chicago: A. C. McClurg, 1903), p. 105.

9. Du Bois, *The Souls of Black Folk*, p. 38.

10. David Firestone, "Many See Their Future in County with a Past," *The New York Times*, April 8, 1999, p. A18.

11. Crowder, *West Africa Under Colonial Rule*, p. 175.

12. According to W.E.B. Du Bois, Liberia had long teetered on the edge of receivership, with Britain and France "on the point of seizing the country," a fate forestalled by the promise of an American loan. "Then suddenly came the World War and smashed all these dreams," he wrote. "Liberia, despite her large German trade, was forced to declare in favor of the Allies. One inducement was a loan promised her by the United States Government. Before this went through, however, the war was over and Congress refused to confirm the loan." See "Liberia, the League and the United States," *Foreign Affairs* 11, no. 4 (1933): p. 683.

13. Danny Hoffman has compellingly argued that barracks remain cardinal features of Monrovia and Freetown today. Although barracks' roots as centers of labor concentration surely lie in the era of barracoons and slave pens, the function and number of colonial barracks buttress his argument. See "The City as Barracks: Freetown, Monrovia, and the Organization of Violence in Postcolonial African Cities," *Cultural Anthropology* 22, no. 3 (2007): pp. 400–28.

14. Hew Strachan, *The First World War: To Arms*, volume 1 (New York: Oxford University Press, 2001), pp. 521–22.

15. Festus Cole, "Sanitation, Disease and Public Health in Sierra Leone, West Africa, 1895–1922: Case Failure of British Colonial Health Policy," *The Journal of Imperial and Commonwealth History* 43, no. 2 (2015): p. 246.

16. That same year, the colony's chief medical officer admitted it was "practically impossible to find a really healthy person in Sierra Leone." Both governor and physician are quoted in Cole, "Sanitation, Disease and Public Health," p. 252.

17. Myron J. Echenberg, "Paying the Blood Tax: Military Conscription in French West Africa, 1914–1929," *Canadian Journal of African Studies* 9, no. 2 (1975): pp. 180, 181.

18. The numbers are, as ever, guestimates. The historian John Barry believes these are conservative ones. See his commentary, "The Site of Origin of the 1918 Influenza Pandemic and Its Public Health Implications," *Journal of Translational Medicine* 2, no. 1 (2004): p. 3. Barry's book-length study is *The Great Influenza: The Epic Story of the Deadliest Plague in History* (New York: Viking, 2004).

19. Emmanuel Akyeampong, "Disease in West African History," in *Themes in West Africa's History*, edited by Emmanuel Akyeampong (Athens: Ohio University Press, 2006), p. 200.

20. Alfred W. Crosby, *America's Forgotten Pandemic: The Influenza of 1918* (Cambridge, U.K.: Cambridge University Press, 1989), p. 37.

21. Barry, "The Site of Origin of the 1918 Influenza Pandemic," p. 3.

22. Sandra M. Tomkins, "Colonial Administration in British Africa During the Influenza Epidemic of 1918–19," *Canadian Journal of African Studies* 28, no. 1 (1994): pp. 62, 63. Emmanuel Akyeampong makes a similar point: "The futility of therapy (both African and Western) created a cognitive crisis in areas of Africa and gave birth to anti-medicine movements" ("Disease in West African History," p. 200).

23. "With the colony situated midway between Simon's Town and the British Isles," writes Festus Cole, "it was also admirably suited for use in war as a rendezvous for convoys of ships on the Cape route, or for those vessels plying the routes between the United Kingdom and West Africa, for mercantile shipping from the U.K., and for those from South American and Australian ports, via Cape Horn, or the Straits of Magellan. The colony also served as a base for replenishing stores and fuel, for repairs, and for effecting changes in personnel." See "In Defence of 'King and Country': Empire Loyalism, Sierra Leone and World War I," *Research in Sierra Leone Studies: Weave* 2, no. 2 (2014): pp. 6–7.

24. Tomkins, "Colonial Administration in British Africa," p. 68.

25. Crosby, *America's Forgotten Pandemic*, p. 37.

26. "HMS *Mantua*—March 1915 to January 1919, 10th Cruiser Squadron Northern Patrol, British Home Waters, Central Atlantic Convoys," *Royal Navy Log Books of the World War 1 Era*, edited by Su Startin, February 11, 2014, naval-history .net/OWShips-WW1-08-HMS_Mantua.htm.

27. Cole, "Sanitation, Disease and Public Health," pp. 259, 256.

28. Another event of note that day concerned the transfer of a medic from a famous battleship to the *Mantua*. Two months later, the *Mantua* would return the favor by rescuing most of HMS *Britannia*'s crew and officers, more than seven hundred souls, in chilly waters off the coast of Spain. Torpedoed on the morning of November 9, 1918, the *Britannia* was the last British ship sunk by German U-boats in that particular war. Like the *Mantua*, the *Britannia* and the *Africa* (another battleship then docked at Freetown) would experience massive outbreaks of the flu in September, losing 1.1 percent and 6.6 percent of their crews, respectively. Two more ships making contact with the *Mantua*—the *Tahiti* and the *Chepstow Castle*—would record mortality rates of 5.7 and 3.1 percent that fall, respectively. (Their sailors were likely infected while lending men to help coal other vessels.) These and other shipborne epidemics are considered in a review by G. Dennis Shanks et al., "Determinants of Mortality in Naval Units During the 1918–19 Influenza Pandemic," *The Lancet Infectious Diseases* 11, no. 10 (2011): pp. 793–99.

29. "HMS *Mantua*—March 1915 to January 1919."

30. A medical historian and a medical geographer, analyzing patterns of spread several decades later, observed that "influenza seemed to rage through sub-Saharan Africa as though the colonial transportation network had been planned in

preparation for the pandemic." See K. David Patterson and Gerald F. Pyle, "The Diffusion of Influenza in Sub-Saharan Africa During the 1918–1919 Pandemic," *Social Science and Medicine* 17, no. 17 (1983): p. 1302.

31. Tomkins, "Colonial Administration in British Africa," p. 68.

32. The medical historian Howard Markel and his colleagues offer a nuanced reread-ing of excess mortality in American cities, concluding that "nonpharmaceuti-cal measures," such as school closings and bans on public gatherings, served to lessen influenza's urban toll when deployed promptly and sustained sufficiently. See "Nonpharmaceutical Interventions Implemented by U.S. Cities During the 1918–1919 Influenza Pandemic," *Journal of the American Medical Association* 298, no. 6 (2007): pp. 644–54.

33. Tomkins, "Colonial Administration in British Africa," p. 62.

34. These were the early years of what the medical historian Scott Podolsky has termed "the turbid age of applied immunology." He further notes (in a second and relevant book) that "during the first decades of the twentieth century, a host of im-munological, microbial, and chemotherapeutic agents—from passive serotherapy and active vaccination, through bacteriophage and lactobacillus therapies, to salvarsan and antiparasitics—were administered and advertised in the name of medical science and commerce." See *Pneumonia Before Antibiotics: Therapeutic Evolution and Evaluation in Twentieth-Century America* (Baltimore: Johns Hop-kins University Press, 2006), p. 22; *The Antibiotic Era: Reform, Resistance, and the Pursuit of a Rational Therapeutics* (Baltimore: Johns Hopkins University Press, 2015), p. 11.

35. Tomkins, "Colonial Administration in British Africa," pp. 62, 65.

36. "Isolation Camp Abekun," *Lagos Standard*, October 2, 1918, p. 6; "Influenza in Lagos," *Lagos Standard*, October 2, 1918, p. 4.

37. Tomkins, "Colonial Administration in British Africa," p. 71.

38. By 2011, the claim of rinderpest eradication was made for the region, the con-tinent, and the world. If not gainsaid, this would mark the second time that a public-health eradication claim proved enduring. (Only smallpox has been erad-icated, although poliovirus might not be far behind.) For instructive reviews, see Peter L. Roeder, "Rinderpest: The End of Cattle Plague," *Preventive Veteri-nary Medicine* 102, no. 2 (2011): pp. 98–106; Peter Roeder, Jeffrey Mariner, and Richard Kock, "Rinderpest: The Veterinary Perspective on Eradication," *Phil-osophical Transactions of the Royal Society B: Biological Sciences* 368, no. 1623 (2013): pp. 1–12. The ecologist C. A. Spinage's book *Cattle Plague: A History* (New York: Kluwer Academic/Plenum Publishers, 2003) presents an elaborate study of rinderpest and its social ramifications; many of its chapters are dedicated to the havoc it wreaked in Africa during the late nineteenth and early twentieth centuries.

39. By 1919, residents of Freetown and districts like Karene were (suggests Ismail Rashid) "energized by a common animus against Syrians who they believed limited their access to food. Local and Creole traders had scores to settle with

Syrians who had edged them out in the rice trade. They had been particularly disaffected at what they perceived as unfair trading practices of European firms and Syrians. Europeans, with their financial resources and strong support of the colonial state, seemed unassailable. The Syrians, who were in closer competition and interaction with African traders and producers, presented easier and more vulnerable targets for local animosity." See "Epidemics and Resistance in Colonial Sierra Leone During the First World War," *Canadian Journal of African Studies* 45, no. 3 (2011): p. 430.

40. Rashid, "Epidemics and Resistance," p. 426.
41. Ismail Rashid, "Patterns of Rural Protest: Chiefs, Slaves and Peasants in Northwestern Sierra Leone, 1896–1956" (Ph.D. dissertation, McGill University, 1998), p. 96.
42. Tomkins, "Colonial Administration in British Africa," p. 76.
43. The "popular riots" in Port Loko and in other large towns across the protectorate laid bare, concludes Rashid, "the desperation of different social groups, and their violent negotiation of relationships of power during a moment when the concurrent crises of economy and disease made their survival and social reproduction tenuous. Peasants, slaves, and other subaltern groups resorted to open confrontation with elite groups not only to defend their interests within a communally justified framework but also to force the colonial state to respond effectively to burdens imposed on them" ("Epidemics and Resistance," pp. 428, 434).
44. Rashid, "Epidemics and Resistance," p. 416.
45. These figures are of course disputed, since European-style censuses were unknown in precolonial Africa. This estimate comes from Daniel Noin and Geneviève Decroix, *People on Earth: The Population of Sub-Saharan Africa* (Paris: UNESCO, 2000).
46. "Predicts Big Rise in Rubber Prices: Harvey S. Firestone Says British Restriction Act May Cost American Tire Users $300,000,000," *The New York Times*, April 5, 1925, p. 14.
47. President Calvin Coolidge's secretary of commerce—a former mining engineer named Herbert Hoover—declared in a 1926 testimony before the U.S. Congress that the British rubber monopoly "threatens not only the sane progress of the world but contains in it great dangers to international good will." See United States Congress, *Crude Rubber, Coffee, Etc.: Hearings Before the Committee on Interstate and Foreign Commerce, House of Representatives, Sixty-Ninth Congress, First Session on H. Res. 59* (Washington, D.C.: U.S. Government Printing Office, 1926), p. 2.
48. Gregg Mitman and Paul Erickson, "Latex and Blood: Science, Markets, and American Empire," *Radical History Review*, no. 107 (2010): p. 48.
49. Du Bois, "Liberia, the League and the United States," p. 684.
50. Mitman and Erickson, "Latex and Blood," p. 52.
51. Richard Strong offered the following regarding this facility: "The Government had selected a two-storied house formerly used as a residence in Monrovia, as a

hospital while we were there, and had placed in it a few beds, several of which were occupied by patients in charge of a poorly qualified Liberian physician and Liberian nurse. This apparently is the only gesture that the Liberians have made with reference to the question of hospitalization and the care of the sick." See "Sanitary and Medical Conditions: Prevailing Diseases," in *The African Republic of Liberia and the Belgian Congo: Based on the Observations Made and Material Collected During the Harvard African Expedition, 1926–1927*, edited by Richard P. Strong, volume 1 (Cambridge, Mass.: Harvard University Press, 1930), pp. 198, 199, 200. According to historian Adell Patton, the doctor on display was the first Liberian to receive medical training in the twentieth century. He studied in the United States—at a historically black school, of course, since America's mainstream medical schools (including Harvard's) were largely closed to blacks and to women. The young man had "actually never practiced medicine because the government made him Secretary of Education" upon his return. See "Liberia and Containment Policy Against Colonial Take-Over: Public Health and Sanitation Reform, 1912–1953," *Liberian Studies Journal* 30, no. 2 (2005): p. 42. Patton has also written about the contributions of historically black U.S. medical schools to addressing the dearth of staff on the African continent. Although seven such medical schools were founded after the Civil War, the release of the *Flexner Report* in 1910 prompted the closure of five of them, leaving just Howard University and Meharry Medical College. At around the same time, the British—worried, surmises Patton, by rising nationalist sentiment among African elites, some of whom were foreign-trained doctors—barred natives of their West African colonies from medical training in London and Edinburgh, rendering Howard and Meharry symbolically important to the aspiring African physician. But one reason Patton's review is brief is that these two schools trained a grand total of two Sierra Leonean doctors and twelve Liberian ones during the first half of the twentieth century. See "Howard University and Meharry Medical Schools in the Training of African Physicians, 1868–1978," in *Global Dimensions of the African Diaspora*, edited by Joseph E. Harris (Washington, D.C.: Howard University Press, 1982), pp. 142–62.

52. See, for example, Kristine A. Campbell, "Knots in the Fabric: Richard Pearson Strong and the Bilibid Prison Vaccine Trials, 1905–1906," *Bulletin of the History of Medicine* 68, no. 4 (1994): pp. 600–638.

53. Richard P. Strong, letter to Harvey S. Firestone, November 30, 1926, on board the SS *Wolfram*, retrieved from "A Liberian Journey: History, Memory, and the Making of a Nation," liberianhistory.org/items/show/3633. The Harvard expedition began its work in Liberia in the summer of 1926, spending several months in various parts of the country, including its rural reaches. The team left Monrovia for the mouths of the Congo on a small German cargo boat on November 21 of that year. It was then that Strong posted one of several fulsome letters to Harvey Firestone.

54. Richard P. Strong, Diary, November 8–21, 1926, p. 147, on board the SS *Wolfram*, retrieved from "A Liberian Journey."

55. Richard P. Strong, "Some Problems Concerning the Welfare of the People," in *The African Republic of Liberia and the Belgian Congo*, volume 1, p. 206.

56. The League found Liberia's president responsible for (in Graham Greene's words) "shipping forced labour to the little dreadful Spanish island, Fernando Po, and for countenancing the mild form of slavery that enabled a man to pawn his children." See *Journey Without Maps*, reprint edition (New York: Penguin Books, 2006), p. 102. The Harvard student newspaper, in reporting on the expedition, was more anodyne: "Conditions closely akin to slavery are existent; but do not present a serious problem. Captives of war are kept in slavery until they are redeemed by ransom." Like the expedition's faculty lead, the students editing the paper were cheerleaders for the Firestone deal. See "'Liberia Would Benefit by American Intervention,' Declares R. P. Strong," *Harvard Crimson*, October 21, 1930, thecrimson.com/article/1930/10/21/liberia-would-benefit-by-american-intervention. For an extended consideration of the slavery scandal, see I. K. Sundiata, *Black Scandal: America and the Liberian Labor Crisis, 1929–1936* (Philadelphia: Institute for the Study of Human Issues, 1980).

57. Raymond Leslie Buell, *The Native Problem in Africa*, volume 2 (New York: Macmillan, 1928), p. 845.

58. Du Bois, "Liberia, the League and the United States," p. 685.

59. Du Bois, "Liberia, the League and the United States," pp. 685–86.

60. Along with a handful of nuns of similar provenance, the Episcopal monks from the Order of the Holy Cross sought (wrote Junge) "to be a nucleus round which helpless and fear-stricken human beings might, as it were, coagulate and crystallize, and also to be a light to lighten that darkness which since time began has brooded beneath the dense forest roof of this part of Liberia." See *African Jungle Doctor: Ten Years in Liberia*, translated by Basil Creighton (London: George G. Harrap, 1952), p. 17.

61. Junge, *African Jungle Doctor*, pp. 16, 33.

62. John Barkham, "A Medico in the Fear-Filled Jungle," *The New York Times*, October 12, 1952, p. BR6.

63. Junge, *African Jungle Doctor*, p. 35.

64. Junge, *African Jungle Doctor*, p. 101. Graham and Barbara Greene missed Werner Junge by a couple of years, but met his shamelessly healthy assistant in Bolahun and again, unexpectedly, in Freetown as he was leaving abruptly for Germany. Barbara Greene attributed his departure to a self-inflicted wound; the Episcopal monk then leading the mission would note only that the younger doctor was "smitten." See Robert Erskine Campbell, *Within the Green Wall: The Story of Holy Cross Liberia Mission, 1922–1957* (West Park: Holy Cross Press, 1957), p. 120.

65. Junge, *African Jungle Doctor*, pp. 86, 96.

66. Matters got worse for W.E.B. Du Bois during the red scares of the fifties and after. Given his massive scholarly output, decades of incisive commentary, and long embrace of pragmatic solidarity, Du Bois should have been treated as the vener-

able old man he was when, in 1961, he "applied for a membership in the Communist Party. Fearing that the state might again restrict his ability to travel, he made plans to move to Accra . . . On his ninety-fifth birthday in February 1963, he became a citizen of Ghana . . . 'largely because the American embassy refused to renew his passport.'" See Bill V. Mullen, *Un-American: W.E.B. Du Bois and the Century of World Revolution* (Philadelphia: Temple University Press, 2015), p. 188.

67. Du Bois, "Liberia, the League and the United States," p. 695.

68. George Schwab, *Tribes of the Liberian Hinterland*, edited by George W. Harley (Cambridge, Mass.: Peabody Museum of American Archaeology and Ethnology, Harvard University, 1947), p. 245. The essentializing and static nature of such observations—the following beliefs are registered among the Grebo and Sapo, these comportments are seen among the Kpelle, Kru, and Mano, et cetera—has been picked apart, sometimes savagely, by subsequent generations of anthropologists.

69. Etta Donner, *Hinterland Liberia*, translated by Winifred M. Deans (London: Blackie & Son, 1939), p. 244.

70. Just about everyone writing about Liberia at the time made reference to cannibalism. Etta Donner, for example, claimed to have "always known that the Kran people were cannibals until recently" (*Hinterland Liberia*, p. 261). Without evident fear of lawsuits, one of the Boston Brahmins from the Harvard expedition was pleased to confide to the grandees of the Royal Geographic Society that he once found "a fresh human thigh-bone lying beside the trail." See George C. Shattuck, "Liberia and the Belgian Congo," *The Geographical Journal* 73, no. 3 (1929): p. 225. There remained a good deal of confusion about the terms of the debate, with "cannibalism" still standing in for accusations of ritual murder. A reflective Catholic like Greene might have referred to his own creed's rituals of body and blood, even if some Protestants remained focused on more literal interpretations. Werner Junge wasn't one of them, even after he was called to perform an autopsy on one young victim, her liver removed with surgical skill uncommon among leopards: the righteous doctor didn't go far in his recounting without referring to Isaac's near miss at the hand of Abraham. For Junge's conclusions about the logic of such murders, see *African Jungle Doctor*, pp. 161–87.

71. The rail was imported, but the platelayers who laid it were local, underpaid, and underfed. "Workers of the World Unite," Greene scoffed upon contemplating this labor force. "I thought of the wide shallow slogans of political parties, as the thin bodies, every rib showing with dangling swollen elbows or pock-marked skin, went by me to the market; why should we pretend to talk in terms of the world when we mean only Europe or the white races? Neither the Independent Labour Party nor Communist Party urges a strike in England because the platelayers in Sierra Leone are paid sixpence a day without their food. Civilization here remained exploitation; we had hardly, it seemed to me, improved the natives' lot

at all, they were as worn out with fever as before the white man came, we had introduced new diseases and weakened their resistance to the old, they still drank from polluted water and suffered from the same worms" (*Journey Without Maps*, pp. 34, 53, 56–57).

72. Americans sent in to dress Liberia's economic wounds did not hesitate to describe themselves as healers. In this respect, they embraced the colonial instrumentalism of tropical medicine, as the historians Gregg Mitman and Paul Erickson note in an extended discussion of the influence of the era's economic ideologies on the Harvard expedition: "These financial missionaries healed 'sick' economies, rid the body politic of inflation, and restored financial order to promote economic health and well-being. Strong similarly expressed the belief that the medical and biological knowledge they gathered—from the pervasiveness of malaria, to the ecology of onchocerciasis (river blindness), to the transmission vectors of yellow fever—would 'bring great benefit to the country and redound to the welfare of its people.' Understanding tropical relations that led to diseased landscapes and people constituted but a first step in reordering those relationships to generate more 'productive' lands" ("Latex and Blood," pp. 53–54).

73. In 1906, the British geographer Harry Johnston termed Liberia "the least known part of Africa." Richard Strong, citing the same source and others, averred the same to be true twenty years later. But a few of the likes of the Greene cousins— upper-crust Britons with a taste for adventure—had written histories or travelogues about the black republic. In 1926, a certain Lady Dorothy Mills, daughter of the Earl of Oxford, published *Through Liberia*. (It was "full of the effortless insouciance of the early white outsider in Africa," according to the journalist Tim Butcher.) The Greenes traveled in a style not unlike Lady Dorothy, who—taking notes while being toted across Liberia in a hammock hoisted by porters—found Liberia's climate to be "quite healthy as long as you have a well proofed and ventilated house, and do not go out in the heat of the day, and do not take a stroke of unnecessary exercise except in the very early morning maybe, or during the hour before sundown to give you zest for your cocktail and cold bath." See Harry Johnston, *Liberia*, volume 1 (London: Hutchinson, 1906), p. 8; Dorothy Mills, *Through Liberia* (London: Duckworth, 1926), p. 170; Tim Butcher, *Chasing the Devil: The Search for Africa's Fighting Spirit* (London: Chatto & Windus, 2010), p. 19.

74. One 770-carat "stone of high quality," was recovered, notes the British geologist J. D. Pollett, from the "rich gravels of the Woyie River" in January 1945. Writing of the real colony, as opposed to Greene's fictional one, Pollett would note with pride that the "production of diamond during the war amounted to nearly 4.75 million carats and of this not a single parcel was lost by enemy action during transit to the United Kingdom." See "The Geology and Mineral Resources of Sierra Leone," *Colonial Geology and Mineral Resources* 2, no. 1 (1951): p. 19. Greene lets history and political economy work their way into the backdrop—like the na-

tives, who carry on separate and mysteriously complex lives, as any colonial police commissioner would know. Scobie placates his wife after learning he will not, after fifteen years in the force, be promoted to police commissioner: "You know, dear, in a place like this in war-time—an important harbour—the Vichy French just across the border—all this diamond smuggling from the Protectorate—they need a younger man." See *The Heart of the Matter* (New York: Viking Press, 1948), pp. 19–20.

75. Greg Campbell, *Blood Diamonds: Tracing the Deadly Path of the World's Most Precious Stones*, revised edition (New York: Basic Books, 2012), pp. 12, 31.

76. British Government Blue Book, quoted in Graham Greene, *Journey Without Maps*, p. 13.

77. Patton, "Liberia and Containment Policy Against Colonial Take-Over," p. 41.

78. The difference did not involve fire, according to the Blue Book, which Graham Greene cites: "The soldiers crept into the banana plantations, which surround all native villages, and poured volleys into the huts. One woman who had that day been delivered of twins was shot in her bed, and the infants perished in the flames when the village was fired by the troops" (*Journey Without Maps*, pp. 13–14).

79. Graham Greene, *Journey Without Maps*, p. 14. On the strength of the slavery claims, see I. K. Sundiata's *Black Scandal*. As for Greene's sarcasm about the "little injustices of Kenya," Caroline Elkins's *Imperial Reckoning: The Untold Story of Britain's Gulag in Kenya* (New York: Henry Holt, 2005) reveals they weren't little at all. Tim Butcher's 350-mile trek, undertaken seventy-five years after the Greenes', is chronicled in *Chasing the Devil*. He retraced the Greenes' steps after the civil wars of the late twentieth century laid waste to many of the villages and towns they described. Turning to the archives of the Anti-Slavery and Aborigines Protection Society, he finds evidence that Greene's trip to Liberia was at least blessed by London's leading abolitionist society. Greene's publisher paid the bills, which were more modest than might be imagined given the size of his entourage.

80. Graham Greene, *Journey Without Maps*, pp. 76, 75–76.

81. It bears noting that the number of helpers was small when compared to the Harvard expedition, which often counted 250 porters. The other practicing physician on the expedition, a Bostonian from a long line of doctors, declared himself astounded by the porters' honesty and by their willingness to be paid with tobacco in lieu of West African shillings. But the private journals of a couple of the gentlemen from Harvard reveal their porters were sometimes physically coerced: forty of them bolted in a single night. Greene's coercion stopped at begging, bribing, and cajoling, and the men in his employ accompanied him through thick and thin, jungle and bush, colony and republic. Werner Junge likewise describes porters as West Africa's unsung heroes, even when he admits to frustration with some of their methods, and their incessant dunning.

82. Paul Theroux, introduction to Graham Greene, *Journey Without Maps*, p. xvi.

83. Graham Greene, *Journey Without Maps*, p. 164.

84. How, then, did George Harley come by at least 391 of these masks? Monni Adams, a former curator at the Peabody Museum, asks a better question about the collection she curated: "Why were people selling their sacred masks in such large quantities during that particular time period, and under what conditions were they selling?" Adams reviews testimony from Harley, his wife, and their son, as well as reports from the thirties and subsequent work of anthropologists who study Liberia. Her sources suggest that conditions were far from propitious for the sellers, who were often desperate for Liberia's official currency in order to pay taxes. Failure to do so entailed severe penalties, which included "beatings, confinement in public stocks in the sun all day, burning down villages." See "Both Sides of the Collecting Encounter: The George W. Harley Collection at the Peabody Museum of Archaeology and Ethnology, Harvard University," *Museum Anthropology* 32, no. 1 (2009): pp. 17, 23.

85. Graham Greene, *Journey Without Maps*, pp. 164, 165, 170. In an essay published by Harvard's Peabody Museum a few years after the Greenes' visit, Harley reported that "initiatory rituals are conducted more or less in secret in a secluded part of the forest, though in some tribes the ceremonies are not only public, but even witnessed nowadays by women." Among other groups, however, Harley alleged that ceremonies were so secret that "both peepers and informers" would likely face the death penalty. See his *Notes on the Poro in Liberia* (Cambridge, Mass.: Peabody Museum of American Archaeology and Ethnology, Harvard University, 1941), pp. 3, 5.

86. The Americo-Liberians, wrote Monni Adams, "pursued a program of destroying the cult houses in the sacred forest grove, where the elders met and where they had stored their masks" ("Both Sides of the Collecting Encounter," p. 27). Such repression failed to eradicate the cults, which had little to do with cannibalism but plenty to do with surviving in difficult environments.

87. "The school and the devil who rules over it are at first a terror to the child," Graham Greene wrote. "It lies as grimly as a public school in England between childhood and manhood" (*Journey Without Maps*, p. 85). Richard Strong drew similar conclusions: "In spite of statements to the contrary, the great majority of adult natives, even in the interior of Liberia, do not stand in great fear or awe of the devil who presides over the boys' bush school, and do not regard him as a supernatural being." See "Tribal Customs," in *The African Republic of Liberia and the Belgian Congo*, volume 1, p. 86.

88. "I am no anthropologist," observed Barbara Greene as she struggled unsuccessfully to pay attention to Harley, "and I could only think, with the same forgetfulness of good English as Alice in Wonderland, that everything was getting 'curiouser and curiouser.'" See *Too Late to Turn Back: Barbara and Graham Greene in Liberia*, reprint edition (London: Settle and Bendall, 1981), pp. 121, 120, 121.

89. Paul Theroux, introduction to Barbara Greene, *Too Late to Turn Back*, p. xxv. Theroux is referring to passages such as one in which Barbara Greene recounts

her attempts to describe her hometown to a scarcely literate rural teacher: "The London I had described of crowds, and hurrying motor vehicles, noise and underground trains, that was terrifying. It all sounded horrible, and I almost felt that I did not want to go back—till, of course, I remembered Elizabeth Arden, my flat, and the Savoy Grill." The whole of Barbara Greene's memoir, reissued in 1981, is without pretense. "I knew perfectly well," she wrote, "that my journey through Liberia would bring no benefit whatsoever to humanity, and that certainly we would contribute nothing new to the scientific world. We were even incapable of describing the birds and plants that we saw, and had no idea if they were really rare and strange" (*Too Late to Turn Back*, pp. 147–48, 43).

90. Barbara Greene, *Too Late to Turn Back*, p. 90.

91. Harley was himself prey to a growing fear of the furtive workings of that gloom, terming these aspects of the Poro and other societies "frightfulness." In the eyes of his successors at the mission, his intense anxiety belied his claims that "the more cruel ceremonies, especially those involving human sacrifice, no longer occurred in the region" (Butcher, *Chasing the Devil*, p. 250). Tim Butcher spent time in the company of one of these successors, a Canadian missionary who also lived in Ganta for decades. He opined that Harley whitewashed his accounts in order to remain in Liberia.

92. Graham Greene, *Journey Without Maps*, p. 103.

93. Werner Junge's young wife, also German, was a rare exception. Her life was likely saved when she received newly developed sulphonamides to treat sepsis stemming from a soft-tissue infection. Junge describes his campaigns to use these miracle drugs to cure gonorrhea and other infections and to discredit those traditional healers who, in his view, bilked the destitute sick. He was especially outraged by deaths during childbirth, and spent years fighting to train local midwives. Although his efforts have been largely forgotten—or supplanted by a disturbing relativism regarding "local" traditions and "traditional" birth attendants—these deaths would have been much reduced by obstetrics and gynecology, had its practitioners (including nurse-midwives) and their supporting staff and stuff been in evidence.

94. When the League of Nations issued a fifty-page report of their investigation of the matter, added Du Bois, "only one-third of a page is devoted to the question of slavery, practically the whole report being on economic conditions and the Firestone contract." If he went a bit far in his defense of the Monrovia elite, the American sociologist cast a gimlet eye on other colonial administrators in West Africa. "Labor supply for modern industry in Africa always tends to approximate slavery because it is bound up with the clan organization of the tribes," Du Bois wrote in 1933. "Black Senegalese troops 'volunteered' for the French Army during the World War; that means that chiefs were induced to designate black soldiers for use in the World War, but it does not mean that these individuals necessarily wanted to go" ("Liberia, the League and the United States," pp. 689, 687). While this strikes the postcolonial reader as spot-on, uncritical support of the Americo-Liberians of the day does not. The political scientist Cedric Robinson explains that "Du

Bois and many other prominent intellectuals drawn from the Black middle class of the late nineteenth and early twentieth centuries recited from the same ideological catechism. With respect to Liberia, however, their most fundamental conceptual error was mistaking it for a nation-state." See "Du Bois and Black Sovereignty: The Case of Liberia," *Race and Class* 32, no. 2 (1990): p. 41.

95. Before his own career as a jungle doctor was cut short by Hitler's war, Junge reported that the League's decline improved his own prospects of collaboration with Liberian officials in efforts to stem yellow fever, smallpox, and leprosy, since failure to stem epidemics had long been cited as another reason for the "international community" of the era—with, in principle, the League of Nations its interwar court of last resort—to take over management of the black republic.

96. The *New York Times* review of his memoir reported Junge to be practicing surgery in Stuttgart, where he "dreams of Bolahun" (Barkham, "A Medico in the Fear-Filled Jungle," p. BR6).

97. John B. West, "United States Health Missions in Liberia," *Public Health Reports* 63, no. 42 (1948): p. 1351.

98. West, "United States Health Missions in Liberia," pp. 1352, 1351.

99. Scobie, the novel's protagonist, is drawn toward a young compatriot widowed on her honeymoon when her ship is sunk by a U-boat far out in the Atlantic. The girl—she looks like a child—is clutching her stamp collection when brought ashore near the border with French Guinea. "Here's a complete set of Liberians surcharged for the American occupation," says a character trying to cheer the widow with a contribution to her soggy collection. "I got those from the Naval Observer" (Greene, *The Heart of the Matter*, p. 166). No need for Greene to belabor the obvious—there's an American occupation next door and Scobie, too, will ply the widow with stamps. She's young enough to be his daughter, the heart of the matter for a father who's lost his own.

100. See Eugene T. Richardson et al., "Biosocial Approaches to the 2013–2016 Ebola Pandemic," *Health and Human Rights* 18, no. 1 (2016): pp. 115–28.

101. Even after the subsequent expulsion of an estimated 45,000 "black foreigners" from Kono District, Koidu town counted 14,309 inhabitants. See Roy Maconachie, "Diamond Mining, Urbanisation and Social Transformation in Sierra Leone," *Journal of Contemporary African Studies* 30, no. 4 (2012): pp. 710–11.

102. Guillaume Lachenal, "Outbreak of Unknown Origin in the Tripoint Zone," *Limn*, January 2015, limn.it/outbreak-of-unknown-origin-in-the-tripoint-zone. Numbers vary, as ever, and there's plenty of evidence—including Thomas Winterbottom's detailed descriptions from 1803—that sleeping sickness was not new to Sierra Leone. See *An Account of the Native Africans in the Neighbourhood of Sierra Leone*, volume 2 (London: C. Whittingham, 1803), pp. 29–31.

103. Although West African trypanosomiasis is epidemiologically and clinically distinct from its East African variant, British officials across the continent were still haunted by memories of the apocalyptic epidemic in Uganda mentioned earlier in this chapter. From 1900 to 1920, it was estimated that more than 250,000

people died in an epidemic that affected the southern part of the country, with the Busoga region particularly hard-hit. See Eric M. Fèvre et al., "Reanalyzing the 1900–1920 Sleeping Sickness Epidemic in Uganda," *Emerging Infectious Diseases* 10, no. 4 (2004): p. 567. In contrast to East African trypanosomiasis, which mostly infects trypanotolerant antelopes and related wildlife—as well as decidedly less tolerant cattle and, as French military veterinarians learned in Morocco, camels—the West African disease predominantly afflicts humans.

104. The history of clinical trials begins much earlier with serotherapies and other biologic agents, as the physician-historian Scott Podolsky notes: "Antipneumo-coccal serotherapy had itself been deemed revolutionary in the very years and months immediately preceding (and often accompanying) the arrival of the sulfa drugs. Founded on the tenets of applied immunology, justified by controlled clinical trials, and grounded in a novel public health ethos, it had supplanted traditional physiology-based supportive therapeutics as the ideal mode of attack on pneumonia. As such, chemotherapeutics and antibiotics, with their own at-tendant dangers and side effects, were perceived as attractive alternative specif-ics rather than as revolutionary approaches to the conquest of pneumonia. Even when the cheaper sulfa drugs ultimately appeared as efficacious as serotherapy, a several-year transition ensued during which serotherapy was placed first along-side chemotherapeutics as a component of a presumably ideal 'combination' ther-apy and later as a critical backup to the sulfa drugs. Only with the widespread advent of penicillin by the end of World War II would antipneumococcal sero-therapy ultimately disappear" (*Pneumonia Before Antibiotics*, p. 7).

105. R. D. Harding and M. P. Hutchinson, "Sleeping Sickness of an Unusual Type in Sierra Leone and Its Attempted Control," *Transactions of the Royal Society of Tropical Medicine and Hygiene* 41, no. 4 (1948): p. 482.

106. The abbreviation FBH is their own, I swear it. The researchers further note that the tsetse flies' other potential snacks, "such as game, crocodiles, and smaller mammals and reptiles suitable for food, are rarely seen and must be largely nocturnal in their habits, while few domestic animals except goats are kept by the local inhabitants. Man is therefore a very important, perhaps the most important, source of food, at any rate at the numerous points of contact adjoining villages and farms" (Harding and Hutchinson, "Sleeping Sickness of an Unusual Type in Sierra Leone," pp. 483, 484). Even if the tsetse fly is not quite so promiscuous in its feeding habits as the British doctors believed, it certainly loves a human blood meal, whether from man or boy. In a later article, the same authors offer a positive update, excepting a couple of new cases of trypanosomiasis among fly-boys as a result of occupational ex-posure. See "Mass Prophylaxis Against Sleeping Sickness in Sierra Leone: Final Report," *Transactions of the Royal Society of Tropical Medicine and Hygiene* 43, no. 5 (1950): pp. 503–512. On the feeding habits of the tsetse fly, see Catherine N. Muturi et al., "Tracking the Feeding Patterns of Tsetse Flies (*Glossina* Genus) by Analysis of Bloodmeals Using Mitochondrial Cytochromes Genes," *PLOS ONE* 6, no. 2 (2011): p. e17284.

107. "At Kailahun there is no railway and no telegraph," wrote Graham Greene. "To communicate with Freetown the Commissioner must send a messenger the eighteen miles to Pendembu. It is difficult to understand what control he has over the border; natives pass freely to and fro; indeed with a little care it would be possible to travel all down West Africa without showing papers from the moment of landing. There is something very attractive in this great patch of 'freedom to travel'; absconding financiers might do worse than take to the African bush" (*Journey Without Maps*, p. 57). Decades later, many shadowy figures in finance and trafficking—of diamonds, other mineral wealth, drugs, weapons, timber, and coerced labor—seem to have reached similar conclusions. So, in a sense, did the Ebola virus.

108. Harding and Hutchinson, "Sleeping Sickness of an Unusual Type in Sierra Leone," p. 486.

109. Lachenal, "Outbreak of Unknown Origin in the Tripoint Zone."

110. Myron Echenberg, *Black Death, White Medicine: Bubonic Plague and the Politics of Public Health in Colonial Senegal, 1914–1945* (Portsmouth, N.H.: Heinemann, 2002), pp. 92, 211.

111. See West, "United States Health Missions in Liberia," p. 1352; Patton, "Liberia and Containment Policy Against Colonial Take-Over," p. 51.

112. Ismail Rashid, "Decolonization and Popular Contestation in Sierra Leone: The Peasant War of 1955–1956," *Afrika Zamani*, no. 17 (2009): p. 116.

113. *Unmasking the State*, the anthropologist Mike McGovern's study of the complex fluidity of Guinean social identity—subtitled *Making Guinea Modern*—is pertinent to understanding these decades. McGovern takes up the task of finding the large-scale in the local, locating in current events the echoes of the Atlantic slave trade and the more recent "competing cosmopolitanisms" of four state powers. The first was a late nineteenth-century polity that developed in the region under the influence of the "conqueror and proselytizer" Samory Touré; the second, the French colonial state; the third, the postcolonial state—declared socialist and pan-Africanist by the long-governing Sékou Touré; the fourth, the postsocialist state led by Colonel Lansana Conté, who took the reins in a 1984 coup d'état and sat in Touré's seat until 2008. See *Unmasking the State: Making Guinea Modern* (Chicago: University of Chicago Press, 2013), pp. 5, 4.

114. The eaves of the forest—the trizone area yet again—became the chief battleground of the culture wars that followed Guinea's declaration of independence. The demystification campaign "focused to a large degree on the polytheistic periphery of a country that had become about 80 percent Muslim and 10 percent Christian by the end of colonialism" (*Unmasking the State*, p. 5). The research on which Mike McGovern's study is based was conducted among Loma speakers in Macenta District, the heart of the rain forest–savanna frontier.

115. Stephen Ellis, *The Mask of Anarchy: The Destruction of Liberia and the Religious Dimension of an African Civil War* (New York: New York University Press, 1999), p. 49.

116. In the political scientist Lansana Gberie's assessment of Margai and his successors, the torch was passed from "a decent leader whose gradualist policy helped the country develop steadily in the 1960s, to the utterly corrupt and destructive Siaka Stevens, whose policies eroded the state's machinery and legitimacy and led to the collapse of much of its institutions, and then to Joseph Momoh, under whose ineffectual leadership the country was plunged into war in 1991." See *A Dirty War in West Africa: The RUF and the Destruction of Sierra Leone* (Bloomington: Indiana University Press, 2005), p. 4. Arthur Abraham paints a similar picture. If the country experienced sustained economic growth and low unemployment in the first decade after independence, "an adverse trend began when Siaka Stevens, leader of the All People's Congress party, in control of the state after winning elections as opposition leader, began assiduously to establish personal rule, eliminating all forms of opposition and over-centralising power in his own hands." See Abraham's essay, "Dancing with the Chameleon: Sierra Leone and the Elusive Quest for Peace," *Journal of Contemporary African Studies* 19, no. 2 (2001): p. 206. Scholars from other disciplines reach similar conclusions. "As diamonds became a strategic political tool for Siaka Stevens' All People's Congress government," observes the political economist Roy Maconachie, "the diamond sector became a sphere of unregulated private enterprise, eventually leading to state collapse and mass internal population displacement" ("Diamond Mining, Urbanisation and Social Transformation," p. 708).

117. See Fred M. Hayward, "The Development of a Radical Political Organization in the Bush: A Case Study in Sierra Leone," *Canadian Journal of African Studies* 6, no. 1 (1972): pp. 1–28.

118. Akyeampong, "Disease in West African History," p. 202.

119. See, for example, Sheik Humarr Khan et al., "New Opportunities for Field Research on the Pathogenesis and Treatment of Lassa Fever," *Antiviral Research* 78, no. 1 (2008): pp. 103–115; Jeffrey G. Shaffer et al., "Lassa Fever in Post-Conflict Sierra Leone," *PLOS Neglected Tropical Diseases* 8, no. 3 (2014): p. e2748; Randal J. Schoepp et al., "Undiagnosed Acute Viral Febrile Illnesses, Sierra Leone," *Emerging Infectious Diseases* 20, no. 7 (2014): pp. 1176–82.

120. Myron Echenberg, *Africa in the Time of Cholera: A History of Pandemics from 1817 to the Present* (Cambridge, U.K.: Cambridge University Press, 2011), pp. 114, 112. Echenberg's works are scholarly, far-ranging, and reliably revelatory.

121. See Donald R. Hopkins et al., "Smallpox in Sierra Leone: I. Epidemiology," *The American Journal of Tropical Medicine and Hygiene* 20, no. 5 (1971): pp. 689–96; Donald R. Hopkins et al., "Smallpox in Sierra Leone: II. The 1968–69 Eradication Program," *The American Journal of Tropical Medicine and Hygiene* 20, no. 5 (1971): pp. 697–704.

122. Donald G. McNeil Jr., "Using a Tactic Unseen in a Century, Countries Cordon Off Ebola-Racked Areas," *The New York Times*, August 12, 2014, nytimes.com /2014/08/13/science/using-a-tactic-unseen-in-a-century-countries-cordon-off

-ebola-racked-areas.html. McNeil, one of the best and most careful medical reporters out there, is referring to the abandonment of such tactics in Europe and North America. The contrary observation regarding West Africa is from Annie Wilkinson and Melissa Leach, "Briefing: Ebola—Myths, Realities, and Structural Violence," *African Affairs* 114, no. 454 (2015): p. 143.

123. See C. Magbaily Fyle, "The State and Health Services in Sierra Leone," in *The State and the Provision of Social Services in Sierra Leone Since Independence, 1961-91*, edited by C. Magbaily Fyle (Dakar: Council for the Development of Social Science Research in Africa, 1993), pp. 44-61.

124. Donald R. Hopkins et al., "Two Funeral-Associated Smallpox Outbreaks in Sierra Leone," *American Journal of Epidemiology* 94, no. 4 (1971): pp. 342, 344.

125. Hopkins et al., "Two Funeral-Associated Smallpox Outbreaks," p. 347.

126. For a piercing analysis of related phenomena elsewhere in Africa, see the volume edited by Jean and John Comaroff, *Millennial Capitalism and the Culture of Neoliberalism* (Durham: Duke University Press, 2001). In a 1999 article in *American Ethnologist*, the Comaroffs observe that "postcolonial South Africa, like other postrevolutionary societies, appears to have witnessed a dramatic rise in occult economies: in the deployment, real or imagined, of magical means for material ends. These embrace a wide range of phenomena, from 'ritual murder,' the sale of body parts, and the putative production of zombies to pyramid schemes and other financial scams. They've led, in many places, to violent reactions against people accused of illicit accumulation." See "Occult Economies and the Violence of Abstraction: Notes from the South African Postcolony," *American Ethnologist* 26, no. 2 (1999): p. 279; their related essay, "Alien-Nation: Zombies, Immigrants, and Millennial Capitalism," *South Atlantic Quarterly* 101, no. 4 (2002): pp. 779-805; and, for some instructive (and entertaining) precursors, historian Luise White's *Speaking with Vampires: Rumor and History in Colonial Africa* (Berkeley: University of California Press, 2000).

127. James Brooke, "Ritual Killing Brings Arrest of 6 Liberians," *The New York Times*, May 4, 1987, p. A11.

128. "The Talk of the Town: Our Own Baedeker," *The New Yorker*, November 29, 1947, p. 36.

129. Fred van der Kraaij, "The Maryland Ritual Murders: Maryland County 1977," *Ritual Killings—Past and Present: From Cultural Phenomenon to Political Instrument*, liberiapastandpresent.org/MarylandRitualMurders02.htm.

130. Fred van der Kraaij, "The Ritualistic Murder of Moses Tweh," *Ritual Killings*, liberiapastandpresent.org/MarylandRitualMurders04.htm. (Formatting altered.)

131. "The crowd kept silent, for at least another 10 minutes," relates van der Kraaij. "Then the people started talking again, louder and louder, until it was back at its normal volume." His description of the ensuing street party has the air of verisimilitude: "There was drumming and dancing in the streets after the public execution of the convicted ritual killers. The crowd was singing and shouting slogans. They thus expressed their sense of happiness and relief." See "The Hanging," *Ritual*

Killings, liberiapastandpresent.org/MarylandRitualMurders09.htm; "After the Hanging," *Ritual Killings*, liberiapastandpresent.org/MarylandRitualMurders10.htm.

132. Van der Kraaij, "After the Hanging."

133. Julius W. Walker, the U.S. chargé d'affaires in Liberia from 1978 to 1981, is quoted in Niels Hahn, "U.S. Covert and Overt Operations in Liberia, 1970s to 2003," *ASPJ Africa and Francophonie* 5, no. 3 (2014): p. 22.

134. In a later declassified cable from the U.S. ambassador to his superiors in Washington, the envoy complains that only four of the thirteen officials were to be executed, but the new government added nine more and "then destroyed the records of the Tribunal." (Ambassador Robert Smith is quoted in Hahn, "U.S. Covert and Overt Operations in Liberia," p. 21.)

135. Ronald Reagan later received Samuel Doe in the White House. The exceedingly pro-American assassin, ostensibly then preparing for the election of a civilian president, seemed not to mind when the absent-minded leader of the free world referred to him as "Chairman Moe." Within two years of the coup, U.S. aid to tiny Liberia had sextupled when compared with what Tolbert had received. By 1985, Doe's Liberia had received an estimated $500 million in U.S. aid—more than any other nation in sub-Saharan Africa.

136. Van der Kraaij, "After the Hanging." Fred van der Kraaij continued formal training in economics after the war pushed him out of Liberia, and spent the rest of his career with Dutch development agencies and at the World Bank. Whether or not he was a believer in the voodoo economics of the day, van der Kraaij's experience in Harper fanned a keen interest in the history of the region, including Dutch participation in the transatlantic slave trade. But more striking to van der Kraaij than remote historical resonances was the unprecedented nature of the arrest, trials, and conviction of such prominent members of the Americo-Liberian elite: "People who seemed to be untouchable were accused, arrested, even convicted, and finally executed. This had never happened before in the Republic" ("Maryland County 1977").

137. Brooke, "Ritual Killing Brings Arrest of 6 Liberians," p. A11.

8. THINGS FALL APART

1. In his study of "how young men in Sierra Leone and Liberia are made available for often violent forms of labor," Danny Hoffman argues that "we should treat the conflict on both sides of the border between Sierra Leone and Liberia as a single, continuous war, one that exceeds the time frames normally cited for these conflicts (1989–1996 and 2000–2003 in Liberia, 1991–2002 in Sierra Leone)." See *The War Machines: Young Men and Violence in Sierra Leone and Liberia* (Durham, N.C.: Duke University Press, 2011), pp. xi, xxi.

2. Richards allows that his "essay on the early part of the war, drafted in January 1993, is guilty of adding some fuel to this anarchist fire." See *Fighting for the Rain Forest: War, Youth and Resources in Sierra Leone* (Oxford, U.K.: James

Currey, 1996), p. xvii. The essay to which he refers is "Rebellion in Liberia and Sierra Leone: A Crisis of Youth?," in *Conflict in Africa*, edited by Oliver Furley (London: Tauris Academic Studies, 1995), pp. 134–70. Greed-versus-grievance frameworks were posited to better understand why these and other conflicts erupted across the continent, from Horn to Cape, during the last quarter of the twentieth century. See, for example, Paul Collier and Anke Hoeffler, "Greed and Grievance in Civil War," *Oxford Economic Papers* 56, no. 4 (2004): pp. 563–95; Mats Berdal and David M. Malone, eds., *Greed and Grievance: Economic Agendas in Civil Wars* (Boulder, Colo.: Lynne Rienner Publishers, 2000).

3. The political scientist Sahr Kpundeh advanced a hybrid case: "Although the insurgency arose because of a deep-seated *grievance* held by the RUF leaders and their 'backers' to rid Sierra Leone of the corrupt and incompetent APC government, *greed* was a major motivating factor for the insurgency because the RUF aspired to wealth through capturing the resources of the country extra-legally, and ultimately the machinery of the government." See his essay, "Corruption and Political Insurgency in Sierra Leone," in *Between Democracy and Terror: The Sierra Leone Civil War*, edited by Ibrahim Abdullah (Dakar: Council for the Development of Social Science Research in Africa, 2004), p. 91. In *Civil War and Democracy in West Africa: Conflict Resolution, Elections and Justice in Sierra Leone and Liberia* (New York: I.B. Tauris, 2012), David Harris offers a book-length consideration of the mixed results of multiparty elections in West Africa during these wars, and explores the greed-versus-grievance framework in some detail. So do Danny Hoffman, in several of the works cited here, and David Keen, in *Conflict and Collusion in Sierra Leone* (Oxford, U.K.: James Currey, 2005). For an overview of these debates, see Yusuf Bangura, "The Political and Cultural Dynamics of the Sierra Leone War," in *Between Democracy and Terror*, pp. 13–40.

4. "The war easily took on an ethnic character," Lansana Gberie explains, "with the Gio and Mano peoples rallying to Taylor's NPFL (even though Taylor himself was a member of the Americo-Liberian elite), and the Krahn and Mandingo peoples rallying to Doe. Ethnic violence and massacres became a commonplace, and by the mid-1990s, the war had killed tens of thousands of Liberians, almost all of them civilians targeted largely because of their ethnicity." See *A Dirty War in West Africa: The RUF and the Destruction of Sierra Leone* (Bloomington: Indiana University Press, 2005), p. 56.

5. "Whether it is based on ethnicity, age, nation, or faction," writes Danny Hoffman, "identity in the Mano River region, as elsewhere in the African postcolony, was flexible enough that most people could comfortably—and productively—inhabit those moments in which identities came into conflict." See "Violence, Just in Time: War and Work in Contemporary West Africa," *Cultural Anthropology* 26, no. 1 (2011): p. 41.

6. The Mano River conflict was not, Danny Hoffman argues, an identitarian war: "To privilege the identity fixing potential in violence risks erasing one of the

most important dynamics in Africa today: the productive ways in which African subjects live with multiple fragmented and often contradictory identities. And it obscures one of the most fascinating—and again, troubling—dynamics of the Mano River war in particular: the identification many militia fighters had with the so-called enemy, identifications that transected lines of ethnicity and solidified around a shared sense that fighters from all factions were marginal youth and political outsiders" ("Violence, Just in Time," p. 37.).

7. Writing in 2000, Sebastian Junger cites the United States Geologic Survey, which estimates Liberian diamond potential at fewer than 150,000 carats a year. The Belgian Diamond High Council—"charged with evaluating diamond imports and certifying their country of origin"—reported exports from Liberia "averaging six million carats a year between 1994 and 1998 alone." See "The Terror of Sierra Leone," *Vanity Fair*, August 2000, vanityfair.com/news/2000 /08/junger200008.

8. Mary H. Moran, *Liberia: The Violence of Democracy* (Philadelphia: University of Pennsylvania Press, 2006), p. 25. Emmanuel Akyeampong handily summarizes the immediate triggers of West Africa's conflicts: "The decline in world prices for African primary exports from the 1960s placed African governments in a weakened financial position, unable to deliver on the promise of rapid economic growth and good health care. Criticism elicited political repression, and in the mid-1960s a wave of military coups overthrew the first democratically elected governments in Togo, Ghana, and then Nigeria. Military adventurism and ethnic tensions have resulted in the current state of political fragility with civil wars having been fought in Nigeria, Liberia, Sierra Leone and Côte d'Ivoire, the last three of them largely post-1990 phenomena, drawing in countries from the entire West African region either as collaborators or as peace keepers." See "Disease in West African History," in *Themes in West Africa's History*, edited by Emmanuel Akyeampong (Athens: Ohio University Press, 2006), p. 203. Many of the best (if partial) accounts of Upper West Africa's conflicts have been written by scholars from West Africa. They include Sylvia Ojukutu-Macauley, Ismail Rashid, Nemata Blyden, Tamba M'bayo, Lansana Gberie, Gibril Cole, Ibrahim Abdullah, Festus Cole, Yusuf Bangura, Jimmy Kandeh, Olu Gordon, 'Funmi Olonisakin, Sahr Kpundeh, and Arthur Abraham.

9. Moran, *Liberia*, p. 20.

10. Herman Cohen, quoted in Niels Hahn, "U.S. Covert and Overt Operations in Liberia, 1970s to 2003," *ASPJ Africa and Francophonie* 5, no. 3 (2014): p. 22. (Formatting altered.)

11. Amos Sawyer, cited in J. Gus Liebenow, *Liberia: The Quest for Democracy* (Bloomington: Indiana University Press, 1987), p. 78.

12. Bryan Bender, "Charles Taylor Claims U.S. Helped Spring Him from Plymouth Jail," *The Boston Globe*, July 16, 2009, bostonglobe.com/2009 /07/16/charles-taylor-claims-helped-spring-him-from-plymouth-jail /1VPRcDmbT45x8h37X5WFBO/story.html. Niels Hahn, of the University of London, spent years conducting research and collecting documents about the

Liberian conflict. "According to Taylor," Hahn reports, "a prison guard escorted him to a minimum-security area from which he escaped through a window and was taken to New York in what he assumes was a U.S. government vehicle" ("U.S. Covert and Overt Operations in Liberia," p. 25).

13. T. Christian Miller and Jonathan Jones, "Firestone and the Warlord," *ProPublica*, November 18, 2014, propublica.org/article/firestone-and-the-warlord-intro.

14. Danny Hoffman has noted that Charles Taylor was a pioneer in using mainstream and digital media in the course of Africa's first large post–Cold War hot war. See "Violent Virtuosity: Visual Labor in West Africa's Mano River War," *Anthropology Quarterly* 84, no. 4 (2011): pp. 949–75.

15. Herman Cohen, quoted in Hahn, "U.S. Covert and Overt Operations in Liberia," p. 27.

16. Miller and Jones, "Firestone and the Warlord."

17. The historian Ibrahim Abdullah writes that the "insurgency force from Liberia was composed of three distinct groups: those who had acquired military training in Libya (predominantly urban lumpens) and had seen action with the NPFL as combatants; a second group of Sierra Leoneans, resident in Liberia, mostly lumpens and criminals recently released from jail; and a third group of hard-core NPFL fighters from Liberia on loan to the RUF." See "Bush Path to Destruction: The Origin and Character of the Revolutionary United Front," in *Between Democracy and Terror*, p. 57.

18. William Reno, "War, Markets, and the Reconfiguration of West Africa's Weak States," *Comparative Politics* 29, no. 4 (1997): p. 502.

19. Reno, "War, Markets, and the Reconfiguration of West Africa's Weak States," p. 502.

20. Rosalind Shaw recalls a jubilant welcome for the young officers who overthrew Momoh and the All People's Congress: "Soldiers—especially young soldiers—enjoyed almost celebrity status as 'our young boys,' the heroes who had rid the country of the corrupt APC regime. Joining the army was, moreover, seen as a young man's only chance of a decent livelihood in the absence of any hope either of succeeding in business in Sierra Leone's depressed economy at that time or of finding an adequately paid job through educational qualifications." See *Memories of the Slave Trade: Ritual and the Historical Imagination in Sierra Leone* (Chicago: University of Chicago Press, 2002), pp. 195–96. Arthur Abraham traces NPRC complicity with the RUF back to the beginning of its tenure, when it could have defeated the insurgents, and nearly did. He knew of what he spoke, having served briefly as minister of education under Captain Strasser.

21. Elizabeth Rubin, "An Army of One's Own," *Harper's Magazine*, February 1997, p. 46.

22. Arthur Abraham, "War and Transition to Peace: A Study of State Conspiracy in Perpetuating Armed Conflict," *Africa Development* 22, no. 3/4 (1997): p. 104. The wrath of the rebels, the historian later observed, wasn't trained on govern-

ment forces or on the ruling party. "In Kailahun district," for example, "the main targets were the chiefs, traditional office-holders, local traders, prosperous farmers and even imams. The people were subjected to public beheadings, open floggings, forced labour and other forms of humiliation, including rape of women and girls." See "Dancing with the Chameleon: Sierra Leone and the Elusive Quest for Peace," *Journal of Contemporary African Studies* 19, no. 2 (2001): p. 207.

23. See, for example, Ismail Rashid, "Student Radicals, Lumpen Youth, and the Origins of Revolutionary Groups in Sierra Leone, 1977–1996," in *Between Democracy and Terror*, pp. 66–89; Lansana Gberie, "The 25 May Coup d'État in Sierra Leone: A Lumpen Revolt," in *Between Democracy and Terror*, pp. 144–63. Danny Hoffman wonders if this Marxian label runs the risk of "overvaluing the economic in what are complex social relations and eclipsing the political and other concerns. Classifying the demographic that constituted both the RUF and Civilian Defense Forces as lumpenproletariat . . . amounts to a rejection of those actors' political subjectivity. For Marx, the lumpen were those unable to be mobilized for participation in the workers' revolution. They constitute instead an underclass." Hoffman further notes that the greed-versus-grievance binary has tended to label the Mano River War as driven by "apolitical, raw economics," protesting "there is nothing in an economically deterministic explanation for the fighting that can account for the strategy of systematically amputating civilians' limbs." See "Disagreement: Dissent Politics and the War in Sierra Leone," *Africa Today* 52, no. 3 (2006): p. 12.

24. Accusations of ritual cannibalism were still a thing during the war, too. "Rumor has it," adds Greg Campbell, that the American commander's "remains were eaten by the RUF. The remainder of the Gurkha force refused to mount a counteroffensive and their contract was quickly canceled." See *Blood Diamonds: Tracing the Deadly Path of the World's Most Precious Stones*, revised edition (New York: Basic Books, 2012), p. 75.

25. Rubin, "An Army of One's Own," p. 47. (Formatting altered.)

26. Hoffman, an astute student of the Kamajors, notes that not all of them were Mende, adding that "national identities could be just as flexible. Many fighters could claim, with more or less equal legitimacy, to be citizens of either Sierra Leone or Liberia. Liberian ex-combatants living for years in Sierra Leone, the children of Sierra Leonean traders who grew up in Monrovia, young men from border communities with parentage in both countries—all of these complex webs of biography made the very idea of a fixed, stable identity absurd." He also labels absurd the assertion that personnel from Executive Outcomes and other security corporations—"unlike the Kamajors, they have no culture"—were the only military subcontractors of note: "The preoccupation with Executive Outcomes and its long-term consequences misses the fact that the real 'private warriors' in the Mano River War were the local militias and the Nigerian-led peacekeeping force, ECOMOG" ("Violence, Just in Time," pp. 40, 52, 51). The subject of the

Kamajors as an invented tradition is carefully dissected in a new book by Mariane Ferme, *Out of War: Violence, Trauma, and the Political Imagination in Sierra Leone* (Oakland: University of California Press, 2018).

27. Rubin, "An Army of One's Own," p. 48.

28. Abraham, "Dancing with the Chameleon," pp. 211, 207, 212.

29. The woman, whom I cite at length in order to avoid interviewing others so maimed and oft-interviewed, continued her story as follows: "We went to our farm, and in the morning we set off for Kabala. We did not reach Kabala that day because of the pain. It took us two days. People in Kabala said we were lucky; the Red Cross was there. After treating us they brought us by helicopter to Freetown here. We were taken to Connaught Hospital. They treated us there. Then we were taken to Waterloo. When the RUF invaded Freetown, we had to flee from Waterloo. We fled to the stadium. From there we were brought to this camp. If you ask me, this is all I know. We were ordinary people, we were farmers, we had nothing to do with the government. Whenever I think about this, and about the time they cut off my hand, and my daughter's hand, only six years of age, I feel so bad. Our children are here now. They are not going to school. Every morning we are given bulgur. Not enough for us. We are really suffering here. We only hope this war will come to an end and that we will be taken back to our own places. If we go back home, we have our own people who will help us." See Michael Jackson, *In Sierra Leone* (Durham, N.C.: Duke University Press, 2004), pp. 65, 66. Kabala is where fellow anthropologist Chris Coulter would later conduct her fieldwork with women and girls abducted by the RUF as "bush wives" and combatants. Her book, *Bush Wives and Girl Soldiers: Women's Lives Through War and Peace in Sierra Leone* (Ithaca, N.Y.: Cornell University Press, 2009), offers important correctives, and not only to our understanding of this war and its aftermath. On the topic of the alleged numbers of amputations, see the correctives offered by Ferme in the chapter "Numbers, Examples, and Exceptions," in *Out of War*, pp. 98–109.

30. Joseph Opala, "What the West Failed to See in Sierra Leone," *The Washington Post*, May 14, 2000, p. B1. Arthur Abraham was also caught up in the moment's optimism, predicting the return of war was unlikely. Because personal fortunes were still to be made from the extralegal peddling of natural resources, and because the sobel alliance used their weapons to take over that trade, the historian was soon forced to revise his views. "However much the people might want a democratically elected government," Abraham conceded from exile a few years later, "the means to protect them and assure them of peace simply did not exist" ("Dancing with the Chameleon," p. 210). Such circumstances were not unique to Sierra Leone but rather one logical outcome, William Reno argues, of the policies and practices of "shadowy states" built on decades of patronage, its roots in the colonial era. He explores the political economy of these conflicts in "War, Markets, and the Reconfiguration of West Africa's Weak States," pp. 493–510; "African Weak States and Commercial Alliances," *African Affairs* 96, no. 383 (1997):

pp. 165–85; and "How Sovereignty Matters: International Markets and the Political Economy of Local Politics in Weak States," in *Intervention and Transnationalism in Africa: Global-Local Networks of Power*, edited by Thomas M. Callaghy, Ronald Kassimir, and Robert Latham (Cambridge: Cambridge University Press, 2001), pp. 197–215. For a review of these matters as related to the electoral process during the civil war, see Jimmy D. Kandeh, "In Search of Legitimacy: The 1996 Elections," in *Between Democracy and Terror*, pp. 123–43.

31. "For the top military officials of the national army and the 'revolutionaries' of the RUF," explain the historians Ismail Rashid and Ibrahim Abdullah, "children represented a cheap and exploitable form of labour." See "'Smallest Victims; Youngest Killers': Juvenile Combatants in Sierra Leone's Civil War," in *Between Democracy and Terror*, p. 242. "To fight was not so much to take on the enemy," adds Danny Hoffman, "as to take up a labor, to work." He interviewed one former member of Taylor's small-boys unit, who pointed to a nearby four-year-old boy to make his point: "If you take a little kid like Opie and you just tell him to carry this cup, that's not training. That's just obeying orders. These are just laborers doing their labor" ("Violence, Just in Time," pp. 41, 49).

32. Hoffman cautions that "the desire to find explanations for what the kamajors became by looking to the ethnographic details of village kamajoisia, early colonial mercenaries, or even to revolutionary youth culture in the postcolony is, I think, misplaced. The kamajors's historical antecedents are not explanatory in the ways we might like them to be" (*The War Machines*, p. 70). This matter is explored in depth by Mariane Ferme in *Out of War*.

33. Drawing on sociologist Max Weber's notion of patrimonialism, the anthropologist William Murphy suggests that youth clientelism—by which young men and women, or boys and girls, become dependent on "big men" able to protect or feed or employ them—was the prewar social logic long at play in both countries: "The political culture of child soldiers is an artifact of an adult social world, which offers power, protection, sustenance, and economic opportunity in exchange for children's combat and labor services." See "Military Patrimonialism and Child Soldier Clientalism in the Liberian and Sierra Leonean Civil Wars," *African Studies Review* 46, no. 2 (2003): pp. 77, 63, 77.

34. Campbell, *Blood Diamonds*, p. 175.

35. "The transformation in warfare brought about by a global economy and the invention of cheap and light-weight but powerful and rapid-fire weapons," observes William Murphy, "made possible the military usefulness even of young, physically immature children" ("Military Patrimonialism and Child Soldier Clientalism," p. 74). Chris Coulter, on the other hand, warns against modern-weapons reductionism, noting that children have been armed with guns since before the American Civil War. Danny Hoffman brought nuance to those debates: "Each faction brought in former soldiers with at least some training to teach new recruits and to operate heavy, technical weapons. But the majority of the violence of this war was done with cheap, lightweight weaponry that required little if any

training—AK-47s and similar assault rifles, rocket propelled grenades, and cut-lasses. The techniques of violence were meant to be spectacular more than they were meant to be precise, so they required little specialized knowledge on the part of combatants" ("Violence, Just in Time," p. 49).

36. Ishmael Beah, *A Long Way Gone: Memoirs of a Boy Soldier* (New York: Sarah Crichton Books, 2007), p. 24. Beah hails from what was once part of the Jong Kingdom, a region in which the British once shelled riverine villages and hanged human leopards. The success of Beah's memoir led to heightened scrutiny, and a couple of journalists from Australia have questioned the veracity of his account. For a review of the argument, see Gabriel Sherman, "The Fog of Memoir: The Feud Over the Truthfulness of Ishmael Beah's *A Long Way Gone*," *Slate*, March 6, 2008, slate.com/articles/arts/culturebox/2008/03/the_fog_of_memoir.html. Both Beah's editor and his college mentor—who encouraged the young man to draw on long-submerged memories—stand by his work, as does he. It's beautifully written and well worth reading.

37. In *Bush Wives and Girl Soldiers*, Chris Coulter—who spent years interviewing former girl soldiers and RUF "bush wives," a new postwar term that stuck—warns against readings of these phenomena that don't place them in the context of the structural violence faced by women and girls before, during, and after the formal cessation of hostilities. Like several of her fellow anthropologists and like the historians Ismail Rashid and Ibrahim Abdullah, Coulter also mistrusts the victims-as-perpetrators paradigm rolled out by diverse players within "the humanitarian community," including those who typically concern themselves with child combatants.

38. Beah, *A Long Way Gone*, pp. 116, 115, 118.

39. Beah, *A Long Way Gone*, pp. 188, 147.

40. Gberie, *A Dirty War in West Africa*, p. 4.

41. Michael Streeter, "Sierra Leone Coup Leader Claims Power," *The Independent*, May 25, 1997, independent.co.uk/news/world/sierra-leone-coup-leader-claims-power-1263627.html.

42. The government, Arthur Abraham reflected a few years later, "erred badly when it ostensibly bowed to pressure from the International Monetary Fund and announced the termination of EO's contract. This blunder provided the political and military space Sankoh needed to manoeuvre and muster the capacity for another military strike" ("Dancing with the Chameleon," pp. 216, 213).

43. William M. Kennedy, "Operation Noble Obelisk: An Examination of Unity of Effort" (Final Report, Naval War College, 2001), p. 10.

44. Will Scully, *Once a Pilgrim: A True Story of One Man's Courage Under Rebel Fire* (London: Headline, 1998), pp. 83–84.

45. Scully, *Once a Pilgrim*, p. 110.

46. James Rupert, "Nigerian Navy Shells Sierra Leone Rebels," *The Washington Post*, June 2, 1997, p. A13.

47. Kennedy, "Operation Noble Obelisk," pp. 13–14. In detailing the history of Sierra Leone's diamond trade and manipulation of its politics, a Canadian NGO named

Partnership Africa Canada dedicates a harsh page to the Mammy Yoko's manager, Roger Crooks. The authors of this report—who include Lansana Gberie—allege that there was more to Crooks "than the hotel business." They cite the London *Sunday Times*, which had previously revealed charges alleging that "Crooks was involved in an attempt to sell 2,000 kilograms of C-4 explosives, Browning machine guns, mines and rocket launchers to contacts in Northern Ireland via Sierra Leone" and reported that Crooks had "owned extensive diamond and mining interests in Sierra Leone." See Ian Smillie, Lansana Gberie, and Ralph Hazleton, *The Heart of the Matter: Sierra Leone, Diamonds, and Human Security* (Ottawa: Partnership Africa Canada, 2000), p. 55. Crooks has denied such allegations, rebutting them with claims of generous service to a country he once described as "great casino." A decade after the attack on the Mammy Yoko, he related his own account of these events to the *Houston Chronicle*: "Rebels attacked the hotel on June 2nd, 1997, firing rocket-propelled grenades, Crooks said. He said he and a handful of fighters took cover on the hotel roof and fired back. A rocket-propelled grenade exploded a few feet from him, leaving him deaf in his left ear." See Dale Lezon, "Lake Conroe Man's Latest African Adventure: Suing Sierra Leone," *Houston Chronicle*, May 7, 2008, chron.com/neighborhood/woodlands-news /article/Lake-Conroe-man-s-latest-African-adventure-Suing-1771962.php. Will Scully's account of these events—*Once a Pilgrim*, published at the height of the war—does not contradict that of Crooks.

48. Madelaine Drohan, *Making a Killing: How and Why Corporations Use Armed Force to Do Business* (Guilford, Conn.: Lyons Press, 2004), p. 238.

49. Campbell, *Blood Diamonds*, p. 85.

50. Ulimo-K shared more than ordnance from their Guinean sponsors, as its fighters showed by launching a brutal echo of Sékou Touré's Demystification Program. "To the outrage of the Loma and Kpelle inhabitants," reports the historian Stephen Ellis, the faction "systematically pillaged the sacred groves of the Poro society, desecrating these holy places and stealing the masks and other religious objects." The Loma and Kpelle in question organized a Lofa Defense Force and so the cycle continued. "This feud had a long history," explains Ellis, "since the area had been at the limit of the conquests of the nineteenth-century Malinke warlord, Samory, whose memory is still alive in the area." As Ellis lays out the macabre and hallucinatory details of the war, and outlines old grievances and religious schisms, he allows that the extractive trades' profits, along with modern weapons, were what kept the blood flowing. Many within ECOMOG were ecumenical about profits from illicit trade, and did (Ellis asserts) "business with every faction at one time or another, trading rubber with Ulimo-J, looted goods and wood with the LPC and palm-oil with the NPFL, while Ulimo-K was trading directly across the northern border with Guinean officers from an army which was a component of ECOMOG." See *The Mask of Anarchy: The Destruction of Liberia and the Religious Dimension of an African Civil War* (New York: New York University Press, 1999), pp. 128, 129, 104.

51. Ambassador William H. Twaddell is cited in Ellis, *The Mask of Anarchy*, pp. 90–91. Charles Taylor, observed the journalist Doug Farah in 2006, "ran this amazingly complex criminal enterprise where the state could provide critical things like diplomatic passports and airplane registration to a range of criminal networks." Farah is cited by Lydia Polgreen in "A Master Plan Drawn in Blood," *The New York Times*, April 2, 2006, nytimes.com/2006/04/02/weekinreview /a-master-plan-drawn-in-blood.html.

52. William H. Twaddell, quoted in Ellis, *The Mask of Anarchy*, p. 138.

53. Ellis, *The Mask of Anarchy*, p. 139.

54. Campbell, *Blood Diamonds*, p. 86.

55. The ECOMOG official is quoted in "Sierra Leone News: January 1999," Sierra Leone Web, January 4, 1999, sierra-leone.org/Archives/slnews0199.html.

56. Junger, "The Terror of Sierra Leone."

57. See the study of ECOMOG by the political scientist 'Funmi Olonisakin, "Nigeria, ECOMOG, and the Sierra Leone Crisis," in *Between Democracy and Terror*, pp. 220–37.

58. Polgreen, "A Master Plan Drawn in Blood."

59. Junger, "The Terror of Sierra Leone."

60. Robert D. Kaplan, "The Coming Anarchy," *The Atlantic Monthly*, February 1994, theatlantic.com/magazine/archive/1994/02/the-coming-anarchy/304670.

61. Several anthropologists have contested claims about a "culture of violence" native to Upper West Africa. Paul Richards, writing from the allegedly isolated rain forest from which anarchy was predicted to metastasize globally, offered *Fighting for the Rain Forest* as a book-length rebuttal to Kaplan's "new barbarism thesis." Rosalind Shaw characterizes "juju journalists" as having their own set of magical beliefs and primeval practices: "When Western media coverage of African wars such as that in Sierra Leone extends beyond discussion of African governments, political and military leaders, peace accords, and international organizations, 'tribalism' and 'juju' tend to be offered up as a recurring duo of inventions. Given that Sierra Leone's rebel war was not (for the main part) characterized by ethnic conflict but did include the use of ritual materials and practices to confer impenetrability or invisibility, these 'magical' techniques of war and defense (often glossed as juju) were prominently highlighted in foreign media coverage." Shaw has little trouble identifying the tribe's paramount chief. "Most notable for its influence," she notes, "is Robert Kaplan's famous 1994 article, 'The Coming Anarchy,' in which he casts Sierra Leone and what he calls its 'juju warriors' as the portents of a growing chaos that threatens to engulf us all." Kaplan's characterization had a wide echo beyond the embassies to which it was faxed, notes Shaw. "'But Kaplan is right—Sierra Leone *is* in a state of anarchy,' scholars I respected would sometimes tell me." But "how prescient," Shaw asks, "did anyone have to be to predict that fighting would continue after the elections in 1996? The Sierra Leonean state still had no resources, the government was still unable to control

its armed forces, and the RUF rebels were still out there." See Shaw's "Robert Kaplan and 'Juju Journalism' in Sierra Leone's Rebel War: The Primitivizing of an African Conflict," in *Magic and Modernity: Interfaces of Revelation and Concealment*, edited by Birgit Meyer and Peter Pels (Stanford: Stanford University Press, 2003), pp. 81, 82, 100. Academic debates aside, and unless profound culture change occurs in the blink of an eye, essentialist claims about Sierra Leone's native barbarism, inevitable tribal strife, and generally poor prospects for salvage were surely undermined after disarmament, if something called the Global Peace Index is correct: Sierra Leone, ranked the second most peaceful country in West Africa in 2015, overtook Ghana to take first place in 2016. See Institute for Economics and Peace, *Global Peace Index 2016: Ten Years of Measuring Peace* (Sydney: Institute for Economics and Peace, 2016).

62. Shaw, *Memories of the Slave Trade*, p. 202. (Formatting altered.)
63. Shaw, *Memories of the Slave Trade*, pp. 202–203.
64. Campbell, *Blood Diamonds*, p. 66.
65. Ismail Rashid, "The Lomé Peace Negotiations," *Accord*, no. 9 (2000): pp. 29, 32.
66. Junger, "The Terror of Sierra Leone."
67. Campbell, *Blood Diamonds*, p. 93.
68. Campbell, *Blood Diamonds*, p. 94.
69. The British journalist Tim Butcher described talisman-free Sankoh as "the talismanic brute who had led the RUF when it established its hallmark of hacking hands and arms from innocent civilians." See *Chasing the Devil: The Search for Africa's Fighting Spirit* (London: Chatto & Windus, 2010), p. 15.
70. See Douglas Farah, "Al Qaeda Cash Tied to Diamond Trade," *The Washington Post*, November 2, 2001, washingtonpost.com/archive/politics/2001/11/02/al -qaeda-cash-tied-to-diamond-trade/93abd66a-5048-469a-9a87-5d2efb565a62.
71. "Despite their differing emphases," observes Danny Hoffman of the Special Court and the Truth and Reconciliation Commission, "the institutions rely on a similar logic: the negotiation of a singular narrative history" ("Disagreement," p. 16).
72. Campbell, *Blood Diamonds*, pp. 144–45, 146.
73. "It was simultaneously frightening, amusing, and depressing to hear ruthless killers complaining that they didn't have movies to watch or balls to play with," relates the journalist. "You were reminded of how young most of the RUF's soldiers were and how fundamentally they'd missed out on childhoods that most people take for granted. The kid who complained to me was probably no older than 13. He had likely killed people and could fire an automatic rifle in combat, but he'd probably never ridden a bike" (Campbell, *Blood Diamonds*, p. 148).
74. Hoffman reminds us that many younger men in these militia had previously served in the RUF. "If there was a marked lack of hostility toward the RUF," he writes of militia members, "by the final years of conflict the tension between the Civilian Defense Forces leadership and the majority of combatants was evident.

From the latter's viewpoint, this was the result of greedy elders' refusing to pass the youth their due" ("Disagreement," p. 9).

75. Complaints and restiveness in Maforki did not let up with the journalists' hasty retreat. "The camp has been the scene of unrest ever since, hosting riots, beatings, and often-repeated threats of further trouble," Campbell observed. "The source of the trouble is always the same: The RUF's contention that the DDR and UNAMSIL have duped them into surrendering by making false promises" (*Blood Diamonds*, p. 149). Danny Hoffman, then working as a journalist, describes similar events during disarmament proceedings in Bo, then the largest city in eastern Sierra Leone. Writing later as an anthropologist concerned to refute "conceptions of violent events as breakdown, as the absence of sociality or the evacuation of meaning." See "Violent Events as Narrative Blocs: The Disarmament at Bo, Sierra Leone," *Anthropological Quarterly* 78, no. 2 (2005): p. 333. Reflecting on the repeated failures of various disarmament campaigns during the Mano River war, Hoffman underlines the primacy of patronage: what the DDR "framework fails to recognize is that the patronage networks which dominate everyday existence have not been replaced in wartime, they have simply become militarized. Ex-combatants remain dependent on their commanders even after disarmament. In both Sierra Leone and Liberia, combatants were required to give up most of the DDR benefits to their patrons/commanders to even secure the opportunity to participate in DDR proceedings. This served to solidify the patron/client relation even further and effectively erased the fresh start that disarmament was supposed to entail. Ironically, disarmament campaigns have helped to create a class of highly mobile young men who can be 'deployed' to the various disarmament proceedings by their patrons in an effort to capitalize on the ever-increasing benefits packages." See "The Meaning of a Militia: Understanding the Civil Defence Forces of Sierra Leone," *African Affairs* 106, no. 425 (2007): p. 660.

76. The chief ceremony marking war's end was held near what remained of Lungi airport, which Hoffman notes to be "an isolated spot far removed from the capital and easy to evacuate." The choice of venue suggested to him that "faith in Sierra Leone's escape from its recent history did not run deep." See "The City as Barracks: Freetown, Monrovia, and the Organization of Violence in Postcolonial African Cities," *Cultural Anthropology* 22, no. 3 (2007): p. 403.

77. *LURD's Political Manifesto*, cited in Hahn, "U.S. Covert and Overt Operations in Liberia," p. 32.

78. "Some form of brokered agreement was critical to averting a transnational disaster," allowed Hoffman while Charles Taylor was still in Nigeria. "Clearly it needed to be one that removed Taylor from power, though the standing indictment meant that he would agree only if shielded from prosecution, making most options impracticable. As it happened, the solution which was eventually reached, exile in Nigeria, was the worst possible arrangement." See "Despot Deposed: Charles Taylor and the Challenge of State Reconstruction in Liberia," in *Legacies of Power: Leadership Change and Former Presidents in African Poli-*

tics, edited by Roger Southall and Henning Melber (Cape Town: HSRC Press, 2006), p. 321.

79. Margaret Novicki, quoted in Campbell, *Blood Diamonds,* p. 206.

INTERLUDE II: THE CRISIS CARAVAN

1. Sharp tongues argued that the poverty of mean aspirations was deepened by these newcomers, pointing to downright perverse outcomes—for example, the notion that providing medical care and social support to amputees sequestered in camps somehow generated increased demand for amputations in Sierra Leone. See Linda Polman, *The Crisis Caravan: What's Wrong with Humanitarian Aid* (New York: Metropolitan Books, 2010).

2. Adia Benton, *HIV Exceptionalism: Development Through Disease in Sierra Leone* (Minneapolis: University of Minnesota Press, 2015), pp. 14, 7, 9, 23.

3. The anthropologist Sharon Abramowitz describes these attempts to narrow the humanitarian gaze by recasting Liberia's social and economic and political turmoil as an essentially psychological and personal affair. "Although there is a growing tendency in the postconflict literature to emphasize social, cultural, and psychological resilience," she warns, "the facts from Liberia show that, prior to 2010, biological resilience often lost out to the postwar context. Most Liberians were not 'getting by'; in fact, population data indicated that Liberians were dying at the beginning and in the middle of their lives relative to the rest of the world's populations." See *Searching for Normal in the Wake of the Liberian War* (Philadelphia: University of Pennsylvania Press, 2014), p. 23.

4. See Joia S. Mukherjee and Regan Marsh, "Excess Maternal Death in the Time of Ebola," *Fletcher Forum of World Affairs* 39, no. 2 (2015): pp. 149–60; Regan H. Marsh et al., "The Challenges of Pregnancy and Childbirth Among Women Who Were Not Infected with Ebola Virus During the 2013–2015 West African Epidemic," in *Pregnant in the Time of Ebola: Women and Their Children in the 2013–2015 West African Epidemic,* edited by David Schwartz, Julienne Ngoundoung Anoko, and Sharon A. Abramowitz (Cham, Switz.: Springer, 2019), pp. 31–51; Elsie G. Karmbor-Ballah et al., "Maternal Mortality and the Metempsychosis of User Fees in Liberia: A Mixed-Methods Analysis," *Scientific African* 3 (2019): p. e00050.

5. See, for example, Agnes Binagwaho et al., "Rwanda 20 Years On: Investing in Life," *The Lancet* 384, no. 9940 (2014): pp. 371–75; Paul Farmer et al., "Reduced Premature Mortality in Rwanda: Lessons from Success," *The British Medical Journal* 346 (2013): p. f65.

6. Chris Coulter, echoing colleagues and citing informants, marvels at the ineffectiveness of these well-intentioned schemes. "It seemed inconceivable that the Sierra Leone local economy could absorb all the gara tie-dyers, tailors, and soap makers being trained," she relates. "When I once asked the managing director of an NGO why they had decided to work with such a limited set of skills, which were also the same skills that all the other organizations were offering, I was told

that he had not really thought about it, but that all their projects were designed by 'the ex-pats in Freetown.'" See *Bush Wives and Girl Soldiers: Women's Lives Through War and Peace in Sierra Leone* (Ithaca, N.Y.: Cornell University Press, 2009), pp. 188, 189.

7. Greg Campbell, *Blood Diamonds: Tracing the Deadly Path of the World's Most Precious Stones*, revised edition (New York: Basic Books, 2012), pp. 246, 253, 253–54, 251, 253.

8. In 1990, when historian Myron Echenberg interviewed elderly villagers in Senegal, he found vivid memories of the approach to plague favored by the authorities during an outbreak in 1944. "French medical policy toward bubonic plague in Senegal continued to be authoritarian, parsimonious, and insensitive to African health perspectives and needs," he summarized. "Quarantine, *cordons*, lazarettos, compulsory vaccination and restriction on travel, undignified burial, even a resettlement scheme for the homeless—all these had become familiar hardships to be endured." See *Black Death, White Medicine: Bubonic Plague and the Politics of Public Health in Colonial Senegal, 1914–1945* (Portsmouth, N.H.: Heinemann, 2002), p. 242.

9. For a review of these budgetary trends, and of their devastating consequences for health-care delivery in Sierra Leone, see C. Magbaily Fyle, "The State and Health Services in Sierra Leone," in *The State and the Provision of Social Services in Sierra Leone Since Independence, 1961–91*, edited by C. Magbaily Fyle (Dakar: Council for the Development of Social Science Research in Africa, 1993), pp. 44–61; Aaron Shakow, Robert Yates, and Salmaan Keshavjee, "Neoliberalism and Global Health," in *The SAGE Handbook of Neoliberalism*, edited by Damien Cahill, Melinda Cooper, Martijn Konings, and David Primrose (London: SAGE Publications, 2018), pp. 511–36. Salmaan Keshavjee's *Blind Spot: How Neoliberalism Infiltrated Global Health* (Oakland: University of California Press, 2014) is a terrific book about the ways in which neoliberal logic has infiltrated charities, humanitarian organizations, and aid agencies.

9. HOW EBOLA KILLS

1. The same professor, however, would warn Piot against a career in infectious diseases, an opinion shared by other mentors at Belgium's Ghent University, where Piot was a medical student. "When, after seven years' study at the medical faculty in Ghent, I broached the idea of specializing in infectious diseases," writes Piot, "the unanimous verdict of my professors was that I would be a fool to do it . . . In general, infectious diseases weren't considered interesting or cutting-edge in 1974." The young doctor ignored them. His résumé—traveling to Zaire in 1976 to help fight the first recorded outbreak of Ebola; characterizing, for the first time, some of Ebola's epidemiological and clinical features; serving as executive director of UNAIDS from its founding in 1995 until 2008; publishing hundreds of scientific papers on HIV, sexually transmitted infections, and Ebola; and now leading the London School of Hygiene & Tropical Medicine—suggests Piot

made the right decision. His memoir relates and reflects on these experiences, and more. See *No Time to Lose: A Life in Pursuit of Deadly Viruses* (New York: W. W. Norton, 2012), pp. 8–9, 6.

2. This definition comes from *Dorland's Illustrated Medical Dictionary*, thirty-second edition (Philadelphia: Saunders, 2012), p. 1396.

3. The 1976 report of the international task force investigating the Yambuku outbreak, published in the WHO's *Bulletin*, is concise, is surprisingly free of jargon, and lays down the boundaries of epidemiological and clinical knowledge about a newly identified disease. Indeed, these boundaries hadn't expanded much by 2013, when the whole chain of events began anew, this time without much in the way of a brake on runaway transmission and scant attention to bringing even 1976-level medical care to bear on case-fatality rates. See "Ebola Haemorrhagic Fever in Zaire, 1976: Report of an International Commission," *Bulletin of the World Health Organization* 56, no. 2 (1978): pp. 271–93.

4. Roosecelis Brasil Martines et al., "Tissue and Cellular Tropism, Pathology and Pathogenesis of Ebola and Marburg Viruses," *The Journal of Pathology* 235, no. 2 (2015): pp. 159, 154.

5. Richard Preston, *The Hot Zone* (New York: Random House, 1994), p. 289.

6. François Lamontagne et al., "Doing Today's Work Superbly Well—Treating Ebola with Current Tools," *The New England Journal of Medicine* 371, no. 17 (2014): p. 1565. (Formatting altered.)

7. In 1976, when "specific" therapies for Ebola were unknown, Peter Piot attempted to rely on working pathophysiological hypotheses to steer his team's clinical decisions. Since hemorrhage was then thought to be the immediate cause of death, Piot learned various hematological lab techniques, with the hope that such training would facilitate the delivery of proper clinical care. "Because this was a hemorrhagic-fever epidemic—which included, by definition, symptoms of bleeding," writes Piot, "I would need to monitor all kinds of blood parameters: the degree of disseminated intravascular coagulation, which causes uncontrollable bleeding; the number of platelets and hematocrits; and so on." Once on the ground, he and his colleagues began drawing blood "to perform a number of blood tests that would guide the decision to prescribe supportive treatment for intravascular coagulation," which they inferred "might be the cause of death in hemorrhagic fever" (*No Time to Lose*, pp. 18, 25–26). I cite this example neither to applaud medical efforts in 1976—the case-fatality rate during the outbreak was 88 percent—nor to correct ideas about the singularity of hemorrhagic symptoms, but to underscore a can-do spirit that sought to connect limited knowledge of Ebola's clinical course with interventions that might have saved lives. This spirit was largely stifled in 2014, giving way instead to an obsession with "specific" therapies and to the therapeutic nihilism fueled by their absence. In a 2015 after-action report, for example, representatives of MSF asserted that the "lack of specific treatment or vaccine for Ebola is a major contributor to the virus's high mortality rate . . . MSF alone cared for 35 per cent of all confirmed cases in this outbreak; a heavy burden for one organisation. With

no cure for Ebola, tragically, despite our best efforts, more than 2,600 of our patients died." See *An Unprecedented Year: Médecins Sans Frontières' Response to the Largest Ever Ebola Outbreak* (Geneva: Médecins Sans Frontières, 2015), pp. 18–19. There's no cure or vaccine for AIDS or diabetes, either, but best efforts to address these afflictions require aggressive efforts to use what tools we do have on hand—and by "on hand," I mean on hand in the global economy to which West Africans have long and often reluctantly contributed.

8. "Fighting Ebola from Day One: Interview with Rob Fowler, a Critical Care Physician from Canada, Who Worked in West Africa Since the First Confirmed Cases of Ebola," World Health Organization, January 2015, who.int/features/2015/ebola-interview-fowler/en. A team in Omaha, Nebraska, has laid out a helpful review of the role of supportive and critical care in the management of Ebola virus disease. See Daniel W. Johnson et al., "Lessons Learned: Critical Care Management of Patients with Ebola in the United States," *Critical Care Medicine* 43, no. 6 (2015): pp. 1157–64.

9. Lamontagne et al., "Doing Today's Work Superbly Well," p. 1566. (Formatting altered.)

10. Dan Bausch, Peter Piot, and Pierre Rollin—infectious-disease specialists whose work and wisdom have been indispensable to this book—are among the exceptions, having long called for a better appreciation of the social forces that determine who dies, and how many die, during outbreaks of filovirus disease. Bausch, for one, has not shied away from criticizing his peers for scanting the biosocial. Writing with a colleague in *The Journal of Infectious Diseases*, he argues that while Ebola scientists may present a "more objective viewpoint" on filoviruses than those advanced by the lay press, they usually do so "with a rather technical focus on identifying epidemiological risk factors and experimental therapies and vaccines. Often lost in the discussion are the human rights elements that consistently underlie large outbreaks of these dangerous viruses." He concludes this commentary with a nod to social medicine: "Health science training in the United States has often presented a false dichotomy that implies that one is either a 'science type' or a 'human rights type,' either a future 'virus hunter' or an 'activist.' As it turns out, if we truly want to make a difference in people's health, we need to pursue social justice as avidly as we do virology." See "Ebola Virus: Sensationalism, Science, and Human Rights," *The Journal of Infectious Diseases* 212, supplement 2 (2015): pp. S79, S83.

11. Deepak Passi et al., "Ebola Virus Disease (The Killer Virus): Another Threat to Humans and Bioterrorism: Brief Review and Recent Updates," *Journal of Clinical and Diagnostic Research* 9, no. 6 (2015): p. LE01. (Formatting altered.)

12. Pardis Sabeti and her colleagues were among those involved in the confusing (and sometimes contested) process of naming and classifying Ebola variants, specifically the one implicated in the West African epidemic and another that circulated during the fall of 2014 in an epidemiologically unlinked outbreak in the Democratic Republic of the Congo. Their consensus is presented in Jens Kuhn et al., "Nomenclature- and Database-Compatible Names for the Two Ebola Virus

Variants that Emerged in Guinea and the Democratic Republic of the Congo in 2014," *Viruses* 6, no. 11 (2014): pp. 4760–99. For a summary of the 2014 Congo outbreak, which caused forty-nine known deaths, see Gaël D. Maganga et al., "Ebola Virus Disease in the Democratic Republic of Congo," *The New England Journal of Medicine* 371, no. 22 (2014): pp. 2083–91.

13. These studies include William E. Diehl et al., "Ebola Virus Glycoprotein with Increased Infectivity Dominated the 2013–2016 Epidemic," *Cell* 167, no. 4 (2016): pp. 1088–98.e6; Richard A. Urbanowicz et al., "Human Adaptation of Ebola Virus During the West African Outbreak," *Cell* 167, no. 4 (2016): pp. 1079–87.e5; Andrea Marzi et al., "Recently Identified Mutations in the Ebola Virus-Makona Genome Do Not Alter Pathogenicity in Animal Models," *Cell Reports* 23, no. 6 (2018): pp. 1806–16.

14. Martines and colleagues make more modest claims of causality by advancing ones from pathologic studies. In comparing species variation in splenic histopathology, their "overall impression is that Zaire Ebola virus infections tend to have greater degrees of lymphoid depletion and necrosis and are found to have comparatively larger amounts of viral antigen by using immunohistochemistry. Bundibugyo virus infection appears to show the least amount of lymphoid depletion and antigen, while the changes seen in Sudan virus cases are somewhat intermediate" ("Tissue and Cellular Tropism, Pathology and Pathogenesis," p. 160). Similar observations are made with respect to the liver in this review.

15. They add a prophecy, one made many times before, but well worth repeating here: "Resolving these issues will require long-term commitment and collaboration from the world community and international partners" (Martines et al., "Tissue and Cellular Tropism, Pathology and Pathogenesis," p. 171). Adam MacNeil and Pierre Rollin have also written, for a different journal, a strong defense of a more broadly biosocial approach: "Those most at risk for Ebola hemorrhagic fever and Marburg hemorrhagic fever are residents of rural central Africa, many of whom are among the bottom billion. Outbreaks of Ebola hemorrhagic fever and Marburg hemorrhagic fever are commonly associated with limited public health surveillance and inadequate medical preventive measures, both partially the result of impoverished conditions." See "Ebola and Marburg Hemorrhagic Fevers: Neglected Tropical Diseases?," *PLOS Neglected Tropical Diseases* 6, no. 6 (2012): p. e1546.

16. C. J. Peters, citing studies conducted largely in nonhuman primates, notes that "possible explanations for the failure to mount an effective immune response in fatal cases include the presence of a putatively immunosuppressive amino acid sequence in the filovirus glycoprotein, the secretion of a soluble glycoprotein by Ebola virus-infected cells, and the extensive lymphoid damage evident in postmortem examination. In addition, Ebola-infected cells have a deficient response to added interferon, induction of the antiviral state, and induction of interferon or activation of downstream pathways. One major filovirus protein, VP35, is known to be responsible for the latter." See "Marburg and Ebola Virus Hemorrhagic

Fevers," in *Mandell, Douglas, and Bennett's Principles and Practice of Infectious Diseases*, seventh edition, edited by Gerald L. Mandell, John E. Bennett, and Raphael Dolin, volume 2 (Philadelphia: Churchill Livingstone, 2010), p. 2262.

17. Preston, *The Hot Zone*, p. 27.
18. When Ebola "emerged in 1976, more-frequent and more-dramatic outbreaks were observed, with larger numbers of infected patients and higher case fatality rates," noted two virologists in 2007: "EBOV was soon found to be endemic in many countries of sub-Saharan Africa, ranging from the Ivory Coast to Sudan. Thus, in general, EBOV was thought to be more dangerous than MARV. However, the outbreaks of MARV infection in the Democratic Republic of the Congo in 1998–1999 and in Angola in 2004–2005 clearly indicated that this view had to be revised. Each outbreak resulted in nearly 200 deaths, and the mortality rate was similar to that attributed to Zaire EBOV. It is also evident that MARV is present in larger areas of Africa than had been previously acknowledged. Thus, MARV has to be considered as big a threat as EBOV." See Werner Slenczka and Hans Dieter Klenk, "Forty Years of Marburg Virus," *The Journal of Infectious Diseases* 196, supplement 2 (2007): p. S134. Regarding the Angolan outbreak of Marburg, see B. Lee Ligon, "Outbreak of Marburg Hemorrhagic Fever in Angola: A Review of the History of the Disease and Its Biological Aspects," *Seminars in Pediatric Infectious Diseases* 16, no. 3 (2005): pp. 219–24; Jonathan S. Towner et al., "Marburgvirus Genomics and Association with a Large Hemorrhagic Fever Outbreak in Angola," *Journal of Virology* 80, no. 13 (2006): pp. 6497–6516. Richard Preston may be forgiven for believing Marburg to be Ebola's gentler sister, since this larger outbreak of Marburg began in Angola a decade after his book was published.
19. "Marburg Outbreak, Angola: When Saving Lives Seems Cruel," Médecins Sans Frontières, July 11, 2005, msf.org/en/article/marburg-outbreak-angola-when-saving-lives-seems-cruel.
20. Armand Sprecher, quoted in "When Saving Lives Seems Cruel."
21. See Daniel B. Domingues da Silva, "The Atlantic Slave Trade from Angola: A Port-by-Port Estimate of Slaves Embarked, 1701–1867," *International Journal of African Historical Studies* 46, no. 1 (2013): 105–122.
22. Daniel S. Chertow et al., "Ebola Virus Disease in West Africa—Clinical Manifestations and Management," *The New England Journal of Medicine* 371, no. 22 (2014): p. 2054.
23. Robert Fowler, quoted in Donald G. McNeil Jr., "Ebola Doctors Are Divided on IV Therapy in Africa," *The New York Times*, January 1, 2015, nytimes.com/2015/01/02/health/ebola-doctors-are-divided-on-iv-therapy-in-africa.html. How many of these Ebola deaths were primarily due to hypovolemic shock and electrolyte imbalances? Not all of them. But "on the occasions when we've been able to obtain basic biochemistry measurements," Fowler and his colleagues report, "we have commonly found extreme serum sodium and potassium abnormalities" (Lamontagne et al., "Doing Today's Work Superbly Well," p. 1566).

24. Armand Sprecher, quoted in McNeil Jr., "Ebola Doctors Are Divided."

25. McNeil Jr., "Ebola Doctors Are Divided."

26. The letter continues by predicting that "the prolonged reluctance of placing IV lines to severely dehydrated patients will remain a symbol of the inadequate clinical care during MSF's Ebola intervention in West Africa." See Manica Balasegaram et al., "Ebola: A Challenge to Our Humanitarian Identity: A Letter to the MSF Movement," December 4, 2014, pp. 3–4. Time will tell if this profound reluctance is acknowledged publicly and its implications widely understood.

27. See the opening chapters of Elin L. Wolfe, A. Clifford Barger, and Saul Benison, *Walter B. Cannon, Science, and Society* (Cambridge, Mass.: Harvard University Press, 2000), pp. 3–44.

28. A comparison of these Latin American epidemics, including a closer look at the biosocial complexities and delivery failures that fueled them, is presented in Jonathan Weigel and Paul Farmer, "Cholera and the Road to Modernity: Lessons from One Latin American Epidemic for Another," *Americas Quarterly* 6, no. 3 (2012): pp. 28–35.

29. Armand Sprecher, quoted in McNeil Jr., "Ebola Doctors Are Divided."

30. Chertow et al., "Ebola Virus Disease in West Africa," p. 2056.

31. Chertow et al., "Ebola Virus Disease in West Africa," p. 2056.

32. Walter B. Cannon, quoted in Wolfe, Barger, and Benison, *Walter B. Cannon*, p. 31.

33. Just days into his first trip to Zaire, Piot became acutely aware of the need to both prevent new infections and care for the sick when prevention failed. A control-over-care paradigm, in other words, would not suffice. After visiting the derelict Yambuku Mission Hospital, a major amplifier of the 1976 epidemic, he and his team were tasked with visiting nearby villages to find new cases, trace their contacts, and learn more about what was then still a mysterious disease. But as the epidemiological investigation chugged along, Piot felt deeply anxious about a virus-hunting mission that did little to reduce villagers' risk of infection and of poor clinical outcomes once infected. "We were all familiar with our terms of mission," he writes. "We were here just for three or four days, to act as scouts in preparation for the arrival of a larger team that would try to set up systems to control the epidemic and break ground for further research. Our job was to document what was going on, sketch out some basic epidemiology, take samples from acutely sick patients, and, if possible, find recovering convalescents who might provide plasma to help cure future sufferers . . . But we knew that from a human point of view this simply wasn't enough. We needed to stop the virus from infecting and killing people" (*No Time to Lose*, pp. 56, 48).

34. A vocal proponent of a minimalist approach put it this way: "If somebody said, what would I love to be able to bring to bear? Dialysis machines? Ventilators? Infusion pumps? No, I would want more person-hours of skilled nursing for patients." But it was largely skilled nurses who were demanding the tools of their

trade. See Denise Grady, "Better Staffing Seen as Crucial to Ebola Treatment in Africa," *The New York Times*, October 31, 2014, nytimes.com/2014/11/01/us /better-staffing-seen-as-crucial-to-ebola-treatment-in-africa.html.

35. Balasegaram et al., "Ebola: A Challenge to Our Humanitarian Identity," pp. 4, 5–6. (Formatting altered.)

36. Wolfe, Barger, and Benison, *Walter B. Cannon*, p. 18.

37. See Paul Farmer, "Pandemic Ebola Virus Disease: Integrating Prevention and Care," Brigham and Women's Hospital, Medical Grand Rounds, October 31, 2014, bwhedtech.media.partners.org/programs/mgr/farmer20141031mgr.

38. These data were presented by Joyce Chang, a nurse directing survivor care efforts for Partners In Health, at a WHO-sponsored Ebola survivors' conference in Freetown; her and others' informative presentations are summarized in the conference report, *WHO Meeting on Survivors of Ebola Virus Disease: Clinical Care of Survivors* (Geneva: World Health Organization, 2015). Other teams also reported ocular complications of Ebola infection—which might have been anticipated and planned for. See, for example, John G. Mattia et al., "Early Clinical Sequelae of Ebola Virus Disease in Sierra Leone: A Cross-Sectional Study," *The Lancet Infectious Diseases* 16, no. 3 (2016): pp. 331–38; Lauren Epstein et al., "Post-Ebola Signs and Symptoms in U.S. Survivors," *The New England Journal of Medicine* 373, no. 25 (2015): pp. 2484–86; Adnan I. Qureshi et al., "Study of Ebola Virus Disease Survivors in Guinea," *Clinical Infectious Diseases* 61, no. 7 (2015): pp. 1035–42. For evidence from previous outbreaks, see Alexander K. Rowe et al., "Clinical, Virologic, and Immunologic Follow-Up of Convalescent Ebola Hemorrhagic Fever Patients and Their Household Contacts, Kikwit, Democratic Republic of the Congo," *The Journal of Infectious Diseases* 179, supplement 1 (1999): pp. S28–S35; Kapay Kibadi et al., "Late Ophthalmologic Manifestations in Survivors of the 1995 Ebola Virus Epidemic in Kikwit, Democratic Republic of the Congo," *The Journal of Infectious Diseases* 179, supplement 1 (1999): pp. S13–S14; Danielle V. Clark et al., "Long-Term Sequelae After Ebola Virus Disease in Bundibugyo, Uganda: A Retrospective Cohort Study," *The Lancet Infectious Diseases* 15, no. 8 (2015): pp. 905–912.

39. Precious few West Africans had, during their illness, anything in the way of a diagnostic workup—no lumbar punctures, of course, but also no noninvasive imaging of the brain or meninges and no sampling of the fluid in the eye. American Patient Four—Ian Crozier—was probably the only survivor to undergo such evaluation, and that was in Atlanta. No direct examination of the central nervous system had ever, to the best of our knowledge, been performed. This even though signs and symptoms of central nervous system involvement have been reported in a larger fraction of recent cases than have frank hemorrhagic symptoms, and tardy sequelae of such involvement, including seizure disorder and ataxia, have been far from rare. See the recent review by Bridgette Jeanne Billioux, Bryan Smith, and Avindra Nath, "Neurological Complications of Ebola Virus Infection," *Neurotherapeutics* 13, no. 3 (2016): pp. 461–70.

40. Pretty much every one of these complications were seen during the Ebola outbreak in West Africa, where they were sometimes described as novel discoveries. Even in the midst of the first documented outbreak of Marburg, medical personnel there (and in Hamburg and Belgrade) documented its clinical course carefully and monitored for sequelae. As in the current Ebola epidemic, gastrointestinal symptoms were dominant early in the course of Marburg disease. This led to misdiagnosis as typhoid, bacillary dysentery, and leptospirosis; hemorrhagic manifestations occurred later and in fatal cases. But the can-do attitude (and staff and stuff and space) that led to Marburg's discovery also led to long-term follow-up and new understandings of its sequelae, as one look back reminds us: "Orchitis, a typical late-stage symptom, appeared in the third week after onset of disease or even at relapse during the fifth week. Mental confusion and paraesthesias were indicative of cerebral involvement. Relapses with hepatitis, orchitis, and uveitis with virus persisting in semen and in the anterior eye chamber were typical during the convalescent phase of both Marburg virus and Ebola virus infections. In one case, a patient transmitted infection to his wife 120 days after onset of his disease, most probably by sexual intercourse" (Slenczka and Klenk, "Forty Years of Marburg Virus," pp. S131–S132).

41. See, for example, J. Knobloch, E. J. Albiez, and H. Schmitz, "A Serological Survey on Viral Haemorrhagic Fevers in Liberia," *Annales de l'Institut Pasteur / Virologie* 133, no. 2 (1982): pp. 125–28. Such serosurveys need not necessarily suggest asymptomatic infection, since it was not the primary concern of the Europe-based researchers to conduct detailed interviews of study subjects, who faced, as did others in the region, repeated bouts of febrile illness. As for Marburg's debut in Europe, "there was no indication of clinically inapparent infection," according to Slenczka and Klenk's review, "Forty Years of Marburg Virus," p. 132. This was not the case with Ebola infection in West Africa, as Eugene Richardson and our colleagues have shown in "Minimally Symptomatic Infection in an Ebola 'Hotspot': A Cross-Sectional Serosurvey," *PLOS Neglected Tropical Diseases* 10, no. 11 (2016): p. e0005087.

42. The 2014 guidelines developed and circulated by a doctor working with MSF were as emphatic as they were discouraging, and offer a textbook example of clinical nihilism. "Present data suggests that maternal mortality remains high (approximately 95 percent) and peri-natal mortality virtually 100 percent for infected pregnant women . . . Fetal monitoring is not advised. The likelihood of a surviving baby is virtually zero. If fetal distress was suspected it would not be advised to undertake any surgical or invasive procedures as these would be of high risk to the staff involved with unlikely benefit to the patient or the fetus . . . In the unlikely event of a live birth the baby must be assumed to be Ebola positive and handled in accordance with full personal protective equipment and safety protocols . . . it should be made clear that the baby is very likely to die in the neonatal period." See Benjamin Black, "Principles of Management for Pregnant Women with Ebola: A Western Context," Royal College of Obstetricians

and Gynaecologists, 2014, rcog.org.uk/globalassets/documents/news/ebola-and
-pregnancy-western.pdf; Médecins Sans Frontières, "Guidance Paper—Ebola
Treatment Centre: Pregnant & Lactating Women," Royal College of Obstetricians and Gynaecologists, 2014, rcog.org.uk/globalassets/documents/news/etc
-preg-guidance-paper.pdf.

43. Rumors about renal failure were later substantiated by surveillance activities
conducted among survivors discharged from Ebola treatment units. One large
study in Guinea found that mortality among survivors during the first year after
discharge was five times higher than that in the general population, and review
of medical records and verbal autopsies suggested that many of these deaths were
due to renal failure. See Mory Keita et al., "Subsequent Mortality in Survivors of
Ebola Virus Disease in Guinea: A Nationwide Retrospective Cohort Study," *The
Lancet Infectious Diseases* 19, no. 11 (2019): pp. 1202–1208. If routine testing
of renal function is performed in the ongoing outbreak in eastern Congo, we will
learn more about the pathophysiology of Ebola than we did in Upper West Africa.

44. TKM-Ebola, a member of a class of drugs called small interfering RNAs, was
evaluated in a clinical trial launched in Port Loko early in 2015, but this trial
was soon halted for lack of demonstrated efficacy. The manufacturer, a Japanese
firm, suspended further work on it. See Gretchen Vogel and Kai Kupferschmidt,
"In Setback for Potential Ebola Drug, Company Halts Trial," *Science*, June 19, 2015,
sciencemag.org/news/2015/06/setback-potential-ebola-drug-company-halts
-trial.

45. Mara Jana Broadhurst et al., "ReEBOV Antigen Rapid Test Kit for Point-of-
Care and Laboratory-Based Testing for Ebola Virus Disease: A Field Validation
Study," *The Lancet* 386, no. 9996 (2015): pp. 867–74. Broadhurst and colleagues
also conducted a field evaluation of another rapid diagnostic, the GeneXpert Ebola Assay, which had 100 percent sensitivity and 95.8 percent specificity; these
results are published in Amanda E. Semper et al., "Performance of the GeneXpert Ebola Assay for Diagnosis of Ebola Virus Disease in Sierra Leone: A Field
Evaluation Study," *PLOS Medicine* 13, no. 3 (2016): p. e1001980.

46. Ana Maria Henao-Restrepo et al., "Efficacy and Effectiveness of an rVSV-
Vectored Vaccine Expressing Ebola Surface Glycoprotein: Interim Results from
the Guinea Ring Vaccination Cluster-Randomised Trial," *The Lancet* 386, no.
9996 (2015): p. 857.

47. Rashid Ansumana et al., "Ebola in Freetown Area, Sierra Leone—A Case Study
of 581 Patients," *The New England Journal of Medicine* 372, no. 6 (2015): pp.
587–88.

48. Pierre Rollin and colleagues noted as much: "While the ability to conduct research
on infectious EBOV and MARV is limited to a small number of high containment
laboratories, extensive funding has been applied to primary research in the past
decade, and progress has been made in understanding the biology of these viruses, as well as toward development of potential therapies. However, from the

perspective of those at most risk of disease, this progress has not been experienced. Large outbreaks of Ebola hemorrhagic fever in the Democratic Republic of Congo in 2007 and 2008, and in Uganda in 2007, have demonstrated the continued potential for prolonged virus transmission in impoverished rural communities" (MacNeil and Rollin, "Ebola and Marburg Hemorrhagic Fevers," p. e1546).

49. The Omaha team's detailed report of standard operating procedures for care of the tiny number of patients transferred to them wouldn't merit publication if the disease in question wasn't Ebola, since they are routine in most ICUs. As in Atlanta, Bethesda, and New York, these procedures made it possible to save these patients' lives without a single secondary infection: "The intensivists systematically donned the following personal protective equipment under close supervision by an experienced biocontainment unit nurse: surgical gown, surgical cap, bouffant cap, face shield, standard patient gloves, impermeable washable shoes, surgical boot covers (over the calf), N-95 respirator mask, long-cuffed nitrile gloves (duct taped to the surgical gown), and splash protection apron. Outer garments consisted of a sterile surgical gown and sterile gloves to ensure adherence to the Centers for Disease Control and Prevention Guidelines for the Prevention of Intravascular Catheter-Related Infections. The outer sterile gloves were upsized by one half size to account for the two pairs of gloves underneath. A nurse and a respiratory therapist were in the room to assist" (Johnson et al., "Lessons Learned," p. 1158).

50. See, for example, Oumar Faye et al., "Use of Viremia to Evaluate the Baseline Case Fatality Ratio of Ebola Virus Disease and Inform Treatment Studies: A Retrospective Cohort Study," *PLOS Medicine* 12, no. 12 (2015): p. e1001908; Jonathan S. Towner et al., "Rapid Diagnosis of Ebola Hemorrhagic Fever by Reverse Transcription-PCR in an Outbreak Setting and Assessment of Patient Viral Load as a Predictor of Outcome," *Journal of Virology* 78, no. 8 (2004): pp. 4330–41.

51. MacNeil and Rollin noted as much in considering a similar list of straightforward interventions: "While logistically challenging, the above interventions are not technologically difficult. These have consistently been applied in outbreaks, and are effective in stopping the chains of transmission" ("Ebola and Marburg Hemorrhagic Fevers," p. e1546).

52. James Surowiecki, "Ebolanomics," *The New Yorker*, August 25, 2014, newyorker.com/magazine/2014/08/25/ebolanomics.

53. "Experts: Ebola Vaccine at Least 50 White People Away," *The Onion*, July 30, 2014, theonion.com/experts-ebola-vaccine-at-least-50-white-people-away-1819576750.

54. Humarr Khan, quoted in Joshua Hammer, "'I Don't Know If I'm Already Infected.' The Controversial Death of Ebola's Unsung Hero," *Matter*, January 12, 2015.

55. See, for example, Sheik Humarr Khan et al., "New Opportunities for Field Research on the Pathogenesis and Treatment of Lassa Fever," *Antiviral Research* 78,

no. 1 (2008): pp. 103–115; Jeffrey G. Shaffer et al., "Lassa Fever in Post-Conflict Sierra Leone," *PLOS Neglected Tropical Diseases* 8, no. 3 (2014): p. e2748; Randal J. Schoepp et al., "Undiagnosed Acute Viral Febrile Illnesses, Sierra Leone," *Emerging Infectious Diseases* 20, no. 7 (2014): pp. 1176–82; Matthew L. Boisen et al., "Multiple Circulating Infections Can Mimic the Early Stages of Viral Hemorrhagic Fevers and Possible Human Exposure to Filoviruses in Sierra Leone Prior to the 2014 Outbreak," *Viral Immunology* 28, no. 1 (2014): pp. 19–31.

56. Daniel G. Bausch, "The Year That Ebola Virus Took Over West Africa: Missed Opportunities for Prevention," *The American Journal of Tropical Medicine and Hygiene* 92, no. 2 (2015): p. 230.

57. Humarr Khan, quoted in Hammer, "The Controversial Death of Ebola's Unsung Hero."

58. Hammer, "The Controversial Death of Ebola's Unsung Hero."

59. "The unfinished shell of the new ward in Kenema still sits collecting rain," reflected Bausch a year after Ebola invaded the rest of the hospital, "a testament to good intentions betrayed by the logistical, bureaucratic, and financial complexities of the world of development, although there are plans now to finally finish it off" ("The Year That Ebola Virus Took Over West Africa," p. 230).

60. Hammer, "The Controversial Death of Ebola's Unsung Hero."

61. Bausch, "The Year That Ebola Virus Took Over West Africa," p. 229.

62. Richard Preston, "The Ebola Wars: How Genomics Research Can Help Contain the Outbreak," *The New Yorker*, October 27, 2014, newyorker.com/magazine/2014/10/27/ebola-wars.

63. The physician, who wishes to remain anonymous, volunteered in the Kailahun unit a couple of months after Khan's death. "We had the staff to do better," he told me. "There were ten expatriate clinicians there, five doctors, and five nurses, along with many local staff. Every night, we would gather for 'vent sessions,' complaining about the lack of aggressive therapy for the disease. One emergency physician said, 'I brought some IOs'"—intraosseous needles—"'and used them to good effect, but was discouraged since it wasn't part of the treatment protocol.' When we brought the issue up in Kailahun, we were told to make no changes and suggest nothing, but to unquestioningly follow protocols set by experts at headquarters." It's clear that professional caregivers working in Kenema and other parts of the clinical desert have long been deprived of the tools of their trade, a lack that quickly proved lethal in the face of a scourge spread in the very act of caregiving. But the reluctance to bring in such tools and put them to good use—which came largely from those who set treatment standards but were far removed from the places in which they were implemented—was also a social mechanism by which Ebola killed. "It was self-evidently unethical to pour resources into research without building a proper platform for delivery of care, as in Kenema," the physician opined, "but also unethical to handcuff clinicians with protocols that would fail to save the majority of patients, as in Kailahun."

64. Hammer, "The Controversial Death of Ebola's Unsung Hero." See also the essays, articles, and tributes by Dan Bausch and colleagues of Humarr Khan.

65. See Gabriel Fitzpatrick et al., "The Contribution of Ebola Viral Load at Admission and Other Patient Characteristics to Mortality in a Médecins Sans Frontières Ebola Case Management Centre, Kailahun, Sierra Leone, June–October 2014," *The Journal of Infectious Diseases* 212, no. 11 (2015): pp. 1752–58. Versions of these data are still being published in various journals, but they all show more or less the same grim outcomes.

66. Hammer, "The Controversial Death of Ebola's Unsung Hero." Hammer also reports that Khan wasn't involved in the decision, which was taken by MSF and the World Health Organization. Richard Preston tells the same story: "The debate quickly centered on ZMapp, which seemed to show more promise than other drugs. Why should Khan, and not other patients, get any experimental drug? What if he died? ZMapp had been tested in some monkeys a few months earlier, but what was the significance of that? It was made from mouse-human antibodies that had been grown in tobacco plants. If such substances enter the bloodstream, a person might have a severe allergic reaction. If something went wrong with the drug, there was no intensive-care unit in Kailahun. The population of Sierra Leone would be furious if the West was seen to have killed Khan, an African scientist and a national hero, with an experimental drug. But if he wasn't given the ZMapp, and he died, people might say that the West had withheld a miracle drug from him" ("The Ebola Wars"). My colleague who later worked in Kailahun put it this way in commenting on the reigning attitude in the ETU: "The dominant logic was about reputational risk. MSF leadership believed that if Khan died after receiving ZMapp, it would decrease what little trust the locals had in us. *We* would take a reputational hit. He ended up getting the shittiest care possible because they made these discussions in the public sphere. And when we later complained about low standards, the party line was, 'You weren't here when it was hard, when we had to make do with what we had.' But, in fact, they came in with these ideas."

67. Lance Plyler, quoted in Preston, "The Ebola Wars."

68. Passi et al., "Ebola Virus Disease (The Killer Virus)," p. LE06.

69. Fitzpatrick et al., "The Contribution of Ebola Viral Load at Admission and Other Patient Characteristics to Mortality," p. 1754.

70. "Speech by MSF International President Joanne Liu to the EU High Level Meeting on Ebola," Médecins Sans Frontières, March 3, 2015, msf.org/speech-msf-international-president-joanne-liu-eu-high-level-meeting-ebola.

71. Bausch, "The Year That Ebola Virus Took Over West Africa," p. 230.

72. Balasegaram et al., "Ebola: A Challenge to Our Humanitarian Identity," pp. 2–3.

73. That agreement, the letter insisted, included clear guidance for any group or individual intervening in the epidemic that began in 2013: "In catastrophic situations that temporarily overwhelm individuals, communities and local health

structures—especially in the absence of other actors—we strive to provide quality medical and other relevant care in order to contribute to the survival and relief of as many people as possible . . . MSF's primary responsibility is to improve the quality, relevance and extent of our own assistance. Obtaining quality clinical results while maintaining respect for the patient must be the major criteria used to evaluate the progress of our medical practice." See "La Mancha Agreement," Médecins Sans Frontières, June 25, 2006, msf.fr/sites/msf.fr/files/2006_06_24 _FINAL_La_Mancha_Agreement_EN.pdf.

74. Balasegaram et al., "Ebola: A Challenge to Our Humanitarian Identity," p. 1.

10. THE SILLY THINGS AND THE FEVER NEXT TIME

1. A few such "flare-ups"—defined as sporadic cases or clusters with no known epidemiological link to ongoing transmission chains—have already occurred. At least half of those detected in West Africa between March 2015 and March 2016 are thought to have originated by sexual transmission from persistently infected survivors. One, registered in Guinea in August 2015, was later found to be a consequence of mother-to-child transmission via infected breast milk: a nine-month-old with no known links to concurrent transmission chains died of Ebola, according to the results of a postmortem oral swab. In searching for the source of her infection, contact tracers tested the baby's parents, neither of whom were ill or suspected of having Ebola. Although blood samples drawn then were Ebola-negative by PCR, both were IgG-seropositive, raising the likelihood of a missed, minimally symptomatic infection in past months. See Daouda Sissoko et al., "Ebola Virus Persistence in Breast Milk After No Reported Illness: A Likely Source of Virus Transmission From Mother to Child," *Clinical Infectious Diseases* 64, no. 4 (2017): pp. 513–16.

2. Many aftermath statements and publications fail to mention a previous countdown—the one a year earlier, in May 2014—when some disease-control experts had deemed Liberia's outbreak over and done. In a report published on May 18, officials from the World Health Organization announced, "The date of isolation of the most recent case is 9 April 2014. It is therefore projected that the Ebola virus disease outbreak could be declared over on 22 May 2014." Within a couple weeks of the latter date, patients sick with its symptoms showed up at a public hospital in Monrovia, becoming the first recorded cases in the capital. Within a couple of months, hundreds of new cases were being diagnosed in the city each week.

3. These cases, which had mostly been registered in Liberia's Margibi County, were later classed as originating from contact with a persistently infected Liberian, rather than reintroduction from an animal reservoir or from neighboring countries. Molecular and conventional epidemiology connected the flare-up with a cluster of cases that had occurred almost a year earlier in the nearby community of Barclay Farm; these investigations are presented in David J. Blackley et al., "Reduced Evolutionary Rate in Reemerged Ebola Virus Transmission Chains,"

Science Advances 2, no. 4 (2016): p. e1600378. There was speculation that the flare-up was linked to a dog from the farm, as five of the seven patients had butchered and consumed it. (This speculation soon died down in epidemiological circles, since there's not any evidence that man's best friend can become infected by or transmit the virus; the dog's remains were nevertheless tested for Ebola and found negative.) Following the Margibi outbreak, Liberia was again declared Ebola-free on September 3, 2015—again, not for the last time.

4. Palo Conteh, quoted in "New Sierra Leone Ebola Cases Frustrate Efforts to End Outbreak," Reuters, September 8, 2015, reuters.com/article/us-health -ebola-leone/new-sierra-leone-ebola-cases-frustrate-efforts-to-end-outbreak -idUSKCN0R81ZZ20150908.

5. Palo Conteh, quoted in "We Will Use Force If . . . NERC Boss," *Awoko*, November 20, 2014, awoko.org/2014/11/20/sierra-leone-news-we-will-use-force-if-nerc -boss. (Formatting altered.)

6. "Stopping Ebola: It Takes Collaboration to Care for a Village," World Health Organization, September 2015, who.int/features/2015/stopping-ebola-in-kambia.

7. "New Sierra Leone Ebola Cases Frustrate Efforts to End Outbreak."

8. Prime Minister Mohamed Saïd Fofana is quoted by Dionne Searcey in "The Last Place on Earth With Ebola: Getting Guinea to Zero," *The New York Times*, November 6, 2015, nytimes.com/2015/11/07/world/africa/the-last-place-on-earth -with-ebola-guineas-fight-to-get-to-zero.html.

9. Searcey, "The Last Place on Earth With Ebola."

10. As regards rinderpest, a large international vaccination effort called Joint Project 15 was launched in 1962 to control the disease in Africa, where it was enzootic in various regions. The project focused first on Cameroon, Chad, Niger, and Nigeria, but was extended in 1965 to Guinea, Liberia, Sierra Leone, and other parts of West Africa, and later to East Africa. With over seventy million head of cattle vaccinated in twenty-two countries by 1976, Joint Project 15 was alleged to eliminate rinderpest from several countries. But incomplete coverage and persistent reservoirs of infection in the pastoral communities of the Senegal River basin—along with dwindling funds and enthusiasm for regional disease-control projects—permitted rinderpest's resurgence in several parts of West Africa. In the early 1980s, reports the ecologist Clive Spinage, a strain moving westward from southern Sudan sparked in Nigeria and abutting regions what he terms "the biggest cattle disaster of the 20th century. One third of cattle belonging to the Fulani died, and many Fulani herdsmen committed suicide, while their relatives were obliged to seek famine-relief camps. In Nigeria alone, 500,000 cattle died, and 2 million were affected." See *Cattle Plague: A History* (New York: Kluwer Academic/Plenum Publishers, 2003), p. 606. Rinderpest's comeback led to the organization of a new eradication effort, known as the Pan-African Rinderpest Campaign, and the last known case was reported in Kenya in 2001. After a decade of surveillance, the world was declared free of rinderpest in 2011.

11. Mainstream estimates had long pegged European mortality during the Black Death at about 20 to 30 percent of the population. These figures were recently interrogated by the Norwegian historian Ole J. Benedictow, whose study of the topic posits that as much as 60 percent of Europe's population (or about fifty million of its eighty million people) perished from the plague and its consequences. In his reappraisal of the prevailing mortality figures, Benedictow suggests that available data largely overlook those who were at greatest risk of disease and death: "The foundation of our knowledge on mortality in the Black Death is the quite numerous data that are based on registers recording taxpaying and rentpaying householders," which were represented overwhelmingly by men of "economically better-off taxable and rentpaying social classes in towns and countryside." In such accounting, he notes, "the poor, destitute, propertyless and landless classes of labourers, sub-tenants, seasonal workers and suchlike people that constituted the proletariat of medieval society are left out, because they could not bear any tax assessment and, consequently, were not worthwhile to record." Accounting for this and other sociodemographic trends—including the likelihood that "the proletarian classes suffered at least significant supermortality as a result of the debilitating effects of malnutrition and undernutrition on the immune system and the higher degree of exposure to rats and rat fleas"—the historian contends that previous estimates of overall mortality ought to be doubled. See *The Black Death, 1346–1353: The Complete History* (Woodbridge, U.K.: The Boydell Press, 2004), pp. 381–82.

12. Laurie Garrett underlines India's fever-diamond connections: "Between 1971 to 1991, the population of Surat grew by an astounding 151.61 percent, with most of that increase representing impoverished migrant workers who toiled in the $600 million textile or $1 billion diamond industries. As the population grew, so did the number of horrendous slums—up from ninety in the 1960s to three hundred by 1994, inhabited by some 450,000 people. There were no formal sewage or water systems in these slums; housing was slapdash lean-tos, even tents; malaria and hepatitis were epidemic; and no one apparently enforced even India's weak labor and safety regulations in the businesses along Ved Road. What drew industry to Surat was precisely the weakness of its government, lack of health and pollution enforcement, an eager, unskilled labor force, and a virtual tax-free environment. By 1994, one out of every three diamonds mined in the world were polished in Surat." See *Betrayal of Trust: The Collapse of Global Public Health* (New York: Hyperion, 2000), p. 23.

13. Many of these debates are summarized (at least from our point of view) in Louise Ivers et al., "Five Complementary Interventions to Slow Cholera: Haiti," *The Lancet* 376, no. 9758 (2010): pp. 2048–51; David Walton, Arjun Suri, and Paul Farmer, "Cholera in Haiti: Fully Integrating Prevention and Care," *Annals of Internal Medicine* 154, no. 9 (2011): pp. 635–37; Paul Farmer et al., "Meeting Cholera's Challenge to Haiti and the World: A Joint Statement on Cholera Prevention and Care," *PLOS Neglected Tropical Diseases* 5, no. 5 (2011): p. e1145; Louise

Ivers, Paul Farmer, and William J. Pape, "Oral Cholera Vaccine and Integrated Cholera Control in Haiti," *The Lancet* 379, no. 9831 (2012): pp. 2026–28; Paul Farmer and Louise Ivers, "Cholera in Haiti: The Equity Agenda and the Future of Tropical Medicine," *The American Journal of Tropical Medicine and Hygiene* 86, no. 1 (2012): pp. 7–8; Jonathan Weigel and Paul Farmer, "Cholera and the Road to Modernity: Lessons from One Latin American Epidemic for Another," *Americas Quarterly* 6, no. 3 (2012); Louise Ivers et al., "Use of Oral Cholera Vaccine in Haiti: A Rural Demonstration Project," *The American Journal of Tropical Medicine and Hygiene* 89, no. 4 (2013): pp. 617–24; Louise Ivers, "New Strategies for Cholera Control," *The Lancet Global Health* 4, no. 11 (2016): pp. e771–e772; Louise Ivers, "Eliminating Cholera Transmission in Haiti," *The New England Journal of Medicine* 376, no. 2 (2017): pp. 101–103.

14. A Nepali source for Haiti's cholera epidemic was suggested at its outset, since it began near the base of the Nepalese battalion of UN peacekeepers stationed in central Haiti. Raw sewage from the base drained into a tributary of the country's largest river, and cholera exploded along its course within days. Formal acknowledgment of this fact was a long time coming from the United Nations. But this was because of defensive legal posturing, not because of faulty epidemiological hypotheses made early in the course of the epidemic. Evidence of the source was first unearthed by investigative journalists and epidemiologists, and later confirmed by molecular and genetic characterization of circulating cholera strains. See Jonathan M. Katz, "UN Worries Its Troops Caused Cholera in Haiti," *NBC News*, November 19, 2010, nbcnews.com/id/40280944/ns/health/t/un-worries -its-troops-caused-cholera-haiti; Jonathan M. Katz, "In the Time of Cholera: How the UN Created an Epidemic—Then Covered It Up," *Foreign Policy*, January 10, 2013, foreignpolicy.com/2013/01/10/in-the-time-of-cholera; Chen-Shan Chin et al., "The Origin of the Haitian Cholera Outbreak Strain," *The New England Journal of Medicine* 364, no. 1 (2011): pp. 33–42; Rene S. Hendriksen et al., "Population Genetics of *Vibrio cholerae* from Nepal in 2010: Evidence on the Origin of the Haitian Outbreak," *mBio* 2, no. 4 (2011): pp. e00157–11; Alejandro Cravioto et al., *Final Report of the Independent Panel of Experts on the Cholera Outbreak in Haiti* (New York: United Nations, 2011). These events are discussed as they were unfolding in *Haiti After the Earthquake* (New York: PublicAffairs, 2011), pp. 188–216.

15. In October 2018, war-torn Yemen surpassed Haiti to become home to the world's largest documented cholera outbreak since the WHO records began a global tally in 1949. Estimates then published by the World Health Organization and the UN Office for the Coordination of Humanitarian Affairs count, respectively, 1.1 million suspected cases to date in Yemen between 2017 and 2018 versus 818,000 suspected cases to date in Haiti between 2010 and 2018.

16. James Surowiecki, "Ebolanomics," *The New Yorker*, August 25, 2014, newyorker .com/magazine/2014/08/25/ebolanomics.

17. Adam Goguen and Catherine Bolten report that "Temne cosmology does not assign the status of living things to anything smaller than the eye can see, which is how most illness is attributed to cosmological maleficence." They go on to explain that "EVD emerged simultaneously as political maneuvering, witchcraft, 'family swears,' and a compendium of familiar physical symptoms that referenced other common diseases. This confounded the initiation of a single 'right' way of understanding its origins, complicating the possibility of breaking transmission through transforming people's beliefs. The intervention was deemed successful when attempts to transform beliefs about disease causation were discarded in favor of mandating temporary behavior change. The legal contours of EVD-specific praxis relieved individuals of contending with challenges to their cosmology, with people able to cite the bylaws that banned most interpersonal practices, and not germ theory, as a reason to reject everyday communion." See "Ebola Through a Glass, Darkly: Ways of Knowing the State and Each Other," *Anthropology Quarterly* 90, no. 2 (2017): pp. 438, 427.

18. Writing at the close of its war, the anthropologist Mariane Ferme recommended "framing a narrative about Sierra Leone in the present by looking at the relationship between traces of historical memory and the potentially occult economy within which the circulation of everyday objects takes place." Ferme underlines "the importance of understanding history not only as a site of causal explanations but also as a source of particular forms—symbolic, linguistic, practical— that social actors deploy to rework the social fabric in response to contingent events." See *The Underneath of Things: Violence, History, and the Everyday in Sierra Leone* (Berkeley: University of California Press, 2001), p. 227. Rosalind Shaw sounds a similar note when she reminds us that "the images that Sierra Leoneans tend to use again and again to express this ambivalence—of the political 'cannibal,' the diabolic diviner, the witch, and the invisible witch city—recapitulate historical connections between witchcraft and the production of human commodities, long-standing representations of slave traders as cannibals, and the human leopards and crocodiles of the legitimate trade." See *Memories of the Slave Trade: Ritual and the Historical Imagination in Sierra Leone* (Chicago: University of Chicago Press, 2002), pp. 266–67.

19. Mariane Ferme, "Hospital Diaries: Experiences with Public Health in Sierra Leone," *Cultural Anthropology*, October 7, 2014, culanth.org/fieldsights/591 -hospital-diaries-experiences-with-public-health-in-sierra-leone. Stories of witchcraft were widespread throughout the western surge. "In the last two weeks," wrote Catherine Bolten that same day, "an even more disturbing set of rumors has emerged from the northern province, where I have worked for over a decade. In several towns where the WHO reported an upswing in Ebola deaths, text messages circulated that these deaths were not due to a virus but to the fact that multiple witch airplanes crashed into densely populated neighborhoods. All the witches onboard were killed, as well as some unlucky souls on the ground. According to my contact in the north, 'This gives new meaning to the phrase air-

borne transmission!'" See "Articulating the Invisible: Ebola Beyond Witchcraft in Sierra Leone," *Cultural Anthropology*, October 7, 2014, culanth.org/fieldsights /596-articulating-the-invisible-ebola-beyond-witchcraft-in-sierra-leone.

20. For evidence of previously undetected infections in the Congo, see Sabue Mulangu et al., "Serologic Evidence of Ebolavirus Infection in a Population with No History of Outbreaks in the Democratic Republic of the Congo," *The Journal of Infectious Diseases* 217, no. 4 (2018): pp. 529–37. Ian Crozier discussed these findings in an accompanying commentary: "Mapping a Filoviral Serologic Footprint in the Democratic Republic of the Congo: Who Goes There?," *The Journal of Infectious Diseases* 217, no. 4 (2018): pp. 513–15.

21. Emily Baumgaertner, "As Aid Workers Move to the Heart of Congo's Ebola Outbreak, 'Everything Gets More Complicated,'" *The New York Times*, June 1, 2018, nytimes.com/2018/06/01/health/ebola-congo-outbreak.html.

22. For a brief overview of the history of the plunder of the Congo, and its current predicament, see Adam Hoschchild's essays, "Congo's Many Plunderers," *Economic and Political Weekly* 36, no. 4 (2001): pp. 287–88; "Blood and Treasure: Why One of the World's Richest Countries Is Also One of Its Poorest," *Mother Jones*, March/April 2010, motherjones.com/politics/2010/03/congo-gold-adam -hochschild. His book-length treatment of these and related matters, *King Leopold's Ghost: A Story of Greed, Terror, and Heroism in Colonial Africa* (Boston: Houghton Mifflin, 1998), is a tour de force.

23. Regan Marsh, the American emergency physician cited here, is unrelated to the Ministry of Health's Ronald Marsh, who shepherded Koidu Government Hospital through this transformation with the help of Jon Lascher, Corrado Cancedda, and Kerry Dierberg, from Partners In Health, and the stellar team from Wellbody Alliance, led by Bailor and Amadu Barrie and others, many of them from Kono District.

24. To be invaded by real and enduring happiness at this time and in this setting, notes the narrator of *The Heart of the Matter* (New York: Viking Press, 1948), might trigger one of Graham Greene's jibes: "Point me out the happy man and I will point you out either egotism, selfishness, evil—or else an absolute ignorance" (p. 128). After surviving the mortars and arson that took out many old buildings, the City Hotel was burned to a crisp in 2000. The power was out, and someone knocked over a candle.

25. This bind is well described by the anthropologist Susan Shepler in "'We Know Who is Eating the Ebola Money!': Corruption, the State, and the Ebola Response," *Anthropology Quarterly* 90, no. 2 (2017): pp. 451–73. The same trap is described in Adia Benton's book, *HIV Exceptionalism: Development Through Disease in Sierra Leone* (Minneapolis: University of Minnesota Press, 2015).

26. "Forgiveness," observed Michael Jackson upon return to Sierra Leone at the close of the war, "implies neither loving those that hate you, nor absolving them from their crime, nor even understanding them ('they know not what they do'); rather, it is a form of redemption, in which one reclaims one's own life, tearing it free from the oppressor's grasp, and releasing oneself from those thoughts of

revenge and those memories of one's loss that might otherwise keep one in thrall to one's persecutor forever." See *In Sierra Leone* (Durham N.C.: Duke University Press, 2004), pp. 71–72, 68.

27. As Catherine Bolten (the anthropologist in question) and Susan Shepler note in their introduction to a special issue of *Anthropology Quarterly* on Ebola, Bolten's gesture, in the eyes of the villagers, "served as confirmation that the larger ethnoprimatology project of which she was a part 'would bring good things.' These were not intellectual things that anthropology brought, but the material gifts of a frightened, grieving anthropologist." But when forced by extreme circumstance and loss to focus on material need, and their own grief, the anthropologists were ambivalent about both. "We acted physically and intellectually, organizing relief and raising money as acts separate from, and often placed in contradistinction to, our intellectual labor," reflect Bolten and Shepler in the epidemic's aftermath. "We did not discuss our 'emotional labor' as though it was a less valid contribution, and we focused instead on being 'experts' rather than emotional individuals who were losing friends and family . . . By inserting ourselves into the conversation as experts—and in doing so questioning the expertise and relevance of local anthropologists and other local professionals—we undermined our own credibility." They conclude this thoughtful essay by insisting that anthropologists ought not only to cultivate knowledge about the people they write about and a hermeneutic of suspicion for the structures that perpetuate suffering among them, but also to nurture oft-suppressed humanitarian impulses to lessen it. See "Producing Ebola: Creating Knowledge in and About an Epidemic," *Anthropology Quarterly* 90, no. 2 (2017): pp. 350–51, 366. For further reflections on pragmatic solidarity and the social sciences in responding to Ebola—and why redistributive efforts should not be seen as less valid than, much less in contradiction to, "intellectual labor"—see "The Second Life of Sickness: On Structural Violence and Cultural Humility," *Human Organization* 75, no. 4 (2016): pp. 279–88.

28. As Iain Wilkinson and Arthur Kleinman have noted, "the difficulty of making adequate sense of suffering makes critics of all of us." See *A Passion for Society: How We Think About Human Suffering* (Oakland: University of California Press, 2016), p. 9. For a thoughtful review of British anthropologists' responses to the West African epidemic, see also the essay by Fred Martineau, Annie Wilkinson, and Melissa Parker, "Epistemologies of Ebola: Reflections on the Experience of the Ebola Response Anthropology Platform," *Anthropology Quarterly* 90, no. 2 (2017): pp. 475–94. Adia Benton discusses the shortcomings of the guild mentality in American anthropology in "Ebola at a Distance: A Pathographic Account of Anthropology's Relevance," *Anthropology Quarterly* 90, no. 2 (2017): pp. 495–524.

29. Emmanuel Akyeampong, "Disease in West African History," in *Themes in West Africa's History*, pp. 187–88.

30. Saidiya V. Hartman, "The Time of Slavery," *South Atlantic Quarterly* 101, no. 4 (2002): p. 763.

EPILOGUE: THE COLOR OF COVID

1. Albert Camus, *The Plague*, translated by Stuart Gilbert (New York: Alfred A. Knopf, 1948).

2. Eugene T. Richardson, "On the Coloniality of Global Public Health," *Medicine Anthropology Theory* 6 (2019): p. 104.

3. Nancy Tomes, "'Destroyer and Teacher': Managing the Masses During the 1918–1919 Influenza Pandemic," *Public Health Reports* 125, supplement 3 (2010): p. 61.

4. Hans-Georg Kräusslich, quoted in Katrin Bennhold, "A German Exception? Why the Country's Coronavirus Death Rate Is Low," *The New York Times*, April 4, 2020, nytimes.com/2020/04/04/world/europe/germany-coronavirus-death-rate.html.

5. Bisola O. Ojikutu's talk is available online: "Race & Place: Is COVID-19 Becoming a Black Disease?," Harvard University Center for AIDS Research, April 14, 2020, cfar.globalhealth.harvard.edu/event/race-place-covid-19-becoming-black-desease-conversations-covid-19-and-black-communities.

6. Edwidge Danticat, "The Ripple Effects of the Coronavirus on Immigrant Communities," *The New Yorker*, April 6, 2020, newyorker.com/magazine/2020/04/13/ripple-effects.

7. Carl Zimmer, "Most New York Coronavirus Cases Came From Europe, Genomes Show," *The New York Times*, April 8, 2020, nytimes.com/2020/04/08/science/new-york-coronavirus-cases-europe-genomes.html.

8. Compare two investigations: Michael D. Shear et al., "The Lost Month: How a Failure to Test Blinded the U.S. to COVID-19," *The New York Times*, March 28, 2020, nytimes.com/2020/03/28/us/testing-coronavirus-pandemic.html; Kevin Sack et al., "How Ebola Roared Back," *The New York Times*, December 29, 2014, nytimes.com/2014/12/30/health/how-ebola-roared-back.html.

9. For more on the initiative, see Ellen Barry, "An Army of Virus Tracers Takes Shape in Massachusetts," *The New York Times*, April 16, 2020, nytimes.com/2020/04/16/us/coronavirus-massachusetts-contact-tracing.html; Martha Bebinger, "Massachusetts Recruits 1,000 'Contact Tracers' to Battle COVID-19," NPR, April 13, 2020, npr.org/sections/health-shots/2020/04/13/832027703/massachusetts-recruits-1-000-contact-tracers-to-battle-covid-19.

10. George A. Soper, "The Lessons of the Pandemic," *Science* 49, no. 1274 (1919): p. 505.

ACKNOWLEDGMENTS

Let me begin a long list of thanks by referring one last time to the fictional protagonist of Albert Camus's *The Plague*. Dr. Rieux refers to the stance of those who came together to fight an outbreak of bubonic plague in a fictional city in Algeria as a "certitude that a fight must be put up, in this way or that, and there must be no bowing down." It's noteworthy, as least in drawing on his pages and on these ones, that many who enlist in such battles do *not* choose between disease control and care, as has happened too often in care-free Upper West Africa in recent years—and as often occurs in response to epidemic disease in settings long stripped of the staff, stuff, space, and systems required to save lives and limit spread.

My deepest thanks, then, to all the caregivers, professional and otherwise, who provided clinical and logistic expertise in a difficult time. *You* did not bow down, and when and if we did, you said, "We gotchu." Most of you are not mentioned in these pages. You're too numerous to count, and I hope that a blanket thank-you will suffice. Short-term volunteers in the fight against Ebola joined West Africans who'd long endured execrable work conditions within dilapidated public-sector institutions. Those commandeered for the care of the afflicted were frayed public hospitals and a series of abandoned structures; hospital or fallow husk, none of them was built for purpose. That meant (for newcomers and for veterans) intermittent or no electricity, long work hours, stockouts of key supplies, and a confusing chain of command. The rewards of working within Sierra Leonean and Liberian institutions will be paid out in the long-term, but some of the risks were immediate. Special thanks are due to Michael Grady, Karin Huster, and all those who returned for multiple tours of duty, and those who returned to stay. We are deeply indebted to our colleagues from Cuba and Haiti, who weathered poor conditions without complaint.

There were many others. Clinicians from around to world responded to the call to stop Ebola, joining new West African colleagues long obliged to confront epidemic disease. Médecins Sans Frontières (and I'm especially grateful to Joanne Liu, Eric Goemaere, and Rachel Cohen) not only showed up early, they also shared expertise with others. So did International Medical Corps (gratitude to Adam Levine and Sean Casey), Emergency, and King's College Partners. Oliver Johnson led us to Connaught Hospital and to the ever-sunny Marta Lado, and they've both become close friends and colleagues. Ian Crozier has been a generous mentor and a friend.

Together, professional caregivers saved many, which allowed survivors of the disease to make their own contributions and to found a growing number of survivors' organizations. Within these groups are those who've shared their stories for this book (and for other projects) and in the process become friends and family: Ibrahim, Yabom, the Chairman (sometimes Michael, sometimes Mohamed), Bai, Hawanatu, Big Ibrahim, Little Ibrahim (and Ibrahim the Truly Big, who was spared Ebola although his wife perished), Hassan, Hafsatu, Kallon, Samba, Mariatu, and Momoh. For leadership in establishing these networks, Gibrilla Sheriff, Gabriel Warren, and Michael Drasher (in Sierra Leone) deserve special thanks. So do Jeffrey Wright, Idris Elba, and Rosario Dawson.

Of course, the chief protagonists of these pages—including the survivors who populate the book—are still working in Upper West Africa, mostly in the countries of their birth. So are several friends and colleagues who hadn't imagined their 2014 itineraries would include places like Port Loko, Koidu, Harper, Freetown, and Monrovia. The "there" there, in this work, is there thanks largely to Partners In Health, and my debt is first and foremost to its leadership. Ophelia Dahl, Ted Philip, Joia Mukherjee, and Sheila Davis (who led the PIH Ebola Response and now leads the entire organization) never wavered once the board signed on to a long-term commitment to Liberia and Sierra Leone; nor did Gary Gottlieb when he transitioned from board member to executive director as the outbreak stuttered on. Ophelia, Jim Yong Kim, and Todd and Anne McCormack—fellow founders of PIH—also helped to keep Ebola front and center in the world of policy makers, famous for attention deficit disorder whenever emergencies are involved. Special thanks to PIH leadership teams in the field, including (in no particular order) Loune Viaud, Maxi Raymonville, Pierre Paul, Jonathan Lascher, Corrado Cancedda, Heather Bedlion, Cate Oswald, Anany Prosper, David Walton, Patrick Ulysse, Maxo Luma, John Welch, Regan Marsh, Katie Bollbach, Jeff Marvin, Jim Ansara, Chelsea Clinton, Wendy Bennett, and many others working in Haiti, Rwanda, and Malawi, and who joined us in a sudden turn toward West Africa. Loving thanks to my friend and confidant Bec Rollins. We will always miss Max Raymond, Jr.

In Sierra Leone, I thank Bailor Barrie, Yusuf Dibba, Amadu Barrie, T. B. Kamara, Matron Rebecca Morlu, Ronald Marsh, Gibrilla Sheriff, A. P. Koroma, Alex Jalloh, Katie Barron, Adikalai Kamara, Dan Kelly, Kerry Dierberg, Edgar Thomas, Joyce Chang, Peter George, Sinead Walsh, Sorie Sesay, Chuck Callahan, Yunus Forna, Abdul Jalloh, Brima Kargbo, Raphy Frankfurter, Gene Richardson (to whom my debts are uncountable), Scott Gordon, Ameet Salvi, Emily Bearse, Emily Gingras, Kumba Tekuyama, Mara Kardas-Nelson, Ambassador John Hoover, and (last but not least) the wonderfully hospitable staff of the Mammy Yoko Hotel, where much of this book was drafted. We are all grateful to our partners in the Ministry of Health, including Dr. Abu Bakarr Fofanah, a gracious host during a time of great tumult and too many guests. Warm thanks to our partner organization in Kono, Wellbody Alliance. This small and valiant group lent local credence and deep familiarity with the district to our efforts to reopen Koidu Government Hospital. It remains our base in Sierra Leone.

In Liberia, I am grateful to Ministers Walter Gwenigale and Bernice Dahn, and to Miatta Gbanya, Elsie Karmbor-Ballah, Vera Musah, Francis Katteh, Tolbert Nyenswa, and our dear friend Moses Massaquoi. Thanks are due to Brian Eustis, Lauren Marcell, the nurses of the TB annex, Chelsea Plyler, and Ambassador Deb Malac. I'm especially partial to our colleagues in Maryland County, who are, again, too numerous to count but include the lone doctor struggling there, Odell Kumeh, and the district health officer, Cyrus Sneh. We would not have ended up there without the gentle push of Ellen Johnson Sirleaf and her cabinet, including the late

Dr. Stephen Kennedy (who never failed to make us laugh even in dark times) and Judeh Tubman. I acknowledge a great debt to Raj Punjabi and his many colleagues at Last Mile Health, including Lynn Black and Josh Albert, and hope to be forgiven for singling out Tracy Slagle, who helped to keep Liberia's Incident Management System rolling during tough times.

Another category of persons to whom I owe thanks includes scholars of West Africa. Although I've lived on that continent for more than a decade, I've done so as a physician, not as an anthropologist; writing about West Africa required more than remedial coaching. Deep thanks to Adia Benton, Emmanuel Akyeampong, Ismail Rashid, Adam (and Arlie) Hochschild, Danny Hoffman, Michael Jackson, Greg Campbell, Jean and John Comaroff, Agnes Binagwaho, Aimé Binagwaho, Drew Faust (a keen student of the aftermath of war), and my inspiring former student Pardis Sabeti. She and her colleagues in West Africa will make sure future epidemics are less lethal.

Infectious-disease experts, including Ebola hands or those who became them, also offered expertise and encouragements. Thanks go to Dan Bausch, Pierre Rollin, Peter Piot, Carlos del Rio, Marshall Lyon, Dan Chertow, Cliff Lane, Ian Crozier, and Steven Yeh. Tony Fauci—friend and mentor and fellow clinician—also took responsibility for the care of patients sick with Ebola. Words won't suffice, Tony. The team of nurses and physicians at the National Institutes of Health may have had a fully equipped biocontainment unit—just of the sort we needed and still need sorely in West Africa— but they also had huge reserves of compassion, kindness, and humility.

At the Brigham and Women's Hospital, many of my colleagues worked to stop an epidemic thousands of miles away. In this category are Betsy Nabel, Joe Loscalzo, Jonathan Gates, Jamie Maguire, Joel Katz, Paul Sax, Sigal Yawetz, Dan Kuritzkes, Howard Hiatt, and Jennifer Goldsmith. Harvard Medical School has been my home for over thirty years, and its deans, faculty, staff, and students unstintingly supported work on Ebola even when some U.S. medical schools discouraged those in its employ from traveling to West Africa. I spent much of 2014–2015 away from Boston and Cambridge (some of it sequestered in quarantine or some strange variant of it), and that would not have been possible without colleagues able to assume clinical, administrative, and teaching responsibilities. Thanks to George Daley, Jeffrey Flier, David Golan, Jules Dienstag, Ed Hundert, Gina Vild (who believed in this book), Emily Bahnsen, Lisa Boudreau, John Sharp, Matt Gardiner, and Jennifer Puccetti. For their "Care for Caregivers" campaign, thanks to the members of my 2014 tutorial group and to my fellow faculty members. Joe Rhatigan, Anne Becker, Salmaan Keshavjee, Arthur Kleinman, Joia Mukherjee, Mercedes Becerra, Scott Podolsky, Allan Brandt, David Jones, and Amartya Sen made it possible for me to participate fully in the events described in these pages, and their scholarship informed my understanding of them. These are both colleagues and dear friends, especially in a pinch. It's hard to thank people by referring to their academic affiliations when we've spent so much time trying to break down walls between institutions. Megan Murray, a colleague at Harvard Medical School and the Brigham, is also the director of research at Partners In Health. She made it possible to be part of a trial for a rapid diagnostic in the hot zone. Without Jennie Block, Jehane Sedky, Abbey Gardner, and Laurie Nuell it's hard for me to imagine commuting between Harvard and West Africa. To get there required Don Bourassa's expertise and Kelly O'Connor's patience; travel within the epidemic zone required the expertise and generosity of Tony Banbury and Mr. Yang Wang.

The *London Review of Books* provided me a forum for observations and reflections, as well as the beginnings of "knowing" (to go back to Camus's formulation); thanks to its editors, and to my lifelong editor in chief, Haun Saussy, and my agent (I've so been wanting to write that), Jay Mandel. At Farrar, Straus and Giroux, Alex Star shaped this project from the very beginning, and always for the better. Thanks, too, to Melinda French, Reed Jobs, Jonathan Galassi, Toby Lester, Ian Van Wye, Cassia van der Hoof Holstein, Cori Stern, Elena Castro, Kevin Savage, Cameron Nutt, Luke Messac, Matt Basilico, and Andrew Boozary, and to the incomparable trio of Ishaan Desai, Vincent Lin, and Gretchen Williams. Most of all, I'd like to thank Katie Kralievits. She entered every edit, checked facts with the rest of us, and endured much travel and long hours as this project was tacked on to our day jobs— these also seemed, at times, too numerous to count. She's family.

Speaking of family, this book would not have been completed if not for the Farmer Fleet (Ginny, Jennifer, Peggy, Jeff, Jim, and especially Katy, who created the beautiful maps and illustrations), Loune Viaud, Jonel Pierre, Emmanuel Pierre, Bryan Stevenson, Andre Ndabarasa, and the Kagames. I'd like to thank my immediate family. Didi, my first *accompagnateur* in this work, was also my companion on my first trip to Freetown. The West African Ebola epidemic was hard on our family. During the plague year, I was often unable (and sometimes unwelcome) to travel directly from West Africa to Rwanda or Haiti or through South Africa to Lesotho. Since we had been living between Harvard and Rwanda, we often had to meet in places as varied as Bangkok, an island off the coast of southern Haiti, Boston, and Miami. Our children, especially Catherine, provided great moral and pragmatic support. The former included a sketch of a medieval plague doctor, but with the familiar beak-shaped mask held in place with very modern-looking plastic straps and other features of a gas mask. In the corner, a quotation from none other than Dr. Rieux: "Desperate times call for desperate measures." I've carried this drawing around with me as a talisman, and can only hope that this account does my family proud.

It would be a mistake to close without acknowledging once more the resources required for staff, stuff, space, and systems, and to acknowledge that we would have had no "there" without the wherewithal required to assemble them. Partners In Health counts thousands of supporters, and many of them directed their donations to West Africa. But we would not have been able to rise to the occasion without the assistance of Wendy and Theo Kolokotrones, Ronda Stryker, Bill Johnson, Cecilia Stone, Laurene Powell, Paul Allen, Larry Page, Michelle Yee, Reid Hoffman, the Sherman Fairchild Foundation, Bill Helman, Mala Goankar, Wes Edens, Chris McKown, Stephen Kahn, Al and Diane Kaneb, Deb Hayes-Stone, Max Stone, Bill and Joyce Cummings, and many others.

I dedicate this book to caregivers who gave their all—as did Bernard Rieux in *The Plague*—to lessen suffering and to cure or stop the plague by enlisting others of good will. In West Africa, those who died trying include Humarr Khan and Martin Salia and close to a thousand other health professionals, but also the thousands of mothers and fathers and sisters and brothers and imams and pastors and priests and nuns and diverse community activists who knew full well they were in harm's way, but who did their best, and without the tools of the trade, to save lives. That, according to Dr. Rieux, is "the most urgent job."

Abdullah, Ibrahim, 419, 592*n*17, 595*n*31, 596*n*37
Abidjan, 261, 562*n*46
Abidjan accords, 377, 399, 412
Abraham, Arthur, 216, 223, 253, 371, 375, 385, 404–405, 548*n*1, 561*n*37, 569*n*73, 570*n*74, 587*n*116, 592*n*20, 592*n*22, 594*n*30, 596*n*42
Abramowitz, Sharon, 601*n*3
Abuja, 399, 403, 411, 416

Adams, John Quincy, 217, 220, 222, 528
Adams, Monni, 582*n*84, 582*n*86
Afghanistan, 358
"Africa and the French Revolution" (Du Bois), 189
African Americans, 282–85, 315, 572*n*6, 573*n*8; African colonization for, 210–12; COVID-19 and, 522; Jim Crow and, 282, 285, 528; lynching of, 231, 283, 572*n*7

African Historical Demography, 280

agriculture, 149–50, 198, 227–28, 498, 544*n*8, 547*n*3; rice, xxiii, 76, 103–106, 110, 149–50, 167, 193–94, 197, 300–304, 321, 553*n*40; in Sierra Leone, 103–105; World War I and, 302–304

AIDS and HIV, xvi, 50–51, 62, 71, 128, 132, 366, 422–24, 465, 470, 495, 514, 524, 604*n*7

Air France, 16, 533*n*10

airline travel, 89–90, 114, 177–78

Akyeampong, Ammanuel, 199, 290, 342, 514, 548*n*4, 566*n*67, 574*n*22, 591*n*8

Alabama, 283, 284, 572*n*6

Algeria, 238, 250

Alldridge, T. J., 254, 272–74, 283, 322

Allen, Paul, 41, 60, 66

Alligator, USS, 213, 217, 220

alligators, human, 74, 213, 271, 274, 326

All People's Congress (APC), 105, 106, 587*n*116, 590*n*3, 592*n*20

al-Qaeda, 363, 412, 416

American colonies, 196–98, 253, 550*n*10, 551*n*14, 551*n*16; war of independence, 206

American Colonization Society, 213, 224, 230, 231, 349; Maryland State Colonization Society, 225–31, 348

American Ethnologist, 588*n*126

American Journal of Epidemiology, 345

American Journal of Public Health, 46

American Revolution, 206

American Way of Death, The (Mitford), xxii

Amistad, 218–23, 528, 555*n*58

amputations, 358, 361, 375–76, 398–99, 406, 594*n*29, 601*n*1

anemia, 444

Anglo-Zulu War, 560*n*29

Angola, 373, 440, 454, 534*n*13; Uíge, 454–55

animals: bats, xx, 7–9, 20, 150, 182, 495–96, 530*n*2; horses, 195, 245, 565*n*59; livestock, 286, 300–301, 549*n*6, 550*n*8, 554*n*48, 575*n*38, 615*n*10; in military, 565*n*59; in models of pathogenesis, 447; primates, *see* primates; rats, 14, 128, 262, 293, 335, 342, 530*n*2

animal-to-human transmission (zoonosis), xx, 51, 262, 286, 437, 495, 523, 549*n*6; AIDS and, 50; Ebola and, xx, 5, 7, 183; Lassa fever and, 14

"Antagonism and Accommodation" (Brandt and Gardner), 46

anthrax, 24

anthropology, anthropologists, xxiv, 147, 317, 317–19, 324, 347, 359, 380, 407, 408, 503, 507, 513, 519–20, 579*n*68, 598*n*61, 620*n*27

Anthropology Quarterly, 620*n*27

antibiotics, 129, 174, 270, 298, 309, 326, 327, 335, 336, 471, 501, 585*n*104

antibodies, 474

apartheid, 568*n*71

armed conflict, *see* war

Ashanti, 238

Atai-Omoruto, Anne, 540*n*12

ataxia, 608*n*39

Atlantic Charter, 329

Atlantic Monthly, The, 407

Atlantic world system, 197

Australia, 36–37

autopsies, 443, 448

Babemba Traoré, 248–50, 257, 287

"'Back to Africa': The Migration of New World Blacks to Sierra Leone and Liberia" (Blyden), 191

baboons, 20

bacteria, 549*n*6

Báez, Felix, 541*n*19

Bah, Chernoh Alpha M., 532*n*3

Bah, Ibrahim, 81–82

Baize, Sylvain, 531n2

Banbury, Tony, 69–70

Ban Ki-moon, 536n23

Bantoro, 148–63, 167, 338, 376, 400–401; initiation in, 152–54

barracks, 287, 573n13

Barrie, Amadu, 619n23

Barrie, Bailor, 55, 58, 70, 74–76, 78, 107, 146–49, 152, 153, 158–61, 165, 166, 169, 170, 172, 175, 176, 391, 393, 403–404, 428, 430, 619n23

Barry, Alpha, 536n22

Barry, John, 573n18

bats, xx, 7–9, 20, 150, 182, 495–96, 530n2

Bausch, Daniel G., 355, 481–85, 491–92, 534n14, 535n19, 604n10

Beah, Ishmael, 381–83, 404, 543n2, 543n4, 596n36

Beatty, Kenneth James, 272–79, 570n88, 571n89

"Beginning of Slavery, The" (Du Bois), 177

Belgium, 235, 239, 265

Benedictow, Ole J., 616n11

Benin, 192, 245

Benson, Stephen Allen, 230

Bentley College, 362, 417

Benton, Adia, 76, 89–90, 189, 355, 423–24

Berlin Conference, 237–42, 255, 258, 281, 305, 306

Bertrand, Didi, 55, 56

Bight of Benin, 216, 266

bilharzia (schistosomiasis), 261, 342, 499

Bill and Melinda Gates Foundation, 536n21

bioterrorism, 24, 51, 479, 481, 534n13

Bismarck, 328

Bismarck, Otto von, 235, 237, 240, 328

Black, Benjamin, 540n13

Black Death (plague), 261–62, 269, 270, 287, 299, 304, 322, 335–36, 431, 456,
499–502, 563n47, 602n8, 616n11; in Dakar, 563n47; vaccine for, 500, 502

bleeding: as Ebola symptom, 14, 43–44, 462, 486, 538n33, 603n7; hemorrhagic fevers, 14, 24, 43, 44, 183, 355, 481

blindness, 332; Ebola and, 133–34, 136, 175–76, 467–68, 476, 494; river (onchocerciasis), 245, 261, 342, 580n72

Block, Mary, 144

Blood Diamonds (Campbell), 321

bloody flux, 194, 207, 214

Blyden, Nemata Amelia, 191

Bolahun, 312–14, 578n64

Bolten, Catherine, 618n17, 618n19, 620n27

bôni hinda, 569n73

borders, 32

borfima, 274, 276

Brandt, Allan, 46

Brantly, Kent, 488–89

Brazil, 196, 306, 455

Brecht, Bertolt, 96

Brigham and Women's Hospital, 457, 461

Brilliant, Larry, 1

Britain, 194, 196–97, 199, 202–208, 210–12, 215–17, 232–35, 237–39, 241–43, 245, 252–57, 262, 264, 285, 305, 310, 312; abolitionism and, 201–203, 210–12, 216–17; Americo-Liberians and, 186–87; apartheid and, 568n71; in First Boer War, 238; Frontier Police of, 255, 257; India and, 199, 208, 233, 235, 238, 239, 250, 270, 568n69, 568n71; influenza epidemic and, 297, 298; rubber latex monopoly of, 306, 327, 576n47; in Sierra Leone, 102–104, 149, 187, 251, 255, 256, 262, 338, 547n3; taxation by, 252–55, 257; in World War II, 330

Britannia, HMS, 574n28

British East India Company, 208, 233, 235

British Medical Journal, 266–67, 563n52
"British Problem in Africa, The"
    (Perham), 189
Brooks, George, 549n5
Brown, Gilbert, 294
bubonic plague, 261–62, 269, 270, 287,
    299, 304, 322, 335–36, 431, 456,
    499–502, 563n47, 602n8, 616n11; in
    Dakar, 563n47; vaccine for, 500, 502
Buchanan, 186, 231
Buck-Morss, Susan, 201, 202, 552n27
Bunce Island, 199, 204, 206, 207, 214,
    217, 321, 412, 552n19
Bundibugyo Ebola virus, 450, 605n14
Bundu initiation, 152–54
Bureh, Bai, 253, 266, 276, 299
burials and funerals, xix–xx, xxii, 18–21,
    23, 36–37, 64, 115–19, 126, 169,
    180–83, 317–18, 336, 431, 473, 497,
    503, 539nn6–7, 544n10, 547n1;
    cremation and, 64, 539n7
Burkino Faso, 245, 363, 394, 409–410
Bush, George H. W., 360
Bush, George W., 416
bush devils, 226, 275, 325
bushmeat, 8, 20, 117, 182, 496, 522,
    530n2
bush schools, 153–54, 313–14, 325
bush wives, 382, 594n29, 596n37
Bush Wives and Girl Soldiers (Coulter),
    596n37
Butcher, Tim, 580n73, 581n79, 583n91

Callahan, Chuck, 130–31
Cameroon, 287, 288
Campbell, Greg, 321, 380–81, 395, 400,
    409–411, 413–15, 427–30, 593n24,
    600n75
Camp Funston, 291, 292, 297
Camus, Albert, 1, 3, 68–69, 433, 515,
    517–18, 525
Canada, 206; Nova Scotia, 206, 208,
    209

Cancedda, Corrado, 70–71, 73, 80–81,
    88–90, 132, 619n23
Candide (Voltaire), 202
cannibalism, 271–72, 275, 315, 319, 325,
    327, 347, 504, 569nn72–73, 570n74,
    571n88, 579n70, 582n86, 593n24
Cannon, Walter B., 457–58, 463, 465–67
Cape Mount, 314
Cape Palmas, 225, 226, 229, 230, 349
Cardew, Frederic, 560n29, 568n69
Caribbean, 195, 196
Carter, Jimmy, 350, 401
cassava, 149–50
cattle, 300–301, 549n6, 575n38, 615n10
CDC (U.S. Centers for Disease Control
    and Prevention), 18, 24, 35, 36, 73,
    89, 438, 444–45, 480, 481, 504–505,
    534n14
Cell, John, 566n67, 567n68, 568n69,
    568n71
cell phones, 112–13
Central America, 195
Central Intelligence Agency (CIA), 360,
    363
central nervous system, 608n39
cesarean section, 30, 54–55
Chairman, the, 99, 100, 127, 148, 164,
    175, 452
Chang, Joyce, 608n38
Chasing the Devil (Butcher), 581n79
Chertow, Dan, 90, 92, 94, 95, 456, 457,
    461
chiefs, 194, 216, 257, 258, 561n37,
    569n72; women as, 256–57, 561n37
chikungunya, 565n62
childbirth, 30, 54–55, 74, 468, 495,
    583n93, 609n42; by cesarean section,
    30, 54–55; mortality and, 426
child soldiers, 358, 361, 379–83, 414–15,
    417, 543n4, 595n31, 595n33, 595n35
China, 340, 350
cholera, xvii, 10, 14, 180, 261, 342–43,
    395, 421, 431, 458–61, 499, 501–502;

in Haiti, 458, 501–502, 617n14; oral rehydration salts for, 458–60; vaccine for, 501, 502; in Yemen, 617n15

Christians, Christianity, 102, 119, 185, 192, 231, 232, 234–35, 544n10, 586n114; missionaries, 31, 224, 226, 235, 252, 312, 314, 420, 439, 578n60; three c's (civilization, commerce, and Catholicism), 234–36, 241

Churchill, Winston, 306, 329, 571n89

CIA (Central Intelligence Agency), 360, 363

Cinque, Joseph (Sengbe Pieh), 217–23, 285, 404, 528, 555n58

circumcision, ritual, 153

cities, xxiii, 54

civil wars (Mano River war), xii, 18, 187, 355–417, 422, 426, 496, 511, 536n21, 581n79, 590nn5–6, 591n8, 600n75; Abidjan accords and, 377, 399, 412; amputations in, 358, 361, 375–76, 398–99, 406, 594n29, 601n1; child soldiers in, 358, 361, 379–83, 414–15, 417, 543n4, 595n31, 595n33, 595n35; Ebola and, 355–56, 358–59, 370; in Liberia, xxiii, xxviii, 10, 60, 71, 83, 158, 183, 186, 355–68, 409, 590n4, 591n8; Liberia and Sierra Leone conflicts as one war, 589n1; Lomé treaty and, 410–12, 415; refugees from, xii, xxiii, 10, 18, 106, 110, 167, 185, 186, 383–84, 421, 532n7; in Sierra Leone, xxiii, 10, 38, 53, 60, 71, 83, 97, 104–110, 113, 136, 148–49, 157–68, 183, 338, 355–60, 368–417, 419, 591n8, 598n61; Special Court and, 415, 416, 422; see also Sierra Leone

Clarkson, John, 207, 211

Clarkson, Thomas, 205, 207, 210–11, 554n43

clinical trials, 332–33, 469, 491, 585n104

Clinton, Bill, 60, 386

Clinton, Hillary, 60

Clinton Foundation, 464

Cold War, 337–39, 343, 345, 349, 350, 356, 360, 361, 363

Cole, Festus, 288, 293, 566n67, 574n23

colonialism, xxii, xxiii, xxvi, xxvii, 103, 149, 183, 185–86, 189, 191–36, 237–79, 280, 304–305, 337, 439, 499, 505, 536n22, 550n9; apartheid and, 568n71; assimilation and, 259–60; Berlin Conference and, 237–42, 255, 258, 305, 306; education systems and, 251–52; European justifications for, 242; extractive trades and, see extractive trades; Great Scramble partition of Africa, xxvi, 236, 237–42, 280, 287, 304, 321; health systems and, xxii, xxvii–xxviii, 19, 44–45, 185, 251–52, 261–71, 280, 431, 438; myths and exoticizing language and, xxii; resistance to, 186, 194, 241–51, 260; and small size of European armies, 250–51; taxation and, see taxation; three c's (civilization, commerce, and Catholicism) in, 234–36, 241; World War I and, 280–81, 286–90; see also specific countries

Columbus, Christopher, 195

Comaroff, Jean and John, 588n126

Communist Party, 350, 579n66, 579n71; Red Scares, 315, 578n66

Conakry, 10–13, 15–17, 20–23, 58, 76, 160, 261, 342–43, 447, 533n10, 534n14, 562n46; evacuation of citizens to, 389–903, 392; Freetown compared with, 562n46, 566n66

condoms, 366

Congo, xxviii, 8, 50, 97, 125, 235, 337–38, 358, 386, 437–38, 478, 505–507, 519, 534n13

Conklin, Alice, 561n42, 562n45

Connaught Hospital, 38–40, 42, 53, 55–58, 67–69, 93, 98, 99, 117, 118, 120–22, 169, 173–74, 403–404, 538n33, 594n29

conquistadors, 195
Conrad, Joseph, 240
Constitution, U.S., 209, 282
containment nihilism, 526–27
Conté, Lansana, 586n113
Conteh, Aniru, 479–81, 483, 485
Conteh, Palo, 494, 497–98
Coolidge, Calvin, 307, 576n47
coronaviruses, 441; COVID-19
    pandemic, xix, xx, xxviii, 33, 45, 498,
    500, 517–28
corvée, 252
Cotton Tree, 209, 223, 321, 341, 383,
    394, 516
Coulter, Chris, 594n29, 595n35, 601n6
cowpox, 549n6
cows, 300–301, 549n6, 575n38, 615n10
cremation, 64, 539n7
Creoles, 232–33, 256, 276, 282, 300,
    302, 304, 338, 560n27
crisis caravan, 419–33, 496–97
Crooks, Roger, 597n47
Crosby, Alfred, 551n16
crowded settings, 441
Crowder, Michael, 204–205, 241, 242,
    244, 245, 251, 260, 286, 558n9,
    559n18, 571n4
"Crown for a Young Marriage" (Block),
    144
Crozier, Ian, 67–69, 93–95, 176, 476,
    608n39
Cuba, 218, 430; clinical workers from, 72,
    75, 88, 127, 140
Cuffe, Paul, 209–212, 217, 228, 554n43,
    554n45
cultural resilience, 19–20, 425
culture of violence, 598n61
curses (swears; sweh), 20, 170–72, 504,
    547n5, 618n17
Cuttington University, 340

Dahl, Ophelia, 65, 74, 75
Dahomey, 245

Dakar, 243, 258, 260–62, 269–70, 281;
    plague in, 563n47
Danticat, Edwidge, 522
Dardanelles, 571n89
Daru, 545n16
Davis, Diana, 565n59
Davis, Sheila, 65, 66, 68, 70, 73, 526
DDT, 270, 336
De Beers, 511
"Declaration" (Smith), 435
Delay, Edward, 33–34
"Demographic Impact of the 1918–19
    Influenza Pandemic in Sub-Saharan
    Africa, The" (Patterson), 280
dengue fever, 565n62
diabetes, 604n7
Diagne, Blaise, 563n47
Diamond, Jared, 195, 531n5, 549n6
diamonds, xxii, 4, 32, 82, 103–106, 149,
    151, 183, 192, 292, 320, 329–31,
    338, 341, 355, 357, 358, 361, 363, 366,
    368–73, 375, 377–79, 395, 397, 399,
    400, 410–12, 416, 428–30, 511–12,
    547n3, 580n74, 591n7; British war
    effort and, 330; environmental
    effects of mining, xxiii; in India, 501,
    616n12
Dierberg, Kerry, 619n23
Dionne, Kim Yi, 189, 355
diphtheria, 297, 421
diseases, 194–96, 213–14, 239–40, 261–62,
    548n4, 554n48; animal-to-human
    transmission in, see animal-to-human
    transmission; lack of immunity to,
    195–96; molecular basis of, 440; World
    War I and, 286–87; see also epidemics
    and pandemics; specific diseases
District Ebola Response Centre (DERC),
    74, 78, 180–82, 547n1
diviners, 170, 200–201, 276, 278, 346,
    431, 559n25; Tongo players, 272–73,
    275, 279
Djenné, 243

Doctors Without Borders, *see* Médecins Sans Frontières

Doe, Samuel Kanyon, *353, 356, 360, 362–66, 370,* 398, 401, 405, 415, 589*n*135

Donner, Etta, 318–19, 324, 325, 579*n*70

Du Bois, W.E.B., 177, 189, 283–86, 315–16, 573*n*8, 578*n*66; Liberia and, 285–86, 307–308, 311, 312, 315, 316, 363, 573*n*12, 583*n*94

Drasher, Michael, 546*n*17

Drayton, Boston J., 229, 230

Dumett, Raymond, 566*n*67

Duncan, Thomas Eric, 35–37, 42, 43, 89, 90, 93

Dutch, 208, 315

Dying Colonialism, A (Fanon), 280

East India Company, 208, 233, 235

Ebola, xi–xxviii, 3–45, 46–95, 113–43, 332, 430–31, 437–93, 494–99, 502–516, 519–21, 523, 527, 530*n*2; bioterrorism threat and, 51, 479, 534*n*13; civil strife as setting the stage for, 355–56, 358–59, 370; consultants and, 19; "cultural resilience" and, 19–20; "Ebola is real" messages, 20, 21, 117, 182; economic impact of, 531*n*1; erroneous and misleading claims about, xxi, 452; exaggerated stories about, 444–45; as filovirus, 14; first months of epidemic, 12; first U.S. case of (Eric Duncan), 35–37, 42, 43, 89, 90, 93; flare-ups of, 495, 497, 614*n*1, 614*n*3; hospital closures due to, 123, 124; hysteria about, 35, 36, 58; identification of, 13–17, 437–38; intercurrent infections and, 128–29; international response to, 12, 17, 19, 61, 65; journalistic accounts of, xx–xxi, 18, 35, 44; racism and racializing and, 90, 477–79; research on, 439–40, 442, 610*n*48; social medicine view of,

437–93; stigma associated with, 18, 98, 139; vaccine for, 28, 31, 90, 470, 479, 495, 502, 506–507, 520, 603*n*7

Ebola complications and sequelae, 129–30, 133–36, 175–76, 467–69, 476, 494, 608*n*39, 609*n*40; blindness, 133–34, 136, 175–76, 467–68, 476, 494; renal failure, 469, 610*n*43; seizure disorders, 130, 134, 136, 138, 467–68, 494, 608*n*39

Ebola containment, xviii, 18, 19–21, 32, 33, 344, 445, 456, 497–99, 500, 535*n*19; ABC (Avoid Body Contact) campaign, 98, 100–101, 120, 126; contact tracing, 19, 21, 64, 84, 173, 465, 500; control-over-care paradigm, 19, 22, 33, 35, 64, 68, 102, 127, 130, 185, 270, 343, 445, 455–56, 457, 463, 477, 499; delayed by bureaucratic obstacles and miscommunication, 15, 17; delayed by lack of identification of Ebola as the culprit, 13–15; failure of, quality of care linked to, 63; intrusive monitoring, 542*n*24; no-touch policies for health-care workers, 30–32; personal protective equipment (PPE), xx, 26, 30, 462, 473, 523, 611*n*49; *réticence* about, 20–21, 33; travel bans and cancellations, 36–38, 89–90, 114, 177–78, 533*n*10

Ebola deaths: autopsies and, 448; in caregivers, xix, 10, 27, 30, 118, 489; from hypovolemic shock, xvi, xvii, 29, 606*n*23; mortality rates, xxv–xxvi, 14, 41–45, 63, 447, 448, 603*n*7

Ebola diagnosis, 14–15, 23, 52; laboratory tests in, xviii, 466, 470

Ebola origins, xxi, 4, 532*n*3; animal-to-human transmission in, xx, 5, 7, 183; Émile as Patient Zero in, 5–12, 24, 25, 42, 495–96, 532*n*6; Eurocentric epistemology in, 532*n*3; reservoirs in, 52, 515

Ebola pathogenesis, 443, 472–77; acquisition of nutrients necessary to survival, 474–75; circumvention of host's innate defenses, 475; entry into human host, 472–73; establishment in the host, 473–74; invasion and replication in those tissues and organs for which it exhibits tropism, 475–76; rapid replication, 475; transmission to new and susceptible hosts, 476–77

Ebola Recovery Tracking Initiative, 541n20

Ebola River, 14

Ebola species, 449–52, 604n10; Bundibugyo, 450, 605n14; clades in, 450; Makona variant, 450, 453; Reston, 444–45, 450, 452; Sudan, 35, 450, 455; Taï Forest, 450; Zaire, xviii, 17, 42, 43, 52, 442, 450, 452, 466, 505, 605n14, 606n18

Ebola survivors, xxiv–xxvi, 116–17, 531n7, 546n17; American and European, xxv–xxvi, 43; dinner gathering of, 97–102, 387; Ibrahim Kamara, 96–143, 174, 178, 152, 164, 169, 175, 180, 185, 294, 368, 387, 442, 452, 471, 477, 489, 516, 528, 540n7, 553n41; Yabom Koroma, 144–76, 180, 185, 368, 376, 380, 387, 400–401, 442, 452, 467, 471, 476, 477, 489, 516, 528, 540n7, 553n41

Ebola symptoms and clinical course, xiii, 14, 52, 451–52, 460, 537n33; bleeding as, 14, 43–44, 462, 486, 538n33, 603n7; dry phase, xiii; fever, 10, 29; most common, 44; wet phase, xiii, xiv, 29; vomiting and diarrhea, xiii, 29, 128, 448, 458, 462

Ebola transmission, xx, 476–77, 530n2; blame and, 13; burial practices and, *see* burials and funerals; containment of, *see* Ebola containment; denial of basic health care services due to fear of, xii;

epidemiology of, 52; national borders and, 32; pattern of, 14; predictions about, 35; social pathways and, xx, 12, 110, 401; superspreaders in, 22–23, 25–26, 347, 483; variable rates of, 41–42

Ebola transmission among caregivers and health professionals, xii, xix, xxvi, 11, 12–13, 18–21, 23, 29, 30, 41–45, 117, 118, 346, 535n19; deaths from, xix, 10, 27, 30, 118, 489; needles and, xvii, 30

Ebola treatment, 31, 52, 446, 447, 469, 471, 479, 603n7; claims of sufferers avoiding, xxi, 18–19; control-over-care approach to, 19, 22, 33, 35, 64, 68, 102, 127, 130, 185, 270, 343, 445, 455–56, 457, 463, 477, 499; costs of developing, 28; critical care in, 29–32, 37, 40–41, 87–88, 444, 456, 470; fluid and electrolyte replacement, xiii–xvii, 28, 29, 40, 100, 124, 129, 174, 448, 456–57, 470–71, 486–87; Hastings protocol, 471; intravenous fluids, xvii, xix, 40, 100, 124, 129, 174, 456–57, 461, 464, 486, 486–87; lack of interest in developing, 90; oral rehydration salts, xiv–xvi, 28, 40, 100, 125, 129, 174, 458–63, 471, 488; Plan A vs. Plan B, 124–27; renal dialysis, xiv, 476; supportive care in, 29–32, 37, 124–27, 442–43, 444, 446, 456, 470, 489; therapeutic nihilism and and, 445, 447–48, 450, 456, 477, 500, 603n7, 609n42; TKM-Ebola, 610n44; ventilatory support, xiv, 476; ZMapp, 28–29, 31, 90, 331, 469, 487–91, 613n66

Ebola treatment unit (ETU), xii–xix, xxvi, 22, 26–27, 29, 34, 35, 39–41, 70, 72–73, 85, 174, 456, 461, 463, 464, 466, 490, 493, 542n21; decontamination in, xviii; home-based care vs., 124–27; isolation vs. treatment in, xiii; rural vs.

urban, 124; zones in, xiii, 529*n*1;
see also specific facilities
Echenberg, Myron, 336, 563*n*47, 602*n*8
ECOMOG (ECOWAS Monitoring
Group), 158–59, 161, 164, 365, 366,
377, 378, 385, 386, 392–94, 399–404,
410, 411, 425, 597*n*50
ECOWAS (Economic Community of
West African States), 158, 365, 394,
398, 401, 410
educational systems, 355, 543*n*4; colonial,
251–52; in Sierra Leone, 151–52
Ellis, Stephen, 597*n*50
"Emergence of Zaire Ebola Virus Disease in
Guinea" (Baize, Pannetier, et al.), 531*n*2
Emergency, 55, 57, 58
Émile (Patient Zero), 5–12, 24, 25, 42,
495–96, 532*n*6
Emory University Hospital, xiv, 31, 68,
89, 489
Enlightenment, 201–202
epidemics and pandemics, xx, 3–4, 10,
245, 261–64, 267, 270, 300, 305,
339, 423, 433, 452; animal-to-human
transmission in, *see* animal-to-human
transmission; emergency fund for,
539*n*5; social drivers of, 449; social
medicine and, 437–93; *see also*
diseases; *specific diseases*
Equal Justice Initiative, 572*n*7
Equiano, Olaudah, 206
Erickson, Paul, 580*n*72
Ethiopia, 235
ethnography, *see* anthropology,
anthropologists
European colonization, *see* colonialism
Executive Outcomes, 373–75, 377–79,
384, 387, 390, 593*n*26, 596*n*42
extractive science, 438
extractive trades, xxii–xxiii, xxvi, xxviii,
4, 188, 192, 305, 317, 499, 510–11;
diamonds, *see* diamonds; gold, xxii,
103, 159, 183, 192–94, 292, 330, 397,

548*n*2; logging, xxi, xxiii, 4, 15, 21,
183, 186, 192, 397, 512; minerals, 4,
103, 104, 106, 149, 151, 183, 186,
192, 292, 330, 339, 341, 379, 409,
410, 512; precious metals, 4, 103, 193;
rubber latex, *see* rubber latex

Falkow, Stanley, 437
family networks, 101, 112, 544*n*8
Fanon, Frantz, 280
Farah, Douglas, 412, 598*n*51
farming, *see* agriculture
Fauci, Anthony, 50–51, 60, 87–89, 90–95,
469, 518, 519, 524, 525
female genital mutilation, 153
Ferme, Mariane, 504–505, 547*n*3, 618*n*18
Fernando Po, 285, 310, 578*n*56
feuds, 216, 231, 242, 251, 300, 356;
see also civil wars; war
fever, febrile illness, xxvii, 9, 10, 15, 24,
52, 81, 194, 195, 197, 200, 204–205,
213–14, 228, 231, 238, 269, 286,
533*n*8, 554*n*49, 566*n*66; in Ebola, 10,
29; hemorrhagic, 14, 24, 43, 44, 183,
355, 481, 603*n*7
Fighting for the Rain Forest (Richards),
357, 589*n*2, 598*n*61
filoviruses, 14, 52, 440–42, 444, 451,
452, 457, 472; autopsies and, 443; as
bioweapons, 24, 51, 534*n*13; differing
virulence among strains of, 449; Ebola
as, 14; Marburg, 12–14, 51, 52, 130,
133, 356, 438, 439, 442, 443, 453–55,
457, 462, 468, 533*n*8, 534*n*13,
605*n*15, 606*n*18, 609*nn*40–41,
610*n*48; pathogenesis of, 451; research
on, 442; social forces and, 604*n*10
Firestone, Harvey, Jr., 309
Firestone, Harvey, Sr., 306–312, 577*n*53
Firestone Tire and Rubber Company,
186–87, 306–312, 316, 317, 322, 327,
340, 349, 350, 360, 361, 364–67, 397,
398, 583*n*94

First Boer War, 238
Flexner Report, 577*n*51
flies, 245; tsetse, 245, 265, 333–34, 585*n*106
Florida, 572*n*6
flu, *see* influenza
fluid and electrolyte replacement, 298; in Ebola treatment, xiii–xvii, 28, 29, 40, 100, 124, 129, 174, 448, 456–57, 470–71, 486–87; *see also* intravenous fluids; oral rehydration salts
Fofanah, Abu Kabarr, 73–75, 77, 81, 100
Fogbo, 545*n*16
Fonnie, Mbalu, 481, 484, 485
foo-foo, 150
Ford, Henry, and Ford Motor Company, 186, 306
Foreign Affairs, 189, 307
forestiers, 4, 10, 20, 21, 536*n*22
forests, 245; logging and deforestation, xxi, xxiii, 4, 15, 21, 183, 186, 192, 397, 512; rain forest, 183
Forten, James, 554*n*46
Fourah Bay College, 232, 234, 252, 338, 368, 379, 391, 402, 404–405
Fowler, Robert, 447–48, 456–57, 606*n*23
Fox, Renée, 465
France, 186, 194, 196, 199, 202, 208, 215, 233–34, 237–39, 241–50, 252, 257–62, 269–70, 285, 305, 337, 340, 559*n*18, 561*n*42, 563*n*47; Enlightenment in, 202; Revolution in, 189, 202; slavery and, 281–82; in World War I, 281, 289–90
Freetown, 26–27, 30, 38–39, 42, 57, 69, 71–77, 80–81, 83, 88, 96–111, 114, 118–20, 123–27, 134–35, 144–47, 151, 167–69, 187, 192, 215–16, 222, 232, 234, 248, 266–67, 272, 273, 282, 338, 396, 413, 415, 426, 428, 503, 524, 533*n*10, 544*n*7, 544*n*10; barracks in, 287, 573*n*13; citizens evacuated from,

386–93; in civil war, 97, 107–108, 158–61, 163–66, 357, 393–95, 400–405, 409; Conakry compared with, 562*n*46, 566*n*66; conference in, 45, 46–49, 53–55; Cotton Tree in, 209, 223, 321, 341, 383, 394, 516; Cuffe in, 210–12; diseases in, 214; Foulah Town, 144–45, 147, 150, 151, 163, 168, 175, 208, 216; founding of, 205–209, 214–15, 217, 223, 266, 553*n*41; France and, 559*n*18; Greene in, 319, 578*n*64; heavy rains in 554*n*41; hills and hill stations of, 266–69, 566*nn*66–67; influenza in, 292–95; Kissy, 159, 216; malaria and, 265–66, 268–69; Mammy Yoko Hotel in, 97–102, 107, 128, 132, 135, 165, 172, 183, 371, 376, 386–93, 399, 404, 413, 597*n*47; Mountain Cut, 145–46, 150, 168, 174–75; Operation No Living Thing in, 164–66, 401–404; Pademba Road Prison in, 109, 113, 341, 368, 370, 371, 378, 384, 402; slavery and, 257, 276, 281, 560*n*27, 560*n*29; smallpox in, 301; Syrians and, 302, 575*n*39; Tower Hill in, 113; workers' strike in, 338
Frenkel, Stephen, 567*n*67
Frontier Police, 255, 257, 561*n*35
Frontline, 532*n*2
Frontline Security Services, 372
fruit, 7, 20, 150
Fula people, 144–45, 147, 159
funerals, *see* burials and funerals
Futa Jallon, 243, 244, 558*n*16

Gabon, 265
Gaddafi, Muammar, 105, 368, 375
Gale, Thomas, 567*n*68
Gambia, 296
Gardner, Martha, 46
Garrett, Laurie, 7, 616*n*12
Garry, Robert, 481, 483, 491
Gates, Bill and Melinda, 60, 536*n*21

Gberie, Lansana, 384, 587*n*116, 590*n*4, 597*n*47

George III, King, 203

Germany, 14, 235, 237–39, 259, 265, 285–87, 292, 305, 312, 520–21, 533*n*8; Nazi, 312, 327

Gettleman, Jeffrey, 125–26

Ghana, 73, 253, 431, 548*n*2, 579*n*66, 591*n*8, 599*n*61

ghom, 170, 171

Glazzard, William, 294

Gleboes, *see* Greboes

Global Peace Index, 599*n*61

Goerg, Odile, 567*n*67

Goguen, Adam, 618*n*17

Gola Forest, 126, 183

gold, xxii, 103, 159, 183, 192–94, 292, 330, 397, 548*n*2

Gold Coast, 193–94, 216, 253, 295, 548*n*2

golf, 199, 412, 552*n*19

Gorée, 199

Gorilla Society, 320

Gottlieb, Gary, 91

Granville Town, 207, 553*n*38

Great Scramble (partition of Africa), xxvi, 236, 237–42, 280, 287, 304, 321

Greboes (Gleboes), 225–30

Greece, ancient, 192

Greene, Barbara, 322–23, 325–26, 331, 578*n*64, 580*n*73, 582*n*85, 582*n*88, 582*n*89

Greene, Graham, 319–26, 329, 331, 334, 444, 578*n*56, 578*n*64, 579*n*71, 580*nn*73–74, 581*nn*78–79, 581*n*81, 582*n*85, 582*n*87, 586*n*107, 619*n*24; *The Heart of the Matter*, 329–30, 584*n*99

Green Parrots (Strada), 539*n*3

Griffith, William Brandford, 277, 278, 571*n*88

Guasco, Michael, 550*n*10

Guéckédou, 6–7, 10, 13, 14, 16, 20, 534*n*14

Guinea, xi, xii, xix, xx, xxiii, xxviii, 15, 22, 23, 31, 33, 42, 47, 49, 63, 72, 85, 86, 109, 110, 126, 136, 148, 159, 160, 166, 178, 183–86, 244, 258, 285, 337, 338, 340, 341, 396, 421, 430, 495, 498, 514, 530*n*2, 541*n*20, 545*n*16, 586*n*114; borders closed in, 53; cholera in, 343; Conakry, *see* Conakry; economy of, 531*n*1; Émile as Patient Zero in, 5–12, 24, 25, 42, 495–96, 532*n*6; Guéckédou, 6–7, 10, 13, 14, 16, 20, 534*n*14; Kissi Triangle, 4, 10–12, 15, 16, 18, 24, 319, 532*n*7; Macenta, 10, 11, 13, 20, 384; McGovern on, 586*n*113; Meliandou, *see* Meliandou; N'Zérékoré, 10, 11, 24, 534*n*14

Guns, Germs, and Steel (Diamond), 531*n*5

Gurkha Security Guards, Ltd., 372, 593*n*24

Hague, The, 416

Hahn, Niels, 591*n*12

Haiti, xxvii, 48, 50, 53, 54, 59, 65, 71–72, 75, 100, 130, 180, 195, 196, 202, 209, 224, 233, 250, 258–59, 286, 312, 315, 316, 522; cholera in, 458, 501–502, 617*n*14; earthquake in, 57, 59–62, 67, 69, 71, 458, 502; hurricanes in, 71; Revolution in, 201–203, 552*n*27

Hall, James, 225–30

Hall, Richard, 226–30

Hammer, Joshua, 486, 488, 613*n*66

Harbel, 312, 327, 364–66, 368, 397

Harding, R. D., 333–34, 585*n*106

Hargreaves, J. D., 560*n*31

Harley, George Way, 324–25, 325–26, 582*nn*84–85, 582*n*88, 583*n*91

Harper, 82–83, 186, 224–29, 231, 348, 350–53, 355, 359, 361, 509, 589*n*136

Harris, Sheldon, 553*n*37

Hartman, Saidiya, 515

Harvard University, 24, 27, 54, 60, 70, 134, 391, 457, 519, 577n51; Liberia expedition of, 307–310, 312, 315, 324, 444, 577n53, 579n70, 580n72, 581n81; Peabody Museum, 317, 325, 582nn84–85

Hastings, 164, 402; treatment unit at, 122, 127, 141, 146, 164, 174–75, 471

Hay, James Shaw, 559n18

healers, traditional, xxviii, 22–23, 346, 431

health systems: "awareness teams" and, 33; black doctors and, 263, 431, 577n51; British doctors' complaints about salaries and time constraints, 263, 563n52; colonialism and, xxii, xxvii–xxviii, 19, 44–45, 185, 251–52, 261–71, 280, 431, 438; community-care centers, 40; control-over-care paradigm in, xxvii, 102, 185, 240, 261, 262, 270, 297–99, 321, 335–36, 344, 345, 424, 431–32, 445, 455–56, 478, 500–502, 505, 520; crisis caravan and, 419–33, 496–97; denial of basic services due to fear of Ebola, xii; disease control linked to profiteering and conflict, 270–71; fee-for-service, 54; immunization, see immunization; insurance and, 54; medical deserts and lack of care, xii, xx, xxii, xxvi, xxviii, 3–5, 18, 21, 22, 24, 32, 42, 50, 54, 59–60, 84, 86, 131, 149, 183, 185, 191, 213, 240, 431, 444, 448–49, 453, 466, 506–508, 510, 536n21, 612n63; programs for strengthening, 7; public health vs. medicine in, 46; religious syncretism and, 111; sanitarians (Pasteurians) in, xxvii–xxviii, 237, 240, 261, 262, 270, 298, 299, 313, 321, 335–36, 344–45, 432, 454, 465, 478, 499, 501, 510, 536n22, 563n47; social context of, 44; surgical care, 53–55, 495, 514; therapeutic nihilism and, 62,

296, 313, 420, 445, 447–48, 450, 500, 526, 527, 603n7, 609n42; vaccines, see vaccines; vertical projects for, 422–23, 425; World War I and, 288–90; see also diseases; epidemics and pandemics

health disparities, understanding, xxiv–xxv

Heart of Darkness, The (Conrad), 240

Heart of the Matter, The (Greene), 329–30, 584n99

Hegel, Georg Wilhelm Friedrich, 201, 552n27

hemorrhagic fevers, 14, 24, 43, 44, 183, 355, 481, 603n7

Herbert, Eugenia, 557n3

herpes, 441

Hickox, Kaci, 37, 80

Hinterland Liberia (Donner), 318

history from below, 184, 547n3

Hitler, Adolf, 328

HIV/AIDS, xvi, 50–51, 62, 71, 128, 132, 366, 422–24, 465, 470, 495, 514, 524, 604n7

HIV Exceptionalism (Benton), 423–24

Hobbes, Thomas, 201

Hochschild, Adam, 202, 203, 206, 207, 552n19, 553n38

Hoffman, Danny, 573n13, 589n1, 590nn5–6, 592n13, 593n23, 593n26, 595nn31–32, 595n35, 599n71, 599n74, 600nn75–76, 600n78

Holland, 199

hookworm, 128

Hoover, Herbert, 311, 316, 576n47

horses, 195, 245, 565n59

Hot Zone, The (Preston), xxv, 43–44, 444–45, 452–53

Howard University, 577n51

human alligators, 74, 213, 271, 274, 326

Human Development Index, 105

human leopards, 271–79, 315, 326, 400, 504, 570n82, 570n88

human trafficking, 320

Hut Tax War, 253–55, 257, 266, 272, 273, 278, 302, 321, 322, 407, 560n31
Hutchinson, M. P., 333–34, 585n106
hypovolemia, hypovolemic shock, xvi, xvii, 29, 40, 44, 456–57, 470–71, 606n23

Iberians, 191–97, 548n2
Ileffe, John, 558n14
immune system and immunology, 296–97, 444, 472, 474, 550n9, 575n34, 585n104, 605n16
immunization: variolation, 240, 289, 523, 557n3; *see also* vaccines
Incan empire, 195
Independent, The, 237
India, 199, 208, 233, 235, 238, 239, 241, 250, 270, 568n69, 568n71; diamonds in, 501, 616n12; plague in, 501; public-health interventions in, 568n71
Indonesia, 342
influenza, 195, 261, 299, 304, 321, 456, 520, 549n6; 1918 pandemic, 280, 290–300, 302–303, 305, 441, 518, 520, 524, 573n18, 574n28, 574n30, 575n32; railways and, 294–95; vaccines for, 290, 296
Inikori, Joseph, 197–98
insects, 549n5; flies, 245; mosquitoes, xxiii, 267–69, 287, 565n62, 567n68, 568n69; tsetse flies, 245, 265, 333–34, intensive care unit (ICU), 28, 30, 40–41, 447, 469, 611n49
International African Association, 237–38
International Monetary Fund (IMF), 348, 546n1, 596n42
"International Political Economy and the 2014 West Africa Ebola Outbreak" (Benton and Dionne), 355
intravenous fluids, 298, 461; in Ebola treatment, xvii, xix, 40, 100, 124, 129, 174, 456–57, 461, 464, 486, 486–87
Isatu, 125–26, 134, 136, 138, 468

Islam, Muslims, 102, 104, 109, 113, 119, 145, 183, 185, 192, 193, 234–35, 238, 240, 241, 244, 275, 543n3, 548n2, 586n114
Islamic College, 111
Israel, 360
Italy, 235, 237, 239
Ivory Coast, 192, 244, 245, 261, 285, 348, 394, 396, 591n8

Jackson, Michael, 115–16, 200, 376, 512, 544n6, 544n8, 619n26
Jalloh, Alex, 135, 137–39, 182–83, 503
Jariatu, 130–33
Jefferson, Thomas, 557n4
Jenner, Edward, 211, 314
Johnson, Oliver, 55–58, 67–68, 99
Johnson, Prince, 365–66
Johnston, Harry, 555n66, 580n73
Jones, David, 549n8, 550n9, 551n16
journalists, xx–xxi, 18, 35, 44; "juju," 598n61
Journal of Clinical and Diagnostic Research, 450
Journal of Infectious Disease, 604n10
Journal of West African History, 419
Journey Without Maps (Greene), 319, 324
Junge, Werner, 312–15, 318, 320, 323–25, 327–28, 331, 333, 337, 344, 578n64, 579n70, 581n81, 583n93, 584n95
Junger, Sebastian, 402, 410, 591n7

Kabala, 376, 594n29
Kabbah, Ahmad Tejan, 157–58, 161, 163, 376–78, 382–84, 391, 394, 395, 399–400, 402, 404, 410, 413, 415
Kailahun District, 15–16, 22, 23, 25–29, 31, 56, 77, 105, 155, 345, 415, 479, 486–87, 490–92, 545n16, 592n22, 612n63
Kalako refugee camp, 167

Kalous, Milan, 569n73
Kamajors, 374–75, 377, 380, 384, 385,
    387, 394, 399–401, 404, 406, 414,
    415, 593n26, 595n32
Kamara, Abdullai, 102–104, 106–109,
    113
Kamara, Hawanatu, 102, 104, 108–111,
    113–15, 117–21, 124
Kamara, Ibrahim, 96–143, 174, 178, 152,
    164, 169, 175, 180, 185, 294, 368,
    387, 442, 452, 471, 477, 489, 516,
    528, 540n7, 553n41
Kamara, T. B., 53–54, 58, 491
Kambia District, 167, 302, 304, 400
Kankan, 243–45
Kanu, James, 155–56
Kaplan, Robert, 407, 598n61, 598n61
Karene District, 301–303, 575n39
Kearsarge, USS, 386, 388, 389, 391, 393
Keltie, John Scott, 237
Kenedougou, 248–49
Kenema District, 30–32, 38, 40, 53, 60,
    77, 81, 118, 378, 384, 395, 423, 480–
    85, 491–92, 496, 534n14, 538n33,
    545n16, 612n63; Kenema Government
    Hospital, 23–27, 42, 43, 56, 67, 69, 93,
    463, 535n16, 535n19
Kenya, 358
Kerry Town, 85
Khan, Humarr, 3, 23–29, 42, 45, 51,
    52, 58, 60, 63, 72, 93, 118, 342, 423,
    440, 451, 480–91, 525, 526, 538n33,
    545n16; death of, 29, 31, 39, 43, 45,
    51, 52, 60, 61, 65, 67, 69, 114, 184,
    333, 479, 489, 490, 493, 514, 526,
    613n66; Salia and, 38
kidney failure, 30, 469, 610n43
Kigali, 47, 48
Kikwit, 535n19
Kim, Jim, 60, 539n5
King, Boston, 553n35
Kingsley, Mary, 214, 554n49
kinship networks, 101, 112

Kissi Teng, 545n16
Kissi Triangle ("trizone" region), 4,
    10–12, 15, 16, 18, 24, 319, 532n7
Kissy Lunatic Asylum, 159, 216, 252, 421
Klain, Ron, 41
Kleinman, Arthur, 620n28
Koidu, xxiii, 32, 82–84, 330–31, 355,
    395, 400, 428, 584n101; hospital in,
    429–30, 508–509
kola nuts, 119, 544n10
Konaré, Alpha, 249
Kono District, Kono people, 22, 74, 77,
    82, 183, 320, 330–31, 338, 341, 358,
    376, 378, 428–30
Koroma, Amadu Mohamed, 149
Koroma, Ernest Bai, 73, 74
Koroma, Fatmata, 149–50, 152, 175
Koroma, Johnny Paul, 384, 394, 398, 399
Koroma, Kadiatu (daughter of Yabom),
    155, 157, 175
Koroma, Kadiatu (sister of Yabom),
    149–52, 154–57, 163, 167, 173, 174
Koroma, Yabom, 144–76, 180, 185, 368,
    376, 380, 387, 400–401, 442, 452,
    467, 471, 476, 477, 489, 516, 528,
    540n7, 553n41
Kpundeh, Sahr, 590n3
Ku Klux Klan, 231, 283

Lachenal, Guillaume, 331–32, 335,
    532n7
Lado, Marta, 55–56, 58, 67–68, 98–99,
    117, 121–22, 174, 526, 538n33
Lagos, 32–33, 269, 295, 297–98, 567n68
Lagos Standard, 297–98
Lamontagne, François, 447, 457
lançados, 197, 299
Lancet, The, 470
Land Benighted (Greene), 326
land mines, 57, 539n3
Lascher, Jon, 65, 66, 78–79, 126, 135,
    138–39, 141, 142, 181, 182, 526,
    542n22, 619n23

Lassa fever, 14, 23–25, 27, 51, 56, 128, 342, 421, 423, 456, 462, 479–84, 509, 514, 534n14

Last Mile Health, 70, 72, 82

Latin America, 306, 308, 550n8, 607n28

Laveran, Charles Louis Alphonse, 565n59

League of Nations, 310, 312, 327, 340, 578n56, 583n94, 584n95

Lebanon, 300, 358

Lend-Lease, 329, 330

leopards, human, 271–79, 315, 326, 400, 504, 570n82, 570n88

Leopold, King, 235

leptospirosis, 128, 195, 549n6

Lesotho, 52, 70

Levantine merchants, 300–304, 321

Lewis, Roy, 544n10

Liberia, xi, xii, xix, xx, xxviii, 15, 17, 22, 23, 31, 33, 42, 47, 49, 60, 61, 63, 66, 70, 72, 82, 85, 86, 95, 105, 126, 136, 142, 157, 161, 178, 183, 186, 191, 214, 223–25, 231–32, 285, 320, 327, 340–41, 348–54, 464, 497, 514, 541n20, 542n21, 546n1, 580n73, 614n2; Americo-Liberians in, 186–87, 213, 224–32, 259, 285, 308–310, 314, 315, 322, 323, 338, 340, 348–50, 352, 353, 362, 365, 582n86; American troops sent to, 34; army of, 34; "black slavery scandal" in, 310–11, 327, 578n56; borders closed in, 53; British Government Blue Books on, 322, 581n78; ceremonial masks in, 325, 582n84, 582n86; civil war in, xxiii, xxviii, 10, 60, 71, 83, 158, 183, 186, 355–68, 409, 590n4, 591n8; cremation in, 64, 539n7; crisis caravan and, 419–33; Doe in, 353, 356, 360, 362–66, 370, 398, 401, 405, 415, 589n135; Donner in, 318–19, 324, 325; Du Bois and, 285–86, 307–308, 311, 312, 315, 316, 363, 573n12, 583n94;

Duncan in, 35–37; economy of, 340, 531n1, 580n72; Firestone Company in, 186–87, 306–312, 316, 317, 322, 327, 340, 349, 350, 360, 361, 364–67, 397, 398, 583n94; founding of, 204, 223–24; Greene in, 320, 322–24, 581n79, 581n81; Harbel, 312, 327, 364–66, 368, 397; Harley in, 324–25, 325–26, 583n91; Harper, 82–83, 224–29, 231, 348, 350–53, 355, 361, 509, 589n136; Harvard expedition to, 307–310, 312, 315, 324, 444, 577n53, 579n70, 580n72, 581n81; health conditions and diseases in, 308–309, 312, 320, 324, 325, 326, 355, 577n51; health plan for, 328–29, 336–37; Junge in, 312–15, 320–25, 578n64, 579n70, 581n81; Kissi Triangle, 4, 10–12, 15, 16, 18, 24, 319, 532n7; Maryland County in, 225–31, 348; missionaries in, 31, 312, 314, 578n60; Monrovia, see Monrovia; National Patriotic Front of Liberia (NPFL) in, 363–64, 366, 396, 397, 398, 590n4, 592n17; native tribes in, 224, 555n66; Open Door Policy of, 339, 340; resilience in, 601n3; Strong in, 307–310, 312, 323, 325; Taylor in, 105, 348, 362–68, 371, 378, 379, 383, 385, 392, 396–98, 400, 401, 403, 405–406, 409–413, 415–17, 421, 590n4, 591n12, 592n14, 598n51, 600n78; Tolbert in, 349–50, 352, 353, 396, 415, 589n135; Tweh's murder in, 350–53; United States and, 186–87, 286, 306–312, 316, 327, 360, 365, 589n135; World War I and, 286, 573n12; World War II and, 327; Zwedru, 82

Libya, 105, 358, 364, 394, 592n17f

Lincoln, Abraham, 282

Little Ibrahim, 133–34, 136, 141, 468

Little Scarcies River, 148, 150

Liu, Joanne, 65, 491, 493

Liverpool Post, 332
livestock, 286, 300–301, 549n6, 550n8,
    554n48, 575n38, 615n10
Livingstone, David, 235, 556n82
Li Wenliang, 525–26
Locke, John, 201, 202
logging and timber, xxi, xxiii, 4, 15, 21,
    183, 186, 192, 397, 512
Lomé treaty, 410–12, 412, 415
London, 206
Long Way Gone, A (Beah), 381–83,
    543n4, 596n36
Lumley, 112–14, 117, 121
Lumumba, Patrice, 338
Lungi, 23, 26, 47–49, 57–58, 88, 401,
    402, 600n76
Lunsar, 168, 176
lynching, 231, 283, 572n7

Mabanta, 102, 103, 110, 118–20, 124,
    125
macaques, 442, 447
MacCormack, Carol, 153, 154
Macenta, 10, 11, 13, 20, 384
MacGregor, William, 567n68
MacNeil, Adam, 605n15, 611n51
Maconachie, Roy, 587n116
Madison, James, 211–12
Maforki, 74–75, 77–81, 83–85, 88, 100,
    123, 124, 127, 128, 130–32, 134, 137,
    138, 140, 141, 178–80, 303, 338,
    413–15, 471, 491, 542n22, 600n75
magnesium, 129
Makeni, 159, 161, 395
malaria, 5, 6, 13–14, 27, 81, 128, 132,
    174, 207, 213, 214, 261, 263, 265–69,
    287, 304, 331, 342, 421, 430, 431,
    456, 470, 499, 514, 554n48, 565n61,
    567n67, 568n69, 580n72; in India,
    568n71; mosquitoes and, 267–69,
    565n62, 567n68, 568n69; quinine
    and, 204, 214, 228, 267–68, 567n68;
    segregation measures as protection

against, 265–66, 269, 273, 321, 567n68,
    568n69
Malawi, 52, 264
Mali, 244, 248, 250, 258
malnutrition, 444
Mammy Yoko Hotel, 97–102, 107, 128,
    132, 135, 165, 172, 183, 371, 376,
    386–93, 399, 404, 413, 597n47
Mane invasions, 193, 548n1
Mange, 162
Manning, Patrick, 196, 201–203, 551n18,
    556n66
Mano River Union Lassa Fever Network,
    534n14
Mano River war, *see* civil wars
Mantua, HMS, 292–94, 302, 330, 524,
    574n28
maps, 9, 246–47
Marburg virus, 12–14, 51, 52, 130, 133,
    356, 438, 439, 442, 443, 453–55, 457,
    462, 468, 533n8, 534n13, 605n15,
    606n18, 609nn40–41, 610n48
Margai, Milton, 341, 587n116
Mariatu, 131–43
Markel, Howard, 575n32
Marsh, Regan, 619n23
Marsh, Ronald, 619n23
Marx, Karl, 372, 395, 593n23
Mary Caroline Stevens, 229–30
Maryland State Colonization Society,
    225–31, 348
MASH (mobile army surgical hospital)
    units, 34, 458
masks, ceremonial, 325, 339, 582n84,
    582n86
Massaquoi, Moses, 464–65, 487, 490,
    492
Mather, Cotton, 551n14
Matthews, John, 552n22
Matweng, 180–82, 303, 547n1
M'bayo, Tamba E., 419
McCormick, Joe, 444–45, 450
McFarlane, Patrick, 294

McGovern, Mike, 586*n*113, 586*n*114
McNeill, William, 548*n*4
measles, 195, 301, 421, 441, 495, 549*n*6
meat, 8, 20, 117, 182, 496, 522, 530*n*2
Médecins Sans Frontières (MSF), 16–17, 21, 22, 27, 28, 56, 61, 62, 65, 67, 72, 114, 420, 454–55, 457, 461, 465–67, 486, 487, 491–93, 529*n*1, 540*n*13, 603*n*7, 607*n*26, 609*n*42, 613*n*66; La Mancha agreement of, 492–93, 613*n*73
Meharry Medical College, 577*n*51
Meliandou, 10, 12, 13, 23, 24, 26, 496, 532*n*2; Émile (Patient Zero) in, 5–12, 24, 25, 42, 495–96, 532*n*6
Memories of the Slave Trade (Shaw), 251
Mende, 218–20, 253, 256–57, 272, 273–76, 406, 407, 541*n*14, 548*n*1, 561*n*37, 569*n*73, 571*n*88; Kamajors and, 374
meningitis, 261, 299
Merewether, E. M., 570*n*82
Merkel, Angela, 520, 521
metals, precious, 4, 103, 193; gold, xxii, 103, 159, 183, 192–94, 292, 330, 397, 548*n*2
Mexico, 196
Migeod, William Hugh, *A View of Sierra Leone*, 76, 541*n*14, 545*n*12
Mills, Dorothy, 580*n*73
minerals, 4, 103, 104, 106, 149, 151, 183, 186, 192, 292, 330, 339, 341, 379, 409, 410, 512
mining, 4, 342, 410, 511; *see also* diamonds; metals, precious; minerals
missionaries, 31, 224, 226, 235, 252, 312, 314, 420, 439, 578*n*60
Mitford, Jessica, xxii
Mitman, Gregg, 580*n*72
mobile army surgical hospital (MASH) units, 34, 458
mobile phones, 112–13
Mobutu Sese Seko, 386
molecular basis of disease, 440

"Molecular Perspective of Microbial Pathogenicity, A" (Relman and Falkow), 437
Momoh (taxi driver), 127–28, 452
Momoh, Joseph Saidu, 151, 156, 368–69, 587*n*116, 592*n*20
monkeys, 8, 14, 44, 182, 447, 487, 496, 530*n*2, 613*n*66
Monrovia, 17, 22, 29, 31, 35, 39, 58, 67, 69–73, 181, 186, 187, 224, 228, 230–32, 259, 285, 286, 309, 322, 327, 328, 336, 361, 363, 396, 412, 426, 463, 465, 486–87, 529*n*1, 534*n*14, 553*n*41, 576*n*51, 583*n*94, 614*n*2; barracks in, 573*n*13; Ebola treatment unit in, xii–xix, xxvi, 456; Freeport complex in, 365; West Point slum in, 34–35
Mora, 287–88, 301
Moran, Mary, 223–26, 359, 360
Morel, Edmund, 561*n*35
mori men, 170
mosquitoes, xxiii, 267–69, 287, 565*n*62, 567*n*68, 568*n*69
Mossi empire, 241, 243
motorcycle accidents, 57
motorcycle taxi drivers (*okada* riders), 110–14
Mukherjee, Joia, 70, 73, 526–28
murders, ritual, 271–73, 276–78, 347, 348, 350–53, 407, 569*n*73, 570*n*74, 579*n*70, 588*n*126
Murphy, William, 595*n*33, 595*n*35
Muslims, Islam, 102, 104, 109, 113, 119, 145, 183, 185, 192, 193, 234–35, 238, 240, 241, 244, 275, 543*n*3, 548*n*2, 586*n*114

Namibia, 259
Napoleon, 202–203, 258, 522
National Association for the Advancement of Colored People, 284
National Ebola Response Centre, 123, 494, 497

National Institute of Allergy and Infectious Diseases (NIAID), 50–51
National Institutes of Health (NIH), 90, 92–94
National Patriotic Front of Liberia (NPFL), 363–64, 366, 396, 397, 398, 590n4, 592n17
National Provisional Ruling Council (NPRC), 370–72, 375, 376, 592n20
Native Americans, 195–96, 213, 224, 227, 550nn8–9, 551n16; Indian removal acts, 210
native business, *see* superstition and witchcraft
Nazi Germany, 312, 327
needles, xvii, 8, 30, 462
neoliberalism, 347–48, 419–21, 501, 505, 508, 539n3
neoslavery, 282–83, 315
nervous system, 608n39
Netherlands, 208, 315
New England, 197–98, 551n16
New England Journal of Medicine, The, 456, 471, 532n2, 536n21, 537n33
New York City, 37, 284, 542n24
New Yorker, The, 349, 479, 485, 522
New York Times, The, 18, 21, 94, 125–26, 250, 284–85, 306, 312–13, 348, 353, 406, 456, 457, 461, 499, 507, 518, 525, 536n23, 572n6, 584n96
Nguyen, Vinh-Kim, 462n46
Niger Bend, 192, 193, 198, 204, 241, 554n48
Nigeria, 32–33, 60, 215, 253, 295, 396, 500, 591n8; civil wars and, 97, 107, 109, 157–58, 161, 162–66, 356, 358, 366, 368, 378, 385, 393, 395, 399, 401, 403–404; Lagos, 32–33, 269, 295, 297–98, 567n68; polio in, 32–33, 60, 536n21
Niger River, 192, 198, 300
nihilism, containment, 526–27

nihilism, therapeutic, 62, 296, 313, 420, 445, 447–48, 450, 500, 526, 527, 603n7, 609n42; Ebola and, 445, 447–48, 450, 456, 477, 500, 603n7, 609n42
9/11 attacks, 24, 51, 358
Njala University College, 404–405
Nova Scotia, 206, 208, 209
Nuremberg trials, 415
nutrition, 444
Nyasaland, 264
N'Zérékoré, 10, 11, 24, 534n14

OAH Magazine of History, 191
Obama, Barack, 34, 37, 38, 41, 80, 536n23; United Nations speech of, 64–65
Observational Interim Care Center, 176
okada riders, 110–14
Olu-Wright, R. J., 553n41
onchocerciasis, 245, 261, 342, 580n72
Onion, The, 31, 479
Opala, Joseph, 222, 377, 379, 553n40, 555n61
Open Society Foundations, 66
Operation Noble Obelisk, 386–93
Operation No Living Thing, 164–66, 401–404
oral rehydration salts (ORS), 458, 461, 462; for cholera, 458–60; for Ebola, xiv–xvi, 28, 40, 100, 125, 129, 174, 458–63, 471, 488
Ouagadougou, 241, 243, 409–410
Ouamouno, Émile (Patient Zero), 5–12, 24, 25, 42, 495–96, 532n6
Ouamouno, Etienne, 8, 532n6
"Outbreak of Ebola Virus Disease in Guinea" (Bausch and Schwarz), 355

Pademba Road Prison, 109, 113, 341, 368, 370, 371, 378, 384, 402
pagan practices, *see* superstition and witchcraft

Pakenham, Thomas, 237
palm oil, 150, 187, 275, 473
pandemics, *see* epidemics and pandemics
Pannetier, Delphine, 531*n*2
parasites, 128, 194, 214, 554*n*48
partition of Africa (Great Scramble), xxvi, 236, 237–42, 280, 287, 304, 321
"Partition of Africa, The" (Keltie), 237
Partners in Health, xxiv, 50, 52–55, 58–62, 65–74, 82–87, 95, 98, 127–28, 130, 133, 142, 175, 178, 225, 228, 348, 388, 413, 453, 458, 464, 503, 508, 511, 526, 527, 546*n*17, 619*n*23; diagnostic test study sponsored by, 469–70; Ebola Response program launched, 66, 68; at Maforki hospital, 74–75, 77–81, 83–85, 88, 100, 123, 124, 127, 128, 130–32, 134, 137, 138, 140, 141, 178–80, 471, 491; *New York Times* article on, 94; at Port Loko hospital, 80–82, 84, 87–95, 123, 124, 127–28, 130–42; vision screening and treatment by, 176
Pasteur, Louis, 437, 449, 450, 453–54
Pasteurians (sanitarians), xxvii–xxviii, 237, 240, 261, 262, 270, 298, 299, 313, 321, 335–36, 344–45, 432, 454, 465, 478, 499, 501, 510, 536*n*22, 563*n*47
pathogenesis, 439, 444; animal models of, 447; of Ebola, *see* Ebola pathogenesis; economic and social terrain and, 449; of filoviruses, 451; mutations and, 451; social medicine and, 437–93
patrimonialism, 595*n*33
patronage and kinship networks, 112
patronage politics, 396; shadowy state and, 594*n*30
Patterson, K. David, 280
Patton, Adell, 577*n*51
Patuxet, 195–96
PCR (polymerase chain reaction) test, xviii, 470

Peabody Museum, 317, 325, 582*nn*84–85
penicillin, 326, 335, 585*n*104
pentamidine, 332–33, 335
Pérez, Jorge, 541*n*19
Perham, Margery, 189
pertussis, 421
Peru, 196
pesticides, 270, 336
Peters, C. J., 605*n*16
Pham, Nina, 91
Philippines, 308
Phoenix, The, 88, 91
phones, 112–13
Pilgrims, 195, 362, 550*n*8, 551*n*16
Piot, Peter, 438, 439, 446, 463, 602*n*1, 603*n*7, 604*n*10, 607*n*33
Pizarro, Francisco, 195
plague, 261–62, 269, 270, 287, 299, 304, 322, 335–36, 431, 456, 499–502, 563*n*47, 602*n*8, 616*n*11; in Dakar, 563*n*47; vaccine for, 500, 502
Plague, The (Camus), 1, 68–69, 517–18, 525
Plymouth, 195, 551*n*16
Plymouth County Correctional Facility, 362
pneumonia, 128, 585*n*104; pneumococcal, 296, 297, 299
poda podas, 109, 120, 151, 394
Podolsky, Scott, 575*n*34, 585*n*104
polio, 32–33, 60, 499, 500, 536*n*21, 575*n*38
Pollett, J. D., 580*n*74
polymerase chain reaction (PCR) test, xviii, 470
Poro society, 272, 273, 275–79, 346, 349, 583*n*91, 597*n*50
Port Loko (town and district), 26, 53, 74–79, 103, 119, 124, 148–49, 158, 161–63, 181, 191, 211, 253, 266, 299–300, 303, 338, 400, 401, 413, 415, 503; Bantoro, *see* Bantoro; history of, 76; influenza in, 302–303; Maforki

Port Loko (town and district) (*cont.*)
　hospital in, 74–75, 77–81, 83–85, 88,
　100, 123, 124, 127, 128, 130–32, 134,
　137, 138, 140, 141, 178–80, 542*n*22;
　Port Loko Government Hospital in,
　80–82, 84, 87–95, 123, 124, 127–28,
　130–42, 179–80; riots in, 303–304,
　576*n*43
Portugal, 191–97, 199, 215, 235, 237,
　239, 260, 266, 455
post-traumatic stress disorder (PTSD),
　425
potassium, 129
poverty, 4, 444, 500
Powell, Richard, 555*n*58
precious metals, 4, 103, 193; gold, xxii,
　103, 159, 183, 192–94, 292, 330, 397,
　548*n*2
pregnancy, 468, 540*n*13; *see also*
　childbirth
Preston, Richard, 485; *The Hot Zone*, xxv,
　43–44, 444–45, 452–53
preventive measures, 441, 501; vaccines,
　see vaccines
primates, 8, 90, 442, 447, 450; baboons,
　20; macaques, 442, 447; monkeys, 8, 14,
　44, 182, 447, 487, 496, 530*n*2, 613*n*66
*Principles and Practice of Infectious
　Diseases*, 437
prostitution, 206, 553*n*37
"psychosocial" category, 139, 425
public health, *see* health systems

Quakers, 205, 210–12, 254
Quigley, David, 572*n*5
quinine, 204, 214, 228, 243, 267–68,
　567*n*68

racism and racialization, 242, 259–60,
　315, 439, 499; COVID-19 and, 522;
　Ebola and, 90, 477–79; Junge on,
　315; in United States, 282–85; white
　supremacy, 204, 233, 259, 286

railways, 261, 543*n*2, 562*n*45, 579*n*71;
　influenza and, 294–95
rain forest, 183
Rambo iconography, 380, 407, 543*n*4
rape, 361
Rashid, Ismail, 302, 303, 304, 338, 410,
　419, 547*n*3, 560*n*27, 560*n*29, 571*n*3,
　575*n*39, 576*n*43, 595*n*31, 596*n*37
rats, 14, 128, 262, 293, 335, 342, 530*n*2
Rats, Lice and History (Zinsser), 324
Reagan, Ronald, 353, 360, 589*n*135
Reconstruction, 231, 282, 528, 572*n*5
Red Cross, 27, 33, 392, 420, 594*n*29
red water (sasswood) ordeals, 200, 227,
　229
refugees, xii, xxiii, 10, 18, 106, 110, 167,
　185, 186, 383–84, 421, 532*n*7
Reid, Richard, 557*n*4
religion, 339; syncretism in, 111;
　tolerance and, 104, 111, 543*n*3; *see
　also* Christians, Christianity; Muslims,
　Islam; superstition and witchcraft
Relman, David, 437
renal dialysis, xiv, 476
renal failure, 30, 469, 610*n*43
Reno, William, 594*n*30
resilience, 19–20, 425, 601*n*3
Reston Ebola virus, 444–45, 450, 452
Revolutionary United Front (RUF),
　105–106, 155, 157, 164–66, 357, 368,
　370–73, 375–77, 379–82, 384–85,
　391, 393, 394–96, 398–402, 404, 410,
　412, 414, 415, 546*n*1, 590*n*3, 592*n*17,
　592*n*20, 593*n*23, 593*n*24, 594*n*29,
　595*n*31, 596*n*37, 599*nn*73–74,
　600*n*75
Rhodesia, 264
Rhône-Poulenc, 332
ribbon developments, 251
rice, xxiii, 76, 103–106, 110, 149–50,
　167, 193–94, 197, 300–304, 321,
　553*n*40
Rice Coast, 208, 553*n*40

Richards, Paul, 36–37, 105, 185, 357, 539nn6–7, 543n4, 544n7, 545n16, 569n73, 589n2, 598n61

Richardson, Eugene, 520, 526

Riley, Stephen, 546n1

rinderpest, 300–301, 304, 321, 499, 549n6, 575n38, 615n10

ring towns, 251, 559n25

river blindness (onchocerciasis), 245, 261, 342, 580n72

Robinson, Cedric, 583n94

Rodney, Walter, 197, 198, 301, 551n17, 558n16

Rollin, Pierre, 443, 451, 604n10, 605n15, 610n48, 611n51

Rollins, Bec, 132, 135, 142–43, 543n1

Roosevelt, Franklin Delano, 316, 327–29, 349, 350, 364

Ross, Ronald, 266–69

Rousseau, Jean-Jacques, 201

Royal African Company (RAC), 202, 233

rubber latex, 4, 183, 186–87, 192, 379, 397, 473, 512; British monopoly on, 306, 327, 576n47; condoms, 366; Firestone Tire and Rubber Company, 186–87, 306–312, 316, 317, 322, 327, 340, 349, 350, 360, 361, 364–67, 397, 398, 583n94

Rubin, Elizabeth, 372–74

Ruiz, Jose, 218, 222

Rwanda, xxiv, 46–49, 52, 55, 58–60, 62, 63, 70–72, 74, 143, 147, 419–20, 417, 420, 539n3

Sabeti, Pardis, 24, 42, 45, 51, 60, 440, 442, 450, 451, 481, 483, 491, 530n2, 604n10

Saint-Domingue, 201, 202

St. John of God Hospital, 168–69

Salia, Martin, 38–43, 54, 56, 58, 85, 93, 98, 423, 526, 537n32; death of, 41, 43, 178, 514, 537n32; Khan and, 38

salmonella, 549n6

Samaritan's Purse, 22

Samory Touré, 243–50, 257, 337, 558n14, 559n18, 586n113

sanitarians (Pasteurians), xxvii–xxviii, 237, 240, 261, 262, 270, 298, 299, 313, 321, 335–36, 344–45, 432, 454, 465, 478, 499, 501, 510, 536n22, 563n47

Sankoh, Foday, 368, 370, 375, 377, 384, 394, 399, 400, 402, 406, 410–13, 415, 416, 596n42

Sanofi, 332

sasswood ordeals, 200, 227, 229

Sawyerr, Harry, 544n10

schistosomiasis, 261, 342, 499

Schwab, George, 317, 579n68

Schwarz, Lara, 355

Schwarzenegger, Arnold, 543n4

Schweitzer, Albert, 265, 565n58

Science, 45, 538n34

Scientologists, 71

Scramble for Africa (partition of Africa), xxvi, 236, 237–42, 280, 287, 304, 321

Scramble for Africa, The (Pakenham), 237

secret societies, 271–79, 318, 320, 325–26, 346, 396, 405, 496, 503, 583n91

seizure disorders, 130, 134, 136, 138, 467–68, 494, 608n39

Sékou Touré, Ahmed, 337, 339, 340, 586n113, 597n50

Sella Kafta, 497–98, 502

Senegal, 234, 258, 259, 270, 431, 501, 563n47, 602n8

Senehun, 256–57, 561n37

Sengbe Pieh (Joseph Cinque), 217–23, 285, 404, 528, 555n58

September 11 attacks, 24, 51, 358

sex workers, 206, 553n37

Shah, Raj, 60

Sharp, Granville, 205, 207

sharps, needles, xvii, 8, 30, 462

Shaw, Rosalind, 200–201, 251, 408, 409, 559n25, 569n72, 592n20, 598n61, 618n18

Shepler, Susan, 620*n*27

Sheriff, Gibrilla, 546*n*17

shock, 457–58, 466–67; hypovolemic, xvi, xvii, 29, 40, 44, 456–57, 470–71, 606*n*23

Sierra Leone, xi, xii, xix, xx, xxvi, xxviii, 12, 15, 17, 22, 23, 25, 31, 35, 42, 46–49, 52, 58, 61, 63, 66, 67, 70, 72–74, 82, 83, 85, 86, 114, 126, 178, 183–86, 191, 197, 208, 209, 217, 232, 238, 244, 248, 278, 304, 330, 338, 341, 356, 497–98, 508, 514–16, 538*n*33, 541*n*14, 541*n*20; Abidjan accords and, 377, 399, 412; agriculture in, 103–105; All People's Congress (APC) in, 105, 106, 587*n*116, 590*n*3, 592*n*20; amputations in, 358, 361, 375–76, 398–99, 406, 594*n*29, 601*n*1; army of, 106, 136, 157, 381, 543*n*4; borders closed in, 53; burials in, 115–19, 539*n*7; British rule in, 102–104, 149, 187, 251, 255, 256, 262, 338, 547*n*3; Cardew in, 560*n*29, 568*n*69; child soldiers in, 358, 361, 379–83, 414–15, 417, 543*n*4, 595*n*31, 595*n*33, 595*n*35; civil war in, xxiii, 10, 38, 53, 60, 71, 83, 97, 104–110, 113, 136, 148–49, 157–68, 183, 338, 355–60, 368–417, 419, 591*n*8, 598*n*61; corruption in, 105, 106; Cotton Tree as symbol of, 209, 223, 321, 341, 516; coups in, 355, 370–71, 378, 383–87, 392–95, 398–99, 401, 412; crisis caravan and, 419–33; Cuffe in, 210–12; diamonds in, *see* diamonds; diseases in, 214; economy of, 4, 104, 151–52, 419, 531*n*1, 546*n*1; educational system in, 151–52; evacuation of citizens from, 386–93; Executive Outcomes in, 373–75, 377–79, 384, 387, 390, 593*n*26, 596*n*42; family networks in, 101, 544*n*8; founding of, 204; Freetown, *see* Freetown; Global Peace Index and,

599*n*61; health care system in, 24–25, 30, 38–41, 53–55, 83, 102, 149, 329, 345, 355, 369, 370, 395, 421, 424, 426; health workers' strike in, 31; Human Development Index ranking of, 105; hut tax in, 253–55, 257, 266, 272, 273, 278, 302, 321, 322, 407, 560*n*31; influenza in, 292–94, 296, 299; Kabbah in, 157–58, 161, 163, 376–78, 382–84, 391, 394, 395, 399–400, 402, 404, 410, 413, 415; Kailahun District, 15–16, 22, 23, 25–29, 31, 56, 77, 105, 155, 345, 415, 479, 486–87, 490–92, 545*n*16, 593*n*22, 612*n*63; Kamajors in, 374–75, 377, 380, 384, 385, 387, 394, 399–401, 404, 406, 414, 415, 593*n*26, 595*n*32; Kambia District, 167, 302, 304, 400; Karene District, 301–303; Kenema District, *see* Kenema District; Kissi Triangle, 4, 10–12, 15, 16, 18, 24, 319, 532*n*7; Koidu, xxiii, 32, 82–84, 330–31, 355, 395, 400, 428; Kono District and people, 22, 74, 77, 82, 183, 320, 330–31, 338, 341, 358, 376, 378; Koroma in, 384, 394, 398, 399; Lomé treaty and, 410–12, 415; Lungi, 23, 26, 47–49, 57–58, 401, 402; Makeni, 159, 161, 395; Mende in, *see* Mende; meritocracy in, 561*n*37; Migeod on, 76, 541*n*14, 545*n*12; Momoh in, 151, 156, 368–69, 587*n*116, 592*n*20; National Provisional Ruling Council (NPRC) in, 370–72, 375, 376, 592*n*20; Port Loko, *see* Port Loko; religious syncretism in, 111; Revolutionary United Front (RUF) in, 105–106, 155, 157, 164–66, 357, 368, 370–73, 375–77, 379–82, 384–85, 391, 393, 394–96, 398–402, 404, 410, 412, 414, 415, 546*n*1, 590*n*3, 592*n*17, 592*n*20, 593*n*23, 593*n*24, 594*n*29, 595*n*31, 596*n*37, 599*nn*73–74, 600*n*75; slavery and abolition in, 252, 310, 558*n*16, 560*n*27; smallpox in, 288, 299, 301, 343–46; sobels in, 107–108, 157, 163, 164–67, 357, 359, 368, 370–72, 375, 377, 384–85, 387, 389, 390, 392–95, 400, 402–404, 409–412, 594*n*30; Special Court for, 415, 416, 422; Stevens in, 106, 151, 209, 341, 368, 370, 543*n*2, 587*n*116; structural adjustment (austerity) programs in, 105, 151–52, 368–70, 546*n*1; teachers' strikes in, 152; Truth and Reconciliation Commission in, 359, 413; "upline" areas of, 102, 543*n*2; World War I and, 287

Sierra Leone Company, 208, 233

Sierra Leone River, 553*n*41

Sierra Rutile, 372

Sikasso, 248–51, 255, 287

silver, 196, 548*n*2

Sirleaf, Ellen Johnson, 33–35, 83, 353, 396, 416

slavery, slave trade, xxii, xxvi, 145, 183, 187, 189, 191, 192, 194, 196–224, 240, 243–46, 258, 259, 271, 275, 280, 305, 321, 347, 439, 455, 515, 528, 547*n*3, 550*n*10, 551*nn*17–18, 552*n*27, 569*n*72; abolitionists and, 201–204, 206, 207, 209–212, 214, 216–17, 220, 224, 281; in America, 203, 220, 222; *Amistad* and, 218–23, 528, 555*n*58; diviners and, 200–201; domestic or internal, 245, 257, 276, 558*n*16, 560*n*27, 560*n*29; France and, 281–82; Haitian Revolution and, 201–203; justification by West Africans involved in, 200; Liberian "black slavery scandal," 310–11, 327, 578*n*56; neoslavery in the American South, 282–83, 315; *non-libre* term and, 281; reversal of fortune between Africa and the Americas caused by, 199, 213, 515; Sierra Leone and, 252,

558*n*16, 560*n*27; slave ships, 202, 203, 212–13; understanding of conflict and misfortune shaped by, 199–200; in United States, 282; witchcraft and, 200–201; World War I and, 281–82

slaves, freed, African colonization for, 210–12; American Colonization Society, 213, 224, 230, 231, 349; Maryland State Colonization Society, 225–31, 348

sleeping sickness (trypanosomiasis), 245, 261, 263–65, 287, 297, 304, 331–35, 342, 343, 431, 455, 456, 499, 558*n*14, 564*nn*54–55, 565*n*58, 566*n*67, 584*n*103, 585*n*106

smallpox, 63, 195, 196, 208, 213, 214, 240, 261, 280, 287, 293, 299, 301, 304, 309, 313–14, 321, 331, 333, 343–47, 431, 455, 456, 499, 514, 549*n*6, 551*n*14, 551*n*16, 557*n*4, 575*n*38; vaccination for, 288–89, 297, 313–14, 343–44, 498; variolation for, 240, 289, 523, 557*n*3

smartphones, 112–13

Smith, Tracy K., 435

snake bites, 149, 150, 324

Snake Society, 318, 324

sobels, 107–108, 157, 163, 164–67, 357, 359, 368, 370–72, 375, 377, 384–85, 387, 389, 390, 392–95, 400, 402–404, 409–412, 594*n*30

social media, 36; Twitter, 17, 34, 36 38, 80, 524, 542*n*24

social medicine, 437–93

sodalities, 153

sodium, 129

Songhai empire, 192

Soper, George, 527

Soros, George, 60, 66

South Africa, 72; apartheid in, 568*n*71

South America, 196

South Carolina, 196

Soviet Union, 24, 337, 340, 342, 350, 534*n*13

sowei, 153

Spain, 196, 197, 199, 215, 217–18, 220, 235, 237, 239, 266, 285, 548*n*2

Spanish flu pandemic, 280, 290–300, 302–303, 518, 520, 524, 573*n*18, 574*n*28, 574*n*30, 575*n*32

Spencer, Craig, 37–38, 43, 80

Spielberg, Steven, 223

Spinage, Clive, 615*n*10

Spitzer, Leo, 566*n*67

"Starvation Camp Near Jaslo" (Szymborska), 144

Stevens, Siaka, 106, 151, 209, 341, 368, 370, 543*n*2, 587*n*116

Strada, Gino, 539*n*3

Strasser, Valentine, 370, 372–74, 546*n*1

streptomycin, 335

Strong, Richard Pearson, 307–310, 312, 323, 325, 576*n*51, 577*n*53, 580*n*73

Sudan, 245, 249, 258, 445

Sudan Ebola virus, 35, 450, 455

Suez Canal, 292

sugar, 196

sulfa drugs (sulphonamides), 335, 336, 583*n*93, 585*n*104

superspreaders, 345–47, 505; Ebola and, 22–23, 25–26, 347, 483

superstition and witchcraft, 20, 111, 180–82, 201, 226–28, 288, 400, 405–406, 412, 478, 496, 502–505, 588*n*126, 598*n*61, 618*nn*17–19; cannibalism, 271–72, 275, 315, 319, 325, 327, 347, 504, 569*nn*72–73, 570*n*74, 571*n*88, 579*n*70, 582*n*86, 593*n*24; diviners, 170, 200–201, 276, 278, 346, 431, 559*n*25; human alligators, 74, 213, 271, 274, 326; human leopards, 271–79, 315, 326, 400, 504, 570*n*82, 570*n*88; Kamajors and, 374; medicine bags, 274, 275; ritual murders, 271–73, 276–78, 347, 348, 350–53, 407, 569*n*73, 570*n*74, 579*n*70, 588*n*126; sasswood ordeals, 200, 227, 229; secret societies, 271–79,

318, 320, 325–26, 346, 396, 405, 496, 503, 583*n*91; slavery and, 200–201; swears (*sweh*; curses), 20, 170–72, 504, 547*n*5, 618*n*17; Tongo players, 272–73, 275, 279

Suret-Canale, Jean, 243, 281, 558*nn*9–10, 571*n*4

surgical care, 53–55, 495, 514

Surowiecki, James, 479

Sutton, William, 294

SWAT teams, 18, 19

swears (*sweh*; curses), 20, 170–72, 504, 547*n*5, 618*n*17

Syria, 233, 300–304, 321, 575*n*39

Szymborska, Sisława, 144

Taï Forest Ebola virus, 450

Tana, 498, 502

taxation, 252–53, 275; hut tax, 253–55, 257, 266, 272, 273, 278, 302, 321, 322, 407, 560*n*31

Taylor, Charles, 105, 348, 362–68, 368, 371, 378, 379, 383, 385, 392, 396–98, 400, 401, 403, 405–406, 409–413, 415–17, 421, 590*n*4, 591*n*12, 592*n*14, 598*n*51, 600*n*78

telegraph, 239, 556*n*2

Temne tribe, 76, 102, 112, 147, 148, 153, 155, 201, 207, 253, 272, 408, 541*n*14, 559*n*25, 618*n*17

tetanus, 297

Theodore Roosevelt, USS, 524

therapeutic nihilism, 62, 296, 313, 420, 445, 447–48, 450, 500, 526, 527, 603*n*7, 609*n*42; Ebola and, 445, 447–48, 450, 456, 477, 500, 603*n*7, 609*n*42

Theroux, Paul, 582*n*89

Thomas, Edgar, 388–89

Thornton, Henry, 205

three *c*'s (civilization, commerce, and Catholicism), 234–36, 241

Through Liberia (Mills), 580*n*73

ticks, 128
Tilling, H., 294
timber and logging, xxi, xxiii, 4, 15, 21, 183, 186, 192, 397, 512
Timbuktu, 241
Time, 86, 493
TKM-Ebola, 610*n*44
Togo, 396, 410, 591*n*8
Tolbert, William, 349–50, 352, 353, 396, 415, 589*n*135
Tomes, Nancy, 520
Tomkins, Sandra, 292, 295–97
Tongo players, 272–73, 275, 279
Touré, Ahmed Sékou, 337, 339, 340, 586*n*113, 597*n*50
Touré, Samory, 243–50, 257, 337, 558*n*14, 559*n*18, 586*n*113
trade, 18, 191–99, 203, 248, 275, 548*n*2, 569*n*72; three *c*'s (civilization, commerce, and Catholicism), 234–36, 241; *see also* extractive trades
Transactions of the Royal Society of Tropical Medicine and Hygiene, 333–35
travel bans and cancellations, 36–38, 89–90, 114, 177–78, 533*n*10
Traveller, 210–11
Treaty of Ghent, 217, 222
Treaty of Versailles, 305
tribes, 184; use of term, 224, 317
Tribes of the Liberian Hinterland (Schwab), 317
True Whig Party, 349, 350, 352, 363
Trump, Donald, 34, 36–38, 80, 178, 518, 524–25, 533*n*10
trypanosomiasis (sleeping sickness), 245, 261, 263–65, 287, 297, 304, 331–35, 342, 343, 431, 455, 456, 499, 558*n*14, 564*nn*54–55, 565*n*58, 566*n*67, 584*n*103, 585*n*106
tsetse flies, 245, 265, 333–34, 585*n*106
tuberculosis, xvi, 128, 132, 261, 331, 342, 495

Tubman, William, 311, 328, 336, 340, 348–54, 405
Tubman University, 348
Tukolor, 241
Turay, Saidu, 146, 156–57, 162–74
Turkey, 300
Turner, Nat, 220
Twaddell, William H., 598*n*51
Tweh, Moses, 350–53
Twitter, 17, 34, 36–38, 80, 524, 542*n*24
typhoid, 14, 214, 261, 267, 331, 395, 421

Uganda, 14, 35, 72, 264; trypanosomiasis in, 584*n*103
Uíge, 454–55
Ulimo-J, 397, 416
Ulimo-K, 397, 416, 597*n*50
Underground Railroad, The (Whitehead), 191
Understanding West Africa's Ebola Epidemic (Abdullah and Rashid), 419
United Fruit, 308
United Nations (UN), 17, 60, 61, 65, 66, 69, 72, 73, 79, 83, 84, 167, 337, 356, 358, 376, 377, 382–84, 410–14, 416, 420, 423, 426, 427, 502, 511, 536*n*23, 541*n*20, 617*n*14; DDR (disarmament, demobilization, and reintegration) program of, 414–15, 600*n*75; Human Development Index of, 105; Mission in Sierra Leone (UNAMSIL), 411, 600*n*75; Obama's speech at, 64–65
United States, 305–306, 358; automobile industry in, 186–87, 327; blacks in, *see* African Americans; civil rights movement in, 284; Civil War in, 53, 231, 282, 577*n*51, 595*n*35; Constitution of, 209, 282; Gilded Age in, 284, 286; Jim Crow in, 282, 285, 528; Liberia and, 186–87, 286, 306–312, 316, 327, 360, 365, 589*n*135; Reconstruction in, 231, 282, 528, 572*n*5; Sierra Leone evacuation

United States (*cont.*)
  by, 386–93; slavery in, 282; State
  Department, 336, 350, 361, 365, 393
United States Geologic Survey, 591*n*7
United States v. Cinque, 219–23
Unmasking the State (McGovern),
  586*n*113
Upper West Africa, xi; maps of, 9, 246–47;
  see also Guinea; Liberia; Sierra Leone
urbanization, xxiii, 54, 544*n*8
USAID (United States Agency for
  International Development), 60, 66

vaccines, 50, 182, 240, 263, 313, 331,
  441, 444, 495, 499, 500, 575*n*34,
  604*n*7; cholera, 501, 502; Ebola, 28,
  31, 90, 470, 479, 495, 502, 506–507,
  520, 603*n*7; influenza, 290, 296;
  plague, 500, 502; polio, 60; and
  resistance to vaccination, 240, 288,
  557*n*4; ring vaccination, 344, 498,
  506; smallpox, 288–89, 297, 313–14,
  343–44, 498
Van Buren, Martin, 220–22
van der Kraaij, Fred, 350–51, 353,
  588*n*131, 589*n*136
Vanity Fair, 406
variolation, 240, 289, 523, 557*n*3
ventilatory support, xiv, 476
veterinarians, 300, 565*n*59
Victoria, Queen, 235, 257
View of Sierra Leone, A (Migeod), 76,
  541*n*14, 545*n*12
viruses, 440–42, 444, 446, 549*n*6; DNA,
  441; economic and social terrain and,
  449; filoviruses, *see* filoviruses; RNA,
  441, 523
vision loss, *see* blindness
Voice of the Negro, The (Du Bois), 177
Voltaire, 201, 202

Wallah, 164, 166
Wampanoag, 195

war, xxi, xxiii, xxiv, 198–99, 243–45,
  356, 419, 439, 551*n*18, 557*n*6;
  health-care systems and, xxviii;
  weapons in, 241, 243, 247, 249, 251,
  253, 359–61, 381, 395–96, 409–410,
  510, 557*n*6, 595*n*35; *see also* civil
  wars
War of 1812, 211, 212; Treaty of Ghent
  and, 217, 222
Warren, Gabriel, 546*n*17
Washington, George, 206, 207
Washington Post, The, 89, 189, 363, 377,
  390, 412
water, stagnant, 194, 549*n*5
weapons, 241, 243, 247, 249, 251, 253,
  359–61, 381, 395–96, 409–410, 510,
  557*n*6, 595*n*35
Weber, Max, 595*n*33
Weil, David, 554*n*48
Wellbody Alliance, 70, 72, 74, 508,
  619*n*23
West Africa, xi; maps of, 9, 246–47;
  see also Guinea; Liberia; Sierra Leone
Western, John, 567*n*67
White, Tom, 59
Whitehead, Colson, 191
white supremacy, 204, 233, 259, 286
Wilberforce, William, 205, 211
Wilhelm II, 235, 259
Wilkinson, Iain, 620*n*28
Winterbottom, Thomas, 263–64, 271–72,
  564*n*54
witchcraft, *see* superstition and witchcraft
women, 428; abducted as "bush wives,"
  382, 594*n*29, 596*n*37; as chiefs,
  256–57, 561*n*37; pregnancy and, 468,
  540*n*13, 609*n*42; vocational training
  for, 428; *see also* childbirth
World Bank, 61, 347, 539*n*5, 546*n*1,
  556*n*66, 589*n*136
World Food Programme, 372
World Health Organization (WHO), 3,
  4, 6, 15–18, 22, 26, 28, 33, 46–47, 61,

67, 343, 447, 448, 480–82, 486, 487, 490, 498, 507, 515, 534*n*14, 603*n*3, 608*n*38, 613*n*66, 614*n*2, 617*n*15, 618*n*19

World Journal of Surgery, 53

"World's One Hope, The" (Brecht), 96

World War I, 300, 304, 305, 328, 347, 414, 458, 465–67, 563*n*47; colonialism and, 280–81, 286–90; Dardanelles campaign in, 571*n*78; diseases and, 286–87; farming and food shortages in, 302–304; health systems and, 288–90; influenza pandemic and, 280, 290–300, 302–303, 518, 520, 573*n*18, 574*n*28; Liberia and, 286, 573*n*12; slavery and, 281–82

World War II, 186, 270, 327–31, 334, 337

Wright, Jeffrey, 543*n*1

Wright, Joseph, 215, 232, 234

Yambuku, 437–39, 446, 463, 478, 505–506, 603*n*3, 607*n*33

yellow fever, 195, 206–207, 214, 261,

269, 287, 293, 299, 304, 309, 322, 331, 499, 562*n*46, 565*n*62, 580*n*72

Yemen, 617*n*15

Yersinia pestis, *see* plague

Yoko, Mammy, 256–57, 275, 277, 561*n*37, 561*n*39

Yoruba, 215, 245

Yugoslavia, 14, 533*n*8

Zaire, 14, 337–38, 386, 437–38, 478; Kikwit, 535*n*19

Zaire Ebola virus, xviii, 17, 42, 43, 52, 442, 450, 452, 466, 505, 605*n*14, 606*n*18

Zambia, 264

Zika, 565*n*62

Zinsser, Hans, 324

ZMapp, 28–29, 31, 90, 331, 469, 487–91, 613*n*66

zoonosis (animal-to-human transmission), xx, 51, 262, 286, 437, 495, 523, 549*n*6; AIDS and, 50; Ebola and, xx, 5, 7, 183; Lassa fever and, 14

Zwedru, 82, 178

A NOTE ABOUT THE AUTHOR

Paul Farmer is the Kolokotrones University Professor and chair of the Department of Global Health and Social Medicine at Harvard Medical School, as well as chief of the Division of Global Health Equity at Boston's Brigham and Women's Hospital and a founding director of Partners In Health. He is also the author of *Partner to the Poor, Pathologies of Power, Infections and Inequalities,* and other books. Among his numerous awards and honors is the Public Welfare Medal from the National Academy of Sciences.